Clinical Applications of VENTILATORY SUPPORT

(Formerly Mechanical Ventilation)

Clinical Applications of VENTILATORY SUPPORT

Edited by

Robert R. Kirby, M.D.
Professor
Department of Anesthesiology
University of Florida College of Medicine
Medical Director
Respiratory Care Services
Shands Hospital
Gainesville, Florida

Michael J. Banner, R.R.T., Ph.D.
Assistant Professor and Coordinator
Anesthesiology Research Laboratory
Department of Anesthesiology
University of Florida College of Medicine
Gainesville, Florida

John B. Downs, M.D.
Professor and Chairman
Department of Anesthesiology
University of South Florida College of Medicine
Tampa, Florida

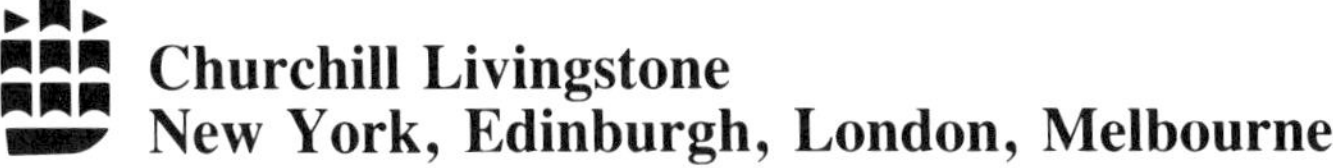
Churchill Livingstone
New York, Edinburgh, London, Melbourne

Library of Congress Cataloging-in-Publication Data

Clinical applications of ventilatory support / edited by Robert R. Kirby, Michael J. Banner, John B. Downs.
p. cm.
Rev. ed. of : Mechanical ventilation. 1985.
Includes bibliographical references.
ISBN 0-443-08613-3
1. Artificial respiration. 2. Respirators. I. Kirby, Robert R. II. Banner, Michael J. III. Downs, John B. IV. Mechanical ventilation.
[DNLM: 1. Respiration, Artificial. 2. Ventilators, Mechanical.
WF 26 C641]
RC87.9.M43 1990
615.8′36—dc20
DNLM/DLC
for Library of Congress 89-13920
CIP

Distributed in the United Kingdom by Churchill Livingstone, Robert Stevenson House, 1–3 Baxter's Place, Leith Walk, Edinburgh EH1 3AF, and by associated companies, branches, and representatives throughout the world.

Accurate indications, adverse reactions, and dosage schedules for drugs are provided in this book, but it is possible that they may change. The reader is urged to review the package information data of the manufacturers of the medications mentioned.

The Publishers have made every effort to trace the copyright holders for borrowed material. If they have inadvertently overlooked any, they will be pleased to make the necessary arrangements at the first opportunity.

Copy Editor: *Bridgett Dickinson*
Production Supervisor: *Christina Hippeli*

Printed in the United States of America

First published in 1990

"If I have seen further . . .
it is by standing upon
the shoulders of giants."
—Sir Isaac Newton

This book is dedicated to Jerome H. Modell, M.D.—physician, teacher, and a dedicated proponent of positive-pressure mechanical ventilation. We have benefited from his knowledge and expert guidance.

Contributors

Michael J. Banner, R.R.T., Ph.D.
Assistant Professor and Coordinator, Anesthesiology Research Laboratory, Department of Anesthesiology, University of Florida College of Medicine, Gainesville, Florida

Tina E. Banner, R.N., M.N., C.C.R.N.
Assistant in Anesthesiology, Department of Anesthesiology, University of Florida College of Medicine, Gainesville, Florida

Lawrence S. Berman, M.D.
Associate Professor, Departments of Anesthesiology and Pediatrics, University of Florida College of Medicine, Gainesville, Florida

Paul Blanch, R.R.T., B.A.
Supervisor, Department of Respiratory Care, Shands Hospital, Gainesville, Florida

Roger C. Bone, M.D.
Chief, Department of Medicine, Rush-Presbyterian-St. Luke's Medical Center, Chicago, Illinois

Reese Clark, M.D.
Director of Research, Department of Neonatology, Wilford Hall USAF Medical Center/SGHP, Lackland Air Force Base, Texas

David A. Desautels, R.R.T., M.P.A.
Technical Director, Hyperbaric Chamber, Shands Hospital, Gainesville, Florida

John B. Downs, M.D.
Professor and Chairman, Department of Anesthesiology, University of South Florida College of Medicine, Tampa, Florida

Orlando G. Florete, Jr., M.D.
Fellow in Critical Care Medicine, Department of Anesthesiology, University of Florida College of Medicine, Gainesville, Florida

Gary W. Gammage, M.D.
Staff Anesthesiologist, Department of Anesthesiology, North Florida Regional Medical Center, Gainesville, Florida

Nikolaus Gravenstein, M.D.
Associate Professor, Departments of Anesthesiology and Neurosurgery, University of Florida College of Medicine, Gainesville, Florida

Robert R. Kirby, M.D.
Professor, Department of Anesthesiology, University of Florida College of Medicine; Medical Director, Respiratory Care Services, Shands Hospital, Gainesville, Florida

Samsun Lampotang, M.E.
Doctoral Student in Mechanical Engineering, Graduate Research Assistant, Department of Anesthesiology, University of Florida College of Medicine, Gainesville, Florida

Neil R. MacIntyre, M.D.
Associate Professor, Department of Medicine, Duke University School of Medicine, Durham, North Carolina

E. Trier Mörch, M.D., Ph.D.
Professor Emeritus, University of Illinois College of Medicine, Chicago, Illinois

Scott Norwood, M.D.
Assistant Professor, Department of Surgery, University of Illinois College of Medicine at Urbana-Champaign; Director, Critical Care and Trauma Service, Carle Foundation Hospital, Urbana, Illinois

Donald Null, M.D.
Chief, Department of Neonatology, Wilford Hall USAF Medical Center/SGHP, Lackland Air Force Base, Texas

Jukka Räsänen, M.D.
Instructor, Department of Anesthesiology, University of South Florida College of Medicine, Tampa, Florida

S. David Register, M.D.
Staff Anesthesiologist, Department of Anesthesiology, Wilford Hall USAF Medical Center/SGHSA, Lackland Air Force Base, Texas; Currently Staff Anesthesiologist, South Georgia Medical Center, Valdosta, Georgia

Howard G. Sanders, Jr., M.S., R.R.T.
Associate Professor, Department of Respiratory Therapy, School of Allied Health Professions, Loma Linda University, Loma Linda, California

Charles B. Spearman, B.S., R.R.T.
Instructor, Department of Respiratory Therapy, School of Allied Health Professions, Loma Linda University, Loma Linda, California

Robert B. Spooner, Ph.D., C.C.E.
Senior Project Engineer, ECRI, Plymouth Meeting, Pennsylvania

M. Christine Stock, M.D.
Assistant Professor, Departments of Anesthesiology and Internal Medicine, Emory University School of Medicine, Atlanta, Georgia

Preface

Clinical Applications of Ventilatory Support represents an update of *Mechanical Ventilation,* published in 1985. The timing of the earlier publication could not have been worse with respect to the almost explosive proliferation of ventilator technology and techniques. For example, microprocessor control of ventilator function was just coming into its own; therapeutic modes, such as pressure support and airway pressure release ventilation, were known only to a very few; and advanced techniques of respiratory monitoring, including pulse oximetry and infrared capnography, were in their infancy. In a sense, the earlier work was obsolete almost from the start.

Bearing in mind that similar advances may be just around the corner, we are, nevertheless, inclined to believe that this effort will be reasonably current into the mid-1990s. Microprocessor technology will continue to evolve, but the modular construction of currently manufactured ventilators allows them to be modified to keep pace. It is possible, but unlikely, that revolutionary new techniques of support will be developed. After all, we still have not decided where the older ones stand (although lack of scientific validation has never stood in the way of aggressive marketing).

Although the emphasis in the following pages is on the mechanical support of ventilation, the overall scope of the text is broader; hence the change in title. The history of mechanical ventilation has not changed appreciably in the five years since *Mechanical Ventilation* was published. However, Dr. Trier Mörch has added more of his personal experiences to his delightful historical chapter. New efforts include a chapter on anesthesia ventilators and the outcome of treatment for acute and chronic respiratory failure. All other chapters have been brought up to the present (and the future). We trust that almost everybody with an interest in respiratory care will find something of value.

Our thanks go to Toni M. Tracy, President of Churchill Livingstone Inc., for her support. If she had not threatened and cajoled, persuaded, and occasionally pleaded, the book never would have happened. Special thanks also to Hope Olivo, our editorial assistant in the Department of Anesthesiology in Gainesville. She was magnificent in her efforts to get everything done on time.

Robert R. Kirby, M.D.
Michael J. Banner, R.R.T., Ph.D.
John B. Downs, M.D.

CONTENTS

1

History of Mechanical Ventilation

E. Trier Mörch

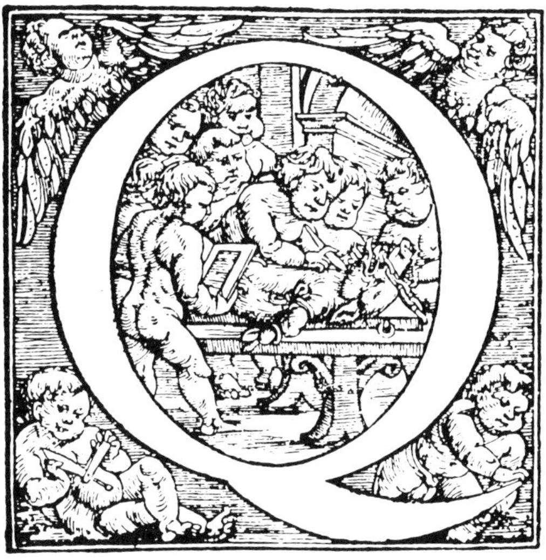

EARLY HISTORY OF RESUSCITATION

The illustrated letter "Q" is copied from Andreas Wesele Vesalius' (1515–1564) *de Humani Corporis Fabrica,* printed in 1555. It depicts chubby cherubs performing a tracheostomy on a sow. In the *Fabrica,* Vesalius was the first to give a detailed report of "modern" resuscitation. He reported:

> But that life may in a manner of speaking be restored to the animal, an opening must be attempted in the trunk of the trachea, into which a tube of reed or cane should be put; you will then blow into this, so that the lung may rise again and the animal take in air. Indeed, with the slight breath in the case of the living animal, the lung will swell to the full extent of the thoracic cavity, and the heart become strong . . . for when the lung, long flaccid, has collapsed, the beat of the heart and arteries appears wavy, creepy, twisting; but when the lung is inflated at intervals, the motion of the heart and arteries does not stop. . . .

It is impressive how well Vesalius understood the "modern" principles of resuscitation and how clearly he described the ventricular fibrillation he saw. Unfortunately, lack of human adaptability delayed extensive application of this same technique for 400 years.

Vesalius was an impetuous genius with an intense desire for correct knowledge and true reporting of anatomy. He was the first to base his anatomic studies on human dissections, which in those days were strictly prohibited by the Church. In so doing, he changed the very principles of the understanding of human anatomy.

The great Greek physician Galen, who lived during the second century AD, based his knowledge of anatomy on dissections of the pig, ape, dog, and ox. He assumed that the structures he found in these animals were identical to those of the human body. For 13 centuries, the human breastbone was thought to be segmented like that of the ape and the liver to be divided into many lobes like that of the hog. The uterus supposedly consisted of two long horns as in the dog, and the hip bones were assumed to be flared as in the ox. Not even the number of bones in the body was accurately known: most often quoted at between 248 and 252, including the bone of Luz. The latter was supposed to be the indestructible nucleus, a sort of seed, from which the body was resurrected. The belief in the bone of Luz and in the missing rib of Adam persisted until Vesalius showed that both were myths. Galen's teaching, accepted by physicians and the Church, had acquired an authority like that of orthodox theology, undebated for 1,300 years. To question Galen was heresy.

Vesalius's demand for truth in anatomy, his impatience, and his hot temper made him take some extreme risks. To obtain a human skeleton, he surreptitiously stole the body of a criminal who had been executed and hanged in chains on exhibit as a lesson to the people. He boiled the body and thus obtained the first complete human skeleton available for study. Had this theft been detected, he would have been executed.

At the age of 23, Vesalius was appointed professor of anatomy in Padua in northeastern Italy. During the next 6 years he secretly conducted painstaking dissections on a number of human cadavers. In 1543, before reaching the age of 29, Vesalius was ready to publish his great work on anatomy in seven volumes. The illustrations were exact and artistic, probably drawn by one of Titian's pupils.

Vesalius completely contradicted Galenic anatomy. The four abdominal muscles of the ape no longer graced man; the multilobed liver disappeared, as did the segmented sternum, the double bile duct, and the horned uterus. Even the bone of Luz, the resurrection bone, was proved a myth, and Adam's missing rib was restored.

The first correct demonstration of the anatomy of the human body was met with a storm of violent protests. Vesalius had dared to cast discredit on Galen—to discard galenic traditions, which were accepted like the Bible. No one had previously had the audacity to doubt them publicly. Intense indignation was aroused among physicians. Even his former teacher Sylvius called Vesalius "an impious madman who is poisoning all of Europe with his vaporings."

To discredit his medical brethren was one thing. It was quite another to offend the clergy, who held strong opposition to dissections because of their belief in material resurrection—that only the whole body would be accepted in heaven.

THE INQUISITION

Started as a tribunal, established by the Catholic church in the darkest days of the Middle Ages, the Inquisition existed for the suppression of heresy. It lasted 800 years, from 1000 to 1800 AD. The name was derived from Latin, *inquirere* ("to inquire") and signified the form of procedure used, that of searching out heretics and other church offenders. In this procedure, the judge presided, received testimony, examined, and absolved or condemned. It was this procedure, *per inquisitionem,* that lay at the heart of the institution we call the Inquisition.

Sworn testimony of two witnesses sufficed to commit the accused to prison. The accused was told of his alleged crimes, but he was never confronted by those who had laid charges and was allowed no legal defense. Artifice, deception, and torture often were used to trap the accused into an admission of guilt. The interrogation of the inquisitors took place on a Sunday. It began with a procession of the ecclesiastic and civil dignitaries and the accused. This pageantry provided a striking display of religious observance that veiled, but thinly, the grim seriousness of the occasion. Following the sermon, the decisions of the inquisitors were read, and sentences were pronounced, all of which were final. This formula was pure fiction, designed to absolve the Church from participation in the shedding of blood.

At first, milder penalties of fines and exile were preferred, until 1200 AD, when the Pope declared that the heretic is guilty of spiritual treason. A tragic example of the subservience of the Inquisition to political purposes was the execution of Joan of Arc, burned at the stake in 1431 in Rouen, France.

Thousands were executed, often following horrible torture, during the Inquisition. This would likely have been the fate of Vesalius. Legend has it that he performed an autopsy on a Spanish nobleman shortly after his *exitus lethalis*. Out of curiosity, he experimentally inflated the lungs through the trachea, and the nobleman's heart started to beat again. This act only outraged his medical associates and the clergy further. The reason he escaped death at the stakes and "only" was condemned to a pilgrimage to the Holy Land was his father's wealth, power, and close ties to Charles V, emperor of both Spain and the Netherlands. Vesalius died during the pilgrimage in a shipwreck on the island of Zante, west of Greece.

The Inquisition cannot be defended or justified; it violated all ideas of freedom and left a legacy of ignorant intolerant fanaticism, which was often to the political and financial advantage of the ruling monarch. However, it must be evaluated within the context of the society that produced it. An accurate appraisal of the tribunal may lead one closer to a realistic understanding of the evolution, or at least the history, of Western civilization and, more specifically, the progress (or lack thereof) of medicine through the Middle Ages.

LATER DEVELOPMENTS

Vesalius's technique of resuscitation was the simplest form of intermittent positive-pressure breathing (IPPB), a form of support that has proved by far the most efficient means of artificial breathing for the past 400 years. One wonders why it has come in and out of vogue so many times. A series of detours have been interspersed, many of which were bizarre and bewildering, although often amusing. Because it was hoped that strong and insulting stimulations would revive patients, they were rolled over barrels, loud bells were rung close to their ears, bright lights were shone into their eyes, they were burned with red-hot irons, or their anuses were dilated and tobacco smoke blown into their rectums. Often they were thrown stomach-down across a trotting horse. Limitless human ingenuity and stupidity of this sort was repeated to an impressive degree over the years.

For 100 years after Vesalius, no progress was made. In 1667 Robert Hooke of London (1635–1703) repeated Vesalius's experiment by fixing a pair of fireside bellows tightly into the cut trachea (*aspera arteria*) of a dog, keeping it alive by regular intermittent inflations.

Another century passed without any publications on resuscitation until in 1744 John Fothergill of England reported a successful case of mouth-to-mouth resuscitation:

> A pair of bellows might possibly be applied with more advantage in these cases, than the blast of a man's mouth; but if any person can be got to try the charitable experiment by blowing, it would seem preferable to the other. . . .

Fothergill, one of the founders of the British Humane Society, was afraid of overdistention of the lungs. He also thought that the warmth of the rescuer's exhaled air might be more beneficial than cold air passing through a bellows.

Because there was a strong prejudice against touching the dead, particularly if the death was due to the criminal offense of suicide, no attempt was made to resuscitate people apparently dead from drowning or other causes of asphyxia until about 1750. Also, a prevalent theory held that drowned people died of apoplexy, and that the lungs collapsed. Therefore, anyone taken from the water was deemed dead and resuscitation was not attempted. Furthermore, if an unknown person was brought into a house and died there, the owner of the house might be liable for the expenses of the funeral.

THE HUMANE SOCIETY

More progressive times began in 1767. To the Dutch belongs the credit for the first serious attempt to take care of the unfortunate citizens who drowned in their many waterways. It was during that year that a group of wealthy merchants in Amsterdam formed a society called *Maatschappy tot Redding van Drenklingen* (the Society for the Rescue of Drowned Persons), also called the Humane Society. Similar societies were formed in England and Denmark, and soon in other European countries as well.

The most important methods employed by members of the Dutch Humane Society were to keep the patient warm and provide mouth-to-mouth ventilation. By compressing the belly and chest with his free hand, the operator brought about an expiratory movement. Several unusual "accessory and useful means" were also recommended, such as fumigation by blowing tobacco smoke into the great bowel (Fig. 1-1). Sometimes all the passengers on a Dutch canal boat might be summoned to assist the operator in administering this treatment if the special instrument, the "Fumigator," was not at hand: "Blood letting by opening the jugular vein" was assumed to be beneficial and particularly necessary as life returned. Vomiting produced by ipecacuanha wine or other emetics was popular, as were sneezing caused by "spirit of quick lime in a rag held in front of the nostrils" and internal stimulants, such as "pouring a gill or two of warm wine into the gullet."

Mouth-to-mouth resuscitation oscillated in popularity with the use of fireside bellows. Other methods were soon condemned, especially by the British and the Danish. In 1776, John Hunter of London advocated the use of a double bellows that he had contrived, so that the first stroke blew fresh air into the lungs and the next stroke, from the other bellows, sucked out the "bad air." He also recommended applying gentle pressure on the larynx against the esophagus to prevent air from going into the stomach (which might be called a "reverse" Sellick maneuver). Hunter advised the use of "dephlogisticated air," or oxygen, and firmly stated that venesection, or blood-letting, should be forbidden.

In 1786 Edmund Goodwyn of London received the gold medal of the Humane Society for his dissertation on the connection between

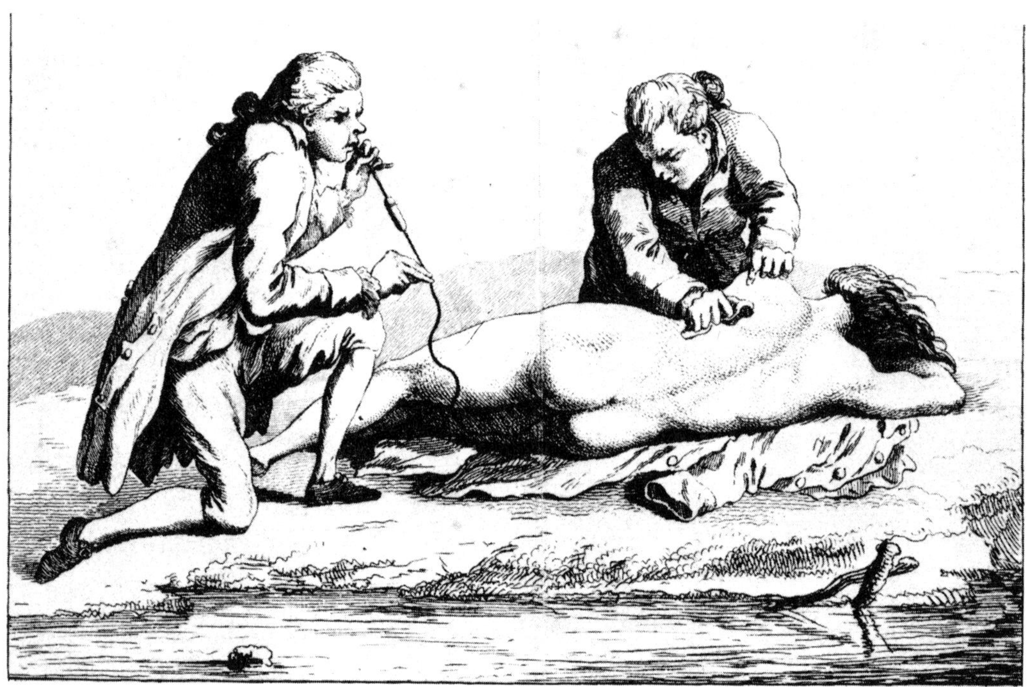

Fig. 1-1. Attempt at resuscitation from drowning by insufflation of tobacco smoke per rectum.

life and respiration. He speculated that respiration enabled a beneficial chemical substance to be transmitted to the blood.

Laymen were encouraged to use artificial respiration as a result of the efforts of Lord Cathcart in Scotland. The method was published, and rewards were offered. A half-crown would go to the messenger who informed the surgeon or minister when a body had been taken out of the water, two guineas to anyone who used the advocated measures for 2 hours, and four guineas if the life was saved. Anyone whose house was used for the rescue was reimbursed all expenses plus one guinea for his trouble.

In 1796 the medical doctor John Daniel Herholdt and the botanist Carl Gottlob Rafn published *Life-Saving Measures for Drowning Persons* in Copenhagen. Together, they took up vital problems for critical analysis and evaluation, reported their findings in a clear and objective style, and pointed the way toward the methods of resuscitation used today (Fig. 1-2). The professor of medicine and physiology and the practical, versatile, scientific government official complemented each other in a way that could well serve as a model! Regretfully, their outstanding work was written in Danish and therefore for all practical purposes was buried until 1960, when Henning Poulsen of Aarhus, Denmark, had it translated and published to celebrate the tenth anniversary of the founding of the Scandinavian Society of Anaesthetists. It has since received wide acclaim and recognition.

E. Coleman from Ayresline, Scotland, later veterinary professor in London, recommended tracheal intubation and used a silver catheter much wider than those previously employed. He suggested using a bellows for insufflation and added that oxygen would be beneficial. He

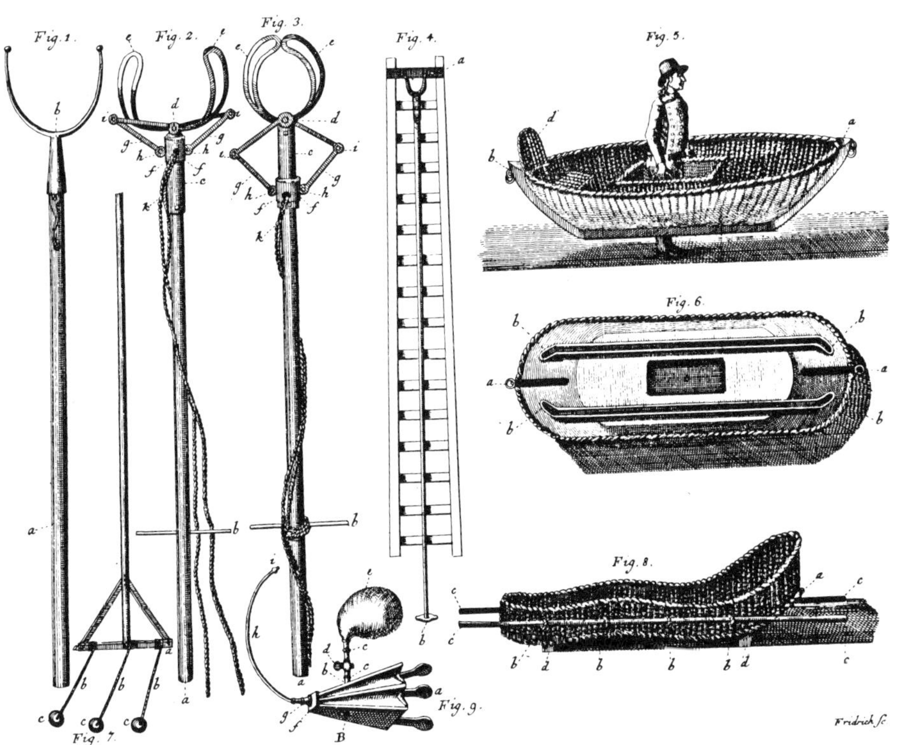

Fig. 1-2. Herholdt and Rafn included this illustration of equipment used to retrieve and resuscitate drowning victims during the late eighteenth century.

also recommended that an electrical current be passed through the heart by means of electrodes placed over the apex and base.

In retrospect, one can only wonder why most of the excellent theories and methods of resuscitation used or advocated by some of the early European workers have been overlooked or completely forgotten, that is, artificial respiration with tracheal intubation, chest compression, and electrical stimulation of the heart.

It is difficult for us to imagine the state of resuscitation 150 years ago. The only instrument used for ventilation was the fireside bellows, an instrument that Vesalius and Hook had demonstrated as lifesaving, but that Leroy d'Etoille in 1827 condemned because, when used incorrectly, it could lead to emphysema and tension pneumothorax. Unfortunately, he forgot to emphasize the benefits when they were used correctly. His discovery led to the abandonment of the bellows. The combined mortality was unacceptably high from the damage caused by incorrect use of the bellows and from overwhelming infections following tracheotomy at a time when antiseptics, asepsis, and antibiotics were unavailable. Even the importance of an open airway was not appreciated.

Discovery of Oxygen

Joseph Priestley, a dissenting minister, was an earnest inquirer into all wonders of nature and philosophy. In 1774 both he and the Swedish chemist Carl Wilhelm Scheele discovered oxygen independently of each other. Priestley called it "pure" or "vital air," or "dephlogisticated air," that is, air from which "phlogiston" (nitrogen) had been removed. He knew that this gas could support life in mice and could cause a candle to burn more vigorously. He wrote: "who can tell but that in time, the pure air may become a fashionable article of luxury; hitherto only two mice and myself have had the privilege of breathing it."

The French chemist Antoine Laurent Lavoisier coined the term *oxygen* and destroyed the phlogiston theory. Simon de Laplace showed that metabolism based on oxidation formed water and carbon dioxide as by-products, and that the lungs take up oxygen and give off carbon dioxide. Lavoisier was condemned as an enemy of the people because of the prerevolutionary royal support of his laboratory. His life was ended in May 8, 1794 by one lightning stroke of the guillotine, and France lost her leading scientist in the prime of his creative career.

Paradoxically, the discovery of oxygen contributed to the disuse of mouth-to-mouth resuscitation; in addition to the indelicacy of the method, it was believed that more oxygen could be given with a bellows than from exhaled air.

Early in the nineteenth century Sir Benjamin Brodie and the Royal Humane Society discontinued attempts to revive drowned people by artificial ventilation. They postulated that no one survived after 4 to 5 minutes under water no matter what was done. Thus the correct ideas of resuscitation were discredited, discontinued, and then forgotten. Again, it took another 100 years before real progress evolved.

NEGATIVE PRESSURE VENTILATION

From the middle of the nineteenth century to the first quarter of the twentieth century, an unbelievable number of devices were introduced that applied subambient, or negative, pressure to the outside of the body. Most of these devices offered the patient only a brief prolongation of a miserable death.

Two excellent reviews of apparatus using negative pressure were published in England by C. H. W. Woolman in 1976. J. H. Emerson of Cambridge, Massachusetts, also published the interesting and informative pamphlet, *The Evolution of the "Iron Lung."* Apparatus using negative pressure on the body surface can be classified in four groups: the tank ventilator, the "iron lung," the cuirass ventilator, and the "differential pressure chamber" of Sauerbruch.

Tank Ventilators

The term *iron lung* is fairly modern; many of the early tank or box ventilators were not made of iron. They were rigid containers big enough to house the entire body except for the head, which protruded through a hole with an airtight collar around the patient's neck. Intermittent negative or alternating negative/positive pressure could be created by mouth or by hand and, therefore, they were useless for prolonged treatments. Subsequently, mechanical drive mechanisms powered by steam, water, or electricity were employed to operate them. Until recent times, electricity was not reliable, especially in the smaller towns, where lightning and mechanical malfunctions could interrupt the electric supply for hours or days.

Physicians believed it was physiologically more beneficial to breathe for a patient by applying negative pressure to the outside of the lungs than to blow positive pressure into the airways. Although this belief is undoubtedly true from an academic (theoretical) point of view, the early machines did not prove it. They were large, cumbersome, awkward, and burdened by innumerable complications. Most of all, in their initial developmental stages they did not work.

In 1838 Dr. John Dalziel of Drumlanrig, Scotland, described a body-enclosing respiratory in which the patient sat upright with his head protruding from the top. A bellows created the pressure changes. A similar iron lung was described by Alfred F. Jones of Lexington, Kentucky, in 1864 (Fig. 1-3). He obtained a patent (U.S. patent no. 44 198) in which he postulated that when properly and judiciously applied it will "cure paralysis, neuralgia, rheumatism, seminal weakness, asthma, bronchitis, and dyspepsia. Also, deafness . . . and . . . many other diseases. . . ."

Describing this tank ventilator in 1876, Ignez von Hauke from Austria noted that the head and neck were enclosed in an elastic cap with the face left uncovered and that negative pressure was generated by a hand-operated mechanism (Fig. 1-4). With the tank ventilator, von Hauke successfully treated a small girl "with great debility and chronic double pneumonia" for 3 months.

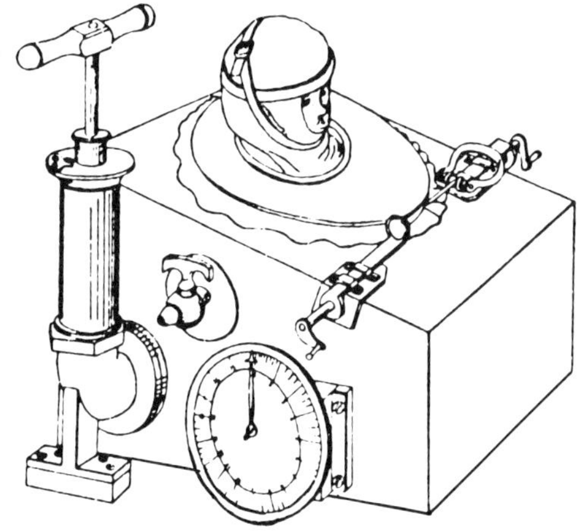

Fig. 1-3. Alfred E. Jones' body-enclosing iron lung (1864). (Courtesy of J. H. Emerson, Esq.)

In 1876 Woillez of Paris built the first workable iron lung, called the "Spirophore," which was very similar to the best of the later models (Fig. 1-5). One unique feature was a rod that rested lightly on the patient's chest and moved up and down, giving visual proof of chest movements.

Some of the other older devices were interesting, although useless. One was described in 1887 by Dr. Charles Breuillard of Paris (Fig. 1-6) in which the patient sat upright in a "bath cabinet." Vacuum was created by a steam ejector, fed by a steam boiler, which was heated by a spirit lamp. The patient was supposed to operate a valve, alternately connecting the cabinet to the vacuum for inhalation and to the atmosphere for exhalation.

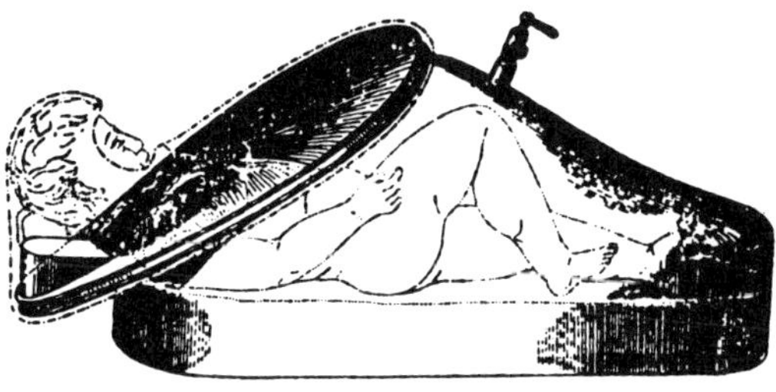

Fig. 1-4. Von Hauke's Pneumatische Apparate (1876).

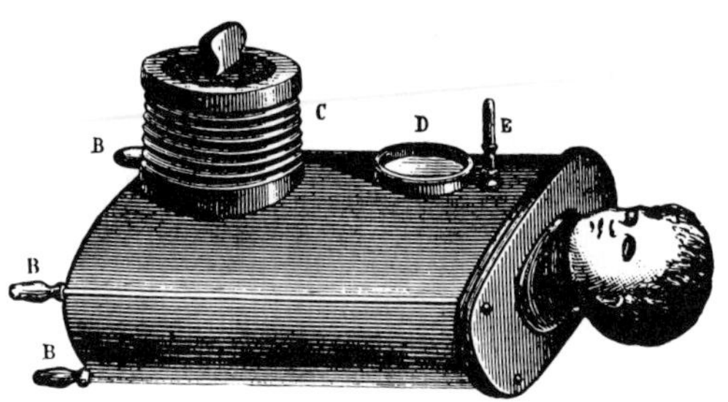

Fig. 1-5. "Spirophore" by Woillez of Paris built in 1876.

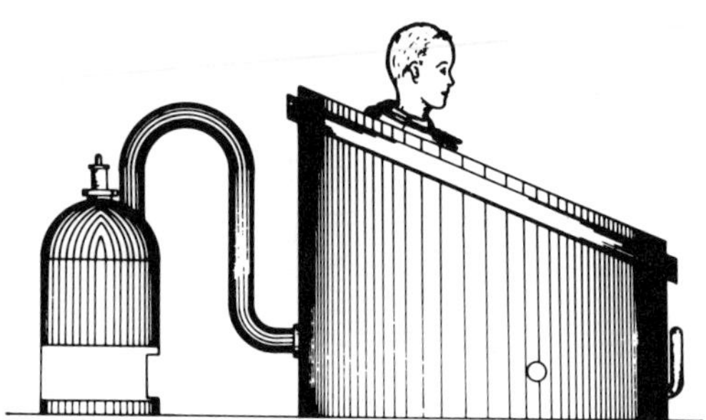

Fig. 1-6. Dr. Charles Breuillard of Paris patented a "bath cabinet" type of respirator in 1877. (Courtesy of J. H. Emerson Company.)

In 1889 Dr. Egon Braun of Vienna described similar machines for resuscitation of asphyxiated children (Fig. 1-7). An infant was placed in a small wooden box supported by a plaster mold, his head was then extended so that the nose and mouth were pressed against a hole in a rubber closure. Pressure and suction were created by the doctor's own breath via a tube going into the box.

In 1905 Dr. William Davenport of London and Dr. Charles Morgan Hammond of Memphis, Tennessee designed iron lungs very similar to that of Woillez. In 1908 Peter Lord of Worchester, Massachusetts, patented a respirator room large enough to allow a nurse to work inside it. Melvin L. Severy of Boston patented an ingenious but hopeless box in 1916 in which the patient had to stand up, pressing his nose and mouth against a triangular opening in the front wall (Fig. 1-8).

The "Barospirator" was introduced in 1920 by Dr. T. Thunberg of Lund, Sweden (Fig. 1-9). The first design had the entire patient enclosed in a tank. Later, it was reconfigured into a room so large that the medical staff could be accommodated as well. It worked on a completely different principle from the rest, being based on the high compressibility of air. An enormously large, motor-driven piston cylinder caused the pressure to vary from 7 kPa (50 mmHg) above atmospheric pressure to 7 kPa below it. When pressure increased, the volume

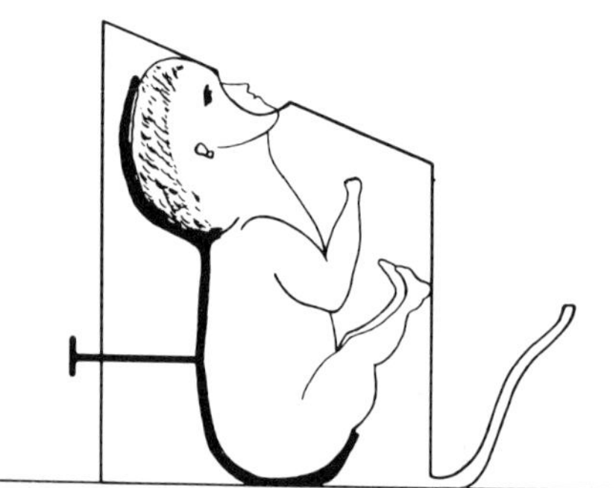

Fig. 1-7. Dr. Egon Braun of Vienna devised a small wooden box in 1889 in which pressure and suction were created by the doctor's own breath (via the tube at the right). This was employed for resuscitating asphyxiated children. (Courtesy of J. H. Emerson Company.)

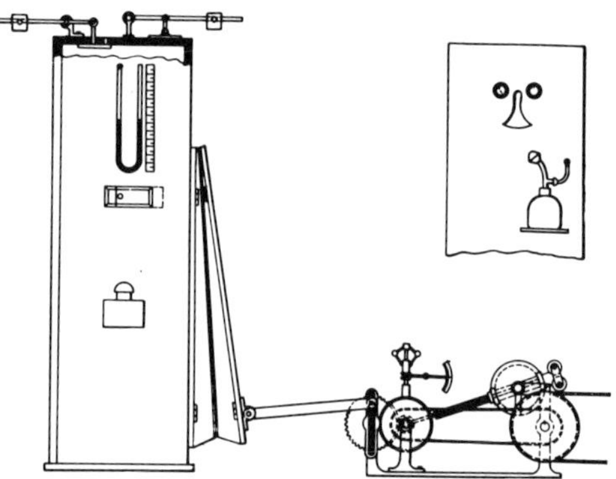

Fig. 1-8. Dr. Melvin L. Severy of Boston created an ingenious mechanical device for ventilation. However, the patient was obliged to stand, pressing his nose and mouth against a triangular aperture below two eye windows. (Courtesy of J. H. Emerson Company.)

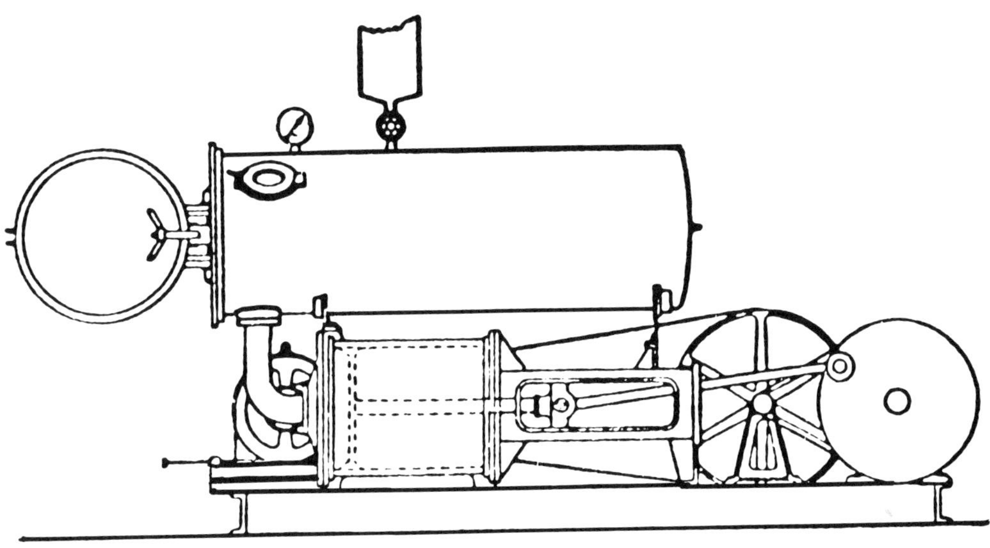

Fig. 1-9. Thunberg's barospirator (1920).

of the air decreased and air flowed into the lungs; the reverse occurred as pressure decreased. By this ingenious technique, artificial respiration was obtained with no respiratory movements of the chest.

In 1926 Wilhelm Schwake of Oranienburg-Eden, Germany patented perhaps the most unusual pneumatic chamber in which the patient had to stand up and create the pressure differences by moving a large bellows with his own hands. Schwake also postulated that "negative pressure upon the skin . . . draws out . . . the gaseous by-products" (Fig. 1-10).

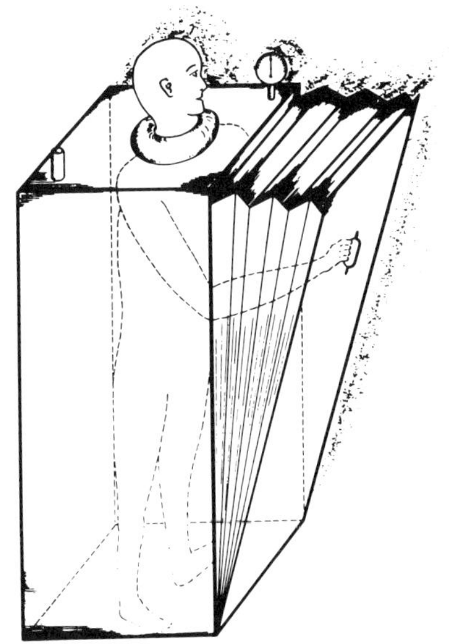

Fig. 1-10. William Schwake of Oranienburg-Eden, Germany, patented a "pneumatic chamber" in 1926. (Courtesy of J. H. Emerson Company.)

Iron Lungs

In 1926 the Consolidated Gas Company of New York documented that an alarming number of their workers were victims of electric shock and gas or smoke inhalation. To treat these afflicted workers, the company retained the services of Dr. C. K. Drinker, professor of physiology at Harvard University School of Public Health. Drinker told the company of the exciting work that his brother, Dr. Phillip Drinker, and his associate, Dr. Louis Agassiz Shaw, were engaged in at Harvard. They placed an anesthetized and curarized cat in an airtight iron box with only the head exposed through a closely fitted rubber collar. The box was connected to a hand-operated cylinder-piston pump; when air was sucked out of the box, the pressure fell and caused the cat to inhale. Alternating inflation and suction kept the cat alive for a long time.

Construction of an adult-sized model followed, composed of a sheet metal cylinder big enough to enclose a patient. It was closed at one end. The patient's head and neck protruded through a hole with an airtight collar in the other end. The sides of the cylinder had portholes for observing the patient, as well as numerous other small sealed outlets for manometers, blood pressure cuffs, stethoscopes, and so forth. An electrically powered pump ran continuously, producing alternating positive and negative pressure in the tank via a system of valves.

In the spring of 1929 the company donated the first fully operational electric iron lung to Bellevue hospital in New York City. Its value was demonstrated immediately when a young woman was brought in unconscious and unable to breathe after accidentally ingesting an unknown drug. The patient was placed in the iron lung, and made a full recovery. Later that year, a student from Harvard University was stricken with poliomyelitis and was ventilated in the iron lung until the polio receded. Gradually he regained the ability to breathe and was eventually weaned from the iron lung. He returned to Harvard, finished his studies, and went on to start a full and useful career.

The enormous potential of the device was immediately recognized, and demand rapidly outpaced supply. Dr. Drinker turned to the Warren E. Collins Company in Braintree, Massachusetts, which manufactured the Drinker Respirator, as the iron lung was more formally named.

The first iron lungs were complicated and bulky, and cost well over $2,000 (enough to buy two automobiles in 1929). In 1931, John Haven Emerson improved, modified, and simplified the iron lung and was able to sell it for $1,000. Emerson added a transparent airtight dome that could be fitted over the patient's head to provide intermittent positive-pressure ventilation (IPPV). With this device, the iron lung could be opened, permitting good and unhurried nursing care to the patient's immobile body.

On a visit to Sir Robert Macintosh's department of Anesthesia at Oxford, Lord Nuffield (William Morris) was shown a film on artificial respiration made under the direction of Dr. C. L. G. Pratt. The British Both Respirator (iron lung) particularly impressed Nuffield. A few days later, he chanced to see a headline in the paper: "Iron Lung Arrives Too Late." It was a story of a young patient whose life might have been saved had a respirator arrived in time. The article said that there were only five iron lungs in England.

On November 24, 1938, after a conference with Macintosh, Lord Nuffield announced in the Oxford Mail that: "It will give me the greatest pleasure to think that his machine will save lives." Nuffield offered to make up 5,000 of them at Cowley, at a cost of some £500,000 (equivalent to $2,500,000) and to donate one to every hospital in the United Kingdom and the dominions.

Nuffield requested that Macintosh's department supervise the distribution of Both respirators and also provided initial instruction in their use. Demonstrations were given daily at the Radcliffe Infirmary to doctors and nurses. This was an enormous task. By the end of 1939, more than 1,600 respirators had been allocated to hospitals throughout the empire.

At one stroke, the engineer-philanthropist resolved a long-standing medical argument and forced physicians to treat developing respiratory failure actively. At the same time, he involved anesthesiologists in this form of therapy, as they were often the only people who knew how the apparatus worked. This event foreshadowed their later involvement in respiratory and critical care medicine. Macintosh in 1940 and Mushin and Faux in 1944 were the first to prevent postoperative lung complications with success; they used the Both iron lung. Although enclosing the patient in a cabinet greatly complicated nursing care, it was not until 1955, when Björk and Engström used positive-pressure ventilation with the Engström ventilator for the same purpose that the latter method became widely popular.

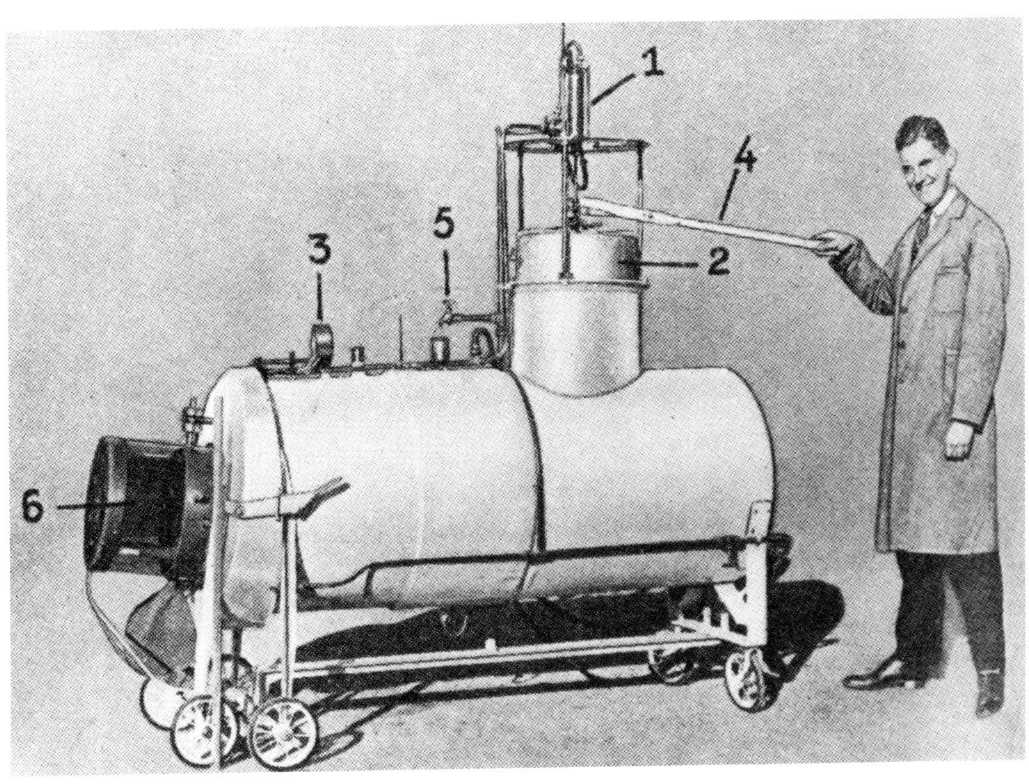

Fig. 1-11. August Krogh's modification of the Drinker "iron lung."

During a visit to New York, the famous Danish physiologist, August Krough, saw the Drinker respirator in use and was immediately impressed by its possibilities as a clinical tool. Upon his return to Copenhagen in 1931, he constructed the first Danish respirator designed especially for clinical use (Fig. 1-11). In principle, it was identical to the Drinker respirator but was improved and simplified. The motor was powered by water from the city piplines. Reciprocating movements were created by leading the water alternatingly to the upper and lower compartments of a piston cylinder, which acted on a large spirometer bell. Among its worthwhile features were a water jacket for regulating the temperature inside the tank, maneuverability that permitted a 15-degree head-down position, and a hood which could be placed over the patient's head to supply him with oxygen or carbogen, a mixture of 95 percent oxygen and 5 percent carbon dioxide which at that time was a popular respiratory stimulant. Krogh also made an infant respirator version and a rocking stretcher.

Inherent Complications of the Iron Lungs

Good nursing care was nearly impossible in the first iron lungs. Simple procedures, such as taking the temperature or blood pressure, counting the pulse, giving a bed bath, or turning the patient to prevent bed sores, were nearly impossible before Emerson developed his transparent dome. Many patients suffered from claustrophobia, disorientation, and loneliness from being encapsulated in the big tank. Visiting relatives, whom they might see approaching upside-down if they were privileged enough to have the necessary mirror, could not even hold their hands. Their necks were always sore from the necessarily tight collar, which in the best of cases felt like a shirt collar two sizes too small. Very often it caused open circular wounds and chronic headaches. It was so constricting that the patients could constantly hear their own pulses.

Perhaps the most important benefit of the iron lung was that it represented a stepping-off point for Emerson. Actually, three generations of the Emerson family have had an enormously beneficial influence on respiratory care advances. In 1909 Grandfather H. Emerson described the influence of artificial respiration on pulmonary edema. His still youthful son, John Haven Emerson, has provided the medical profession with an endless number of intelligently designed and usable pieces of equipment. Finally, George P. Emerson seems to be following the same line. He has been of great help to this author.

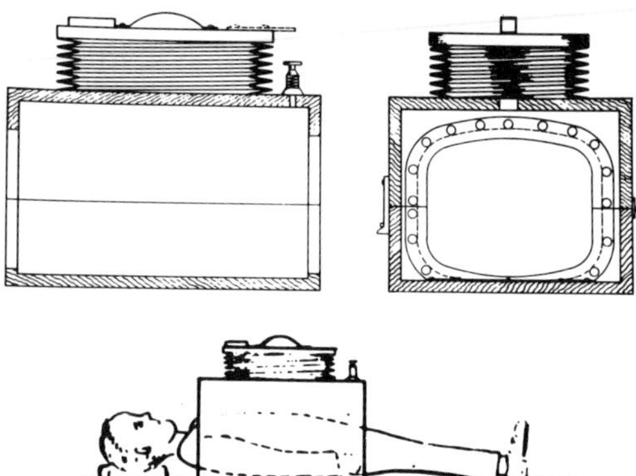

Fig. 1-12. In 1901 Rudolf Eisenmenger of Piski, Hungary patented a portable respirator which consisted of a "simple, two-part box" enclosing only the patient's chest. (Courtesy of J. H. Emerson Company.)

Cuirass Ventilators

The word *cuirass* dates back to the fifteenth century and means a piece of armor covering the chest. Cuirass ventilators were also rigid, intermittent negative-pressure containers. However, they covered only the patient's chest or chest and abdomen, leaving the extremities and pelvis accessible. Two additional advantages over the iron lungs were their economy and portability.

According to Woollam, the first cuirasses were made by Ignez von Hauke of Austria in 1874, by Alexander Graham Bell in 1882, and by Rudolph Eisenmenger of Piski, Hungary in 1901 (Fig. 1-12). In 1927 the "Dr. Eisenmenger Biomotor," a motor-driven version, was patented in the United States. It was reported to be an "extraordinary success." A great number of cuirasses are described in Woollam's excellent thesis, most of them developed in the United Kingdom, United States, France, or Sweden.

Eventually, Collier and Affeldt compared cuirasses with tank respirators. They found that if they took the tidal volume produced by the tank as 100 percent, the thoracoabdominal cuirass produced 61 to 63 percent but the thoracic cuirass only 47 percent. Bryce-Smith and Davis found that the cuirass required much more negative pressure to produce the same tidal volume as the tank. In 1948 in a preliminary report of 827 cases of poliomyelitis, Bergman reported with pride the results of use of the Swedish "Sahlin-Stille" cuirass. Fifteen percent of the patients survived, which "by far exceeds the general Swedish mortality. Those—indeed many—cases we cannot save by the respirators are at least spared the torments of suffocation." He suggested, however, that "only 2 percent of all treated cases could be saved for a useful social life."

In 1955 Pask stated that:

> It is very much to be hoped that further development will occur in this field, for the cuirass respirators must surely embarrass the circulation less than nearly all other types. . . . IF it can be made comfortable enough for continuous use over long periods, IF it can be made capable of producing really adequate ventilation in all patients, and IF it can be so modified that it be possible to nurse the patient in the

prone position, then surely the future for this-type of respirator must be very important.

Professor Pask's three "IFs" accurately summed up the problems of cuirass ventilation.

In 1953 Toker, and later Green and Coleman, described a completely new use for the cuirass when he successfully used a "Kifa" cuirass to ventilate patients during general anesthesia for bronchoscopy and laryngoscopy, a procedure which previously had presented a very difficult problem for the anesthetist. Wallace and his associates produced the longest single series of 248 such patients. They failed to ventilate only 16 of these adequately because of poor fit of the shell, obesity, or chronic lung disease. I have found that the Emerson wrap-around "raincoat" ventilator driven by a vacuum cleaner may be the best for these difficult cases because the rigid metallic supporting shell and the covering raincoat adapt better to patients with unusual shapes (Fig. 1-13).

A few users still advocate tank respirators in the acute stages of some respiratory disease and for some cases of chronic paralysis in special chronic hospital units. There are also a considerable number of patients living at home whose lives depend on the use of the cuirass respirator. Some have used it for more than 25 years.

From an educational viewpoint, I must agree with Woollam that "It is unfortunate that a generation of anaesthetists is being trained who have little or no knowledge of the tank or cuirass."

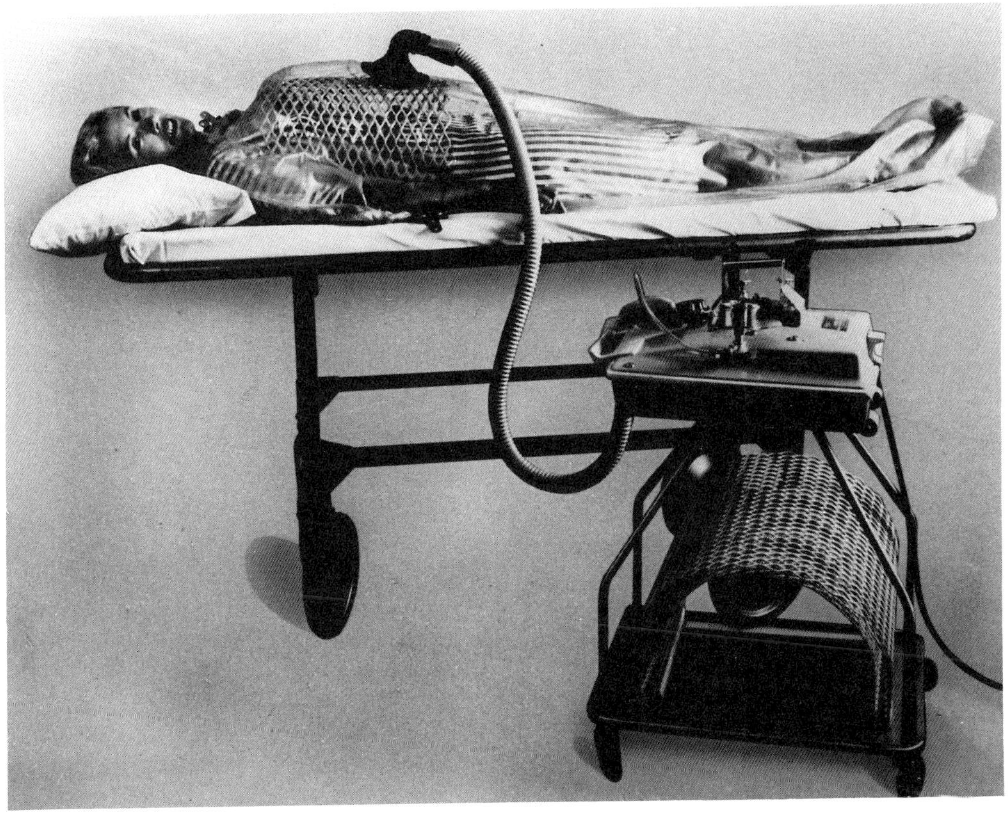

Fig. 1-13. An Emerson chest respirator that employed a light garment ("raincoat") over the patient to effect the air seal and a shell over the chest and abdomen to hold the plastic garment away from the body. Intermittent negative pressure was developed inside the shell by a vacuum cleaner. (Courtesy of J. H. Emerson Company.)

Sauerbruch's Differential Pressure Chamber

Sauerbruch's differential pressure chamber appeared in 1904, when Ernst Ferdinand Sauerbruch, assistant to von Mikulicz in Breslau, Germany, published his dramatic experimental work, *The Pathology of Open Pneumothorax and the Basic Principle of My Method of Eliminating It.* Unfortunately, this treatise represented a significant deviation from the sequential ventilator development pattern that had preceded its publication. Sauerbruch transformed the operating room into a sort of enlarged pleural space (Fig. 1-14). He constructed a small airtight operating room where the patient's body and the surgeons were inside, and the patient's head outside. The hole around the patient's neck was airtight. By continuous suction, Sauerbruch created a subatmospheric pressure inside the operating room equal to the pleural pressure, and the patient's head and upper airways were exposed to atmospheric pressure. In this way, he expanded the lungs during open thoracotomy and theorized that the patient could breathe spontaneously while receiving inhalation anesthesia.

Sauerbruch's "pneumatic chamber," as this contraption was called, solved a theoretical problem from the physiological point of view. However, even the most technically perfect chamber broke down during clinical use for several reasons: the surgeon and his assistants had

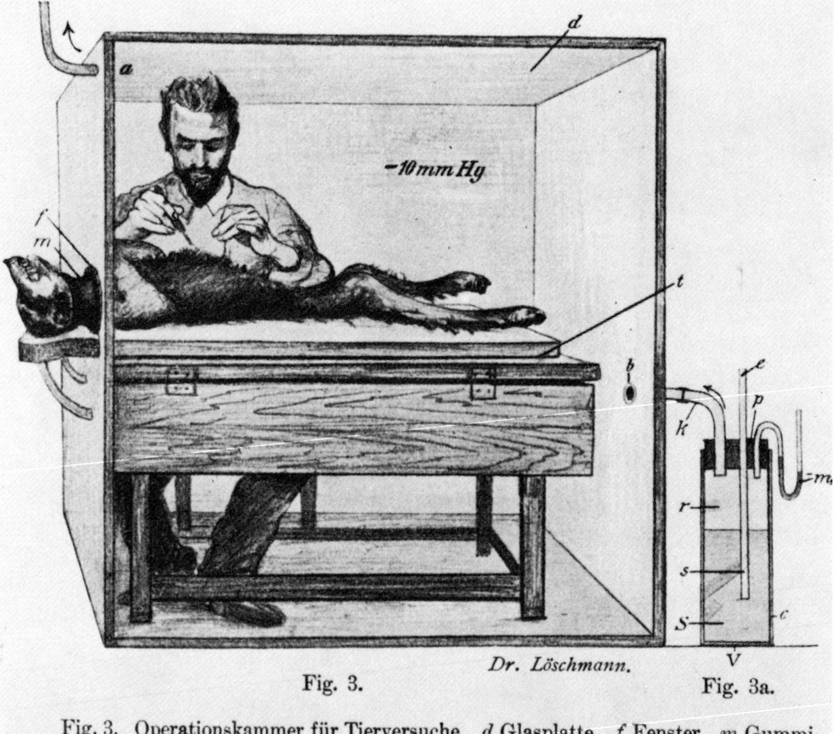

Fig. 1-14. Ernst Ferdinand Sauerbruck of Breslau, Germany developed a differential pressure chamber in 1904.

very little room for movement; the heat was almost unbearable; and it was extremely difficult to communicate satisfactorily with the anesthetist outside the chamber. For these and other reasons, the differential pressure method was abandoned and today is nothing more than a historical curio. Sauerbruch's assistant, R. Nissen, later professor of surgery a Basel, said that Sauerbruch's refusal to recognize modern anesthesia and its physiological approach delayed the advance of thoracic surgery by more than 25 years.

I experienced a remnant of this attitude when I visited the leading surgeon at the University of Heidelberg during the 1950s. Grand rounds took place whenever it suited the professor. The procession was based on rank only, with the professor in the front of a pyramid-shaped flock of first assistants, most often overtrained, underpaid, subservient surgeons in their 40s. Behind

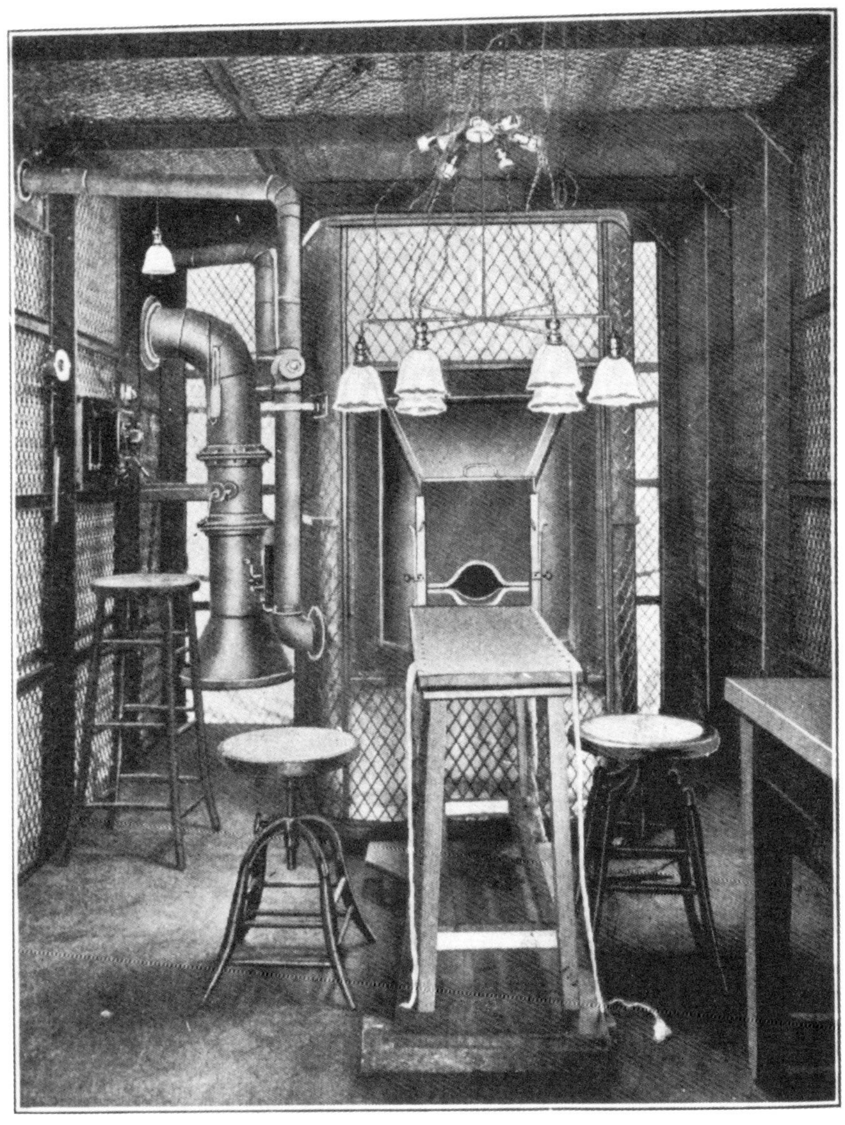

Fig. 1-15. In 1909 Dr. Willy Meyer of New York constructed a differential pressure chamber in which to perform thoracic surgical procedures.

them came second and third assistants, residents, interns, students, and last, because after all they were only female, the nurses.

As a visiting professor, I was allowed to walk a half step behind the professor. I saw him walk right into a closed door, screaming and stamping, convulsing, and swearing because none of his humble servants had jumped ahead of him to open the door. Finally, we reached the large ward with 20 or more patients, all lying flat on their backs, in military attention position, with all the sheets folded in a perfect continued, interrupted line from bed to bed. The professor never talked directly to the patients or mentioned them by name. Remarks about "the gallbladder in bed 17" were delivered to the shivering head nurse.

The use of differential pressure chambers was never popular in the United States except with one surgeon, Willy Meyer, at the German Hospital in New York. In 1909 he and his brother Julius constructed a chamber for positive and/or negative differential pressure (Fig. 1-15). It was composed of an outer negative chamber, which served as the operating room, and a positive inner pressure chamber, in which the anesthetist remained. Thus, the surgeon could operate under negative pressure around the thorax or under positive pressure around the patient's head. A combination could also be employed, and a change from one to the other was possible during the same operation.

BACK TO THE DIRECT APPROACH

As early as Vesalius in 1542, Robert Hooke in 1667, Fothergill in 1744, Meltzer in 1892, and Matas in 1899, controlled breathing had been practiced by physiologists who kept their curarized animals alive by this means. Conditions of controlled breathing were clearly described in Meltzer's work *Respiratory Changes of Intrathoracic Pressure,* which he published in 1892. The tubes employed were introduced through a tracheotomy. Apparently no one noticed the difference when Auer and Meltzer introduced oral intubation in 1909. Today controlled ventilation has become an integral part of general anesthesia, and physicians and respiratory therapists find it difficult to believe that a mystique still enshrouded tracheal intubation as late as 1950.

During the last decade of the nineteenth century, knowledge of respiration and the support thereof was more than adequate for the purpose of open chest surgery. It included understanding basic physiologic principles, tracheal intubation with cuffed tubes, oxygen compressed in tanks, ventilators, devices for producing continuous positive pressure or intermittent positive pressure with retard of expiration, and apparatus for the administration of general anesthesia. In 1899 Rudolph Matas of New Orleans wrote: "The procedure that promises the most benefit is . . . rhythmic maintenance of artificial respiration by a tube in the glottis" (Fig. 1-16).

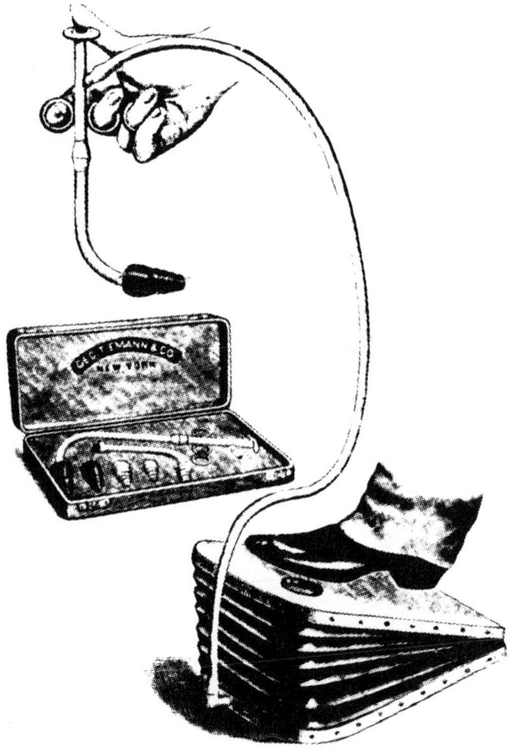

Fig. 1-16. In 1899 Rudolph Matas of New Orleans described a procedure of artificial respiration achieved with endotracheal intubation and manual insufflation of air using the Fell-O'Dwyer Bellows.

On the European continent, the simplest direct approach, combining artificial respiration with tracheal intubation, was presented by Franz Kuhn in Kassel, Germany in 1905. He was the first to pass a suction catheter through an endotracheal tube. In 1910 Läwen and Sievers, in Friederich Trendelenburg's department in Leipzig, reported a piston ventilator that applied alternating positive and negative pressure, with supplemental oxygen through an endotracheal tube (Fig. 1-17).

The period from 1880 to 1910 was one of high hopes and a flurry of activity for thoracic surgeons. However, it failed because of a lack of antibiotics and blood transfusions. Mortality from sepsis and hemorrhage was high. Surgical techniques were often not sufficiently developed, bronchi and vessels being ligated en bloc. Biilau's underwater drain was forgotten. The chest was closed airtight, with sudden deaths resulting from bronchial leak and tension pneumothorax. For these reasons, and *not* because of failures to support ventilation, clinical activities decreased and experimental work increased.

For many decades, the dangers of pneumothorax were overestimated because no apparent distinction was made between open and tension varieties. One of the mistakes involved the application of observations made in animals directly to humans. Not until the second decade of this century did the French surgeon Duval point out the fundamentally different nature of human and animal mediastina. In humans the mediastinum is sufficiently firm to prevent spontaneous tearing if only one pleural space is opened. By contrast, because of the dog's delicate mediasti-

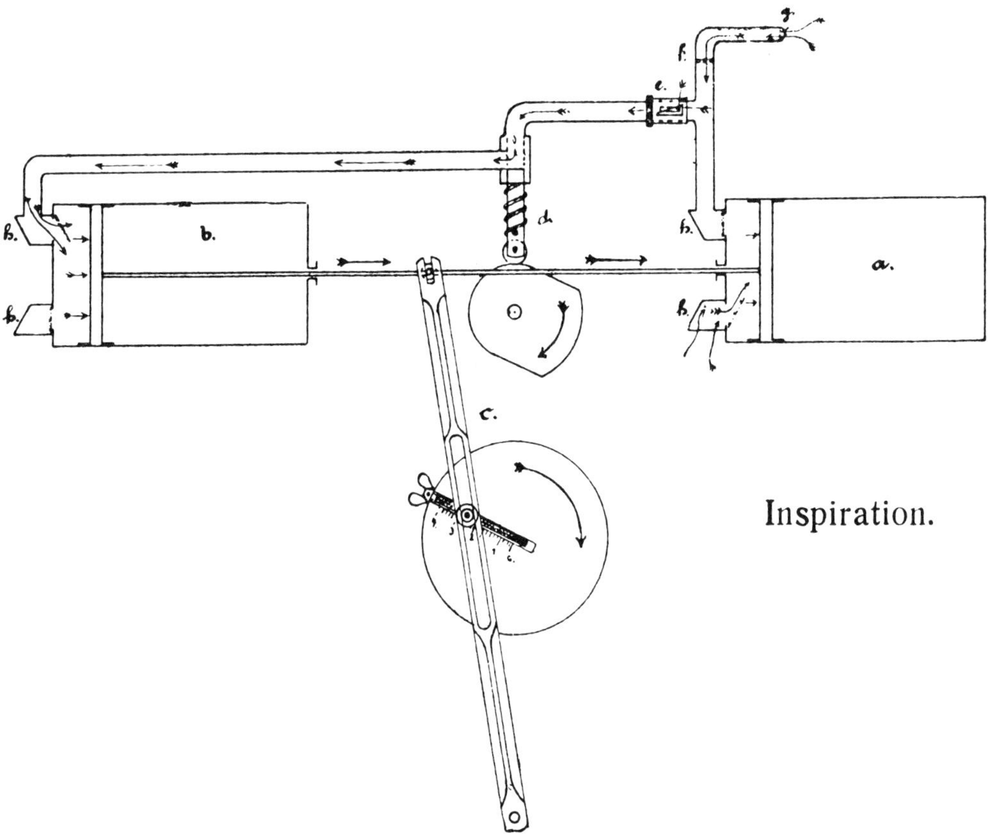

Fig. 1-17. Läwen and Sievers of Leipzig, Germany developed a double-piston respirator in 1910. It provided mechanical inspiration and facilitated exhalation in intubated patients.

nal septum, a unilateral open pneumothorax at once becomes bilateral.

Experimental Thoracic Surgery

From 1910 to 1930, significant advances occurred in experimental surgical and physiological laboratories. Negative- and positive-pressure cabinets never became popular among American surgeons. Instead, they developed a variety of intralaryngeal tubes for direct introduction of air into the lungs from pumps especially devised for this purpose. In 1920, for example, the Philadelphia surgeon George Morris Dorrance and the New York surgeon C. A. Elsberg, as well as Läwen and Sievers from Trendelenburg's department in Liepzig, all published outstanding works on these procedures. In 1913 Henry H. Janeway of New York described an ingenious machine for anesthesia and artificial respiration (Fig. 1-18) with a cuffed endotracheal tube ("a little rubber occluding bag with double wall, pulled over the end of the intratracheal catheter"), exactly the shape of the ones used today. Janeway also developed the first modern laryngoscope:

> The back of the tongue is touched with 10 percent cocaine; the patient is then anesthetized, preferably by chloroform, in the usual manner and the catheter inserted into the trachea. This may be accomplished by means of the Jackson direct laryngoscope so modified that it is deficient at the side in a manner permitting of the withdrawal of the instrument without the necessity of pushing the catheter through it—without detaching it from—the gas bag.

This laryngoscope was the first to use batteries in the handle. Janeway also appreciated the potentially adverse effects of positive pressure on the circulation. In many respects, he was 20 to 30 years ahead of his time.

Unfortunately, as so often happens, these bril-

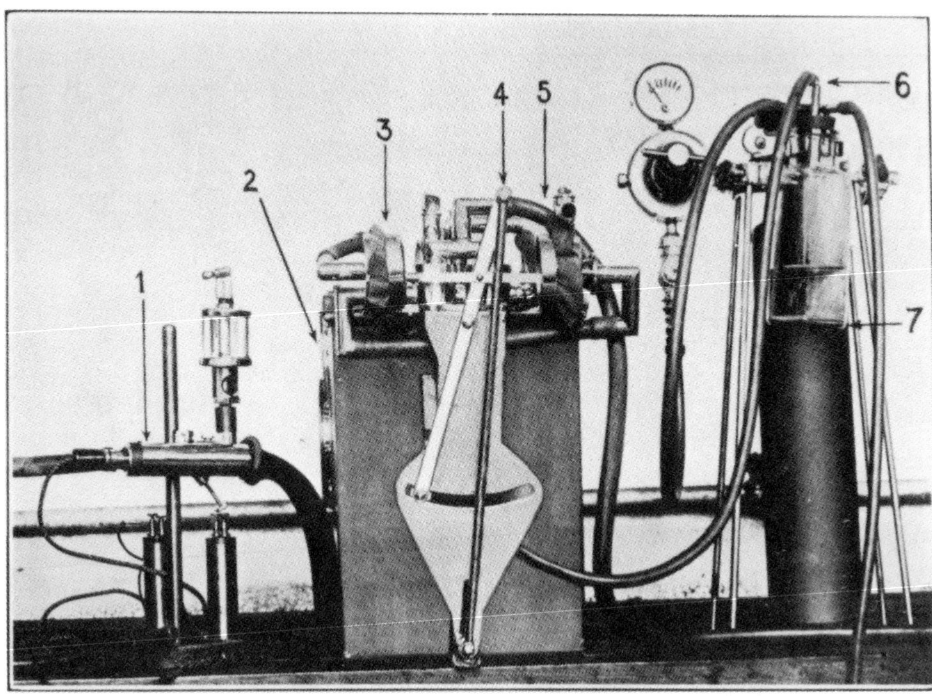

Fig. 1-18. Janeway's anesthesia machine, which was constructed about 1910 at Columbia University. 1, rebreathing valve; 2, aluminum box; 3 and 5, tambours controlling position of valves; 4, spring controlling height of pressure within box; 6, nitrous tank with reducing valve attached; 7, wash bottle measuring the flow of nitrous oxide and oxygen.

liant experimental surgeons evolved satisfactory solutions to the anesthetic and respiratory problems they faced while they were young, enthusiastic, and idealistic, but they did not follow up their developments. Few interested assistants were available; anesthetic techniques were crude, poorly taught, and practiced by members of the house or nursing staff who were unenthusiastic but could not avoid administering anesthesia for the next (not infrequently fatal) case. Perhaps the inventors did not try to persuade others of their ideas; or maybe as they grew older they saw that there was no money in research and much to be had in the treatment of patients. Their brilliant ideas languished and withered with nobody to follow up on them. Janeway left the field in 1914 to become a pioneer in radiotherapy. His respiratory machine was available at Presbyterian Hospital, but it was deemed too complicated to use and it never became popular (Fig. 1-18). Elsberg, one of the few surgeons who learned laryngoscopy for tracheal intubation and who developed the clinical application of Meltzer's and Auer's insufflation methods, made a much better living as a neurosurgeon.

Small Portable Resuscitators

In 1907 the idea of using positive airway pressure during resuscitation was rediscovered by Heinrich Dräger of Lübeck, Germany. His famous "Pulmotor" was a small apparatus built into a suitcase. It consisted of two small concertina bags and a very stiff spring-and-toggle mechanism which activated a valve, giving a mixture of oxygen and air, sometimes with 5 percent carbon dioxide, at 3 kPa (20 mmHg) pressure during inspiration. During expiration, a subatmospheric pressure of −3 kPa was applied, a dangerously low level that could easily cause airway collapse in certain patients.

The Pulmotor was designed for resuscitation in mines and gained great popularity over the next 40 years, particularly with fire departments and police rescue units. The general medical standard of resuscitation during the mid-1930s is illustrated by the fact that as a medical student I observed surgeons calling the fire department to bring their Pulmotor to treat patients in hospitals that had absolutely no means of resuscitation.

I have tried breathing with the Pulmotor. It requires an enormous and unpleasant pressure to stop the mechanical inspiratory flow rate, and I found the suction, or negative pressure, during exhalation most unpleasant before the pulmotor switched back to the brutally high inspiratory flow. I estimate that airway pressure was higher than the commonly quoted value of ±3 kPa (20 mmHg), probably closer to ±7 to 10 kPa (50 to 75 mmHg). Drinker and McKhann found the Pulmotor unsatisfactory following a case in which it was used to provide life support for 2 days. A rupture of the esophagus and stomach developed, and gastric contents were found in the mediastinum.

A great number of other smaller, hand-held resuscitators gained popularity during the many years before ventilators became commonly used. A few examples are the Kreiselman resuscitator (about 1940); Neff inflation valve (1945); Burn valve, especially designed for the Air Force (1946); Mushin and Hillard "Cardiff" valve (1953); Fink valve (1954); Digby-Leigh valve (1956); Frumin nonrebreathing valve; and Reed "Dewsbury" inflation valve (1959).

Undoubtedly the most popular hand-operated resuscitator is the Ambu-bag designed in 1954 by Henning Ruben of Copenhagen. It is a simple, reliable instrument used for manual resuscitation in the emergency room and during transportation inside and outside the hospital—a resuscitator so good it has been copied dozens of times by other manufacturers. Today, rightfully so, it is found in most hospitals throughout the world.

Tracheal Intubation

Although Chevalier Jackson of Pittsburgh devoted his life to instructing anesthesiologists in "the technique of inserting intratracheal insufflation tubes," few paid any attention to the advantages of the technique. Positive-pressure methods that did *not* require intubation were preferred—tracheal intubation was still considered very difficult and very dangerous.

Nevertheless, improvement in methodology was achieved during the First World War by Ivan Whiteside Magill and E. S. Rowbotham of London while they served as anesthetists with the British Army plastic surgery unit in France. They modified, simplified, and publicized tracheal intubation. To them goes our gratitude for intubation as we know it today.

While studying in London in 1947, I had the privilege and great pleasure to listen to and learn from these two physicians. Magill was a technical master in anesthesia, charming and delightful to observe but somewhat less accomplished as a teacher. Rowbotham was a better teacher (and showman), who demonstrated his points in a direct, dry way. He was a chain smoker and always smoked while giving anesthesia. While demonstrating that explosions only happened to those who did not know what they were doing, he enjoyed observing our reactions as he rested his lit cigarette on the ether vaporizer during anesthesia.

MODERN VENTILATORS

The evolution of present-day ventilators has been described in such a masterly fashion by Mushin, Rendell-Baker, Thompson, Mapleson, and Hillard that I refuse to even try to compete with them; instead, I prefer to quote them extensively, especially in the following pages.

Modern ventilators can, in fact, be traced back to Scandinavian initiatives taken in 1915 by Holder Mølgaard of Copenhagen, T. Thunberg of Lund, and especially by K. H. Giertz of Stockholm, in 1916. However, these three outstanding scientists all made the same unforgivable mistake. They published in Danish or Swedish, which in the scientific community was similar to writing in water. The data were hidden, lost, and forgotten almost as soon as it was written.

Giertz, formerly one of Sauerbruch's assistants, showed experimentally that artificial ventilation obtained through positive-pressure rhythmic insufflation was superior to every form of constant differential pressure breathing. He enlisted the help of the skilled ear, nose, and throat surgeon Paul Frenckner to evolve a series of endotracheal tubes. He also convinced the experimental engineer Emil Anderson of the AGA Company to develop an air-driven ventilator, the "Spiropulsator." Its essential valve was the AGA flasher for automatic sea buoys, designed to send out precisely timed flashes of burning acetylene. Clarence Crafoord used the Spiropulsator while working on the technical problems of pneumonectomy. The first commercial model of the Spiropulsator was offered in 1940; Mushin et al. write:

> Crafoord found the interest of his American colleagues lukewarm, at best, when he demonstrated the "Spiropulsator" during operations on their patients. Among the exceptions were the experimental cardiac surgeons, Beck and Mautz of Cleveland, who had already made their own similar version in 1939.

Unfortunately, Crafoord's demonstration in the United States ended with a loud bang when the cyclopropane found it's way back to the source of the compressed air created by a vacuum cleaner with a sparking motor.

At the beginning of World War II, I was unable to import a Spiropulsator from Sweden and was compelled, therefore, to commence the design and construction of my first piston ventilator in German-occupied Denmark (Fig. 1-19). Ole Lippmann of the medical instrument company of Simonsen and Weel had an excellent workshop in Copenhagen with several highly skilled mechanics. The mechanic who did most of my work was Arne Fin Schram, later the founder and owner of the competing instrument firm "Dameca." Because of the war, materials were scarce. The piston and cylinder, for example, had to be made from a discarded piece of dirty old sewer pipe from the streets of Copenhagen. The ventilator rate was changed by a rheostat acting on an old electric brush motor that sent out a continuous shower of sparks during the administration of nitrous oxide and ether.

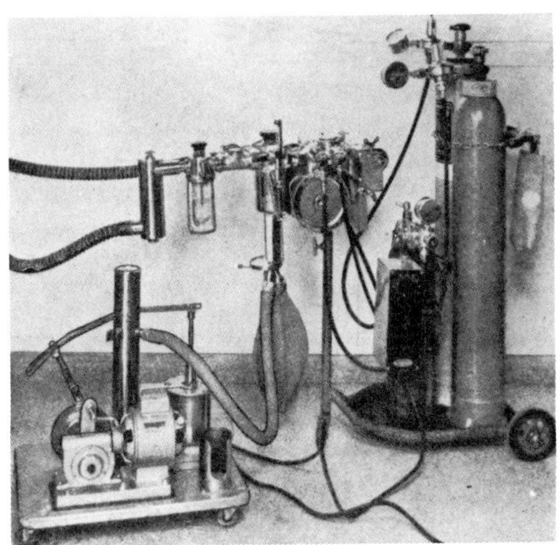

Fig. 1-19. In 1940 Ernst Trier Mörch designed his first piston ventilator.

This, the first clinically proven volume ventilator, was used in a great number of thoracic operations performed by Erik Husfeldt, Tage Kjaer, and Jens Lyn Hansen between 1940 and 1949 in Denmark.

At a relatively early stage in my new career as anesthesiologist in Denmark, Henry Beecher from Harvard visited Copenhagen. After one of his lectures, he was asked about his technique for thoracic surgery anesthesia. He told the bewildered audience that he rarely used endotracheal tubes, never used a mechanical respirator. There I was, a young, unproved candidate for a new and important job, using all the commodities the "prophet" from Harvard had just condemned. My only defense was that most of my patients survived.

During 1946 and 1947 I was privileged to study anesthesia under Sir Robert Macintosh and William W. Mushin; I have never met better teachers. My first meeting with Sir Robert Macintosh was in the winter of 1945 when I applied for a position in his and Mushin's masterly teaching program. I went to his office, and his secretary informed me that the professor was out skating on the meadows of Oxford. She asked me if I could skate, and when I answered affirmatively she gave me a pair of Sir Robert's skates. Thus we met while executing turns and pirouettes; both he and Mushin were elegant skaters.

At this point, I cannot resist the temptation to relate why Macintosh was chosen as Lord Nuffield's favorite and only candidate for the chair of anesthetics at Oxford University, as told by Jennifer Beinart. Lord Nuffield, then William Morris, was the successful founder and the ingenious owner of the Morris automobile factory in Cowley, near Oxford. He had bought the golf club at Huntercombe, halfway between London and Oxford, and used the residential quarters at his country house. He also continued to run it as a private golf club, particularly favored by a group of doctors, including Macintosh, from Guy's hospital in London. He and his wife often joined the Guy's doctors at the communal table, and apparently enjoyed listening to the doctors' shop talk. Macintosh later remarked: "that's where all his medical benefactions came from."

Nuffield mentioned at one of the convivial Huntercombe suppers that he had been approached on behalf of the Oxford University to consider giving a very sizeable sum: "They have opened their mouths widely this time." The university had projected three chairs, in medicine, surgery, and obstetrics. According to Macintosh, there was a lull in the conversation and he remarked casually, "I see they have forgotten anesthetics again," rather to fill in the pause than with any serious intent.

It became clear that Macintosh was the man Nuffield had earmarked for the job. As was the case with most of his contemporaries, Macintosh doubted that anesthetics merited a professorial appointment. He also had qualms on financial grounds about taking the chair. It meant abandoning his share in the highly successful anesthetics practice—the first joint practice of its kind, which he had built up in London with two outstanding anesthetists, W. S. McConnell and Bernard Johnson. Nuffield made it clear that he wanted Macintosh in the chair. Macintosh's wife, Marjorie, a friend of Lady Nuffield, possibly supported Nuffield's plan in spite of the inevitable interruption in the Macintoshes' elegant West End lifestyle. Macintosh secured the agreement of his partners in the "Mayfair Gas, Fight and Choke Company," as it was popularly known among London doctors, to keep his place in the partnership open for 1 year so that, if he disliked Oxford, he could return to his former life. However, once in Oxford, he never seriously contemplated going back to London. It seems certain that it was Morris' initiative, and his insistence, that secured the University's acceptance of the chair of anaesthetics.

Three overlapping suggestions for Nuffield's concern about anesthetics can be put forward. First was his personal experience with anesthetics. As a young man he twice suffered terrifying anesthetic ordeals, vivid memories of which remained with him throughout the rest of his life. One of the watersheds between the old and the new in anesthesia was the method of induction. The only procedure available before the late 1930s was mask inhalation, a technique disliked by all and dreaded by most. Around the turn of the century, Nuffield underwent the older style of induction, twice for multiple dental extractions, each time experiencing nightmares of suffocation. Later, when he was due to have a small operation in London he dreaded the anesthetic. However, Macintosh, who was the anesthetist, used Evipan, the precursor of sodium thiopental, as the induction agent: "a little prick in the arm and you go to sleep." When Nuffield awoke, he looked at his watch and inquired why the operation had been postponed. This experience clearly made a deep impression on Nuffield, and it may have fueled his determination that anesthesia was a subject crying out for research and teaching.

Second, Nuffield's familiarity with medical matters stemmed from his warm relations with the Guy's doctors who spent practically every other weekend at Huntercombe. He had a particularly cordial regard for Macintosh and may have taken a special interest in the fascinating details of his calling and his spirit of inquiry. From Macintosh's account, it is clear that Lady Nuffield and Mrs. Macintosh were on close terms and that in itself probably encouraged sociability between the two men.

Third, the technical side of anesthesia may have had an appeal for the ex-motor mechanic. Certainly, Nuffield derived great satisfaction from his tours of the anesthesia laboratory and workshops. His interest in this subject was later demonstrated by his generous gift of Both respirators to every hospital in Britain and the Dominions that requested one, and by the mass production of the Oxford Vaporizer developed at the Cowley-Morris Motor Plant during the Second World War. Later, a thermostatic valve routinely used in the engines of his Morris cars was incorporated into the Epstein-Macintosh Oxford Vaporizer.

Nuffield strongly supported Macintosh's idea, that one of the reasons for the backward state of anesthesia in Britain and elsewhere, except the United States, was that it was not recognized as a specialty. Macintosh strongly felt the advantage that a professorship at Oxford would bring to the status of anesthesiology.

In December 1936, Nuffield donated £2,-000,000, at that time equivalent to $10,000,000 (when an automobile could be bought for $1,000), to the University of Oxford for the chairs in the three "important" old fields of medicine, surgery, and obstetrics, and in the new field of anesthesia. Macintosh was the first professor of anesthesiology in the world, and kept his chair for nearly 30 years, from February 1, 1937 to 1965.

Here again, I wish to quote from the masterpiece by Mushin et al:

> When Trier Mörch in a paper to the Royal Society of Medicine in London in 1947 enthusiastically advocated mechanical controlled respiration, he found in his audience some eager to try this new approach, one of them being Cecil Gray. By this time, surgeons in many European countries no longer needed to be convinced that the abolition of spontaneous respiration greatly eased their work within the chest and ensured excellent oxygenation and carbon dioxide elimination. The work of Ralph Waters of Madison on the carbon dioxide absorption and the use of cyclopropane was familiar to British anesthetists, and these methods were in widespread use by the time the

> war broke out. In 1941, Nosworthy described controlled respiration with cyclopropane for thoracic surgery. However, automatic apparatus for controlled respiration was at this time virtually unknown in the field. In Britain, the ready availability of skilled anesthetists, trained to meet the needs of the armed forces but back in civilian life, meant that increasingly, the surgeons left these problems to their colleagues.

The good reception of Mörch's advocacy of ventilators was in marked contrast to that accorded to Janeway and Jackson by an earlier generation of doctors. (This, however, was probably due as much to the advancements in blood transfusion, antibiotics, and surgical techniques as it was to timing and luck.)

A pharmacologist, Dennis E. Jackson of Cincinnato, Ohio, had repeatedly demonstrated the first commercially available anesthesia machine with a built-in ventilator and carbon dioxide absorption apparatus as early as 1927. Exasperated by their lack of acceptance, he wrote:

> 378 years ago Vesalius had demonstrated what artificial respiration may often accomplish. . . . It would appear, however, that the interval of time required for artificial respiration in the dog to evolute into artificial respiration in man may be almost as great as that required for an animal comparable to the dog to evolute into a man.

In 1944 K. B. Pinson of Manchester devised an automatic ventilator, "the pulmonary pump" (Fig. 1-20). He incorporated many refinements, but the apparatus consisted essentially of two piston pumps: One took over respiration, and the other employed suction to evacuate secretions or pus from the trachea and bronchial tree. Observing this very unusual and interesting ventilator in use was a pleasure. Dr. Pinson

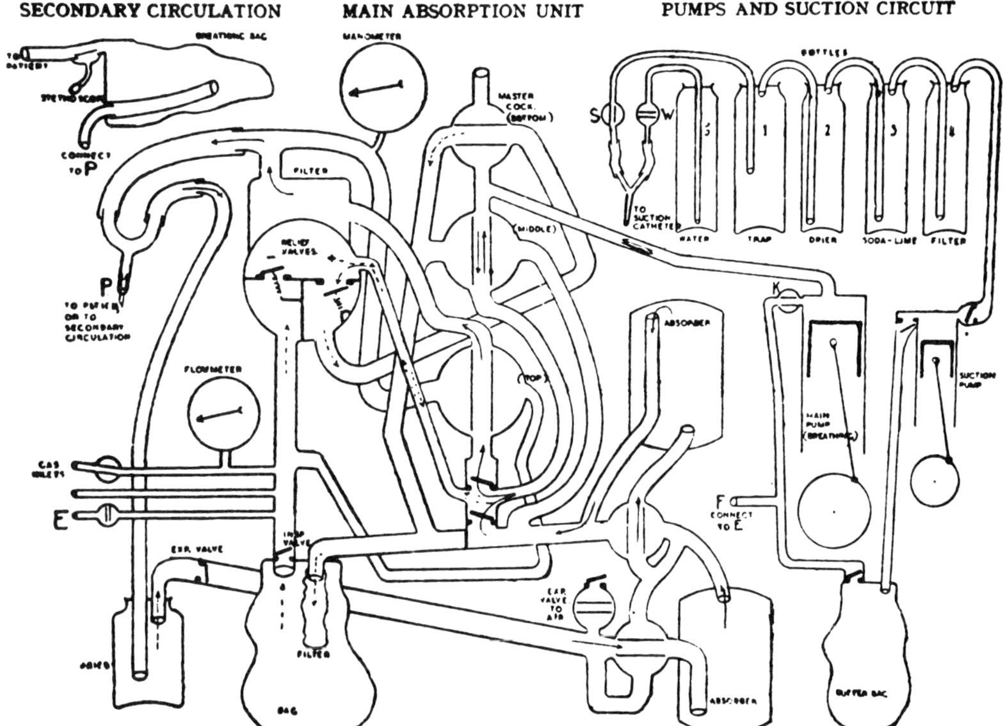

Fig. 1-20. A "simplified" illustration of "the pulmonary pump" devised in 1944 by K. B. Pinson of Manchester.

had come to the hospital the evening before surgery and assembled the pump in the operating room corridor. The next morning, however, it was discovered that the pump was too large to fit through the door to the operating room. The case was postponed until the following day, the pump disassembled and then reassembled inside the operating room. Indeed, it worked very well!

During the Second World War, a motorcycle engineer, J. H. Blease of London, produced an anesthetic apparatus for a local physician. When the physician suddenly died, Mr. Blease found himself pressed into providing emergency anesthesia during the air raids on Merseyside. Put off by

> . . . the drudgery of manually controlled ventilation for thoracic surgery, in 1945 he built the first prototype of what was to become the ''Pulmoflator.'' Though the reception of this prototype by some was skeptical, the convenience provided was especially appreciated when the introduction of curare during surgery necessitated artificial respiration throughout many other operations besides thoracic ones.

Blease's efforts were followed by designs of Esplen's ''Aintree'' ventilator in 1952 and the ''Fazakerley'' ventilator in 1956.

ANESTHESIOLOGY PRINCIPLES IN RESPIRATORY CARE

One of the most revolutionary changes in respiratory care was attributable to the anesthesiologist Bjørn Ibsen of Copenhagen. In 1952 Scandinavia was struck by a poliomyelitis epidemic of unprecedented severity, and thousands of patients were hospitalized. From July 24, to December 3, the Hospital for Communicable Diseases in Copenhagen admitted 2,722 polio patients, 315 of whom required respiratory support. Early in the epidemic, all patients were treated by the one tank and six cuirass respirators available. Uncuffed tracheostomy tubes were used to secure an open airway. Adeqaute humidification of inspired gas was not available. Effective chest physical therapy was hampered by body-enclosing respirators. Of the first 31 patients with respiratory paralysis admitted, 27 died within 3 days. When the 32nd patient, a 12-year-old girl was nearing a terminal state of respiratory insufficiency, Ibsen was consulted, and a tracheotomy was promptly performed, followed by insertion of a cuffed tracheostomy tube and initiation of manual artificial ventilation with a conventional Water's to-and-fro system. Improved oxygenation and correction of respiratory acidosis were followed by shock, but blood transfusions reestablished adequate circulation. Thus the patient had been improved by the measures usually carried out by the anesthetist in the operating theater.

The therapeutic principles demonstrated by Ibsen now became the accepted methods for management of respiratory paralysis throughout Northern Europe. Teams of ''ventilators'' consisting of nurse-anesthetists, interns, and medical students provided manual artificial ventilation and respiratory care in shifts during the epidemic. For several months the medical school in Copenhagen closed to allow its students to volunteer as ''ventilators.'' At the peak of the epidemic, such teams were able to ventilate 75 patients simultaneously.

At first, professor H. C. A. Lassen was faced with a seemingly hopeless situation. About 500 patients were already in the hospital, and 50 to 60 new cases were coming in every day. However, with Ibsen's help, he quickly created an organization that worked extremely well. To give an impression of the magnitude of the task, Ibsen stated that within each 24-hour period the teams included 260 extra nurse auxillaries, 250 medical students, and 27 technicians just to handle the 250 large gas cylinders. A team of epidemiologists, ear-nose-throat specialists, and anesthesiologists worked with an excellent laboratory staffed by two full-time specialists and 15 technicians. Eventually, x-ray technicians and physiotherapists joined in as well. I cannot resist mentioning three of my now American friends who participated as anesthesiologists in this stupendous epoch: Henrik H. Bendixen (Columbia University, New York),

Henning Pontoppidan (Massachusetts General Hospital, Boston), and Christian C. Rattenborg (University of Chicago).

The importance of care during transportation was demonstrated by many early tragic experiences when lay people alone accompanied the patients in the ambulance to the hospital. Aspiration often occurred, and on arrival at the hospital many patients were found to be moribund, some even dead.

Ibsen stressed that equipment for emergency respiration and suction must be available, even in the patient's home. He wanted help to come to the patient, not for the patient to go to the help. Thus teams went all over the country, by ambulance or by plane, to ensure safe patient transportation. When suctioning and ventilation, with either a bag and mask or a bag connected to an oral endotracheal or tracheostomy tube, were performed by trained personnel, a striking difference in results was noted in Copenhagen. Regional centers were soon established all over the country, and the overall mortality rate of patients with respiratory paralysis was reduced from 87 percent to less than 30 percent.

Most of the essential principles of positive-pressure mechanical ventilation and airway care were implemented during the 1952 Danish epidemic. Chest physical therapy with meticulous attention to postural drainage, manual assistance to coughing, and tracheobronchial aspiration of secretions were now universally applied. Inspired gas with partial rebreathing was humidified, albeit incompletely, in the to-and-fro system. More effective bypass humidifiers soon became available. Oxygen toxicity was avoided by using mixtures of nitrogen and oxygen. Orotracheal intubation preceded tracheotomy, thus eliminating the hazard of emergency tracheotomy without airway control. Large-bore cuffed tracheostomy tubes were used to facilitate controlled ventilation and airway protection. Because blood gas and pH measurements were not available, adequacy of oxygenation was judged by clinical observation, measuring arterial oxygen saturation, or oximetry. Intermittent pulmonary hyperinflation, a forerunner of the "sighing" described in 1959 by Mead and Collier, were empirically applied to overcome the complaint of dyspnea commonly expressed by patients with ventilatory failure, despite what seemed to be adequate oxygenation and ventilation. As the patient's ability to breathe spontaneously improved, weaning was accomplished by gradual reduction in the number of assisted breaths, the forerunner of present-day intermittent mandatory ventilation (IMV). In many respects, and on an entirely empirical basis, the ventilation pattern provided by an "educated hand" proved to be physiologically superior to that provided by early mechanical ventilators. Toward the end of the epidemic, when a few Engström, Lundia, and Bang ventilators became available, they were often referred to as "mechanical students."

Similar experiences were reported in the United States. During a minor poliomyelitis epidemic in Kansas during 1951 to 1952, I treated a few patients with intermittent positive-pressure ventilation (IPPV) from my first American-made piston ventilator. Van Bergen of Minneapolis adopted Ibsen's methods of treatment during the polio epidemics in Minnesota and Western Canada in 1952 and developed his own ventilator. The New England region was struck by a severe epidemic of paralytic poliomyelitis in 1955. Anesthesiologists again assumed an important role in the care of patients with respiratory paralysis (Pontoppidan). At the Massachusetts General Hospital, an entire floor was converted to a poliomyelitis respiratory failure unit. At the height of that epidemic, 49 patients were mechanically ventilated at one time: 46 were in tank respirators, and 3 were on the Jefferson ventilator, an early version of a volume-preset device capable of providing controlled ventilation. Once again, the superiority of IPPV was demonstrated, as it had been in 1899 by Matas, in 1905 by Kuhn, in 1910 by Läwen and Sievers, in 1916 by Giertz, in 1948 by Bower and colleagues and in 1952 by Ibsen. However, complications from inadequate humidification and tracheal trauma from tracheostomy tubes with high-pressure cuffs were still evident. Measurement of arterial oxygen saturation was the only clinically available method for assessing the adequacy of oxygenation at that time.

In 1960 one of my more memorable experiences was thrust on me when I suddenly became responsible for the care of Alon P. Winnie, recently Chairman of the Department of Anesthesiology at the University of Illinois but then a surgical intern at Cook County Hospital in Chicago, who was rotating through the anesthesia service. At 7 AM one morning, he walked in complaining of a severe headache. Knowing that he was a popular party man, I presumed that he just had a hangover, so I gave him two aspirins and asked him to get going. An hour later, he looked and was really sick, so I released him from work. I have never seen any case of bulbospinal poliomyelitis so violent and fulminant. By 4:00 PM, I had performed a tracheostomy on him and connected him to a Mörch piston respirator placed under his bed.

(Winnie has an unusual sense of humor. One of his favorite fables was his admiration for my taking care of "the whole patient." On the evening of his admission, he had a date with a beautiful young student nurse. Realizing that he would not be able to fulfill this obligation, I took her out dancing in the Pump Room at the Ambassador Hotel. Now this is Winnie's version!)

Ancillary Use of a Mechanical Ventilator

Finally, after several months of serious, paralytic poliomyelitis, Al Winnie was discharged from Cook County Hospital. In gratitude, Al threw a party in his third floor apartment near the hospital for all the interns and residents who had cared for him. The main beverage streamed merrily from two large kegs of beer until at midnight the party was in grave danger when the pump failed, and beer would no longer leave the keg.

Unseen by the rest of the party, Trier Mörch sneaked out, returned to the hospital, found the very ventilator which had been breathing for Winnie only a few months earlier and dragged it across the street, and up the long, steep stairway. After a few on-the-spot modifications, Mörch adjusted the machine to run at low volume, high speed and high pressure to pump air into the kegs, and—*mirabile dictu*—the beer was again streaming down the throats of an appreciative crowd. Never did one mechanical ventilator save so many "patients" at one time!

Tracheobronchial Suction

Infection around the tracheostomy tube is always present. One of the many means to keep the infection to a minimum is careful, gentle aspiration with a sterile catheter (to be done as rarely as possible). It is difficult for our younger colleagues to realize how such care was carried out a score or more years ago.

In those days, before disposable plastic suction catheters were introduced, suction was performed with one red rubber urethral catheter of the type used on old prostatic men. In better hospitals the catheter was changed at least once daily! After use, it was "cleansed" by sucking saline (which also had been sterile in the early morning) through it; it was then stored in a container with some old cloudy alcohol, hoping that this procedure would resterilize it. When needed next time, it was taken from the solution and introduced into the trachea, which now also suffered the additional chemical irritation of the alcohol.

At Cook County Hospital, we never had enough nurses; very often one nurse alone would look after 40 sick patients. To the irritation and consternation of these dedicated but badly overworked nurses, I insisted on 10 red rubber catheters, preferably of the coudé type, for each patient daily. Each catheter was wrapped in a separate towel and sterilized. I was undoubtedly the first, at least in the Middle West, to use sterile catheters for each suctioning. I still have not completely accommodated to today's expense and waste of beautiful, sterile, disposable catheters.

Piped-In Artificial Ventilation

The recovery room at Cook County Hospital in Chicago had space for 50 patients in 2 large rooms. In a corner of each room was a Mörch Piston Respirator connected to a 25-mm (1-inch) pipe, which was mounted on all the walls. At each patient station was an outlet with a stopcock. Rhythmic pulses of compressed air could thus be available at each station without moving the respirator. From the stopcock, a rubber hose could guide the air to a plastic cylinder surrounding a concertina shaped bag. The humidified air-oxygen mixture inside the concertina bag could then be directed to the patient at the desired volume and pressure. In this way one, two, or three patients could be ventilated from the same respirator.

THE END OF POLIOMYELITIS ANTERIOR ACUTA

The introduction of the Salk and the Sabin poliomyelitis vaccines and their use in mass immunization campaigns in the United States practically eradicated poliomyelitis. The National Foundation for Infantile Paralysis shifted its attention to other fields, and the polio respirator centers it had supported closed about 1960. As a result, the use of mechanical ventilators declined sharply during the next few years. Those few patients requiring ventilator support were cared for on general hospital wards. Complications and mortality rates were high, in large measure because of inexperience of the personnel and mechanical failure of airway equipment or ventilators. For the most part, only a few patients with potentially reversible neuromuscular diseases or drug-induced coma, particularly from barbiturates, were treated successfully.

Eventually, an increase in the number of patients requiring mechanical ventilation prompted the reestablishment of respiratory units, now most often called intensive or critical care units.

INTERMITTENT POSITIVE-PRESSURE BREATHING

Intermittent positive-pressure breathing (IPPB) was described by Irwin Ziment of the University of California at Los Angeles. In 1937 Barach, Eckman, and Ginsburg and in 1945 Motley, Cournand, and Werkö, all of Columbia University in New York, were among the first to suggest that IPPB had therapeutic indications other than the maintenance of artificial respiration in completely apneic subjects. Barach and co-workers treated patients with pulmonary edema and other pulmonary diseases. Their studies found important application in the methods of oxygen delivery to pilots flying at high altitudes during World War II. Motley and colleagues treated a number of conditions, including respiratory insufficiency caused by barbiturates, carbon monoxide, or alcohol; paralysis caused by central nervous system pathology; acute asthmatic attacks; and postoperative thoracic surgery cases. They used the "Burns pneumatic balance resuscitator" developed for the Air Force.

Around that time, V. Ray Bennett developed the "Bennett clinical research model (Ben X-2) valve" which permitted intermittent delivery of oxygen under pressure during inspiration; subsequently the Bennett family of respirators was introduced into pulmonary medicine as a result of the studies of Motley and his colleagues. By 1950 IPPB had started its meteoric use as a major type of therapy for various disorders of the lung. Shortly thereafter, entry of Bird pressure-cycled respirators into the medical field led to a form of competition in which the operational characteristics of the rival instruments became the major consideration, overshadowing the questionable therapeutic value of IPPB.

Nevertheless, for many years the Bird equipment was very popular in the United States and abroad. Bird nebulizers were superior and were used extensively in the treatment of chronic obstructive pulmonary disease (COPD). Forrest Bird maintained an attractive school for inhalation therapy and provided a free IPPB clinic in Palm Springs, California at a time when very few such facilities existed.

Many other ventilators subsequently were introduced, some of which received enthusiastic commendations, although little evidence suggested that there was any one outstanding model or even that IPPB was clinically efficacious.

A major turning point in development occurred in 1954 when Engström introduced his excellent and highly sophisticated piston ventilator, which the following year was used by Björk and Engström for postoperative support of pulmonary resection patients. This therapy, which they pioneered, is still widely accepted for cardiac surgical patients, as well as for many other individuals who have undergone a variety of major operative procedures.

CRUSHING INJURIES OF THE CHEST

During the 1950s, the treatment of severe crushed chest injuries was directed for the first time toward the maintenance of adequate ventilation. N. K. Jensen of Minneapolis used what was later described as positive end-expiratory pressure (PEEP) in 1952, and in 1953 tracheostomy was advocated by Carter and Guiseffi. In June 1954 an acute emergency led A. E. Avery, D. W. Benson and me to devise a new management technique for this problem.

A husky 51-year-old worker was directing a pack train in a Chicago steel mill. As the train approached, he stepped back, forgetting that he stood in front of a furnace. He was slowly crushed and rolled into an 8-inch "sausage." Upon admission to the hospital, he was moribund and in deep shock, with multiple bilateral fractures of all ribs, costochondral separations, bilateral tension hemopneumothoraces, fractures of the sternum, clavicles, and pelvis, crushing injuries of the liver and genitourinary tract, paralytic ileus, and acute gastric dilatation.

His chest wall was partially stabilized with soft tissue traction by the method of Hudson; long metal pins were passed under the pectoralis and serratus anterior muscles; spreader bows were attached, and traction was applied from an overhead frame. In spite of all efforts, he was slowly dying from shock, pulmonary edema, and respiratory acidosis. We then realized that his major problem was inadequate ventilation and that we had to breathe for him. An Ambu-bag and later a Mörch piston ventilator were attached to his tracheostomy tube. The patient improve minute by minute from a semicomatose state with respiratory acidosis to a comfortable and alert state with respiratory alkalosis.

The two most important factors in this treatment were: First, *no* active muscular movements of the ribs were allowed at all, because this would displace the many fragments. This state was achieved by deliberate overventilation until apnea occurred. (Only if acidosis was present was it necessary to give sedatives or narcotics.) Second, *no* negative pressure was applied in the chest in order to prevent paradoxical respirations.

We were amazed to observe how rapidly the numerous rib fragments moved back into place under the influence of IPPV. Because the force of air pressure on each fragment was proportional to the underlying pulmonary area, the lungs acted as splints. The patient was kept overventilated in respiratory alkalosis for 30 days. CO_2 and pH of the blood were checked twice daily. He was discharged from the hospital 51 days after the injury and returned to work. Since that case in 1954, this therapy has been preferred for severe cases of crushed chest.

The Mörch piston ventilator (Fig. 1-21) used in this case was the first modern volume unit and became very popular during the mid-1950s. It was simple to use, having only two variants: rate and volume. The cylinder was an 8-inch (20-cm) diameter sleeve from a large diesel engine, and the piston rings were made of Teflon, which is nearly indestructible. Rate selection was controlled by a robust mechanism built originally for antiaircraft guns in the U.S. Navy. A stainless steel 12-mm (0.5-inch) ball in the exhalation valve was from a ball bearing.

The cylinder assembly was the only part in

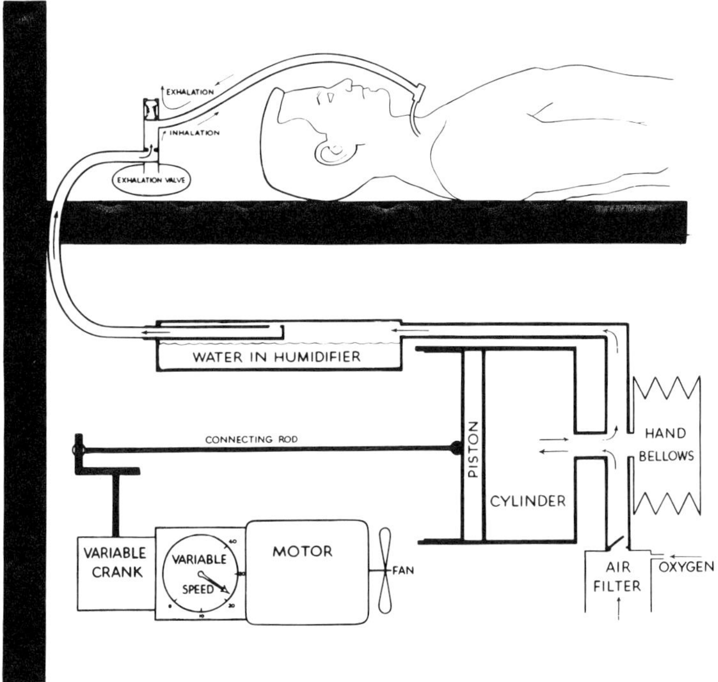

Fig. 1-21. Diagram of the Mörch III piston ventilator.

contact with air going to the patient and could be sterilized easily by boiling, autoclaving, or treating with chemicals. The entire unit was so low it could be placed under the patient's bed; thus it did not take up any additional floor space, an important consideration because most hospital rooms were small. It was a very reliable machine which required almost no maintenance. The chief physician at the largest "respirator center" in Chiacago tried all the ventilators. When I asked him why he used the Mörch so rarely, he answered, "Oh, we keep the Mörch in reserve for when the other machines fail."

SAGA OF THE UNCUFFED TRACHEAL TUBE

In Kansas City in 1952 I was treating a polio patient using a cuffed tracheostomy tube and the Mörch piston ventilator. One night the occlusive cuff ruptured. The nurse called me, and I was afraid we might lose the patient before I could get there (I lived 15 minutes from the hospital). However, she told me to take my time because she had simply increased the volume until the chest moved normally. This episode convinced me that we did not need a cuff at all. Any leak which was present depended on the ratio of the diameters of the trachea and the tracheal tube and on several other factors. We found empirically that the correct volume was about three times the tidal volume; thus if an adult patient needed 500 ml tidal volume but the leak around the tube was 1,000 ml, the ventilator had to be set to deliver a 1,500-ml tidal volume. Many patients could tell us the correct volume as well as when they had bronchial obstruction (often delineating which side the obstruction was on). In patients with polio who had normal or even decreased lung thorax compliance, the volume of air moving down the tracheal tube at a high velocity was greater than that lost even in the presence of a sizable leak.

This uncuffed system was described in 1956

by Mörch, Saxton and Gish. Possible advantages included the absence of tracheal pressure necrosis, a real risk if the cuff was overinflated; improved pumonary toiletry as the leaking air blew particulate matter or secretions up into the pharynx, where the patient or nursing staff could remove them; the ability to talk—even if it was—only the time while—the machine was—blowing the air—between the vocal cords. To be able to talk at all was a major improvement.

I treated a patient in Michigan who broke his neck diving in a gravel pit in 1960, and today he is still alive and talking—synchronously with the ventilator inflation. In most patients, however, it is desirable to use a cuff on the endotracheal or tracheostomy tube. Ideally, the cuff should be inflated until there is a "microscopic" annular space between its wall and the trachea; one should be able to hear a tiny leak, big enough to prevent pressure damage to the mucosa but so small it does not interfere with effective ventilation.

Motion of the tracheostomy tube transmitted from the rhythmic inflation and deflation of the connecting tubes can be decreased by positioning a swivel connector between the tracheal tube and the ventilator circuit. I invented the first such swivel adaptor and described it with Saxton in 1956.

ADVANCES IN THORACIC SURGERY

By 1930, after two decades of relative inactivity, thoracic surgeons were getting ready for another attempt at open chest surgery. Several crucial developments had taken place. The various blood types had been described and transfusions were now a clinical reality. The beginning of antibiosis was coming, first in the form of sulfa drugs, later penicillin. Tracheal intubation had been improved, mostly because of the influence of Magill and Rowbothen during World War I. Surgical techniques had been improved to include individual ligation of pulmonary vessels, closure of the bronchial stump, and underwater drainage of the chest. The surgical pioneers, include Beck, Blalock, Brunn, Churchill, Crafoord, Gibbon, Graham, Nissen, and many others.

Any physician trained in anesthesiology today would naturally assume that the principles of tracheal intubation and IPPB, which had been understood and technically available since the turn of the century, would be put into service in anesthesia for thoracic surgery. Such, however, was not the case. At most centers, the continuous positive-pressure technique with spontaneous ventilation, the modern-day equivalent to continuous positive-airway pressure (CPAP), and often with a tightly fitting mask, was the predominant approach. Beecher described the principles of anesthesia using continuous positive-pressure breathing during pulmonary surgery in 1938. As antiquated as the technique sounds today, it was not without effectiveness. He reported 117 lobectomies with a 6.8 percent overall mortality, and no deaths attributed directly to anesthesia. He was among the most outspoken of that era's anesthesiologists in the defense of spontaneous ventilation.

A pivotal point was the inability to assess with precision the depth of anesthesia once respiration was controlled. The modern anesthesiologist cannot readily appreciate how important spontaneous ventilation was as an index by which the depth of anesthesia could be assessed with precision. If ventilation was controlled, or assisted effectively, the depth of anesthesia could no longer be estimated with sufficient accuracy to make deep single-agent anesthesia safe.

At a few centers, the approach to thoracic surgery included controlled mechanical ventilation. Mautz and Beck in 1939 in the United States designed a ventilator for use during thoracic surgery (Fig. 1-22). The foremost advocate of this technique was Crafoord in Sweden (1940). He based his approach on the observations by Giertx in 1916, that IPPB was more physiologic, and better tolerated, than continuous positive-pressure breathing. Frenckner, an otolaryngologist (who also worked on tracheal intubation techniques), and the engineer, Anderson, built the first "Spiropulsator" ventilator,

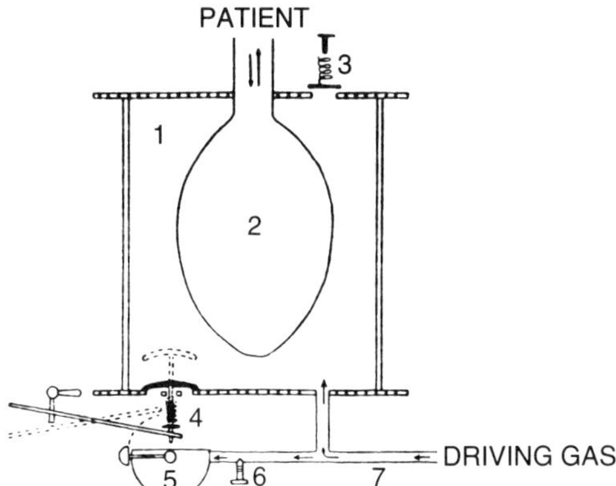

Fig. 1-22. Diagram of the Mautz ventilator.

using a "flasher" from a sea buoy made by the Swedish company AGA. The Spiropulsator was used by Crafoord's team, including Torsten Gordh, for approximately 15,000 patients. Interesting is the fact that this took place before the era of curarization and arterial blood gas analysis. Also, there were difficulties with some patients fighting the ventilator when the induced apnea technique failed, probably because of metabolic acidemia.

THE ERA OF "ASSISTED" VENTILATION

In the United States, unlike Scandinavia, Britain, and some other countries of Europe, the value of controlled respiration during anesthesia—to say nothing of automatic ventilation—was strongly disputed as late as the 1950s. Although puzzled over the occurrence of both metabolic and respiratory acidosis, both surgeons and anesthesiologists doubted the value of automatically controlled ventilation. The dangers of explosion and the unsatisfactory pulmonary ventilation sometimes produced by stubborn anesthesiologists who did not learn to use the machines appropriately were thought to outweigh any possible advantages. Instead, they preferred:

> respiration carefully assisted by the anesthetist, by squeezing the bag just as the patient inspires . . . feeling that this . . . gives the most effective type of ventilation. [One anesthesiologist commented that he] did not mean to imply that we have a closed mind about ways of improving the situation. [Maybe] it would be desirable for the surgeons to consider the possibility of other operating positions for these cases. We anesthetists, on our side, must find improved ways of *assisting respiration*.

As late as 1951, when I became head of the Department of Anesthesia at the University of Chicago, I was told by a surgeon on the staff "*No* endotracheal tube, *no* controlled respiration, *no* curare, and—naturally—*no* automatic breathing machines!" When I objected, it was hesitatingly conceded that only in extreme emergency situations would I be permitted to do whatever I deemed best for the patient. Shortly thereafter, an "emergency situation" occurred followed by others in slowly increasing numbers until we practiced the type of anesthesia I was used to. There were no objections (because the patients were doing better than previously).

Many anesthesiologists in the United States insisted that assisted ventilation was safer than controlled ventilation. They resisted the introduction of ventilators which, as a result, were quite rare in American operating rooms during the 1950s and early 1960s. The impetus for their adoption and increasing use came from cardiac surgeons involved in a concerted attack on the problems of open heart surgery.

CONTROLLED VENTILATION

Surgical pioneers (e.g., Beck and Blalock of Johns Hopkins; Brunn, Churchill, and Crafoord of Stockholm; Graham of St. Louis; and Nissen of Basel, Switzerland) and cardiac surgeons (including Albritten and Gibbon, the pioneer of pump oxygenators, of Philadelphia; and Dennis of New York), like Läwen, Sievers, and Mautz before them, showed that mechanical artificial ventilation enhanced the results of their work by providing more efficient CO_2 elimination and oxygenation.

The cardiac surgeon, F. R. Mautz of Cleveland, constructed a simple and reliable ventilator in 1939. A bag-in-a-bottle arrangement was the basic design (Fig. 1-22). An automobile windshield wiper driving motor powered by compressed air was used in the ventilator. An anesthesia breathing bag was enclosed in a transparent plastic cylinder into which compressed air was blown continually. The resultant increasing pressure within the cylinder compressed the breathing bag and thus, deliver a mechanical inhalation. When a certain pressure was reached, the windshield wiper motor was activated and opened a valve in the cylinder, allowing pressure to escape. As a result, the breathing bag expanded, and passive exhalation ensued. When the pressure in the cylinder decreased to ambient pressure, the motor closed the valve, and the ventilator once again reverted to the mechanical inhalation phase.

One of the first commercially available anesthesia ventilators in the United States resulted from efforts in Philadelphia. Beck's technical assistant, Kenneth Wolfe, with the help of the engineer H. J. Rand, produced a simple and sturdy successor to the Mautz ventilator for everyday use in cardiac surgery in 1950. John Gibbon's brother, who was the president of an engineering company, and his engineer Chris Andreason improved it and produced the widely used "Jefferson ventilator." The benefits of automatic ventilation slowly became recognized by surgeons and anesthesiologists alike, and other anesthesia ventilators became commercially available, including the Mörch surgical ventilator (1955), the Stephenson "CRU" (1956), the Bennett ventilator (1957), and the Bird Mark 4 ventilator (1959).

The Mörch anesthesia ventilator incorporated several unique features: (1) it was the first ventilator in the United States to have a concertina-shaped bellows, an idea taken from the Blease and Oxford ventilators (Fig. 1–21) (this feature permitted a reading of the tidal volume); (2) it was available as a separate unit or as a built-in component of several popular anesthesia machines; (3) it was the first ventilator in which all the parts in contact with the inspired gas could easily be cleaned or even sterilized; (4) it was the first ventilator that could be used either as a pressure-sensitive assistor or as a volume-controlled ventilator; and (5) most of the controls could be operated by foot.

The working principle was that of an air pressure amplifier based on two commercially available valves made by Johnson Control, Inc. (Milwaukee, WI). The first was an air-driven switch intended as a remote control for an electrical switch to enable its use in areas with flammable or explosive gases and liquids. This switch was activated by a large diaphragm in the ventilator and thus was sensitive to small variations in pressure. It regulated the air to a second three-way valve with larger openings for the air or oxygen that acted on the concertina breathing bag.

A bewildering array of ventilators for use in and out of the surgical suite have since been produced, some of which seem to have pursued sophistication as an end in itself. Often we have to decide whether to sacrifice reliability and simplicity for the sometimes dubious advantages that a highly sophisticated piece of apparatus may provide. Many of the newer ventilators are described elsewhere in this book.

EXPANDED FIELDS FOR SUPPORTIVE VENTILATION

Until the mid-1950s, ventilation had been applied only in 1909 by H. Emerson for the treatment of pulmonary edema in the field of resuscitation, for poliomyelitis, and in a few pioneering cases of anesthesia. By the late 1960s, however, mechanical ventilation was used widely in other areas, and new/rediscovered techniques appeared.

Idiopathic Respiratory Distress Syndrome

The idiopathic respiratory distress syndrome (IRDS) occurs primarily in premature infants. Infants so affected need resuscitation because each breath requires an extraordinary effort.

With progression of the disease, they become tachypneic, often with alternating periods of apnea. If left untreated, they die. Yet careful support, from simple increases of inspired oxygen to fully controlled mechanical ventilation, is associated with a better than 80 percent survival.

Adult Respiratory Distress Syndrome

Adult respiratory distress syndrome (ARDS) usually is caused by serious pulmonary injury or illness. Most of the patients have no history of previous pulmonary or cardiac illness. Symptoms and signs vary but usually include severe dyspnea, tachypnea, bloody sputum, cyanosis, and elevated minute ventilation. The lungs become ''stiff'' with patchy alveolar infiltrates and may require 40 to 60 cm H_2O inspiratory pressure (or more) to achieve adequate tidal volumes. Without adequate treatment, death may occur within 24 to 48 hours.

Pulmonary dysfunction of this type has been known since World War I and has been called shock lung, wet lung, Da Nang lung, and post-traumatic pulmonary insufficiency. It has been the focus of extensive research and treatment because of the high rates of associated morbidity and mortality, which still occur. Prolonged artificial ventilation is still a mainstay of support.

Positive End-Expiratory Pressure

More than four decades ago, Barach and associates recognized that breathing with an elevated airway pressure was often therapeutic in the resolution of pulmonary edema associated with congestive heart failure. They increased airway pressure with a motor-driven blower and an expiratory valve, both connected to the patient's airway through a face mask. This technique—constant (or continuous) positive-pressure breathing—was used in 1952 by H. K. Jensen of Minneapolis to treat pulmonary contusion in spontaneously breathing patients with crush injuries of the chest.

In 1959 Frumin, Bergman, Holaday, et al. found that their patients' arterial oxygen tension was improved by adding positive end-expiratory pressure (PEEP). This observation was later confirmed by Ashbaugh et al. from Denver and McIntyre et al. from Toronto in the treatment of ARDS.

PEEP may prevent alveolar collapse by maintaining positive airway pressure throughout the respiratory cycle. A higher functional residual capacity and better overall ventilation/perfusion ratio results. Other potential benefits include a reduction in pulmonary blood flow and capillary stasis and congestion.

Intermittent Mandatory Ventilation

Weaning of patients from prolonged mechanical ventilation may present difficult problems. Several measurable variables have been used to predict whether ventilator support can be discontinued (Bendixen et al., 1965; Pontoppidan et al., 1970). Trial-and-error methods often were resorted to, with their inherent dangers of hypoventilation, hypoxia, undue stress, and anxiety.

Some of these problems were lessened when Kirby et al. introduced IMV as a treatment mode for neonates with IRDS in 1971; and Downs et al. from the University of Florida in Gainesville, proposed IMV as an aid to wean adult patients from mechanical ventilatory support.

IMV requires a system in which the patient may breathe spontaneously from a reservoir while the ventilator provides positive-pressure (mandatory) breaths of adjustable volume and timed intervals. As the patient's ability to breathe improves, the number of mandatory breaths is gradually reduced until completely spontaneous ventilation is achieved. Other variables (e.g., V_T, F_IO_2) may be maintained constant during the period of rate adjustment.

One potential shortcoming of IMV is that the positive-pressure inflation may be out of phase with the patient's spontaneous ventilation.

To avoid the possibility of poor coordination between patient and ventilator, synchronized IMV (SIMV), also called intermittent demand ventilation (IDV) or intermittent assisted ventilation (IAV), has been popularized by several investigators, including Svein Harboe at the University of Olso, Norway. Harboe used a new, improved model 900B of the Siemens-Elema Servo ventilator, which produced patient-triggered sighs during spontaneous breathing. The expired minute volume (EMV) was displayed continuously on the panel during spontaneous breathing as well as during controlled ventilation, with or without PEEP or CPAP.

IMV and SIMV have many alleged advantages. For example, the patient starts quickly to train his own respiratory muscles, which may prevent the irregular breathing patterns frequently seen after prolonged disuse with controlled mechanical ventilation (Pontoppidan et al., 1970). In addition, regular "sighing" offered by IMV/IAV may prevent atelectasis (Bendixen et al., 1964).

FLUIDIC-CONTROLLED VENTILATORS

Fluidic-controlled ventilators have become popular in many countries because they are less sensitive to outside interferences, such as temperature fluctuation, vibration, and electricity. Also there are no moving mechanical parts. Fluidic systems utilize moving streams of liquid or gas for sensing, logic, amplification, and controls. Most elements operate either on wall attachment or beam deflection principles.

When a high-speed stream of air or other fluids emerge from a nozzle, air is entrained from all sides (the Bernouilli effect). When a wall is placed close to the jet on one side, less air enters from that side, causing pressure to fall even more here and the jet to be "sucked" over against the wall. This is called the surface or wall attachment effect. As is often the case, the basic phenomenon is by no means new. It was reported in 1800 by Thoman Young and is also called the "Coanda effect" after a Romanian aeronautic engineer, Dr. Henri Coanda, who designed, built, flew, and in 1910 destroyed the first jet-propelled aircraft in Paris.

Coanda's first, last, and only test flight took place at the Issy-les-Moulineaux airport, just outside the old walls around Paris. To start his test, Coanda took his flying machine to the end of the field farthest away from the Paris wall. At the start, the airplane emerged from a sheet of flame and a cloud of smoke, flying straight for the Paris wall. Coanda reported:

> apparently I had given it too much fuel—when I looked over the side, I saw raw flames shooting out, and that should not be. Not with my wooden wings full of petrol. I ducked inside to adjust matters. A moment later, things felt very differently. I looked outside again to find myself many feet in the air. Straight ahead of me was the Paris wall. I didn't know what to do. I pulled on the control wheels, the machine went up on one wing and I was thrown out. The machine crashed right at the foot of the wall.

Fortunately, Coanda was not seriously hurt, but the plane was burnt and nobody was interested in his jet engine. To his dismay, Coanda noted that the mica deflector plates, intended to deflect the exhaust away from the fuselage, actually had pulled the flames toward it. Later, he invented a flying saucer as well as improved burners for central heating furnaces, and developed a revolutionary new agricultural insecticide spray, but he did nothing further that related to fluidic controls.

Today's knowledge of fluidic systems is based mainly on the systematic and ingenious teamwork around 1959 of Billy M. Horton, Raymond W. Warren, and Ronald E. Bowles at the Army's Harry Diamond Laboratories in Washington, D.C. The first fluidic ventilator was designed for the Army in 1964 by Barila, Meyer, and Mosley and other anesthesiologists from the Walter Reed Army Institute for Research working with engineers from the Harry Diamond Laboratories.

Commercial versions of the U.S. Army's simple resuscitators and ventilators have since been designed and built by several companies, such as Bowles Fluidic Corporation, in cooperation with the Rectec Company in Portland, Oregon (1967); Senko Medical (Japan), Mine Safety Appliance Company (United States), and French companies that made the ventilators called "Airox R" and "VP 2000," which utilized pure fluidic components in 1969 for resuscitation and respiratory therapy. The first versatile complex, commercial fluidic ventilator, the "Hamilton Standard PAD," appeared in 1970 and was very similar to the Corning's ventilator described in 1973 by R. K. Smith. This was followed by the "Monaghan 225" in 1973, the "Ohio Medical 550" in 1974, and the North American Dräger in 1975.

HIGH-FREQUENCY VENTILATION

Few techniques for ventilatory support have excited the minds and the imagination as much as has high-frequency ventilation (HFV). HFV may be defined as very fast ventilatory frequencies with tidal volumes sometimes smaller than dead-space volume.

Nature has several examples of HFV. The best known example is the panting dog who ventilates at high frequencies to regulate temperature and to get rid of excess heat while still satisfying gas exchange requirements. In the hummingbird and in several insects, repiration is timed with the beat of their wings, which can be as rapid as 80 beats/sec or 80 Hz (1 cycle per second equals 1 Hz).

As early as 1667, Robert Hooke reported to the Royal Society in London:

> I formerly tryed of keeping a Dog alive after his Thorax was all display'd by cutting away of the Ribbs and Diaphragme; and after the Pericardium of the Heart also was taken off—the Dog being kept alive by the Reciprocal blowing of the Lungs with Bellows, and they suffered to subside, for the space of an hour or more, after his Thorax had been so display'd and his Aspera arteria cut off just below the epiglottis, and bound on upon the nose of the Bellows.

The exact function of the lungs was at that time in some doubt, and Hooke reported that:

> Some eminent Physitians had affirm'd that the Motion of the Lungs was necessary to Life upon the account of promoting the Circulation of the Blood, and that it was conceiv'd, the Animal would immediately be suffocated as soon as the Lungs should cease to be moved.

Hooke did not believe this and to disprove it carried out another experiment which he describes as follows:

> I caused another pair of Bellows to be immediately joyn'd to the first, by a contrivance, I had prepar'd, and pricking all the outer-coat of the Lungs with the slendar point of a very sharp pen-knife, this second pair of Bellows was mov'd very quick, whereby the first pair was alwayes kept full and alwayes blowing into the Lungs; by which means the Lungs also were alwayes kept very full, and without any motion; there being a continual blast of Air forc'd into the Lungs by the first pair of Bellows, supplying it as fast, as it could find its way quite through the Coat of the Lungs by the small holes priked in it, as was said before. This being continues for a pretty while, the Dog lay still—and his Heart being very regularly. . . .

Hooke foreshadowed future oxygenators when he reported that:

> I shall shortly try, whether suffering the Blood to circulate through a vessel, so as it may be openly exposed to the fresh Air, will not suffice for the life of an Animal.

In 1915 Henderson and Chillingworth reported their experimental research on HFV. On March 2, 1955, J. H. Emerson of Arlington, Massachusetts, applied for a United States patent, later granted as No. 2,913,197: Apparatus For Vibrating Portions of a Patient's Airway.

> This invention pertains to an apparatus for treating a patient by vibrating a column of gas which is in communication with his airway at a rate which is greater than a patient's normal rate—from 100 to more than 1,500 vibrations per minute—vibrating the column of gas doubtless causes the gas to diffuse more rapidly within the airway and therefore aiding in the breathing function by circulating the gas more thoroughly to and from the walls of the lungs.

Modern-era HFV was introduced in 1967 and widely publicized by Ulf Sjöstrand and co-workers in Sweden during studies of the cardiac sinus reflex. These investigators used HFV as a means to maintain sufficient respiratory gas exchange without major changes in intratracheal and intrapleural pressure or thoracic volume and with no negative effects on circulation.

Clinicians hope that HFV will minimize cardiovascular impairment in patients with severely compromised ventilatory and/or cardiovascular systems. It has been used successfully in surgery of the airways, where an endotracheal tube may interfere with the operative procedure, and in microvascular surgery of the brain.

An impressive amount of research in the area of HFV has been, and still is being, performed. It is difficult to compare the different investigations because of the variability in technique (high-frequency positive-pressure ventilation, high-frequency jet ventilation, and high-frequency oscillation), inspiratory time and flow waveform, ventilatory frequency (most often 1 to 20 Hz), tidal volume, power source, airway pressure profile, humidity, airway temperature, system impedance, bias-flow, and other factors. Recently, Banner and colleagues found that high-frequency jet ventilation might comprise one or more physiologic variables at certain combinations of frequency and percent of inspiratory time.

The future role of HFV is impossible to predict for several reasons: There is incomplete knowledge and understanding of how HFV works and of its physiologic effects and potential complications. There are almost as many different systems for delivery of HFV as there are investigators. This makes comparisons of various studies difficult. HFV is still a fascinating technique in search of applications.

THE FUTURE

Fifty years from now, future colleagues may review our current efforts and wonder at primitive and bewildering changes in concepts, theories, and practices of mechanical ventilation. Indeed, in this area no previous time has been as restlessly changing and as interesting as our own. Improvements will continue; for example, the era of servo and computerized equipment has just begun. Adaptation of the servo control method was attempted by Frumin and Lee in 1957 with their "Autoanestheton," in which end-expired CO_2 was sampled and the results used to adjust the ventilator through a feedback circuit. Similar concepts may be based on the oxygen tension, pH, or brain activity, as was reported during the 1940s by Albert Faulconer at the Mayo Clinic. More recently, the Siemens-Elema Servo 900 series of ventilators have been developed to compensate for changes in the patient's airway resistance or compliance.

Large numbers of ventilators, monitors, and other "gadgets" have been invented, and some are even useful! A good ventilator gives us a third hand, so that we can better observe and treat the patient. There will always be a need for well-educated, conscientious physicians, nurses, and respiratory therapists who understand the monitors and who use them well in our most important task: to safeguard those who sleep and those whose lives and very survival are in our hands.

ADDENDUM

I thank the editors for inviting me to write this chapter. I am old enough to be part of history, to have been in the midst of this wonderful and progressive century. Many of the personalities mentioned are or were my teachers, many my friends, and I thank y'all!

BIBLIOGRAPHY

Abel FL, Waldhausen JA: Effects of anesthesia and artificial ventilation on caval flow and cardiac output. J Appl Physiol 25:479, 1968

Abel FL, Waldhausen JA: Respiratory and cardiac effects on venous return. Am Heart J 78:266, 1969

Abrahams N, Fisk GC, Vonwiller JB, Grant GC: Evaluation of infant ventilators. Anaesth Intensive Care 3:6, 1975

Adams H, Ellis BN, Kaye G: A new respiratory pump. Aust J Exp Biol Med Sci 28:657, 1950

Adams AP, Eronomides AP, Finlay WEI, Sykes MK: The effects of variations in inspiratory flow waveform on cardio-respiratory function during controlled ventilation in normo-, hypo-, and hypervolemic dogs. Br J Anaesth 42:818, 1970

Adamson TM, Collins LM, Delan M, et al: Mechanical ventilation in newborn infants with respiratory failure. Lancet 2:227, 1968

Adelman MH, Berman RA, Touroff ASW: A new method of automatic controlled respiration. J Thorac Surg 19:817, 1950

Adelman MH, Berman RA, Touroff ASW: Automatic controlled respiration. Anesthesiology 10:673, 1949

Adelman MH, Megibow SJ, Blum L: A method of controlled respiration for anesthesia in the dogs. Surgery 28:1040, 1950

Agostoni E, Miserocchi G: Vertical gradient of transpulmonary pressure with active and artificial lung expansion. J Appl Physiol 29:705, 1970

Agostino R, Orzalesi M, Nodari S, et al: Continuous positive airway pressure (CPAP) by nasal cannula in the respiratory distress syndrome (RDS) of the newborn. Pediatr Res 7:50, 1973

Ahlgren EW and Stephen CR: Mechanical ventilation of the infant. Anesthesiology 27:692, 1966

Ahlström H, Jonson B, Svenningsen NW: Continuous positive airway pressure with a face chamber in early treatment of idiopathic respiratory distress syndrome. Acta Paediatr Scand 62:433, 1973

Allbritten FF, Haupt GJ, Amadeo JH: The change in pulmonary alveolar ventilation achieved by aiding the deflation phase of respiration during anesthesia for surgical operations. Ann Surg 140:569, 1954

Almeida JJ Cabral de: Novo método de respiração controlada mecânicamente. Rev Bras Anestesiol 1:117, 1951

Amaha K, Liu P, Weitzner SW, et al: Effects of constant chest compression on the mechanical and physiological performance of different ventilators. Anesthesiology 28:498, 1967

Ambiavagar M, Jones ES: Resuscitation of the moribund asthmatic; use of intermittent and positive pressure ventilation, broncheal lavage and intravenous infusion. Anaesthesia 22:375, 1967

Andersen EW, Ibsen B: The anaesthetic management of patients with poliomyelitis and respiratory paralysis. Br Med J 1:786, 1954

Andersen MN, Kuchinbak K: Depression of cardiac output with mechanical ventilators. J Thorac Surg 54:182, 1967

Andersen E, Crafoord C, Frenckner P: A new and practical method of producing rhythmic ventilation during positive pressure anesthesia. Acta Otolaryngol (Stockh) 28:95, 1939

Angrist SW: Fluid control devices. Sci Am 211:81, 1964

Ankeney JL, Hubay CA, Hackett PR, et al: The effect of positive and negative pressure respiration on unilateral pulmonary blood flow in the open chest. Surg Gynecol Obstet 98:5, 1954

Arp JL, Dillon RE, Humphries TJ, et al: A new approach to ventilatory support of infants with respiratory distress syndrome. Part I. The Arp infant respirator. Anesth Analg 48:251, 1969

Arp JL, Dillon RE, Humphries TJ, et al: A new approach to ventilatory support of infants with respiratory distress syndrome. Part II. The clinical applications of the Arp infant respirator. Anesth Analg 48:517, 1969

Arthur DS, Mathur AK, Nisbet HIA, et al: The effect of artificial ventilation on functional residual capacity and arterial oxygenation. II. Comparison of spontaneous respiration and artificial ventilation at similar arterial carbon dioxide tensions, tidal volume, and inspiratory gas flow rates. Can Anaesth Soc J 22:432, 1975

Ashbaugh DG: Effect of ventilatory methods and patterns on physiologic shunt. Surgery 68:99, 1970

Ashbaugh DG, Bigelow DB, Petty TI, et al: Acute respiratory distress in adults. Lancet 2:319, 1967

Ashbaugh DG, Petty TL: Positive end-expiratory pressure: Physiology, indications and contraindications. J Thorac Cardiovasc Surg 65:165, 1973

Ashbaugh DG, Petty TL, Bigelow DB, et al: Continuous positive pressure breathing (CPPB) in adult

respiratory distress syndrome. J Thorac Cardiovasc Surg 57:31, 1969
Asmussen E, Nielsen M: Efficacy of artificial respiration. J Appl Physiol 3:95, 1950
Astrup P, Goetzche H, Neukirk F: Lab investigation during treatment of patients with poliomyelitis and respiratory paralysis. Br Med J 1:780, 1954
Avery AE, Mörch ET, Benson DW: Critically crushed chests: a new method of treatment with continuous hyperventilation to produce alkalotic apnea and internal pneumatic stabilization. J Thorac Surg 32:291, 1956
Babinski M, Klain M, Smith RB: High frequency jet ventilation. American Society of Anesthesiology Annual Meeting, New Orleans, 1977 (abstract)
Baker AB: Artificial respiration, the history of an idea. Med Hist 15:344, 1971
Baker AB: Physiological responses to artificial ventilation. Thesis, University of Oxford, 1971
Bang C: A new respirator. Lancet 1:723, 1953
Banner MJ, Gallagher TJ, Banner TE: Frequency and percent inspiratory time for high frequency jet ventilation. Crit Care Med 13:395, 1985
Barach AL: Principles and Practices of Inhalation Therapy, JB Lippincott, Philadelphia, 1944, p. 52
Barach AL, Barach B, Echman M, et al: An appraisal of intermittent positive breathing as a method of increasing altitude tolerance. CAM Reports No. 399, November 1944
Barach AL, Bickeman HA, Petty TL: Perspectives in pressure breathing. Resp Care 20:627, 1975
Barach AL, Eckman M, Ginsburg E, et al: Studies on positive pressure respiration. J Aviat Med 17:290, 1946
Barach AL, Fen WO, Ferris, et al: The physiology of pressure breathing. J Aviat Med 18:73, 1947
Barach AL, Martin J, Eckman M: Positive pressure respiration and its application to the treatment of acute pulmonary edema. Ann Intern Med 12:754, 1938
Barach AL, Martin J, Eckman M: Positive pressure respiration and its application to the treatment of acute pulmonary edema. Proc Soc Clin Invest 16:664, 1937
Baratz RA, Ingraham RC: Renal hemodynamics and antidiuretic hormone release associated with volume regulation. Am J Phisiol 198:565, 1960
Baratz RA, Philbin DM, Patternson RW: Plasma antidiuretic hormone and urinary output during continuous positive pressure breathing in dogs. Anesthesiology 34:510, 1971
Barker E, Singer R, Elkinton J, et al: The renal response in man to experimental respiratory alkalosis and acidosis. J Clin Invest 36:515, 1957
Barnes CH: Bristol Aircraft Since 1910. Putnam, London, 1964, p. 20
Barrie H: Simple method of applying continuous positive airway pressure in respiratory distress syndrome. Lancet 1:776, 1972
Bates DV, Macklem PT, Christie RV: Respiratory Function in Disease: An Introduction to the Integrated Study of the Lung. WB Saunders, Philadelphia, 1971, p. 441
Baumeister J, Blood MJ, Marsh A, et al: The use of tracheotomy, intermittent positive pressure, and sedation treatment in children with poliomyelitis. J Kans Med Soc 53:281, 1952
Beaver RA: Pneumoflator for treatment of respiratory paralysis. Lancet 1:977, 1953
Beckman M, Norlander O: Pulmonary ventilation during thoracic surgery. Acta Chir Scand [Suppl] 245:27, 1959
Beecher HK: Principles of anesthesia for lobectomy and total pneumonectomy. Acta Med Scand [Suppl] 90:146, 1938
Beecher HK, Murphy AJ: Acidosis during thoracic surgery. J Thorac Surg 19:50, 1950
Behress CW: What is fluidics. Appliance manufacture, July 1968
Beinart J: A History of the Nuffield Department of Anesthetics. Oxford University Press, Oxford, 1987
Bendixen HH: Respirators and respiratory care. Acta Anaesth Scand 26:279, 1982
Bendixen HH, Bullwinkel B, Hedley-Whyte J: Atelectasis and shunting during spontaneous ventilation in anesthesia patients. Anesthesiology 25:297, 1964
Bendixen HH, Egbett LD, Hedley-Whyte J, et al: Respiratory Care. CV Mosby, St. Louis, 1965
Bendixen HH, Hedley-Whyte J, Laver MB: Impaired oxygenation in surgical patients during general anesthesia with controlled ventilation: A concept of atelectasis. N Engl J Med 269:991, 1963
Bendixen HH, Kinney JM: History of intensive care. p. 1. In Kinney J, Bendixen H, Powers S (eds): Manual of Surgical Intensive Care. WB Saunders, Philadelphia, 1977
Bendixen AH, Smith GM, Mead J: Pattern of ventilation in young adults. J Appl Physiol 19:195, 1964
Bergen FHV, Buckley JJ, Weastrehead DSP, et al: A new respirator. Anesthesiology 17:708, 1956
Bergman NA: Effects of different pressure breathing

patterns on alveolar-arterial gradients in dogs. J Appl Physiol 18:1049, 1963

Bergman NA: Effects of varying respiratory waveforms on gas exchange. Anesthesiology 28:390, 1967

Bergman NA: Intrapulmonary gas trapping during mechanical ventilation at rapid frequencies. Anesthesiology 37:626, 1972

Bergman R: Eight hundred cases of poliomyelitis treated in the Sahlin respirator. Acts Paediatr Scand 36:470, 1948

Berneus B, Carlsten A: Effect of intermittent positive pressure ventilation on cardiac output in polio. Acta Med Scand 152:19, 1955

Berry PR, Pontoppidan H: Oxygen consumption and blood gas exchange during controlled and spontaneous ventilation in patients with respiratory failure. Anesthesiology 29:177, 1968

Binda RE, Cook DR, Fischer CG: Advantages of infant ventilators over adapted adult ventilators in pediatrics. Anesth Analg 55:769, 1976

Birnbaum GL, Thompson SA: The mechanism of asphyxial resuscitation. Surg Gynecol Obstet 75:79, 1942

Bjerager K, Sjöstrand U, Wattwil M: Long-term treatment of two patients with respiratory insufficiency with IPPV/PEEP and HFPPV/PEEP. Acta Anaesth Scand [Suppl] 64:55, 1977

Björk VO: Principles and indication for treatment of ventilatory insufficiency. Bull Soc Int Chir 15(3):249, 1956

Björk VO, Engström CG: Notre expérience de la respiration artificielle en chirurgie thoracique. Anesth Analg (Paris) 12:1955

Björk VO, Engström CG, The treatment of ventilatory insufficiency after pulmonary resection with tracheotomy and prolonged artificial respiration. J Thorac Cardiovasc Surg 30:356, 1955

Björk VO, Engström CG, Friberg O, et al: Ventilatory problems in thoracic anaesthesia: A volume-cycling device for controlled respiration. J Thorac Surg 31:117, 1956

Blaisdell FW, Lewis FR: Respiratory Distress Syndrome of Shock and Trauma. WB Saunders, Philadelphia, 1977

Blaisdell FW, Schlobohm RM: The respiratory distress syndrome: a review. Surgery 74:251, 1973

Bland RD, Kim MH, Light MJ, et al: High-frequency mechanical ventilation of low-birth weight infants with respiratory failure from hyaline membrane disease: 92% survival. Pediatr Res 11:531, 1977

Bland RD, Kim MH, Light MJ, et al: Mechanical ventilation at high respiratory frequencies in severe hyaline membrane disease—an alternative treatment? Crit Care Med 8:275, 1980

Bohm DJ, Miyasaka K, Marchak B, et al: Ventilation by high frequency oscillation. J Appl Physiol 48:710, 1980

Borg U, Eriksson I, Lyttkens L, et al: High-frequency positive-pressure ventilation (HFPPV) applied in bronchoscopy under general anaesthesia—an experimental study. Acta Anaesth Scand [Suppl] 64:69, 1977

Borg U, Lyttkens L, Nilsson LG, et al: Physiologic evaluation of the HFPPV pneumatic valve principle and PEEP—an experimental study. Acta Anaesth Scand [Suppl] 64:37, 1977

Boros SJ, Matalon SV, Ewald R, et al: The effect of independent variations in inspiratory-expiratory ratio and end-expiratory pressure during mechanical ventilation in hyaline membrane disease. J Pediatr 91:794, 1977

Bower AG, Bennett VR, Dillon JB, et al: Investigation of the care and treatment of poliomyelitis patients. Ann West Med Surg 4:561, 1950

Brauer L: Die ausschaltung der Pneumothorax folgen mit Hilfe des Überdruckverfahrens. Mitt Grenzgeb Med Chir 8:583, 1904

Braun E: Apparatus for resuscitating asphyxiated children. Boston Med Surg J 120:9, 1889

Braunwald E, Binion JT, Morgan WL, et al: Alteration in central blood volume and cardiac output induced by positive pressure breathing and counteracted by metaraminol. Circ Res 5:670, 1957

Breathing Machines and Their Use in Treatment: Report of the Respirators (Poliomyelitis) Committee. Medical Research Council, London, November 22, 1939

Breathing Mechanics for Medical Use. Proposed JSO Standard Specifications. International Standards Organization Technical Committee 121, Boston, 1972

Brecker GA: Venous Return. Grune & Stratton, New York, 1956

Breivik H, Grenvik A, Miller E, et al: Normalizing low atrial CO_2 tension during mechanical ventilation. Chest 63:525, 1973

Briscoe WA, Forster RE, Comroe JH: Alveolar ventilation at very low tidal volumes. J Appl Physiol 7:27, 1954

Brown EB Jr: Physiological effects of hyperventilation. Physiol Rev 33:445, 1953

Browne AGR, Pontoppidan H, Chiang H: Physiological criteria for weaning patients from prolonged artificial ventilation. American Society of Anesthesiolgists Annual Meeting, 1972

Brundin T, Hendenstierna G, McCarthy G: Effect of intermittent positive pressure ventilation on cardiac systolic time intervals. Acta Anaesth Scand 20:278, 1976

Bryce-Smith R, Davis HS: Tidal exchange in respirators. Anesth Analg 33:73, 1954

Bryce-Smith R, Mitchell JV, Parkhouse J: The Nuffield Department of Anaesthesia. Oxford University Press, Oxford, 1937–1962

Bull PR: A water driven respirator. Med J Aust 34:238, 1947

Bunnell J, Karlson K, Shannon D: High frequency positive pressure ventilation in dogs and rabbits. Am Rev Respir Dis 117:289, 1978

Burger EJ Jr, Macklem PT: Airway closure: demonstration of breathing 100 percent oxygen at low lung volumes and by N_2 washout. J Appl Physiol 25:139, 1968

Burke JF, Pontoppidan H, Welch CE: High output respiratory failure: an important cause of death ascribed to peritonitis or ileus. Ann Surg 158:581, 1963

Burns HL: A pure fluid cycling valve for use in breathing equipment. Inhal Ther 14:11, 1969

Burns HL: Pneumatic balance resuscitator. Air Surg Bull 2:306, 1945

Burns HL: Specifications: RETEC Automatic Respirator Model A-30, RETEC Inc., Portland, OR, 1967

Burton CG, Gee GN, Hodgkin JE: Respiratory Care. JB Lippincott, Philadelphia, 1977

Bushman JA, Askill S: An adjustable annular fluid logic ventilator. Br J Anaesth 43:1197, 1971

Bushnell LS, Pontoppidan H, Hedley-Whyte J, et al: Efficiency of different types of ventilation in longterm respiratory care: mechanical versus spontaneous. Anesth Analg 45:696, 1966

Butler J, Smith BH: Pressure-volume relationships of the chest in the completely relaxed anaesthetized patient. Clin Sci 16:125, 1957

Butler WJ, et al: Ventilation by high frequency oscillation in humans. Anesth Analg 59:577, 1980

Campbell DI: A compact versatile, fluidic controlled ventilator. Anaesth Intensive Care 4:7, 1976

Campbell EJM, Nunn JF, Peckett BW: A comparison of artificial ventilation and spontaneous respiration with particular reference to ventilation-blood flow relationships. Br J Anaesth 30:166, 1958

Carden E: Positive-pressure ventilation during anaesthesia for bronchoscopy: a laboratory evaluation of two recent advances. Anesth Anal Curr Res 52:402, 1973

Carden E, Burns WW, McDevitt NB, et al: A comparison of venturi and side-arm ventilation in anaesthesia for bronchoscopy. Can Anaesth Soc J 20:569, 1973

Carden E, Chir B, Schwesinger WB: The use of nitrous oxide during ventilation with the open bronchoscope. Anesthesiology 39:551, 1973

Carden E, Crutchfield W: Anaesthesia for microsurgery of the larynx (a new method). Can Anaesth Soc J 20:378, 1973

Carden E, Ferguson GB: A new technique for microlaryngeal surgery in infants. Laryngoscope 93:691, 1973

Carden E, Trapp WG, Oulton J: A new and simple method for ventilating patients undergoing bronchoscopy. Anesthesiology 33:454, 1970

Carlon GC, Fay C, Klain M, et al: High frequency positive pressure ventilation in management of patients with bronchopleural fistula. Anesthesiology 52:160, 1980

Carr DT, Essex HE: Certain effects of positive pressure respiration on the circulatory and respiratory system. Am Heart J 31:53, 1946

Cartwright RY, Hargrave PR: Pseudomonas in ventilators. Lancet 1:40, 1970

Chakrabarti MK, Sykes MK: Cardiorespiratory effects of high frequency positive pressure ventilation in the dog. Br J Anaesth 52:475, 1980

Cheney FW, Wayne EM: Effects of continuous positive pressure ventilation on gas exchange in acute pulmonary edema. J Appl Physiol 30:378, 1971

Civetta JM, Barnes JA, Smith LO: Optimal PEEP and intermittent mandatory ventilation in the treatment of acute pulmonary failure. Respir Care 20:551, 1975

Civetta JM, Brous R, Gabel JC: A simple and effective method of employing spontaneous positive pressure ventilation. J Thorac Cardiovasc Surg 63:312, 1972

Civetta JM, Hudson J, Kirby RR, et al: Mechanical ventilatory support. Crit Care Med 3:114, 1977

Clowes GHA, Cook WA, Vujovic V, et al: Pattern of circulatory responses to the use of respirators. Circulation 31(suppl I):157, 1965

Coanda H: Keynote address to the Third Fluid Amplification Symposium, October 26, 1965. Kindly provided by JM Kirshner, Harry Diamond Laboratories, Washington, DC, 1965

Coleman E: Dissertation on Natural and Suspended Respiration. 2nd Ed. Cox, London, 1802

Collier CR, Affeldt JE: Ventilatory efficiency of the

cuirass respirator in totally paralyzed chronic polio patients. J Appl Physiol 6:531, 1954

Comroe JH Jr, Dripps R: Artificial respiration. JAMA 130:381, 1946

Conway CM: Haemodynamic effects of pulmonary ventilation. Br J Anaesth 47:761, 1975

Conway CM, Payne JP: Hypoxemia associated with anaesthesia and controlled respiration. Lancet 1:12, 1964

Cooper JD, Grillo HC: The evaluation of tracheal injury due to ventilatory assistance through cuffed tubes: a pathologic study. Ann Surg 169:334, 1969

Corbet AJS, Ross JA, Beaudry PH, et al: Effect of positive-pressure breathing on a-ADO_2 in hyaline membrane disease. J Appl Physiol 38:33, 1975

Cornwell JB, Davis HN: Historical perspective, current applications of the chest cuirasse. Respir Ther 9:879, 1979

Cournand A: Recent observations on the dynamics of the pulmonary circulation. Bull NY Acad Med 23:27, 1947

Cournand A, Motley HL, Werkö L: Mechanism underlying cardiac output change during intermittent positive pressure breathing. Fed Proc 6:92, 1947

Cournand A, Motley HL, Werkö L, et al: Physiological studies of effects of intermittent positive pressure breathing on cardiac output in man. Am J Physiol 152:162, 1948

Courtois MLH: Mémoire sur les asphyxie, avec la description d'un nouvel instrument propre à rappeler le méchanism de la respiration. J de Med Chir Pharm 82:361, 1790

Cox LA, Chapman EDW: A comprehensive volume cycled lung ventilator embodying feedback control. Med Biol Eng 12:160, 1974

Crafoord C: On the technique of pneumonectomy in man. Acta Chir Scand [Suppl 64] 81:1, 1938

Crafoord C: Pulmonary ventilation and anesthesia in major chest surgery. J Thorac Surg 9:237, 1940

Crafoord C: Thirty-five years experience with controlled ventilation in thoracic surgery. Int Anesthesiol Clin 10:1, 1972

Craig DB, McCarthy DS: Airway closure and lung volumes during breathing with maintained airway positive-pressures. Anesthesiology 36:540, 1972

Crampton Smith, A: Effect of mechanical ventilation on the circulation. Ann NY Acad Sci 121:733, 1965

Cross DA: A variation of the intermittent mandatory ventilation assembly. Anesthesiology 44:182, 1976

Cullen SC, Comroe JH Jr, Brown EB, et al: Problems in ventilation. Anesthesiology 15:416, 1954

Cullen W: A letter to Lord Cathcart, President of the Board of Police in Scotland concerning the recovery of persons drowned and seemingly dead. London, 1776. Quoted in Herholdt JD, Rafn CG: An Attempt at an Historical Survey of Life-Saving Measures for Drowning Persons and Information of the Best Means by Which They Can Again Be Brought Back to Life. H Tikiob, Copenhagen, 1796.

Cumarasamy N, Nussli R, Vischer D, et al: Artificial ventilation in hyaline membrane disease: the use of positive end-expiratory pressure and continuous positive airway pressure. Pediatrics 51:629, 1973

Cutler EC: The origin of thoracic surgery. N Engl J Med 208:1233, 1933

Daily WJR, Meyer HPP, Sunshine P, et al: Mechanical ventilation of the newborn infants, III, IV, V. Anesthesiology 34:119, 1971

Daily WJR, Smith PC: Mechanical ventilation of the newborn infant. Curr Probl Pediatr 1:1, 1971

Daily WJR, Sunshine P, Smith PC: Mechanical ventilation of the newborn infant: five year experience. Anesthesiology 34:132, 1971

Dalziel J: On Sleep and an Apparatus for Promoting Artificial Respiration. British Association for Advancement of Science Report No. 2, p. 127, 1838

Dameron JT, Greene DG: Use of the Burns valve as a simple respirator for intrathoracic surgery in the dog. J Thorac Surg 20:706, 1950

D'Avignon P, Sundell L, Werneman H: Treatment in cuirass and/or positive pressure respirator: primary lethality, invalidity, and physical fitness of respirator patients after one year. Acta Med Scand 154:316, 1956

Dehan FH: La respiration mecaniquement controlée en chirurgie thoracique. Acta Chir Belg 49:938, 1950

deLemos R, Mclaughlin GW: Technique of Ventilation in the Newborn: the Use of IMV. Physiologie Appliquèe de la Ventilation Assistée Chez le Nouveau-née. Report of Colloquium. Pont-a-Moussou, France, September 27–28, 1973, pp. 173–178

deLemos RA, Armstrong RG, Kirby RR, et al: A new pediatric volume ventilator evaluation in

90 newborn infants (abstract). Am Thorac Soc, 1971

deLemos RA, McLaughlin GW, Robison EJ, et al: Continuous positive airway pressure as an adjunct to mechanical ventilation in the newborn with respiratory distress syndrome. Anesth Analg 52:328, 1973

deLemos RA, Wolsdorf J, Nachman R, et al: Lung injury from oxygen in lambs; the role of artificial ventilation. Anesthesiology 30:609, 1969

Dennis C, Karlson KE, Eder WB, et al: A simple, efficient respirator and anesthesia bag for open chest surgery. Surg Forum 583, 1950

Desautels D: Ventilator classification: a new look at an old subject. Curr Rev Respir Ther 1:82, 1979

Desautels D, Bartlett JL: Methods of administering intermittent mandatory ventilation (IMV). Respir Care 19:187, 1974

Dickinson DG, Wilson JL, Graham BG: Studies in respiratory insufficiency. I. Carbon dioxide and oxygen studies in early respiratory paralysis in poliomyelitis. Am J Dis Child 3:265, 1953

Dobkin AB: Ventilators and Inhalation Therapy. Little, Brown, Boston, 1972

Doctor NH: A device for mechanical ventilation suitable for newborn and infants during anaesthesia. Br J Anaesth 36:259, 1964

Donald I: Augmented respiration; emergency positive-pressure patient-cycled respirator. Lancet 1:895, 1954

Dorrange GM: On the treatment of traumatic injuries of the lungs and pleura: with the presentation of a new intratracheal tube for use in artificial respiration. Surg Gynecol Obstet 11:160, 1910

Downes JJ: CPAP and PEEP: a perspective. Anesthesiology 44:1, 1976

Downes JJ: Mechanical ventilation of the newborn. Anesthesiology 34:116, 1971

Downes JJ, Nicodemus HF, Pierce WS, et al: Acute respiratory failure in infants following cardiovascular surgery. J Thorac Cardiovasc Surg 59:21, 1970

Downs JB, Block AJ, Vennum KB: Intermittent mandatory ventilation in the treatment of patients with chronic obstructive pulmonary disease. Anesth Analg 53:437, 1974

Downs JB, Douglas ME, Sanfelippo PM, et al: Ventilatory pattern, intrapleural pressure and cardiac output. Anesth Analg 56:88, 1977

Downs JB, Klein EF, Desautels D, et al: Intermittent mandatory ventilation—a new approach to weaning patients from mechanical ventilators. Chest 64:331, 1973

Downs JB, Klein EF, Modell JH: The effect of incremental PEEP on PaO_2 in patients with respiratory failure. Anesth Analg 52:210, 1973

Downs JB, Mitchell LA: Intermittent mandatory ventilation following cardiopulmonary bypass. Crit Care Med 2:39, 1974

Downs JB, Perkins HM, Modell JH: Intermittent mandatory ventilation: an evaulation. Arch Surg 109:519, 1974

Downs JB, Perkins HM, Sutton WW: Successful weaning after five years of mechanical ventilation. Anesthesiology 40:602, 1974

Drinker CK: Development of the school of public health (at Harvard University). Harvard Med Alumni Bull 10:9, 1935

Drinker CK: Pulmonary Edema and Inflammation. Harvard University Press, Cambridge, MA, 1945

Drinker P, McKhann CF: The use of a new apparatus for the prolonged administration of artificial respiration in a fatal case of poliomyelitis. JAMA 92:1658, 1929

Drinker P, Shaw LA: An apparatus for the prolonged administration of artificial respiration. J Clin Invest 7:229, 1927

Drury DR, Henry JP, Goodman J: Effects of continuous pressure breathing on kidney function. J Clin Invest 26:945, 1947

Duffin J: Fluidics and pneumatics principles and applications in anaesthesia. Can Anaesth Soc J 24:126, 1977

Dunn PM: Continuous positive airway pressure (CPAP) using the Gregory box. Proc R Soc Med 67:245, 1974

E & J resuscitator: Report from Council of Physical Therapy. JAMA 121:1219, 1943

Egan DF: Fundamentals of Oxygen Therapy. CV Mosby, St. Louis, 1977

Eger EI II, Hamilton WK: Positive negative pressure ventilation with a modified Ayre's T-piece. Anesthesiology 19:611, 1958

Elam JO, Brown ES, Janney CD: Ventilator. Anesthesiology 17:504, 1956

Elam JO, Kerr JH, Janney CD: Performance of ventilators—effect of changes in lung-thorax compliance. Anesthesiology 19:56, 1958

Elliott LS: A pictorial history of mechanical devices. Respir Ther 9:52, 1979

El-Naggar M: "Weaning." Middle East J Anaesthesiol 3:401, 1972

Elsberg CA: Clinical experiences with intratracheal insufficiency (Meltzer) with remarks upon the value of the method for thoracic surgery. Ann Surg 52:23, 1910

Elsberg CA: The value of continuous intratracheal insufflation of air (Meltzer) in thoracic surgery: with description of an apparatus. Med Rec 77:493, 1910

Emerson H: Artificial respiration in the treatment of edema of the lungs. Arch Intern Med 3:368, 1909

Emerson JH: Respiratory problems in poliomyelitis. Presented at the National Foundation for Infantile Paralysis Conference, Ann Arbor, MI, March 1952, p. 11

Emerson JH: The Evolution of "Iron Lung." JH Emerson Co., Cambridge, MA, 1978

Emerson resuscitator: Report from Council of Physical Therapy. JAMA 119:414, 1942

Enghoff E: Konstgjord Andning. Almqvist & Wiksell, Uppsala, 1956, p. 19

Enghoff H: Bemerkungen zur Frage des Schädlischen Raumes. Uppsala Läkarföreningens Forhandlinge 44:191, 1938

Enghoff H: Der Barospirator: Untersuchungen über seine Wirkungsweise mit besonderer Berüchsichtigung die Pneumographischen Methodik. Scand Arch Physiol 51:1, 1927

Engström CG: Respirator enligt nyt princip. Svensk Läkartidn 50:545, 1953

Engström CG: The clinical application of prolonged controlled ventilation. Acta Anaesth Scand [Suppl] 13:25, 1963

Engström CG: Treatment of severe cases of respiratory paralysis by the Engström universal respirator. Br Med J 2:666, 1954

Engström CG, Herzog P: Ventilation nomogram for practical use with the Engström respirator. Acta Anaesth Scand 6:49, 1959

Engström CG, Herzog P, Norlander OD, et al: Ventilation nomogram for the newborn and small childrento be used with the Engström respirator. Acta Anaesth Scand 6:175, 1962

Engström CG, Norlander OD: A new method for analysis of respiratory work by measurement of actual power as a function of gas flow, pressure, and time. Acta Anaesth Scand 6:49, 1962

Epstein RA: The sensitivities and response times of ventilatory assistors. Anesthesiology 34:321, 1971

Eriksson I: The role of the conducting airways in N_2-washout during high frequency mechanical ventilation. Anesthesiology 55(suppl):354, 1981

Eriksson I, Heijman L, Sjöstrand U: High-frequency positive-pressure ventilation (HFPPV) in bronchoscopy during anaesthesia. Opusc Med 19:14, 1972

Eriksson I, Jonzon A, Sedin G, et al: The influence of the ventilatory pattern on ventilation, circulation, and oxygen transport during continuous positive-pressure ventilation—an experimental study. Acta Anaesth Scand [Suppl] 64:149, 1977

Eriksson I, Lyttkens L, Nilsson LG, et al: The importance of frequency and relative insufflation time in ventilation during bronchoscopy under general anaesthesia. Svenska Läkarsällskabets Handlingar Opusc Med 21:142, 1976

Eriksson I, Nilsson LG, Nordström S, et al: High-frequency positive pressure ventilation (HFPPV) during transthoracic resection of tracheal stenosis and during perioperative bronchoscopic examination. Acta Anaesth Scand 19:113, 1975

Eriksson I, Sjöstrand U: A clinical evaluation of high-frequency positive-pressure ventilation (HFPPV) in laryngoscopy and under general anaesthesia. Acta Anaesth Scand [Suppl] 64:101, 1977

Eriksson I, Sjöstrand U: Effects of high frequency positive-pressure ventilation (HFPPV) and general anaesthesia on intrapulmonary gas distribution in patients undergoing diagnostic bronchoscopy. Anesth Analg 59:585, 1980

Eriksson I, Sjöstrand U: Experimental and clinical evaluation of high-frequency positive-pressure ventilation (HFPPV) and the pneumatic valve principle in bronchoscopy under general anesthesia. Acta Anaesth Scand [Suppl] 64:83, 1977

Eriksson I, Sjöstrand U: High frequency positive-pressure ventilation (HFPPV) during laryngoscopy. Opusc Med 19:278, 1974

Erlanson P, Lindholm T, Lindquist B, et al: Artificial respiration in severe renal failure with pulmonary insufficiency. Acta Med Scand 166:81, 1960

Esplen JR: A new apparatus for intermittent pulmonary inflation. Br J Anaesth 24:303, 1952

Esplen JR: Differential pressure respiration in thoracic operations. Br J Anaesth 23:214, 1951

Esplen JR: The Fazakerley respirator. Br J Anaesth 28:176, 1956

Fairley HB: Respiratory insufficiency. Int Anesthesiol Clin 1:351, 1963

Fairley HB, Britt BA: The adequacy of the air-mix

control in ventilators operated from an oxygen source. Can Med Assoc J 90:1394, 1964

Fairley HB, Hunter DD: Mechanical ventilators: an assessment of two new machines for use in the operating room. Can Anaesth Soc J 10:364, 1963

Fairley HB, Hunter DD: The performance of respirators used in the treatment of respiratory insufficiency. Can Med Assoc J 90:1397, 1964

Fairley HB, Schlobohm RM, Singer MM, et al: The appropriateness of intensive respiratory care. Crit Care Med 1:115, 1973

Falke KJ, Pontoppidan H, Kumar A, et al: Ventilation with end-expiratory pressure in acute lung disease. J Clin Invest 51:2315, 1972

Falor WH, Kelly TR, Reynolds CW: Mechanical elimination of respiratory acidosis during open thoracic procedures. Surg Forum 5:536, 1954

Fanaroff AA, Klaus MH: Evaluation and care of the newborn infant. p. 30. In Lough MD (ed): Pediatric Respiratory Therapy, Year Book Medical Publishers, Chicago, 1974

Faridy EE, Perman HS, Riley RL: Effect of ventilation on surface forces in excised dogs' lungs. J Appl Physiol 21:1453, 1966

Feeley TW, Hedley-Whyte J: Current concepts: weaning from continuous ventilatory supplemental oxygen. N Engl J Med 292:903, 1975

Feeley TW, Saumaurez R, Klick JM, et al: Positive end-expiratory pressure in weaning patients from continuous ventilation: a prospective randomized trial. Lancet 2:725, 1975

Fell GE: Artificial respiration. Surg Gynecol Obstet 10:572, 1910

Fell GE: Forced respiration in opium poisoning. Buffalo Med Surg J 28:145, 1887

Fenn WO, Chadwick E: Effect of pressure breathing on blood flow through the finger. Am J Physiol 151:270, 1947

Fenn WO, Otis AB, Rahn H, et al: Displacement of blood from the lungs by pressure breathing. Am J Physiol 151:258, 1947

Ferris BG, Mead J, Whittenberger JL, et al: Pulmonary function in convalescent poliomyelitis patients. III. Compliance of the lungs and thorax. N Engl J Med 247:390, 1952

Flaum A: Experience in the use of a new respirator (Sahlin type) in the treatment of respiratory paralysis in poliomyelitis. Acta Med Scand [Suppl] 78:849, 1936

Fleming WH, Bowen JC; A comparative evaluation of pressure-limited and volume-limited respirators for prolonged post-operative ventilatory support in combat casualties. Ann Surg 176:49, 1972

Fleming WH, Bowen JC: Early complications of long-term respiratory support. J Thorac Cardiovasc Surg 64:729, 1972

Fletcher PR, Epstein MAF, Epstein RA: Alveolar pressure during high frequency ventilation (HFV). Fed Proc 39:576, 1980

Fletcher PR, Epstein MAF, Epstein RA: A new ventilator for physiologic studies during high frequency ventilation. Respir Physiol 47:21, 1982

Fletcher PR, Epstein RA: A high frequency ventilator for physiologic studies. Anesthesiology 53:399, 1980

Fletcher PR, Epstein RA: Experimental studies in high-frequency ventilation. Anesthesiology 53: 401, 1980

Fletcher PR, Epstein RA: Measurement of alveolar pressure during HFV. Anesthesiology 55 (suppl):358, 1981

Folkow B, Pappenheimer JR: Components of the respiratory dead space and their variation with pressure breathing and with bronchoactive drugs. J Appl Physiol 8:102, 1955

Fothergill J: A case published in the last volume of Medical Essays of recovery of a man dead in appearance, by distending the lungs with air. In Lettsam JC (ed): The Works of John Fothergill, M.D. C Dilly, London, 1784

France EM: Some eighteenth century authorities on resuscitation of the apparently drowned. Anaesthesia 30:530, 1975

Frank I, Noack W, Lunkenheimer PP, et al: Light- and electronmicroscopic investigations of pulmonary tissue after high-frequency positive-pressure ventilation (HFPPV). Anaesthesist 24:171, 1975

Fredberg JJ: Augmented diffusion in the airways can support pulmonary gas exchange. J Appl Physiol 49:232, 1980

Fredberg JJ, Mean J: Impedance of intrathoracic airway models during low frequency period flow. J Appl Physiol 47:347, 1979

French-Brevet d'Invention (patent) P.V. No. 956,441, No. 1 386.37, entitled: Appareils distributeurs à membranés, granted December 14, 1964

Frenkner P: Bronchial and tracheal catheterization. Acta Otolaryngol Scand [Suppl] 20:97, 1934

Frost GT, Dupuis YG, Bain JA: A modification of the Bird Mark VIII ventilator to deliver continuous positive pressure breathing and intermittent mandatory ventilation. Can Anaesth Soc J 22:719, 1975

Frumin MJ: Clinical use of a physiological respirator producing N_2O amnesia-analgesia. Anesthesiology 18:290, 1957

Frumin MJ, Bergman NA, Holaday DA, et al: Alveolar arterial O_2 differences during artificial respiration in man. J Appl Physiol 14:694, 1959

Frumin MJ, Lee ASJ: A physiologically oriented artificial respirator which produces N_2O-O_2 anesthesia in man. J Lab Clin Med 49:617, 1957

Frumin MJ, Lee ASJ, Papper EM: Intermittent positive-pressure respirator. Anesthesiology 21:220, 1960

Frumin MJ, Lee ASJ, Papper EM: New valve for nonrebreathing systems. Anesthesiology 20:383, 1959

Gagge AP, Allen SC, Marborger JP: Pressure breathing. J Aviat Med 16:2, 1945

Galen: De usum partium corpus humani. Lib VII cap. IV. Translated by M T May. Cornell University Press, Ithaca, NY, 1908, p. 339

Gallagher TJ, Civetta JM, Kirby RR, et al: High level PEEP, cost vs value. Annual Meeting of American Society of Anesthesiologists, 1976, (abstract)

Galloon S: The Toronto ventilating laryngoscope. Br J Anaesth 45:912, 1973

Galloon S, Rosen N: Changes in airway resistance and alveolar trapping with positive-negative ventilation. Anaesthesia 20:429, 1965

Gammanpila S, Bevan DR, Bhudu R: Effect of positive and negative expiratory pressure on renal function. Br J Anaesth 49:199, 1977

Garzon AA, Seitzer B, Karlson KE: Physiopathology of crushed chest injuries. Ann Surg 168:128, 1968

Gauer OH, Henry JP, Sieker HO, et al: Effect of negative pressure breathing on urine flow. J Clin Invest 33:287, 1954

Gett PM, Sherwood-Jones JG, Shepherd GF: Pulmonary oedema associated with sodium retention during ventilator treatment. Br J Anaesth 43:460, 1971

Gibbon JH, Haupt GJ: The need for adequate pulmonary ventilation during surgical operation. Surg Clin North Am 35:1553, 1955

Gibbon JH, Stayman JW, Allbritten FF: Controlled respiration in thoracic and upper abdominal operations. Minn Med 33:1031, 1950

Giertz HK: Studier över tryckdifferensandning enligt Sauerbruch och över konstgjord andning (rytmisk luftinblåsning vid intrathoracala operationer). Ups Läkareför Forh 22 (suppl):1, 1916

Gillick JS: The inflation-catheter technique for ventilation during bronchoscopy. Anesthesiology 40:503, 1974; Can Anaesth Soc J 23:534, 1976

Gioia FR, Harris AP, Hamburger C, et al: Peripheral circulatory changes with high frequency ventilation. Anesthesiology 55(suppl):357, 1981

Gioia FR, Rinehart G, Parke SD, et al: Pulmonary blood flow during high frequency ventilation. Anesthesiology 55(suppl):356, 1981

Giordano J, Harken A: Effect of continuous positive pressure ventilation on cardiac output. Am Surg 41:221, 1975

Glover DW: Model No. 110, Kreiselman Resuscitator. Respir Care 22:203, 1977

Gold MI: Impedance in anoxia. Anesthesiology 30:663, 1969

Goldstein DH, Slutsky AS, Ingram RH, et al: CO_2 elimination by high frequency ventilation (4–10 Hz) in normal subjects. Am Rev Respir Dis 123:251, 1981

Goodwyn E: Dissertatio Medica Inauguralis de Morbo Morteque Submersorum Investigandis. Edinburgh, 1786

Goodwyn E: La Connexion de la Vie Avec la Respiration. Paris, An VI, 1798

Goodwyn E: The connexion of life with respiration; or an experimental inquiry into the effects of submersion, strangulation, and several kinds of noxious airs, on living animals; with an account of the nature of disease they produce; its distinction from death itself; and the most effectual means of cure. Printed by T. Spilsbury, Snow-hill. For J. Johnson, in St. Paul's Church-yard, 1788

Gordh T: Postural circulatory and respiratory changes during ether and intravenous anesthesia: experimental analysis of significance of postural changes during anesthesia with special regard to value of head down posture in resuscitation. Acta Chir Scand 92 (suppl 102):1, 1945

Gordh T, Linderholm H, Norlander O: Pulmonary function in relation to anesthesia and surgery evaluated by analysis of oxygen tension of arterial blood. Acta Anaesth Scand 2:15, 1958

Gordon AS, Frye CW, Langston HT: The cardiorespiratory dynamics of controlled respiration in the open and closed chest. J Thorac Surg 32:431, 1956

Gorham J: A medical triumph: the iron lung. Respir Ther 9:71, 1979

Gotoh F, Meyer J, Takagi Y: Cerebral effects of hyperventilation in man. Arch Neurol 12:419, 1965

Green NW: The positive pressure method of artificial respiration. Surg Gynecol Obstet 2:512, 1906

Greenfield LJ, Ebert PA, Benson DW: Effect of positive pressure ventilation on surface tension properties of lung extracts. Anesthesiology 25:312, 1964

Greer JR, Donald I: A volume controlled patient-cycled respirator for adults. Br J Anaesth 30:3236, 1958

Gregory GA: Respiratory care of newborn infants. Pediatr Clin North Am 19:311, 1971

Gregory GA, Kitterman JA, Phibbs RH, et al: Treatment of the idiopathic respiratory distress syndrome with continuous positive airway pressure. N Engl J Med 184:1333, 1971

Grenard S, et al: Advanced Study in Respiratory Therapy. Glenn Educational Medical Services, Monsey, NY, 1971

Grenvik A: Acute respiratory failure; with special reference to current management of life threatening failure in an intensive care unit. In Current Therapy. WB Saunders, Philadelphia, 1983

Grenvik A: Respiratory, circulation, and metabolic effects of respiratory treatment: a clinical study in post-operative thoracic surgical patients. Acta Anaesth Scand [Suppl] 19:1, 1966

Gunkler WA, Mahoney EG: A respirator for use in intrathoracic surgery in the dog. Surgery 26:821, 1949

Gwathmey JT: Anesthesia. Appleton. New York, 1914

Haddad C, Richards CC: Mechanical ventilation of infants: significance and elimination of ventilator compression volume. Anesthesiology 29:365, 1968

Haggard HW: Devils, Drugs and Doctors. Pocket Books, New York, 1959

Haglund G, Waldinger A: En ny övertrycksrespirator. Nord Med 53:804, 1955

Hardy MJ: The de Havelland Mosquito. p. 20. Arco, New York

Harris AP, Gioia F, Hamburger C, et al: Peripheral circulatory changes with high frequency ventilation. Anesthesiology 555(suppl): 357, 1981

Harrison VC, Heese H de V, and Klein M: The effects of intermittent positive pressure ventilation on lung function in hyaline membrane disease. Br J Anaesth 41;908, 1969

Hedenstierna G, McCarthy G, Bergström M: Airway closure during mechanical ventilation. Anesthesiology 44:114, 1976

Hedley-Whyte J, Laver MB: O_2 solubility in blood and temperature correcting factors for PO_2. J Appl Physiol 19:901, 1964

Hedley-Whyte J, Pontoppidan H, Morris MJ: The response of patients with respiratory failure and cardiopulmonary disease to different levels of constant volume ventilation. J Clin Invest 45:1543, 1966

Heese H de V, Harrison VC, Klein M, et al: Intermittent positive pressure ventilation in hyaline membrane disease. J Pediatr 76:183, 1970

Heifetz M, DeMyttenaere S, Rosenberg B: Intermittent positive pressure inflation during microscopic endolaryngeal surgery. Anaesthesist 26:11, 1977

Heijman K, Heijman L, Jonzon A, et al: High-frequency positive-pressure ventilation during anaesthesia and routine surgery in man. Acts Anaesth Scand 16:176, 1972

Heijman K, Sjöstrand U: Treatment of the respiratory distress syndrome—a preliminary report. Opusc Med 19:235, 1974

Heijman K, Sjöstrand U: Treatment of the respiratory distress syndrome by HFPPV and PEEP and by CPAP. p. 336. In Stembera ZK (ed): Perinatal Medicine. Thieme, Stuttgart, 1974

Heijman L, Nilsson LG, Sjöstrand U: High-frequency positive-pressure ventilation (HFPPV) in neonates and infants during NLA and routine plastic surgery, and in postoperative management. Acta Anaesth Scand [Suppl] 64:111, 1977

Heijman L, Sjöstrand H: Some anaesthetic techniques in operations for cleft lip and palate. Abstract of the Society of Anaesthiae Sueciae, Karlskoga-Kristineham, 1974

Heironimus T: Mechanical Artificial Ventilation. Charles C Thomas, Springfield, IL, 1970

Hellsten H: Lundia respiratorn. Svensk Lakartidn 50:1512, 1953

Henderson Y, Chillingworth TP, Whitney JL: The respiratory dead space. Am J Physiol 38:1, 1915

Herholdt JD, Rafn CG: An attempt at an historical survey to live-saving measures for drowning persons and information on the best means by which they can again be brought back to life. Printed at Tikiob Booksellers with M. Seest, Copenhagen, 1796. Re-edited by Henning Poulsen; English translation by DW Hannah and A Rousing, 1960. Scan Soc Anaest

Herzog P: Advice and practical instruction for use

of the Engström respirator. Opusc Med (Stockh) 9:280, 1964

Herzog P, Norlander OP: Distribution of alveolar volumes with different types of positive pressure gas-flow patterns. Opusc Med 13:3, 1968

Hewitt PB, Chamberlain JH, Seed RF: The effect of carbon dioxide on cardiac output on patients undergoing mechanical ventilation following open heart surgery. Br J Anaesth 45:1035, 1973

Hewlett AM: Artificial ventilation. p. 573. In Gray TC, Utting JE, Nunn JF (eds): General Anesthesia. Vol I. Butterworth, London, 1980

Hill DW: Recent developments in the design of electronically controlled ventilators. Anaesthesia 15:234, 1966

Hill DW, Moore V: The action of adiabatic effects on the compliance of an artificial thorax. Br J Anaesth 37:19, 1965

Hill JD, Main FB, Osborn JJ, et al: Correct use of respirator on cardiac patients after operation. Arch Surg 91:775, 1965

Hirsch H: Uber künstliche Atmung durch Ventilation der Trachea. Thesis, University of Giessen, Germany, 1905

Hjalmarson O: Mechanics of breathing in newborn infants with pulmonary disease. Thesis, University of Gothenburg, Sweden, 1974

Holaday DA, Rattenberg CC: Automatic lung ventilators. Anesthesiology 23:493, 1962

Holmdahl M: The effect on inadequate gaseous interchange in the postoperative period upon the circulation. Acta Chir Scand 113:402, 1957

Hubay CA, Brecher GA, Clement FL: Etiological factors affecting pulmonary arterial flow with continuous respiration. Surgery 38:215, 1955

Hubay CA, Waltz RC, Brecher GA, et al: Circulatory dynamics of venous return during positive-negative pressure respiration. Anesthesiology 15:445, 1954

Hudson LD: The use of positive end-expiratory pressure in the adult respiratory distress syndrome. p. 472. In Fontoni A (ed): Atti del 2° Corso Naziole di Aggiornamento in Rianimazione, Napoli, 1974

Humphreys GH, Moore RL, Barkley H: Studies of the jugular, carotid, and pulmonary pressures of anesthetized dogs during positive inflation of the lungs. J Thorac Surg 8:553, 1939

Humphreys GH, Moore RL, Maier HC, et al: Studies of the cardiac output of anesthetised dogs during continuous and intermittent inflation of the lungs. J Thorac Surg 7:438, 1938

Hunsinger DC: Respiratory Technology: a Procedure Manual. Prentice-Hall, Reston, VA, 1973

Hunter AR: The classification of respirators. Anaesthesia 16:231, 1961

Hunter J: Observation on certain parts of the animal oeconomy. Philos Trans R Soc Lond 66:1776

Hunter J: Proposals for the recovery of people apparently drowned. Philos Trans R Soc Lond 66:412, 1776

Ibsen B: From anaesthesia to anaesthesiology. Acta Anaesth Scand [Suppl] 61:65, 1975

Ibsen B: The anaesthetist and positive pressure breathing. p. 14. In Lassen HCA (ed): Management of Life-Threatening Poliomyelitis. Livingstone, Edinburgh, 1956

Ibsen B: The anesthetist's viewpoint on the treatment of respiratory complications in poliomyelitis during the epidemic in Copenhagen in 1952. Proc R Soc Med 47:72, 1954

Ibsen B: Treatment of respiratory complications in poliomyelitis. Dan Med Bull 1:9, 1954

Ingestedt S, Jonson B, Nordström L, et al: A servo-controlled ventilator measuring expiratory minute volume, airway flow and pressure. Acta Anaesth Scand [Suppl] 47:9, 1972

Inkster JS, Lunn JN: A device for mechanical ventilation suitable for newborn and infants during anesthesia. Br J Anaesth 38:381, 1964

Inkster JS, Pearson DT: Some infant ventilator systems: a description of their characteristics and functions. Br J Anaesth 39:667, 1967

Jackson C: The Life of Chevalier Jackson, An Autobiography. Macmillan, New York, 1938

Jackson C: The technique of insertion of intratracheal insufflation tubes. Surg Gynecol Obstet 17:507, 1913

Jackson DE: A universal artificial respiration and closed anesthesia machine. J Lab Clin Med 12:998, 1927

Jackson DE: The use of artificial respiration in man, report of a case. Cinc J Med 11:515, 1930

Jacobs HJ: The burns pneumatic balance resuscitator. J Aviat Med 18:436, 1947

James NR: A automatic machine for controlled respiration. Med J Aust 6:325, 1950

Janeway HH: An apparatus for intratrachcal insufflation. Ann Surg 56:328, 1912

Janeway HH: Intratracheal anaesthesia by nitrous oxide and oxygen under conditions of differential pressure. Ann Surg 58:927, 1913

Janeway HH, Green NW: Experimental intrathoracic esophagus surgery. JAMA 53:1975, 1909

Jansson L, Jonson B: A theoretical study on flow patterns of ventilators. Scand J Respir Dis 53:237, 1972

Jardine AD, Harrison MJ, Healy TEJ: Automatic flow interruption bronchoscope: a laboratory study. Br J Anaesth 47:385, 1975

Jensen HK: Recovery of pulmonary function after crushing injuries of the chest. J Dis Chest 22:319, 1952

Johannson H: Studies on inspiratory gas flow patterns during artificial ventilation. Linkoping Univ Med Diss 18:24, 1974

Johansson L, Silander T: Twenty-one years of thoracic injuries: a clinical study of 313 cases. Acta Chir Scand [Suppl] 245:91, 1959

Johnston RP, Donovan DJ, MacDonnell KF: PEEP during assisted ventilation. Anesthesiology 40:308, 1974

Jonzon A: High-frequency positive-pressure ventilation and carotid sinus nerve stimulation. Acta Univ Upsaliensis 138:1972

Jonzon A: Phrenic and vagal nerve activities during spontaneous respiration and positive-pressure ventilation. Acta Anaesth Scand [Suppl] 64:29, 1977

Jonzon A, Öberg Å, Sedin G, et al: High frequency low tidal volume positive pressure ventilation. Acta Physiol Scand 80:21A, 1970

Jonzon A, Öberg Å, Sedin G, et al: High-frequency positive-pressure ventilation by endotracheal insufflation. Acta Anaesth Scand [Suppl] 43:1, 1971

Jonzon A, Sedin G, Sjöstrand U: High-frequency positive-pressure ventilation (HFPPV) applied for small lung ventilation and compared with spontaneous respiration and continuous positive airway pressure (CPAP). Acta Anaesth Scand [Suppl] 53:23, 1973

Joyce JW, Woodward KE, Barila T: A fluid amplifier-controlled respirator. p. 20. In Proceedings of the Conference on Engineering in Medicine and Biology, Vol. 7. Abstract 145. Institute of Electrical and Electronic Engineers, New York, 1965

Junger T, Laurent B: The polio epidemic in Stockholm 1953. XI. Biochemical laboratory investigation. Acta Med Scand [Suppl] 316:71, 1956

Kadosch M, Paulin C, Gilbert J, et al: Appareil de respiration artificielle basé sur le principe des commutateur fluides, sans pièce mobile. J Fr Med Chir Thorac 20:5, 1966

Kattwinkel J, Fleming D, Cha CC, et al: A device for administration of continuous positive airway pressure by the nasal route. Paediatrics 52:131, 1973

Keats AS: A simple and versatile mechanical ventilator for infants. Anesthesiology 29:591, 1968

Keiskamp DHG: Automatic ventilation in paediatric anaesthesia using a modified Ayre's T-piece with negative pressure during expiratory phase. Anaesthesia 18:46, 1963

Keith A: The mechanism underlying the various methods of artificial respiration. Lancet 1:745, 1909

Kellcher WH, Kinnier Wilson AB, Ritchie RW, et al: Notes on curiass respirator. Br Med J 2:413, 1952

Kelman GR, Nunn JF: Computer Produced Physiological Tables for Calculations Involving the Relationships Between the Blood Oxygen Tension and Content. Butterworth, London, 1968

Kelman GR, Prys-Roberts C: Circulatory influences of artificial ventilation during nitrous oxide anaesthesia in man. I. Introduction and methods. Br J Anaesth 39:523, 1967

Kenney LJ, Schosser RJ: Severe crushing injury of the chest: management with the Mörch respirator. J Mich Med Soc 57:225, 1958

Kety SS, Schmidt CF: The effects of altered arterial tensions of carbon dioxide and oxygen on cerebral blood flow and cerebral oxygen consumption in normal young men. J Clin Invest 27:484, 1948

Khambatta HJ, Sullivan SF: Effects of respiratory alkalosis on oxygen consumption and oxygenation. Anesthesiology 38:53, 1973

Kilburn KH: Shock, seizures, and coma with alkalosis during mechanical ventilation. Ann Intern Med 65:977, 1966

Kilburn KH, Sieker HO: Hemodynamic effects of continuous positive and negative pressure breathing in normal man. Circ Res 8:660, 1960

Kirby RR: High levels of positive end-expiratory pressure (PEEP) in acute respiratory insufficiency. Chest 67:156, 1975

Kirby RR: Intermittent mandatory ventilation in the neonate. Crit Care Med 5:18, 1977

Kirby RR: Is intermittent mandatory ventilation a satisfactory alternative to assisted and controlled ventilation. American Society of Anesthesiology Refresher Course Lecture, 1975

Kirby RR: High-frequency positive-pressure ventilation (HFPPV): what role in ventilatory insufficiency. Anesthesiology 52:109, 1980

Kirby RR, Desautels D, Smith RA: Mechanical ventilation. p. 556. In Burton GG, Hodgkin JE (eds): Respiratory Care: A guide to Clinical Practice. JB Lippincott, Philadelphia 1984

Kirby RR, Downs JB, Civetta JM, et al: High level positive end-expiratory pressure (PEEP) in acute respiratory insufficiency. Chest 67:156, 1975

Kirby RR, Graybar GB (eds): Intermittent mandatory ventilation. Int Anesthesiol Clin 18:1, 1980

Kirby RR, Perry JC, Calderwood HW, et al: Cardiorespiratory effects of high positive end-expiratory pressure. Anesthesiology 43:533, 1975

Kirby RR, Robison EJ, Schulz J, et al: A new pediatric volume ventilator. Anesth Analg 50:533, 1971

Kirby RR, Robison EJ, Schulz J, et al: Continuous flow ventilation as an alternative to assisted or controlled ventilation in infants. Anesth Analg 51:871, 1972

Kirschner JM: Fluid Amplifiers. McGraw-Hill, New York, 1966

Kirschner JM: Fluidics. I. Basic Principles. TR-1498, Harry Diamond Laboratory (U.S. Army), Washington, DC, 1968

Kirschner JM, Horton BM: A brief history of fluidics (from the viewpoint of the Harry Diamond Laboratories). Presented at the Seventh National Fluidics Symposium, Tokyo, 1972

Kite C: On submersion of animals; its effects on the vital organs; and the most probable method of removing them. Mem Med Soc London III:215, 1792

Klain M, Smith RB: Fluidic technology. Anaesthesia 31:750, 1976

Klain M, Smith RB: High frequency percutaneous transtracheal jet ventilation. Crit Care Med 5:280, 1977

Klein RL, Safar P, Grenvik A: Respiratory care in blunt chest injury: retrospective review of 43 cases. p. 145. In Abstracts of Scientific Papers, Annual Meeting of ASA, New York, October 17–21, 1970

Kolton M, Cattran C, Bryan AC, et al: High frequency oscillation and mean lung volume. Anesthesiology 55 (suppl 3A):353, 1981

Komesaroff D, McKie B: The "bronchoflator": a new technique for bronchoscopy under general anaesthesia. Br J Anaesth 44:1057, 1972

Kotheimer TG, Dickie KJ, DeGroot WJ: Mechanical determinants of inspiratory oxygen concentration in a pressure-cycled ventilator. Am Rev Respir Dis 103:679, 1971

Kreiselman J: New resuscitation apparatus. Anesthesiology 4:608, 1943

Kristensen HS, Lunding M: Two early Danish respirators designed for prolonged ventilation. Acta Anaesth Scand [Suppl] 67:96, 1978

Krogh A: En respirator efter Philip Drinker's princip. Hosp Tidende 75:629, 1932

Kuhn F: Perorale intubation mit Überdrucknarkose. Dtsch Z Chir 76:148; 78:467, 1905, 1907

Kumar A, Falke KJ, Geffin G, et al: Continuous positive-pressure ventilation in acute respiratory failure—effects on hemodynamics and lung function. N Engl J Med 283:1430, 1970

Kumar A, Pontoppidan H, Baratz RA, et al: Inappropriate response to increased plasma ADH during mechanical ventilation in acute respiratory failure. Anesthesiology 40:215, 1974

Kumar A, Pontoppidan H, Falke KJ, et al: Pulmonary barotrauma during mechanical ventilation. Crit Care Med 1:181, 1973

Kuwabara S, McCaughey TJ: Artificial ventilation in infants and young children using a new ventilator with the T-piece. Can Anaesth Soc J 13:576, 1966

Lassen HCA: A preliminary report of the 1952 epidemic of poliomyelitis in Copenhagen. Lancet 1:37, 1953

Lassen HCA: The Management of Respiratory and Bulbar Paralysis in Poliomyelitis. Monograph Series No. 26. World Health Organization, Geneva, 1955, p. 157

Laver MB: Prevention of post-operative respiratory complications. p. 31. In Saidman LJ, Moya F (eds): Complications of Anesthesia. Charles C Thomas, Springfield, IL, 1970

Laver MB, Morgan J, Bendixen HH, et al: Lung volume compliance and arterial oxygen tension during controlled ventilation. J Appl Physiol 19:725, 1964

Läwen, Sievers: Zur Praktischen Anwendung der instrumentellen künstlichen Respiration am Menschen. MMW 57:2221, 1910

Lawler PGP, Nunn JF: Intermittent mandatory ventilation. Anaesthesia 32:138, 1977

Lecky JH, Quinsky AJ: Postoperative respiratory management. Chest 62:503, 1972

Lee CJ, Lyons JH, Konisberg S, et al: Effects of spontaneous and positive pressure breathing of ambient air and pure oxygen at one atmosphere pressure on pulmonary surface characteristics. J Thorac Cardiovasc Surg 53:759, 1967

Lee ST: A ventilating bronchoscope for inhalation

anesthesia and augmented ventilation. Anesth Analg 52:89, 1973

Lee ST: A ventilating laryngoscope for inhalation anaesthesia and augmented ventilation during laryngoscopic procedures. Br J Anaesth 44:874, 1972

Lehr J: Circulating currents during high frequency ventilation. Fed Proc 39:576, 1980

Lenaghan R, Silva YJ, Walt AJ: Hemodynamic alterations associated with expansion rupture of the lung. Arch Surg 99:339, 1969

Lenfent C, Howell BJ: Cardiovascular adjustments in dogs during continuous pressure breathing. J Appl Physiol 15:425, 1960

Leroy J: Recherches sur l'asphyxie. J Physiol (Paris) 8:97, 1828

Leroy J: Second mémoire sur l'asphyxie. J Physiol (Paris) 8:97, 1828

Levine M, Gilbert R, Auchincloss JH Jr: A comparison of the effects of sighs, large tidal volumes, and positive end-expiratory pressure in assisted ventilation. Scand J Respir Dis 53:101, 1972

Little DM Jr: The methodology of controlled respiration. Ann NY Acad Sci 66:939, 1957

Llewellyn MA, Swyer PR: Assisted and controlled ventilation in the newborn period: effect on oxygenation. Br J Anaesth 43:926, 1971

Llewellyn MA, Swyer PR: Positive expiratory pressure during mechanical ventilation in the newborn. p. 224. Proceedings of the Society of Pediatric Research, 1970

Loredo MA, Avila JD, Gonzales CG: Apparatus for effortless inhalation anesthesia. Curr Res Anesth Analg 28:352, 1949

Lough MD, Doershuk CF, Stern RC: Pediatric Respiratory Therapy. Year Book Medical Publishers, Chicago, 1974

Lucas BGB: A portable resuscitator. Br J Med 1:541, 1949

Luedke J, Kosmatka A: A new method of weaning from respiratory support. Respir Care 18:561, 1973

Lunkenheimer PP, Frank I, Ising I, et al: Intrapulmonaler Gaswechsel unter simulierter Apnoe durch transtrachealen, periodischen intrathorakalen Druckwechsel. Anaesthesist 22:232, 1973

Lunkenheimer PP, Raffenbeul W, Keller H, et al: Application of transtracheal pressure-oscillations as a modification of "diffusion respiration." Br J Anaesth 44:627, 1972

Lunn JN, Mapleson WW, Chilcoat RT: Effects of changes of frequency and tidal volume of controlled ventilation: measurements at constant arterial P_{CO_2} in dogs. Br J Anaesth 47:2, 1975

Lutch JS, Murray JF: Continuous positive pressure ventilation—effects on systemic oxygen transport and tissue oxygenation. Ann Intern Med 76:193, 1972

Lyager S: Influence of flow pattern on the distribution of respiratory air during intermittent positive pressure ventilation. Acta Anaesth Scand 12:191, 1968

Lyager S: Ventilation/perfusion ratio during intermittent positive pressure ventilation—importance of no-flow interval during the insufflation. Acta Anaesth Scand 14:211, 1970

Lyons J, Moore F: Posttraumatic alkalosis—incidence and pathophysiology of alkalosis in surgery. Surgery 60:93, 1966

Maloney JV, Affeldt JE, Sarnoff SJ, et al: Electrophrenic respiration. 9. Comparison of effects of positive pressure breathing on the circulation during hemorrhage and barbiturate poisoning. Surg Gynecol Obstet 92:672, 1951

Maloney JV, Derrick WS, Whittenberger JL: A device producing regulated assisted respiration. Surg Forum 588, 1950

Maloney JV, Derrick WS, Whittenberger JL: Device producing regulated assisted respiration: prevention of hypoventilation and mediastinal motion during intrathoracic surgery. Anesthesiology 13:23, 1952

Maloney JW, Elam JO, Handford SW, et al: Importance of negative pressure phase in mechanical respirator JAMA 152:212, 1953

Maloney JV, Elam JO, Handford SW, et al: Response to intermittent positive and alternating positive-negative pressure respirations. J Appl Physiol 6:453, 1954

Maloney JV, Whittenberger JL: The direct effects of pressure breathing on the pulmonary circulation. Ann NY Acad Sci 66:931, 1957

Mannino FL, Feldman BH, Heldt GP, et al: Early mechanical ventilation in RDS with a prolonged inspiration. Pediatr Res 10:464, 1976

Mapleson WW: Physical aspects of automatic ventilators: basic principles. p. 42. In Mushin WW, Rendell-Baker L, Thompson PW (eds): Automatic Ventilation of the Lungs. Blackwell, Oxford, 1959

Mapleson WW: The effect of changes of lung characteristics on the functioning of automatic ventilation. Anaesthesia 17:300, 1962

Mapleson WW: Volume-pressure characteristic of

the "one gallon" reservoir bag. Br J Anaesth 26:11, 1954

Marcotte RJ, Phillips FJ, Adams WE, et al: Differential intrabronchial pressure and mediastinal emphysema. J Thorac Surg 9:346, 1940

Margand PMS, Chodoff P: Intermittent mandatory ventilation; an alternative weaning technique: a case report. Anesth Analg 54:41, 1975

Markland E, Boucher RF: A Guide to Fluidics. Macdonald, London, 1971, p. 2

Martin AM Sr, Simmons RL, Heisterkamp CA III: Respiratory insufficiency in combat casualties. I. Pathologic changes in the lungs of patients dying of wounds. Ann Surg 170:30, 1969

Masud KZ, Byoan M, Hoffman R, et al: Hemodynamic effects of IMV and HFV in patients with acute respiratory failure. Anesthesiology 55 (suppl):355, 1981

Matas R: Artificial respiration by direct intralaryngeal intubation with a modified O'Dwyer tube and a new graudated air-pump in its application to medical and surgical practice. Am Med 3:97, 1902

Matas R: Intralaryngeal insufflation for the relief of acute surgical pneumothorax: its history and methods with a description of the latest devices for this purpose. JAMA 34:1468, 1900

Matas R: On the management of acute traumatic pneumothorax. Ann Surg 29:409, 1899

Matilla MAK: The role of the physical characteristics of the respirator in artificial ventilation of the newborn. Acta Anaesth Scand [Suppl] 56:1, 1974

Matilla MAK, Suntarinen T: Clinical and experimental evaluation of the Loosco baby respirator. Acta Anaesth Scand 15:229, 1971

Mautz FR: A mechanism for artificial pulmonary ventilation in the operating room. J Thorac Surg 10:544, 1941

Mautz FR: Mechanical respirator as adjunct to closed system anesthesia. Proc Soc Exp Biol 42:190, 1939

Mautz FR: Surgery: thoracic, physical consideration. p 1514. In Glasser O (ed): Medical Physics. Year Book Medical Publishers, Chicago, 1944

Mautz FR, Beck CS, Chase HF: Augmented and controlled breathing in transpleural operation. J Thorac Surg 17:283, 1948

Mead J: The distribution of gas flow in the lungs. p. 204. In Ciba Foundation Symposium: Circulatory and Respiratory Mass Transport. Churchill, London, 1969

Mead J, Collier C: Relationship of volume of lungs to respiratory mechanisms in anesthetized dogs. J Appl Physiol 14:669, 1959

Mead J, Whittenberger JL: Lung inflation and hemodynamics. p. 477. In Fenn WO, Rahn H (eds): Handbook of Physiology, Section 3: Respiration. Vol I. American Physiological Society, Washington, DC, 1964

Meier A, Baum M: The influence of the internal compliance of a respirator on the alveolar gas distribution. Acta Anaesth Scand [Suppl] 63:1, 1976

Meltzer SJ: Der gegenwärtige Stand der intratracehealan Insufflation. Berl Klin Wochenschr 51:677, 743, 1914

Meltzer SJ: History and analysis of the methods of resuscitation. Med Rec 92:190, 1939

Meltzer SJ, Auer J: Continuous respiration without respiratory movements. J Exp Med 11:622, 1909

Merlis JK, Degelman J: Improved artificial respirator for animal experimentation. Science 114:692, 1951

Meyer JA, Joyce JW: The fluid amplifier and its application in medical devices. Anesth Analg 47:710, 1968

Meyer W: Anesthesia in differential pressure chambers, cabinets, and other apparatus for thoracic surgery. p. 953. In Keen WW (ed): Surgery, Its Principles and Practice. WB Saunders, Philadelphia, 1913

Meyer W: Pneumonectomy with the aid of differential air pressure. JAMA 53:1978, 1909

Minkowski A, Monset-Couchard M, Amiel-Tison: Symposium on artificial ventilation. Biol Neonate 16:1, 1970

Modell JH: Intermittent mandatory ventilation in the treatment of patients with chronic pulmonary disease. Anesth Analg 54:119, 1975

Modell JH: Ventilation/perfusion changes during mechanical ventilation. Dis Chest 55:447, 1969

Mölgaard H: Fysiologisk Lungekirurgi. Gyldendal, Copenhagen, 1915, p. 1

Monckcom W, Patterson RW: Ventilation-perfusion inequalities resulting from hypocapnic changes in lung mechanics. J Thorac Cardiovasc Surg 63:577, 1972

Moore FD, Lyon JH, Peirce EC, et al: Post-Traumatic Pulmonary Insufficiency: Pathophysiology of Respiratory Failure and Principles of Respiratory Care after Surgical Operations, Trauma, Hemorrhage, Burns and Shock. WB Saunders, Philadelphia, 1969, p. 12

Moore RL, Humphreys GH, Wreggit WR: Studies on the volume output of blood from the heart in anesthetized dogs before thoracotomy and after thoracotomy and intermittent or continuous inflation of the lungs. J Thorac Surg 5:195, 1935

Morales ES, Krumperman LW: The effects of instrumentation on gas flows during bronchoscopy using the Sanders ventilating attachment. Anesthesiology 38:197, 1973

Mörch ET: Anaesthesi. Munksgaard, Copenhagen, 1949 p. 405

Mörch ET: Anaesthesien under intrapleurale operationer. Nord Med 36:2234, 1947

Mörch ET: Controlled respiration by means of special automatic machines as used in Sweden and Denmark. Proc R Soc Med 40:39, 1947

Mörch ET:Et nyt obstetrisk analgesi-apparat. Ugeskr Laeger 110:856, 1948

Mörch ET, Avery E, Benson DW: Hyperventilation in the treatment of crushing injuries of the chest—problems in pulmonary physiology and pathology. Surg Forum 6:270, 1955

Mörch ET, Benson DW: Automatic artificial respiration during anesthesia. p. 30. In Proceedings of the Third Congress of the Scandinavian Society of Anaesthesiologists, Copenhagen, 1954

Mörch ET, Engel R, Light GA: Effects of pressure breathing on the preipheral circulation: motion picture observations in the bat wing and rabbit ear chamber. Arch Surg 79:493, 1959

Mörch ET, Saxton GA: Tracheostomy tube connectors. Anesthesiology 17:366, 1956

Mörch ET, Saxton GA, Gish G: Artificial respiration via the uncuffed tracheostomy tube. JAMA 160:864, 1956

Morgan BC, Crawford EW, Guntheroth WG: The hemodynamic effects of changes in blood volume during intermittent positive pressure breathing. Anesthesiology 30:297, 1965

Morgan BC, Crawford EW, Hornbein TF, et al: Hemodynamic effects of changes in arterial carbon dioxide tension during intermittent positive pressure ventilation. Anesthesiology 28:866, 1967

Morgan BC, Crawford EW, Winterscherd LC, et al: Circulatory effects of intermittent positive pressure ventilation. Northwest Med 67:149, 1968

Morgan BC, Martin WE, Hornbein TF, et al: Hemodynamic effects of intermittent pressure respiration. Anesthesiology 27:584, 1966

Morgan WL, Binion JT, Sarnoff SJ: The circulatory depression induced by high level of positive pressure breathing counteracted by metaraminol. J Appl Physiol 10:26, 1957

Morton JHV: Respiratory patterns during surgical anaesthesia. Anaesthesia 5:112, 1950

Motley HL: Physiological and clinical studies on man with the pneumatic balance resuscitation "Burns model." Memorandum Report TSEAL-3-660-49. O, AAF Hedgs. ATSC, Engineering Div, Aero Med Lab Wright Field, August 23, 1945

Motley HL, Cournand A, Eckman M, et al: Physiology studies on man with pneumatic balance resuscitator "Burns model." J Aviat Med 17:431, 1946

Motley HL, Cournand A, Werkö L, et al: Intermittent positive pressure breathing. JAMA 137:370, 1948

Motley HL, Cournand A, Werkö L, et al: Observation on the clinical use of intermittent positive pressure. J Aviat Med 18:417, 1947

Motley HL, Cournand A, Werkö L, et al: Physiological and clinical studies of intermittent pressure respirators and manual methods for producing artificial respiration in man. Report No. TSEEA-697-79-F. Army Air Forces, Engineering Division. Memorandum, September 6, 1946

Motley HL, Cournand A, Werkö L, et al: Physiological studies on man with pneumatic balance resuscitator "Burns model." J Aviat Med 17:431, 1946

Motley HL, Lang LP, Gordon B: Use of intermittent positive pressure breathing combined with nebulization in pulmonary disease. Am J Med 5:853, 1948

Mousel LH, Stubbs D, Kreiselman L: Anesthetic complications and their management. Anesthesiology 7:69, 1946

Moylan FMB, Walker AM, Kramer SS, et al: The relationship of bronchopulmonary dysplasia to the occurrence of alveolar rupture during positive pressure ventilation. Crit Care Med 6:140, 1978

Munson ES, Eger EI II: Continuous ventilaton in the newborn. Anesthesiology 24:871, 1963

Murdaugh HV, Seiker HO, Manfredi F: Effect of altered intrathoracic pressure on renal hemodynamics, electrolyte excretion, and water clearance. J Clin Invest 38:834, 1959

Murphy FT: A suggestion for a practical apparatus for use in intrathoracic operations. Boston Med Surg J 152:428, 1905

Musgrove AH: Controlled respiration in thoracic surgery: a new mechanical respirator. Anaesthesia 7:77, 1952

Mushin WW, Faux N: Use of the Both respirator to reduce postoperative morbidity. Lancet 2:685, 1944

Mushin WW, Mapleson WW, Lynn JN: Problem of automatic ventilation in infants and children. Br J Anaesth 34:514, 1962

Mushin WW, Rendell-Baker L: Modern automatic respirators. Br J Anaesth 26:131, 1954

Mushin WW, Rendell-Baker L: Principles of Thoracic Anaesthesia. Blackwell, Oxford, 1953

Mushin WW, Rendell-Baker L: The Principles of Thoracic Anaesthesia Past and Present. Charles C Thomas, Springfield, IL, 1953, p. 172

Mushin WW, Rendell-Baker L, Thompson PW: Automatic Ventilation of the Lungs. Blackwell, Oxford 1959, 1980; FA Davis, Philadelphia, 1969

MacDonnell K, Lefemine AA, Moon HS, et al: Comparative hemodynamic consequences of inflation hold, PEEP, and interrupted PEEP. Ann Thoracic Surg 19:552, 1975

Macintosh RR: New use of Both respirator. Lancet 2:745, 1940

MacNaughton FI: Catheter inflation ventilation in tracheal stenosis. Br J Anaesth 47:1225, 1975

Macrae J, McKendrick GDW, Claremont JM, et al: Positive-pressure respiration: management of patients treated with Clevedon respirator. Lancet 2:21, 1954

Macrae J, McKendrick GDW, Claremont JM, et al: The Clevedon positive-pressure respirator. Lancet 2:971, 1953

McIntyre RW, Laws AK, Ramachandran PR: Positive expiratory pressure plateau: improved gas exchange during mechanical ventilation. Can Anaesth Soc J 16:477, 1969

McLaughlin GW, Kirby GG, Kemmerer WT, et al: Indirect measurement of blood pressure in infants using doppler ultrasound. J Pediatr 79:300, 1971

McLellan L: Resuscitation apparatus. Anaesthesia 36:307, 1981

McMahon SM, Halpin GM: Modification of intrapulmonary blood shunt by end-expiratory pressure application in patients with acute respiratory failure. Chest 59:27S, 1971

McPherson SP: Respiratory Therapy Equipment. CV Mosby, St. Louis, 1977

McPherson SP, Glasgow GD, William AA, et al: A circuit that combines ventilator weaning methods using continuous flow ventilation (CFV). Respir Care 20:261, 1975

Naess K: A simple apparatus for artificial respiration, built of a vacuum window wiper. Acta Physiol Scand 22:376, 1951

Nash G, Blennerhassett JB, Pontoppidan H: Pulmonary lesions associated with oxygen therapy and artificial ventilation. N Engl J Med 276:368, 1967

Nash G, Bowen JA, Langlinais PC: "Respirator lung": a misnomer. Arch Pathol Lab Med 91:234, 1971

National Fluid Power Association: Recommended Standard Graphic Symbols for Fluidic Devices and Circuits. NFPA/T3.7.2–1968. National Fluid Power Association, Thiensville, WI, 1968

National Fluid Power Association: What You Should Know About Fluidics. National Fluid Power Association, Thiensville, WI, 1972

Nause FP: Crushed chest, treatment using a mechanical respirator. Wis Med J 59:697, 1960

Neff W, Phillips W, Gunn G: Anesthesia for pneumonectomy in man. Anesthesiology 3:314, 1942

Nennhaus HP, Javis H, Julian OC: Alveolar and pleural rupture: hazards of positive pressure respiration. Arch Surg 94:136, 1967

Nicotra MB, Stevens PM, Viroslav J, et al: Physiologic evaluation of positive end-expiratory pressure ventilation. Chest 64:10, 1973

Nightingale DA, Richards CC, Glass A: An evaluation of rebreathing on a modified T-piece system during continuous ventilation for anaesthesia in children. Br J Anaesth 37:762, 1965

Nilsson E: On treatment of barbiturate poisoning. Acta Med Scand [Suppl] 253:1, 1951

Nilsson LG, Lyttkens L, Sjöstrand U, et al: Positive end-expiratory pressure (PEEP)—an experimental study on dogs. Opusc Med 21:117, 1976

Nisbet HIA, Dobbinson TL, Steward DJ, et al: The effect of artificial ventilation on FRC and arterial oxygenation. Can Anaesth Soc J 21:215, 1974

Nissen R: Historical development of pulmonary surgery. Am J Surg 89:9, 1955

Nordenström B: Contrast examination of the cardiovascular system during increased intrabronchial pressure. Acta Radiol Scand [Suppl] 200:1, 1960

Nordström L: Haemodynamic effects of intermittent positive-pressure ventilation with and without an end-inspiratory pause. Acta Anaesth Scand [Suppl] 47:29, 1972

Nordström L: On automatic ventilation. Acta Anaes Scand [Suppl] 47:1, 1972

Nordström S, Eriksson I, Nilsson LG, et al: High frequency positive pressure ventilation (HFPPV) during transthoracic resection of tracheal stenosis and during preoperative bronchoscopic examination. Acta Anaesth Scand 19:113, 1975

Norlander O: Anaesthesiologische Gesichtspunkte der Handhabung Thoracchirurgischer Fälle während und nach der Operatioń. Thoraxchirurgie 6:162, 1958

Norlander O: Functional analysis of force and power of mechanical ventilation. Acta Anaesth Scand 8:57, 1964

Norlander O: Management of respirator and anesthesia patients: monitoring and developments. Med Prog Technol 3:15, 1974

Norlander O, Björk VO, Crafoord C, et al: Controlled ventilation in medical practice. Anaesthesia 16:285, 1961

Norlander O, Herzog P: An Engström respirator designed for high frequency ventilation. Opusc Med 18:74, 1973

Norlander O, Holmdahl MH, Matell G, et al: Clinical experience with a new modular Engström care system (ECS 2000) ventilator. p. 516. In Arias A, Llaurado R, Nalda MA, Lunn JN (eds): Recent Progress in Anaesthesiology and Resuscitation. Excerpta Medica, Amsterdam, 1975

Norlander O: The use of respirators in anesthesia and surgery. Acta Anaesth Scand [Suppl] 30:1, 1968

Norlander O, Pitzela S, Edling N, et al: Anaesthesiological experience from intracardiac surgery with the Crafoord-Senning-heart-lung machine. Acta Anaesth Scand 2:181, 1958

Northrup WP: Apparatus for artificial forcible respiration. Med Surg Rep Presbyterian Hosp (NY) 1:127, 1896

Northway WR Jr, Rosal RC, Porter DY: Pulmonary disease following respiratory therapy of hyaline membrane disease: bronchopleural dysplasia. N Engl J Med 276:357, 1967

Nosworthy MD: Anaesthesia in chest surgery. Proc R Soc Med 34:479, 1941

Nunn JF: Physiological aspects of artificial ventilation. Br J Anaesth 29:540, 1957

Nunn JF, Bergman NA, Coleman AJ: Factors influencing the arterial oxygen tension during anaesthesia with artificial ventilation. Br J Anaesth 37:898, 1965

Nystrom G, Blalock A: Contribution to the technique of pulmonary embolectomy. Thorac Surg 5:169, 1936

Obdrzalek J, Kay JC, Noble WH: The effects of continuous positive pressure ventilation on pulmonary oedema, gas exchange, and lung mechanics. Can Anaesth Soc J 22:399, 1975

O'Donoline W Jr, Baker JP, Beil GM, et al: The management of acute respiratory failure in a respiratory intensive care unit. Chest 58:603, 1970

O'Dwyer J: Fifty cases of croup in private practice treated by intubation of the larynx, with a description of the method and of the dangers incident thereto. Med Res 32:557, 1887

O'Dwyer J: Intubation of the larynx. NY Med J 32:145, 1885

Okmian L: Artificial ventilation by respirator for newborn and small infants during anaesthesia. Acta Anaesthesiol Scand [Suppl] 20:1, 1966

Opie LH, Smith AC, Spalding JMK: Conscious appreciation of the effects produced by independent changes of ventilator volume and of end-tidal P_{CO_2} in paralyzed patients. J Physiol (Lond) 149:494, 1959

Opie LH, Spalding JMK, Smith AC: Intrathoracic pressure during intermittent positive pressure respiration. Lancet 1:911, 1961

Orth OS, Wilhelm RL, Waters RM: The question of pulmonary drainage with artificial respiration. J Thorac Surg 14:220, 1945

Orton RH: Controlled respiration. Med J Aust 2:255, 1947

Oulton JL, Donald DM: A ventilating laryngoscope. Anesthesiology 35:540, 1971

Parham FW: On the management of acute traumatic pneumothorax. Ann Surg 29:409, 1899

Parham FW: Thoracic resection for tumor growing from the bony wall of the chest. Trans South Soc Anesthet 11:223, 1898

Parson EF, Travis K, Shore N, et al: Effect of positive pressure breathing on distribution of pulmonary blood flow and ventilation. Am Rev Respir Dis 103:356, 1971

Patterson JR, Russell GK, Pierson DJ et al: Evaluation of a fluidic ventilator: a new approach to mechanical ventilation. Chest 66:706, 1974

Peck CH: Intratracheal insufflation anesthesia (Meltzer-Auer): observation on a series of 216 anaesthesiae with the Elsberg apparatus. Ann Surg 56:192, 1912

Pedersen B: Respirator treatment of neonates. Acta Anaesth Scand 16:38, 1972

Perea EJ, Criado A, Moreno M, et al: Mechanical ventilators as vehicles of infection. Acta Anaesth Scand 19:180, 1975

Peslin RL: Étude sur modèles de la distribution aérienne au cours de la ventilation instrumental. Bull Physiol Pathol Respir 2:253, 1966

Peslin RL: The physical properties of ventilators in the inspiratory phase. Anesthesiology 30:315, 1969

Peters RM: The Mechanical Basis of Respiration. J Churchill, London, 1969

Peters RM, Hutchin P: Adequacy of available respirations to their tasks. Ann Thorac Surg 3:414, 1967

Petrén K, Sjövall E: Eine studie über die tödliche akute Form der Poliomyelitis. Acta Med Scand 64:260, 1926

Petty TL: IMV vs IMC. Chest 67:630, 1975

Petty TL: Intensive and Rehabilitative Respiratory Care. Lea & Febiger, Philadelphia, 1974

Petty TL, Ashbaugh DG: The adult respiratory distress syndrome. Chest 60:233, 1971

Petty TL, Bigelow DB, Broughton JO: A new volume cycled ventilator. Respir Ther 2:33, 1972

Petty TL, Nett LM, Ashbaugh D: Improvement in oxygenation in the adult respiratory distress syndrome by positive end-expiratory pressure (PEEP). Respir Care 16:173, 1971

Phillein DM, Baratz RA, Patterson RW: The effect of carbon dioxide on plasma antidiuretic hormone levels during intermittent positive pressure breathing. Anesthesiology 33:345, 1970

Pierce HF: An artificial respiration and ether apparatus for use with compressed air. J Lab Clin Med 9:197, 1923

Pilcher J: Prolonged orotracheal intubation without tracheostomy for respiratory failure. Br J Dis Chest 61:95, 1967

Pinson KB: Mechanically controlled respiration in thoracic surgery. Anaesthesia 4:79, 1949

Pinson KB, Bryce AG: Constant suction in thoracic surgery: description of an anaesthetic apparatus. Br J Anaesth 19:53, 1944

Plum F, Lukas DS: An evaluation of the cuirass respirator in acute poliomyelitis with respiratory insufficiency. Am J Med Sci 221:417, 1951

Plum F, Wolff HG: Observations on acute poliomyelitis with respiratory insufficiency. JAMA 146:442, 1951

Plut HG Jr, Miller WF: New volume ventilator. Inhal Ther 13:91, 1968

Poisvert M, Cara M: Un nouveau concept en ventilation artificielle: la cellule logique. Ann Anesthesiol Fr 8:411, 1967

Poling HE, Wolfson B, Siker ES: A technique of ventilation during laryngoscopy and bronchoscopy. Br J Anaesth 47:382, 1975

Pontoppidan H: Mechanical aid to lung expansion in non-intubated surgical patients. Am Rev Respir Dis 122:109, 1980

Pontoppidan H: Pneumonia treated by extracorporeal member oxygenation. N Engl J Med 292:1174, 1975

Pontoppidan H, Berry PR: Regulation of the inspired oxygen concentration during artificial ventilation. JAMA 201:11, 1967

Pontoppidan H, Geffin B, Lowenstein E: Acute respiratory failure in the adult. N Engl J Med 287:690, 743, 799, 1972

Pontoppidan H, Hedley-Whyte J, Bendixen HH, et al: Ventilation and oxygen requirements during prolonged artificial ventilation in patients with respiratory failure. N Engl J Med 273:401, 1965

Pontoppidan H, Laver MB, Geffin B: Acute respiratory failure in the surgical patients. Adv Surg 4:163, 1970

Pontoppidan H, Wilson RS, Rie MA, et al: Respiratory intensive care. Anesthesiology 47:96, 1977

Poulsen H, Skall-Jensen J, Staffeldt I, et al: Pulmonary ventilaton and respiratory gas exchange during manual artificial respiration and expired-air resuscitation on apnoeic normal adults. Acta Anaesth Scand 3:129, 1959

Powers SR Jr, Mannal R, Neclerio M, et al: Physiologic consequences of positive end-expiratory pressure (PEEP) ventilation. Ann Surg 128:265, 1972

Price HL, Conner EH, Dripps RD: Some respiratory and circulatory effects of mechanical respirators. J Appl Physiol 6:517, 1954

Price HL, Conner EH, Elder JD, et al: Effect of sodium thiopental on circulation response to positive pressure inflation of lung. J Appl Physiol 4:629, 1952

Prys-Roberts C, Kelman GR, Greenbaum R, et al: Circulatory influences of artificial ventilation during nitrous oxide anesthesia in man. II. Results: the relative influences of mean intrathoracic pressure and arterial carbon dioxide tension. Br J Anaesth 39:533, 1967

Pyle P, Darlow M, Firman JE: A treated ultra-high-efficiency for mechanical ventilators. Lancet 1:136, 1969

Qvist J, Pontoppidan H, Wilson RS, et al: Hemodynamic response to mechanical ventilation with PEEP: the effect of hyperventilation. Anesthesiology 42:45, 1975

Radford EP: Ventilation standards for use in artificial respiration. J Appl Physiol 7:451, 1955

Ramanathan S, Sinha K, Arismendy J, et al: Bronchofiberscopic high frequency ventilation. Anesthesiology S5(suppl 3A):352, 1981

Randall HT, McPherson RC, Haller JA, et al: Treatment of flail chest injuries with a piston respirator. Am J Surg 104:22, 1962

Rattenborg CC: Clinical Use of Mechanical Ventilation. 2nd Ed. Year Book Medical Publishers, Chicago, 1989

Reba I: Applications of the Coanda effect. Sci Am 214:84, 1966

Rees GJ, Owen-Thomas JB: A technique of pulmonary ventilation with a nasotracheal tube. Br J Anaesth 38:901, 1966

Reicher J: Pulmonary suck and blow as respiratory analeptic. Arch Surg 53:77, 1946

Reynolds EOR: Methods of mechanical ventilation for hyaline membrane disease. Proc R Soc Med 67:10, 1974

Reynolds EOR: Pressure waveform and ventilator settings for mechanical ventilation in severe hyaline membrane disease. Int Anesthesiol Clin 12:259, 1974

Reynolds EOR, Taghizadeh A: Improved prognosis of infants mechanically ventilated for hyaline membrane disease. Arch Dis Child 49:505, 1974

Reynolds JA: A method of recording pulmonary ventilation. J Sci Instrum Ser 2:1, 1968

Reynolds RN: A pulmonary ventilator for infants. Anesthesiology 25:712, 1964

Richardson B: Artificial respiration. In Druitt R (ed): The Surgeons Vade Mecum. 10th Ed. Churchill, London, 1870

Robinson S: A classical cone with a rubber drum over the base of dog's face. Ann Surg 47:184, 1908

Robinson S: Experimental surgery of the lungs. I. Thirty animal operations under positive pressure. Ann Surg 47:184, 1908

Robinson S, Leland GA: Survey of the lungs under positive and negative pressure. Surg Gynecol Obstet 9:255, 1909

Rochford J, Welch RF, Winks DW: An electronic time-cycled respirator. Br J Anaesth 30:23, 1958

Rogers EJ: Physics vs physiology in infant ventilation. Respir Ther 2:1, 1972

Roos A, Thomas LJ, Nagel EL, et al: Pulmonary vascular resistance as determined by lung inflation and vascular pressure. J Appl Physiol 16:77, 1961

Rossing TH, Slutsky AS, Lehr JL, et al: Tidal volume and frequency dependence of carbon dioxide elimination by high frequency ventilation. N Engl J Med 305:1375, 1981

Rotherman EB Jr, Safar P, Robin ED: CNS disorder during mechanical ventilation in chronic pulmonary disease. JAMA 189:993, 1964

Ruben H: A new nonrebreathing valve. Anesthesiology 16:643, 1955

Russell WR, Schuster E: Respiration pump for poliomyelitis. Lancet 2:707, 1953

Russell WR, Schuster E, Smith AC, et al: Radcliffe respiration pump. Lancet 1:539, 1956

Safar P: Long term resuscitation in intensive care units. Anesthesiology 25:216, 1964

Safar P: Respiratory Therapy. FA Davis, Philadelphia, 1965

Safar P, Berman B, Diamond E, et al: Cuffed tracheostomy tube vs. tank respirator for prolonged artificial ventilation. Arch Phys Med 43:487, 1962

Safar P, Davis G: Modified Mörch piston respirator. Anesthesiology 25:81, 1964

Safar P, Grenvik A: Critical care medicine: organizing and staffing intensive care units. Chest 59:535, 1971

Safar P, Grenvik A: Multidisciplinary intensive care. Mod Med 39:92, 1971

Safar P, Kunkel HG: Prolonged artificial ventilation. Clin Anesth Respir Ther 1:93, 1965

Safar P, Nemoto EM, Severinghaus JW: Pathogenesis of central nervous system disorder during artificial hyperventilation in compensated hypercarbia in dogs. Crit Care Med 1:15, 1973

Sahlin B: En ny respiratortyp. Hygeij Revy 20:129, 1931

Sahlin B: Zehn Fälle von Atemlähmung mit dem Barospirator Behandelt. Acta Med Scand 79:75, 1932

Sahn SA, Lakshmenarayan S, Petty TL: Weaning from mechanical ventilation. JAMA 235:2208, 1976

Saklad M: Inhalation Therapy and Resuscitation. Blackwell, Oxford, 1953

Saklad M, Wickliff D: Functional characteristics of

artificial ventilators. Anesthesiology 28:718, 1967

Sanders RD: Two ventilating attachments for bronchoscopes. Del Med J 39:170, 1967

Sandison JW, McCormick PW, Sykes MK: Intermittent positive pressure respiration after open heart surgery. Br J Anaesth 35:100, 1963

Sarnoff SJ, Maloney JK, Whittenberg JL: Electrophrenic respiration. V. Effect on the circulation of electrophrenic respiration and positive pressure breathing during the respiratory paralysis of high spinal anesthesia. Ann Surg 132:921, 1950

Sauerbruch EF: Ueber die physiologischen und physikalischen Grundlagen bei intrathoracalen Eingriffen in meiner pneumatischen Operations—Kammer. Arch Klin Chir 73:977, 1904

Sauerbruch EF: Master Surgeon. Cromwell, New York, 1953

Sauerbruch EF: Zur Pathologie des öffennen Pneumothorax und die Grundlagen meines Verfahrens zu seiner Ausshaltung. Mitt Grenzgeb Med Chir 8:399, 1904

Scales JT, Kinnier Wilson AB, Holmes Sellors T, et al: Cuirass respirators: their design and construction. Lancet 1:671, 1953

Schmid ER, Knopp TJ, Rehder K: Intrapulmonary gas transport and perfusion during high frequency oscillation. J Appl Physiol 51:1507, 1981

Schwerma H, Ivy AC: Safety of modern alternating positive and negative pressure resuscitation. JAMA 129:1256, 1945

Scott DB, Stephen GW, Davie IT: Haemodynamic effects of a negative (subatmospheric) pressure expiratory phase during artificial ventilation. Br J Anaesth 44:171, 1972

Scullin G: The jet propelled genius and his mighty blow. Time Magazine 36:41, 1950

Secher O, Wandall HH, Clemmesen T, et al: The Mölgaard positive-pressure anaesthetic apparatus. Acta Chir Scand [Suppl] 283:8, 1961

Sedin G, Heijman K, Heijman L, et al: High-frequency positive-pressure ventilation during anaesthesia in man. Opusc Med 18:82, 1973

Selmeyer JP, Liberatore JM: Respiratory distress syndrome and continuous positive airway pressure. Lancet 2:1422, 1972

Severinghaus J, Swenson E, Finley T, et al: Unilateral hypoventilation producccd in dogs by occluding one pulmonary artery. J Appl Physiol 16:53, 1961

Shaw LA, Drinker P: An apparatus for the prolonged administration of artificial respiration. J Clin Invest 8:33, 1929

Shinnick JP, Johnston RF, Oslick T: Bronchoscopy during mechanical ventilation using the fiberscope. Chest 65:613, 1974

Simonds AK, Sawicka NC, Branthwaite MA: Use of negative pressure ventilation to facilitate the return of spontaneous ventilation. Anaesthesia 43:216, 1988

Singer MM: Intermittent mechanical ventilation in the treatment of patients with chronic obstructive pulmonary disease. Anesth Analg 53:441, 1974

Sjöberg A, Engström CG, Svanborg N: Diagnostiska och kliniska ron vid behandling av bulbospinal polio-myelit (med film och demonstration av ny respirator). Nord Med 47:536, 1952

Sjöstrand U: Anesthésie générale et bronchoscopie. Ann Anesth Fr 17(8):871, 1976

Sjöstrand U: Pneumati systems facilitating treatment of respiratory insufficiency with alternative use of IPPV/PEEP, HFPPV/PEEP, CPPB or CPAP. Acta Anaesth Scand [Suppl] 64:123, 1977

Sjöstrand U: Review of the physiological rationale for and development of high-frequency positive-pressure ventilation—HFPPV. Acta Anaesth Scand [Suppl] 64:165, 1977

Sjöstrand U: Summary of experimental and clinical features of high-frequency positive-pressure ventilation—HFPPV. Acta Anaesth Scand [Suppl] 64:165, 1977

Sjöstrand U (ed.): Experimental and clincial evaluation of high-frequency positive-pressure ventilation (HFPPV). Acta Anaesth Scand [Suppl] 64:1, 1977

Sjöstrand U, Eriksson I, Heijman L, et al: High-frequency positive-pressure ventilation (HFPPV) in bronchoscopy under general anaesthesia: preliminary communication. Opusc Med 21:113, 1976

Sjöstrand U, Jonzon A, Sedin G: Ventilazione a pressione positiva con alta frequenza: studio sperimentale ed espereinza clinica. p. 13. In Fantoni A (ed): Atti del 3° Corso Nazionale di Aggiornamento in Rianimazione. Piccin Editore, Padua, 1973

Sjöstrand U, Jonzon A, Sedin G, et al: High-frequency positive-pressure ventilation. Opusc Med 18:74, 1973

Skillmann JJ, Malhorta JV, Pallotta JA, et al: Detriments of weaning from continuous ventilation. Surg Forum 22:198, 1971

Sladen A, Laver MB, Potoppidan H: Pulmonary complications and water retention in prolonged me-

chanical ventilation. N Engl J Med 279:448, 1968
Sliom CM: Infant ventilator systems. Br J Anaesth 40:306, 1968
Slocum HC, Hayes GW, Laezman BL: Ventilator techniques of anesthesia for neurosurgery. Anesthesiology 22:143, 1961 (abstract)
Slutsky AS, Brown R, Lehr J, et al: High-frequency ventilation: a promising new approach to mechanical ventilation. Med Instrum 15:229, 1981
Slutsky AS, Drazen J, Ingram RH, et al: Effective pulmonary ventilation with small volume oscillation at high frequency. Science 209:609, 1980
Smith C: Continuous ventilation employing a modified Ayre's technique. Anesth Analg 44:842, 1965
Smith RA: Respiratory Care. p. 1379. In Miller RD (ed): Anesthesia. Churchill Livingstone, New York, 1981
Smith RB, Babinski M, Petruscak J: A method for ventilating patients during laryngoscopy. Laryngoscope 84:553, 1974
Smith RB, Lindholm CE, Klain M: Jet ventilation for fiberoptic bronchoscopy under general anaesthesia. Acta Anaesth Scand 20:111, 1976
Smith RB, MacMillan BB, Petruscak J, et al: Transtracheal ventilation for laryngoscopy. Ann Otol 82:347, 1973
Smith RE: Modified Both respirators. Lancet 1:679, 1953
Smith RK: Respiratory care application for fluidics. Respir Ther 3:29, 1973
Smith-Clarke GT: Mechanical breathing machines. Proc Inst Mech Eng 171:52, 1957
Smith-Clarke GT, Galpine JF: Positive-negative pressure respirator. Lancet 1:1299, 1955
Soper RL: The pneumatic balance valve and its applications: a preliminary repott. Br Med J 4733:717, 1951
Spalding JMK: Pressure and duration of inspiration during artificial respiration by intermittent positive pressure. Lancet 1:1099, 1955
Spalding JMK, Crampton Smith A: Clinical Practice and Physiology of Artificial Respiration. FA David, Philadelphia, 1963
Spalding JMK, Crampton Smith A: Clinical Practice of Artificial Respiration with Some Physiological Observations. Blackwell, Oxford, 1963
Spearman CB: Control of inspiratory oxygen concentration and addition of PEEP or CPAP with the Bourns pediatric ventilator. Respir Care 18:405, 1973
Speidel BD, Dunn PM: Effect of continuous positive airway pressure on breathing pattern of infants with respiratory-distress syndrome. Lancet 1:302, 1975
Spenser FC: Use of a mechanical respirator in the management of respiratory insufficiency following trauma or operation for cardiac or pulmonary disease. J Thorac Cardiovasc Surg 38:758, 1959
Speranza V, Beckman M, Norlander O: Il tratamento del insufficienza ventilatoria con la ventilazione artificiale a mezzo del respiratore di Engström. Chir Gen 9:417, 1957
Speranza V, Beckman M, Norlander O: L'insufficienza ventilatoria in chirurgia. Chir Gen 7:498, 1959
Spoerel WE, Greenway RE: Technique of ventilation during endolaryngeal surgery under general anesthesia. Can Anaesth Soc J 20:369, 1973
Sporel We, Narayanan PS, Singh NP: Transtracheal ventilation. Br J Anaesth 43:932, 1971
Stahlman MT, Malan AT, Shepard FM, et al: Negative pressure assisted ventilation in infants with hyaline membrane disease. J Pediatr 76:174, 1970
Stange G, Gebert E, Van de Loo C: Intubationslose Narkose bei direkter Laryngoscopie. Laryngol Rhinol 53:339, 1974
Steen SN, Lee ASJ: Prevention of inadvertent excess pressure in closed system. Anesth Analg 39:264, 1960
Steigman AJ, Rumph PH: The positive pressure respirator dome. Am J Nurs 52:311, 1942
Steinbereithner K, Baum M, Meier A: The influence of a respirator internal compliance on "pendelluft." Excerpta Med Int Congr Ser 387:163, 1976
Sterling GM: The mechanism of bronchoconstriction due to hypocapnia in man. Clin Sci 34:377, 1968
Steuart W: Demonstration of apparatus for inducing artificial respiration for long periods. Med J South Afr 13:147, 1918
Stone JG, Sullivan SF: Failure of shallow ventilation to produce pulmonary shunting in the anesthetized dog. Anesthesiology 32:338, 1970
Straub H, Meyer JA: An evaluation of a fluid amplifier, face mask respirator. p. 309. In Proceedings of the Third Fluid Amplification Symposium, Vol. 3, 1965
Styles J, Robinson JS, Jones JG: Continuous ventilation and oedema. Br J Anaesth 42:522, 1970
Sugarman HJ, Olofsson KB, Pollack TW, et al: Continuous positive pressure end-expiratory pressure ventilation (PEEP) for the treatment of diffuse

interstitial pulmonary edema. J Trauma 12:263, 1972

Sugerman JH, Rogers RM, Miller LD: Positive end-expiratory pressure (PEEP): indications and physiological considerations. Chest 62:86, 1972

Suter PM, Fairley HB, Isenberg MD: Optimum end-expiratory airway pressure in patients with acute respiratory failure. N Engl J Med 292:284, 1975

Suwa K, Bendixen HH: Change in $PaCO_2$ in the mechanical dead space during artificial ventilation. J Appl Physiol 24:556, 1968

Suwa K, Geffin B, Pontoppidan H, et al: A monogram for deadspace requirement during prolonged artificial ventilation. Anesthesiology 29:1206, 1968

Swensson A: Artificial respiration in general surgery. Acta Chir Scand 113:417, 1957

Swensson A: Artificial respiration in severe abdominal disease. Arch Dis Child 37:149, 1962

Swyer PR: Methods of artificial ventilation in the newborn (IPPV). Biol Neonate 16:3, 1970

Sykes MK, Adams AP, Finlay WEI, et al: The effects of variations in end-expiratory inflation pressure on cardiorespiratory function normo- hypo- and hypervolemic dogs. Br J Anaesth 42:669, 1970

Sykes MK, Lumley J: The effect of varying inspiratory:expiratory ratios on gas exchange during anaesthesia for open-heart surgery. Br J Anaesth 41:374, 1969

Sykes MK, McNicol MW, Campbell EJM: Respiratory Failure. FA Davis, Philadelphia, 1969

Sykes MK, Young WE, Robinson BE: Oxygenation during anesthesia with controlled ventilation. Br J Anaesth 37:314, 1965

Taylor G, Gerbode F: Observations on the circulatory effects of short duration positive pressure pulmonary inflation. Surgery 30:56, 1951

Thatcher VS: History of Anesthesia. JB Lippincott, Philadelphia, 1953

Thompson SA: The effect of pulmonary inflation and deflation upon the circulation. J Thorac Surg 17:323, 1948

Thompson SA, Lange K, Rocky EE: The use of fluorescein to demonstrate the effect of artificial respiration upon the circulation. J Thorac Surg 16:710, 1947

Thompson SA, Quimby EH, Smith BC: The effect of pulmonary resuscitative procedures upon the circulation as demonstrated by the use of radioactive sodium. Surg Gynecol Obstet 83:387, 1946

Thompson SA, Rockey EE: The effect of mechanical artificial respiration upon maintenance of circulation. Surg Gynecol Obstet 84:1059, 1947

Thunberg T: Andning utan andningsrörelser. Hygiejnisk Revy, Uppsala Sweden 13:147, 1924.

Thunberg T: Der Barospirator: Ein neuer apparat für künstliche Atmung nach einem neuen Prinzip. Skan Arch Physiol 48:80, 1926

Tiegel M: Ein einfacher apparat zur Überdrucknarkose. Zbl Chir 22:679, 1908

Todd HM, Toutant SM, Shapiro HM, et al: Intracranial pressure effects of low and high frequency ventilation. Anesthesiology 53:196, 1980

Tossack W: Medical Essays and Observations. Vol. V. Part 2. p. 605. Society of Gentlemen of Edinburgh, Edinburgh, 1744

Trier-Mörch E: *see* Mörch ET

Trimble C, Smith DE, Rosenthal MH, et al: Pathophysiological role of hypocarbia in posttraumatic pulmonary insufficiency. Am J Surg 122:633, 1971

Trippenbach T: Effects of vagal blockade in artificially ventilated rabbits. Acta Physiol Pol 24:491, 1973

Tuffier T, Hallion L: Opérations intrathoracique avec respiration artificielle per insufflation. C R Soc Biol 48:951, 1896

Ueda H, Neclerio M, Leather RP, et al: Effect of positive end-expiratory pressure ventilation on renal function. Surg Forum 23:209, 1972

Ulf B, Eriksson J, Lyttkens L, et al: High frequency positive-pressure ventilation (HFPPV) applied in bronchoscopy under general anesthesia. Acta Anaesth Scand [Suppl] 64:69, 1977

Urban BJ, Weitzner SW: The Amsterdam infant ventilator and the Ayre's T-piece in mechanical ventilation. Anesthesiology 40:423, 1974

Uzawa T, Ashbaugh DG: Continuous positive pressure breathing in acute hemorrhagic pulmonary edema. J Appl Physiol 26:427, 1969

Van Bergen FH, Buckley JJ, Weatherhead DSP, et al: A new respirator. Anesthesiology 17:708, 1956

Vandam LD: Ten years ago: re-evaluation of critically crushed chests. Surv Anesthesiol 1:523, 1966

Van Vliet PKJ, Fisk GC, Gupta JM: Artificial ventilation in respiratory failure in the newborn. Med J Aust 2:648, 1971

Vesalius A: de Humani Corporis Fabrica Libra Septem. Basel, 1555

Vidyasagar D, Chernick V: Continuous positive transpulmonary pressure in hyaline membrane disease. Pediatrics 48:296, 1971

Vidyasagar D, Pildes RS: Use of the Amsterdam infant ventilator for continuous positive pressure breathing. Crit Care Med 2:89, 1974

Vilee CA, Vilee DB, Zuckerman J: Respiratory Distress Sydnrome. Academic Press, New York, 1973

Visscher MB: The physiology of respiration and respirators with particular reference to poliomyelitis. p. 156. In National Foundation for Infantile Paralysis Round Table Conference. Minneapolis, October 1947

Volgyesi G, Misbet HIA: A new position ventilator for use in respiratory studies. Can Anaesth Soc J 19:662, 1972

Volhardt F: Ueber Künstliche Atmung durch Ventilation der Trachea und eine einfache Vorrichtung zur rhytmischen, künstlichen Atmung. MMW 55:209, 1908

Volpitto PP, Woodburg RA, Abreu BE: Influence of different forms of mechanical artificial respiration on the pulmonary and systemic blood pressure. JAMA 126:1066, 1944

Von Hauke I: Neue pneumatische Apparat und ihre Anwendung in der Kinderpraxis. W. Braunmüller, Vienna, 1876

Von Hauke I: Der Pneumatische Panzer. Beitrage zur "mechanischen Behandlung der Brustkrankheiten." Wein Med Presse 15:785, 1874

Waltz RC, Hubay CA, Ankeney JL, et al: Experimental study of pulmonary histopathology following positive and negative pressure respiration. Surg Gynecol Obstet 99:5, 1954

Watrous WG, Davis FE, Anderson BM: Manually assisted and controlled respiration: a review. Anesthesiology 12:33, 1951

Watson WE: Observation on physiological dead space during intermittent positive pressure respiration. Br J Anaesth 34:504, 1962

Watson WE: Some observations on dynamic lung compliance during intermittent positive pressure breathing. Br J Anaesth 34:274, 1962

Watson WE, Smith AC, Spalding JMK: Transmural central venous pressure during intermittent positive pressure breathing. Br J Anaesth 34:274, 1962

Weenig CS, Pietak S, Hickey RF, et al: Relationship of pre-operative closing volume to functional residual capacity and alveolar-arterial oxygen difference during anesthesia with controlled ventilation. Anesthesiology 41:3, 1974

Weil H, Shubin H: The new practice of critical care medicine. Chest 59:473, 1971

Weil H, Williams TB, Burk RH: Laboratory and clinical evaluation of a new volume ventilator. Chest 67:14, 1975

Weitzner SW, Urban BJ: A new ventilator utilizing fluid logic. JAMA 207:1126, 1969

Weitzner SW, Urban BJ: Fluid amplifiers: a new approach to the construction of ventilators. p. 1068. In Proceedings of the Fourth World Congress on Anesthesiology. Excerpta Medica, Amsterdam, 1968

Werkö L: The influence of positive pressure breathing on the circulation in man. Acta Med Scand [Suppl] 193:1, 1947

Werl H, Williams TB, Buck RH: Laboratory and clinical evaluation of a new volume ventilator. Chest 67:14, 1975

West JB: Ventilation/Blood Flow and Gas Exchange. Blackwell, Oxford, 1970

Whittenberger JL: Artificial respiration. Physiol Rev 35:611, 1955

Whittenberger JL (ed): Artificial Respiration. Harper & Row, New York, 1962

Whittenberger JL: Medical progress: resuscitation and other uses of artificial respiration. Part I. N Engl J Med 251:775, 1954

Whittenberger JL: Medical progress: resuscitation and other uses of artificial respiration. Part II. N Engl J Med 251:816, 1954

Whittenberger JL: Respiratory problems in poliomyelitis. p. 10. In National Foundation for Infantile Paralysis Conference. Ann Arbor, MI, March 1952

Whittenberger JL, McGregor M, Berglund E, et al: Influence of state of inflation of the lung on pulmonary vascular resistance. J Appl Physiol 5:878, 1960

Whittenberger JL, Sarnoff EJ: Physiological principles in the treatment of respiratory failure. Med Clin North Am 34:1335, 1950

Wiggers CJ: The dynamics of lung inflation. p. 422. In Wiggers CJ (ed): Physiology in Health and Disease. 5th Ed. Lea & Febiger, New York, 1949

Williams MH Jr, Shin CS: Ventilatory failure: etiology and clinical forms. Am J Med 48:477, 1970

Williams TM: An automatic breathing attachment to Boyle's apparatus. Br J Anaesth 24:222, 1952

Wilson JL: The Use of the Respirator in Poliomyelitis. National Foundation of Infantile Paralysis, New York, 1942

Wilson RF, Gibson D, Percivel AT, et al: Severe alkalosis in critically ill surgical patients. Arch Surg 105:197, 1972

Wilson RS, Pontoppidan H: Respiratory care. Mod Med 39:100, 1971

Woillez EJ: Du spirophore, appareil de sauvetage pur le traitment de l'asphyxie et principalement de l'asphyxie des noyes et des nourveaunes. Bull Acad Méd Paris 5:611, 1876; also Dict Encyclopedique Sci Méd Paris Series 13:609, 1876

Woollam CHM: The development of apparatus for intermittent negative pressure respiration. Anaesthesia 31:537, 666, 1976

Woollam H, Smith TC, Stephan G, et al: Effects of extremes of respiratory and metabolic alkalosis on cerebral blood flow in man. J Appl Physiol 24:60, 1968

Wood DW, Downes JJ, Lecks HI: The management of respiratory failure in childhood status asthmaticus: experience with 30 episodes and evolution of a technique. J Allerg 42:261, 1968

Wyche MQ, Teichner RL, Kallo ST, et al: Effects of continuous positive pressure breathing on functional residual capacity and arterial oxygenation during intra-abdominal operations: studies in man during nitrous oxide and d-tubocurarine anesthesia. Anesthesiology 38:68, 1973

Yakaitis RW, Cooke JE, Redding JS: Re-evaluation of relationship of hyperkalemia and P_{CO_2} to cardiac arrhythmias during mechanical ventilation. Anesth Analg 50:368, 1971

Young J, Crocker D: Principles and Practice of Respiratory Therapy. Year Book Medical Publishers, Chicago, 1976

Zapol WM, Snider MT, Schneider RC: Extracorporeal membrane oxygenation for acute respiratory failure. Anesthesiology 46:27, 1977

Ziment I: Intermittent positive pressure breathing. p. 546. In Burton GG, Gee GN, Hodgkin JE (eds): Respiratory Care. JB Lippincott, Philadelphia, 1977

2

Physical Principles and Functional Designs of Ventilators

Charles B. Spearman
Howard G. Sanders, Jr.

PHYSICAL PRINCIPLES OF VENTILATORS

The physical characteristics of mechanical ventilators are important to the clinician because they establish the framework within which most mechanical ventilatory support is provided. Physiologic parameters (e.g., minute ventilation, distribution of inspired air, alveolar gas exchange, distribution of pulmonary blood flow, venous return and cardiac output, oxygen consumption, and work of breathing) can all be affected by the physical characteristics and available modes of the ventilator. A basic understanding of the physical aspects of ventilators is essential to their proper clinical application. Most ventilators in common use today have similar operational characteristics. The classification that follows is intended to provide a basic overview to prepare the reader for later chapters on clinical use of ventilatory support and individual ventilator descriptions. Specific ventilators are mentioned only as examples of the principles discussed. Terminology for the variety of ventilatory support modes is also introduced in this chapter.

Positive Versus Negative Pressure Ventilation

Normally, movement of air into the lungs is provided by contraction of the respiratory muscles, producing a "negative" or subatmospheric intrapleural and intra-alveolar pressure. A pressure gradient is thereby established between the upper airway (atmospheric) and alveoli (subatmospheric), and air flows into the lungs. During expiration, which is usually passive, the natural recoil of the lung tissue causes an increase in alveolar pressure so that the pressure gradient is reversed (positive intra-alveolar pressure to atmospheric upper airway pressure), and air flows out of the lungs.

Mechanical support of air movement into the lungs can be provided either by applying a subatmospheric pressure around the chest or by generating a positive pressure above atmospheric pressure to the upper airway. The necessary pressure gradient develops because the alveoli are at atmospheric pressure just before inspiration. As intra-alveolar pressure rises during positive-pressure ventilation, intrapleural pressure also rises to levels potentially above atmospheric pressure. When gas flow into the upper airway ceases, the lungs usually deflate passively. Upper airway pressure is equal to atmospheric pressure and the higher intra-alveolar pressure causes the air to flow out of the lungs. Intrapleural pressure also falls during this time and returns to a subatmospheric level if alveolar pressure is allowed to return to atmospheric pressure.

Mechanical ventilatory support by negative-pressure ventilation can be provided by three basic types of ventilators[1–4]: those that completely surround the patient's entire body, often referred to as "tank ventilators" or "iron lungs"; those that fit only around the chest; and those that fit around the abdomen.[5] The chest and abdominal units are called cuirass ventilators, the chest unit being the most common. The abdominal unit pulls the abdominal wall forward and the diaphragm downward during inspiration. Although negative-pressure ventilators are still used to provide support for patients with various neuromuscular disorders, they are seldom employed in the critically ill patient with respiratory failure. The remainder of this chapter is devoted to positive-pressure ventilation systems.

Ventilator Power and Control Systems

The power source required to operate mechanical ventilators is provided by either compressed gases, electricity, or both. The control system refers to the decision-making or logic component which starts and stops inspiration and expiration. Ventilators may be controlled by electronic, pneumatic, or fluidic means, or by combinations of the three.

Pneumatic Ventilators

Pneumatic ventilators require some source of compressed gas in order to provide a positive-pressure breath. The gas may be compressed air and/or oxygen and is usually pressurized to 50 psig. Internally, this pressure is regulated by mechanisms that include reducing valves (e.g., Bennett PR-2) or a highly resistant needle valve or venturi mechanism (e.g., Bird Mark 7).[1,2] All controls are influenced by gas pressure and are therefore considered pneumatic in nature.

Some pneumatic ventilators use more refined fluidic controls.[1,2,6] These components have no moving parts and depend solely on gas flow and pressure to function. A ventilator that requires a compressed gas source to operate and uses fluidic logic for its decision-making is referred to as pneumatically powered and fluidically controlled. The Monaghan 225/SIMV volume ventilator is an example of such a unit.

Electronic Ventilators

Ventilators which require only an electrical source to provide mechanical ventilation are referred to as electronically powered and controlled. Compressed oxygen is required only to provide a fraction of inspired oxygen (F_{IO_2}) greater than that of room air but is not required as a driving or controlling force. These ventilators continue to provide positive-pressure ventilation with room air even when oxygen failure occurs. The primary logic systems for controlling inspiration and expiration are provided by electrical components. Examples of electronically powered and controlled ventilators include the Emerson 3-PV and Bennett MA-1. The Emerson uses an electrical motor to drive a piston in a cylinder, and this piston provides the positive inspiratory pressure. In the MA-1, an electrical compressor provides the compressed air necessary to drive a bellows system during inspiration.

Combined Power Ventilators

Certain ventilators use both pneumatic and electrical power sources. Compressed air and oxygen are often required to provide a variable F_{IO_2} and the driving force during mechanical inspiration. Most often the electrical power is used for timing, phasing, and monitoring. Because these ventilators cannot provide mechanical inspiration with only one of the two sources, they are considered to be *both* pneumatically and electronically powered.

Some pediatric ventilators provide a continuous flow of gas into their delivery circuit while using either electronic or a combination of electronic and fluidic components for controlling inspiratory and expiratory phasing. The BEAR CUB BP 2001 is an example of a pneumatically and electrically controlled infant ventilator. The Sechrist IV-100B is pneumatically and electrically powered and is controlled by a combination of electronic and fluidic components.

The Servo 900 series ventilators by Siemens are units that also require pneumatic and electrical power sources. The pneumatic source is part of the driving system, whereas the logic functions are primarily electronic. Therefore, these ventilators are classified as being pneumatically and electrically powered and electronically controlled.

Drive Mechanisms

Each mechanical ventilator must have a system that provides the *force* with which the positive-pressure gas flow is generated. The mechanism providing this force is considered the driving system. A knowledge of driving systems is important because each general type suggests certain performance characteristics. The general categories presented here are simplified but cover the most commonly used drive mechanisms.

Single and Double Circuit Systems

Driving systems can be broadly subdivided into *single-circuit* and *double-circuit* types. If the gases within the driving mechanism go directly to the patient, the device is considered a single-circuit device. If gas from the driving mechanism is used to compress another system (e.g., a bag or bellows) which in turn delivers gas to the patient, the unit is considered a double-circuit device.

A common example of a single-circuit ventilator system is shown in Figure 2–1. Here the drive system is a piston within a cylinder. When the piston moves forward (to the right), it expels gas from the cylinder directly into the tubing system connected to the patient. Other sources can also be used to provide a single-circuit drive mechanism, including pneumatic systems and spring-driven bellows. Examples of single-circuit ventilators using a piston include the Emerson 3-PV and 3-MV models. Pneumatically driven single-circuit units are represented by the Bird Mark series and Bennett PR series ventilators. The Siemens Servo 900 series are examples of single-circuit, spring-loaded bellows ventilators.

Figure 2–2 shows a double-circuit system. In this example, a piston is again used to provide the driving power. However, gases from the piston are not sent directly to the patient. Instead, these gases pressurize a chamber and

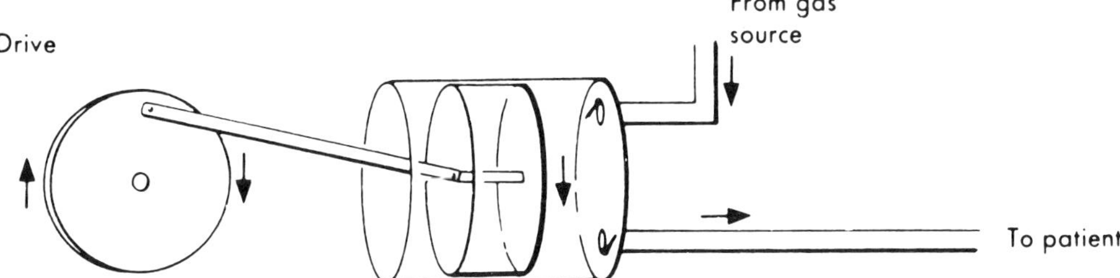

Fig. 2–1. Single-circuit drive mechanism. In this example, gas passes directly from the cylinder to the patient circuit. The drive mechanism is a rotary-driven piston. (From Spearman et al.,[10] with permission.)

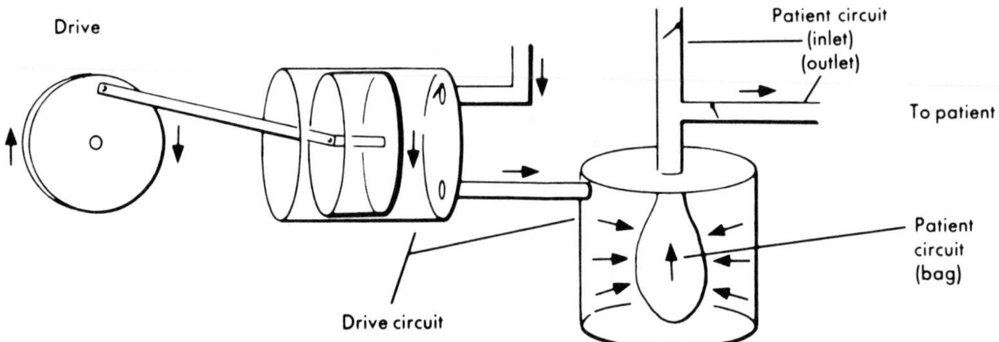

Fig. 2–2. Double-circuit drive mechanism using a rotary-driven piston. Gas passes from the cylinder to a rigid cannister and compresses a bag. Gas contained within the bag is then delivered into the patient circuit. The two gas sources are separate. A collapsible bellows may be substituted for the bag in the patient circuit. (From Spearman et al.,[10] with permission.)

compress a bag which contains gas the patient is to receive. The piston is considered the driving circuit, and the bag and connecting tubing comprise the patient circuit. A collapsible bellows or concertina bag can be used instead of the bag as part of the patient circuit, and other driving sources can be used in place of the piston. Engström 150 and 300 series ventilators are piston-driven, double-circuit ventilators which produce unique pressure and flow patterns partly because of their double-circuit design. Bennett MA-1 and Monaghan 225/SIMV ventilators are double-circuit ventilators using a collapsible bellows.

Piston-Driven Ventilators

A piston moving back and forth through a cylinder has provided a convenient method for providing positive-pressure ventilation for several decades.[2] Pistons are coupled to one of two basic components that provide the to-and-fro movement: a rotary drive or a linear drive mechanism.

Rotary-Driven Piston

A rotary-driven piston is one that is connected to the edge of a wheel which is, in turn, powered by an electrical motor. As the piston moves back, one-way valves allow fresh gas to fill the cylinder. On the forward stroke these gases are then pushed into the patient's circuit, causing inspiration (single-circuit, as shown in Fig. 2–1).

The flow pattern from a rotary-driven, single-circuit piston is unique and is shown in Figure 2–3. As the rotary wheel turns, the piston is moved through the cylinder in an accelerating, then decelerating fashion, producing a similar pattern of airflow. This flow profile occurs because at the beginning of inspiration the movement of the piston's connecting rod is mostly upward rather than forward. Subsequently, the motion is transferred to a more forward direction as the wheel continues to rotate, and gas flow out of the cylinder accelerates. When the wheel is one-quarter through its rotation, the piston has moved one-half its total forward distance and peak flow is reached. The remainder of inspiration occurs with the forward motion of the piston being transferred progressively in a downward direction, causing a deceleration of inspiratory flow. This accelerating then decelerating inspiratory flow pattern is often termed sinusoidal, or like a sine wave, although it is more precisely one-half of a sine wave. During the remainder of the cycle, the wheel continues its rotation and pulls the piston backward through the cylinder, which is refilled with fresh gas for the next breath. The patient is not affected by this refilling because of the one-way valve

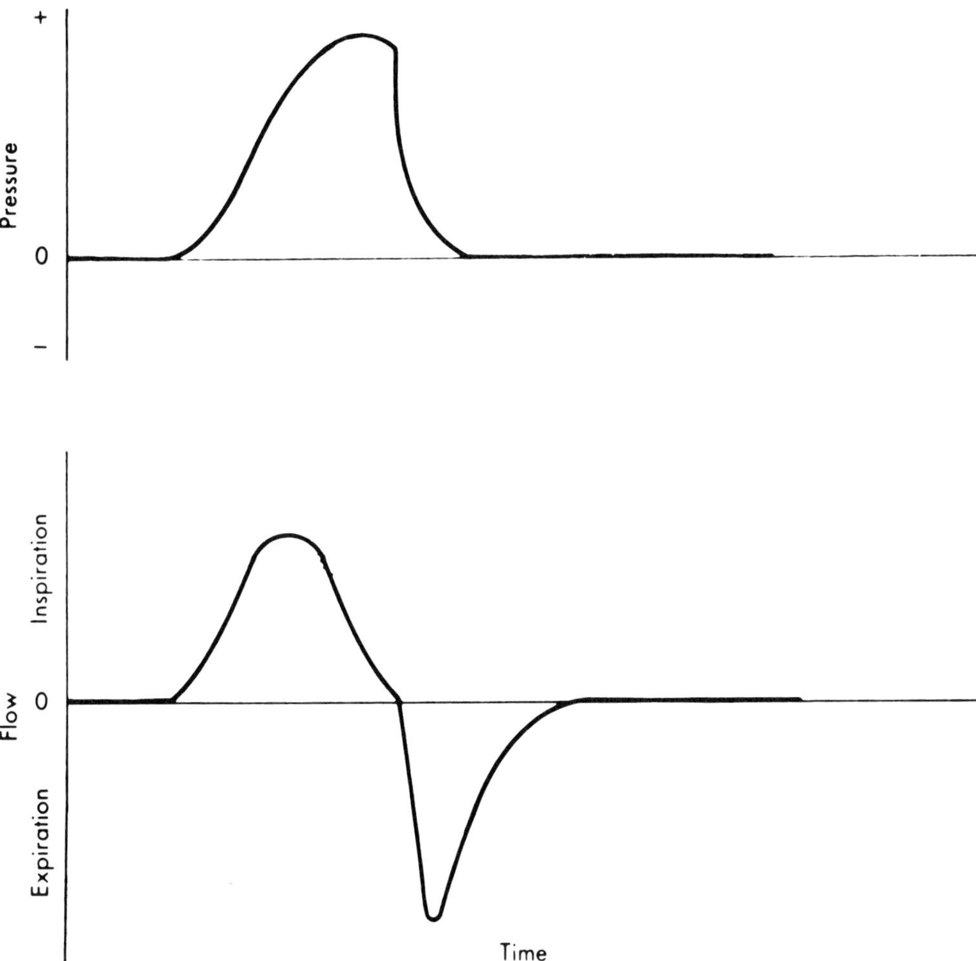

Fig. 2–3. Pressure (sigmoidal) and flow (sinusoidal) waveforms associated with a rotary-drive piston mechanism (Fig. 2–1). (From Spearman et al.,[10] with permission.)

system that interrupts the ventilator-airway communication during exhalation. The patient's exhalation occurs independent of the piston stroke, and the waveform produced for expiratory flow (Fig. 2–3) is primarily a function of the lung-chest wall compliance, airway resistance, and tubing circuit resistance (not shown).

The Emerson models 3-PV and 3-MV ventilators are examples of rotary-driven piston devices. Because these ventilators use a rather powerful electrical motor to turn the rotary wheel, relatively high pressures can be generated at the airway with very little influence on the inspiratory flow pattern. This sine-wave flow pattern is similar to that produced during typical spontaneous breathing and may have some theoretical advantages over other flow patterns.

Linear-Driven Piston

Piston ventilators may also use a driving system that moves the piston at a constant rate of speed throughout the inspiratory phase. Thus the movement is said to be linear. These devices can be powered in several ways, two of which are depicted in Figure 2–4. A rotating gear connected to the piston's rod by cogs or teeth can

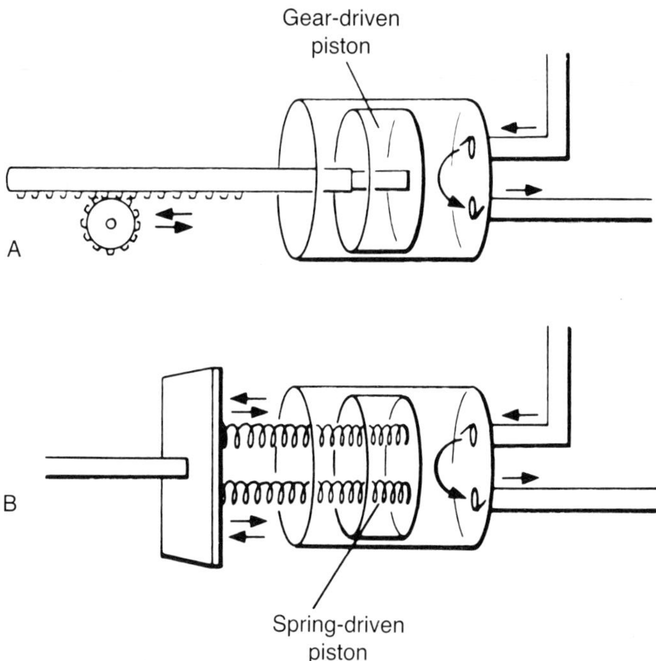

Fig. 2–4. Piston-drive mechanisms. **(A)** Single-circuit gear. **(B)** Spring-loaded. (From Spearman et al.,[10] with permission.)

produce a constant piston movement and therefore a constant flow. High-tension springs can also be used to drive the piston at a relatively constant rate. This constant flow is often described as a square wave, and is discussed later in this chapter.

The Bourns LS 104–150 Infant Ventilator uses a gear system to provide a linear-driven piston, and the no longer manufactured Searle VVA unit used a relatively high spring tension drive system with its piston-like component.[1,2]

Pneumatically Driven Ventilators

Numerous ventilators use compressed gases as the primary driving force during inspiration. Various methods are used to control the amount and pattern of both pressure and flow in pneumatically driven ventilators, and three are presented here.

High-Pressure Drive with High Internal Resistance

The simplest form of a pneumatic drive system can be constructed from a high-pressure source gas (3 to 50 psig oxygen or compressed air), incorporating an adjustable resistance to control pressure and flow rate. These driving forces equal 200 to over 3,500 cm H_2O and represent 2 to 35 times the typical maximum pressure developed at the airway. To avoid sudden pressurization in the patient with these high-pressure systems, a highly resistant valve is used. This "needle valve" adjusts the size of an orifice at the outlet of the high-pressure source and therefore controls the flow rate.

The flow pattern produced by this type of system is generally constant or square wave in nature because the driving force is relatively high. It can exist in either a single- or double-circuit configuration (Fig. 2–5). In a single-circuit device, the driving source passes through

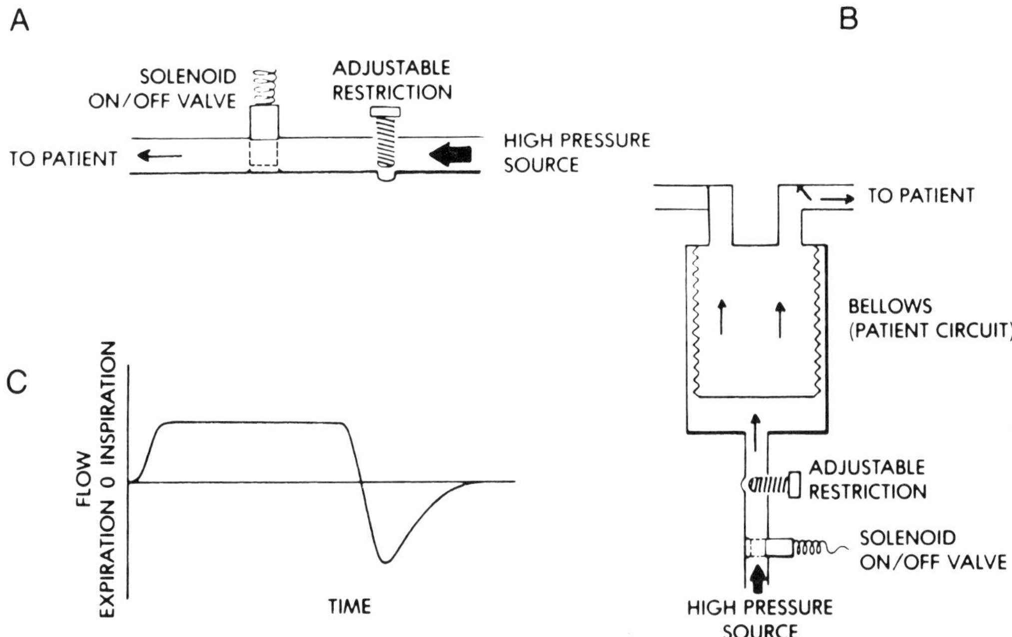

Fig. 2–5. High-pressure pneumatic drive systems with high internal flow resistance. **(A)** Single-circuit. **(B)** Double-circuit. Adjustable restrictions control flow from high-pressure source gas. Electrical solenoids open (solid line drawings) and close (dashed line drawings), creating inspiration and expiration, respectively. **(C)** Constant inspiratory flow pattern typical of these systems.

its high internal resistor directly into the patient. In a double-circuit system, the driving source compresses a bag or bellows containing gases for the patient. An example of a single-circuit ventilator with a high-pressure pneumatic drive system is the Bird Mark 7 on its "100 percent" setting, as the Venturi mechanism is bypassed. The Monaghan 225/SIMV ventilator is a double-circuit unit that uses a high-pressure drive system.[1]

Low-Pressure Drive System

Another pneumatic drive system is one that regulates the pressure to a relatively low level, for example, 60 cm H_2O pressure or less. A number of mechanisms may incorporate this principle, two of which are described here.

Some ventilators use a Venturi or injector as their driving force. Generally, a high-pressure source of compressed air and/or oxygen is used to drive the jet of the Venturi. The pressure applied to the small orifice of the jet establishes a high forward velocity, and air is entrained by this gas.[7] The amount of pressure that can be generated by the Venturi is proportional to, but much less than, the pressure applied to the jet, assuming that the entrainment area is left open and without valves.

Pressure-reducing valves are also used in ventilators with a low driving pressure.[1] In these systems, adjustment of the spring tension within the reducing valve establishes the desired driving pressure.

The flow pattern created by low-pressure drive systems of the Venturi or reducing valve types is quite similar. Both systems are susceptible to backpressure caused by increased airway resistance, decreased lung-thorax compliance, etc., such that flow decreases as pressure in the patient system increases. As an example, a ventilator using a low-pressure drive is set to produce 20 cm H_2O driving pressure. At the beginning of inspiration, if the pressure in the patient's airway is 0 cm H_2O, the gradient between the ventilator and the patient is 20 cm H_2O (20 cm H_2O drive − 0 cm H_2O patient) and flow begins at its highest level. As pressure increases in the patient's airway through inspiration, this pressure gradient progressively decreases until finally the airway pressure equals the driving pressure. Concomitantly, flow also decreases progressively until it finally reaches 0. Figure 2–6 shows theoretical airway pressure and flow patterns produced by a ventilator with a low-pressure drive mechanism. Examples of devices using a low-pressure Venturi drive mechanism include the Hand-E-Vent from Ohio Medical Products and Bird Asthmastik from Bird Corp. The Bennett PR-1 and PR-2 ventilators are examples of low-pressure drive units that use an adjustable reducing valve.

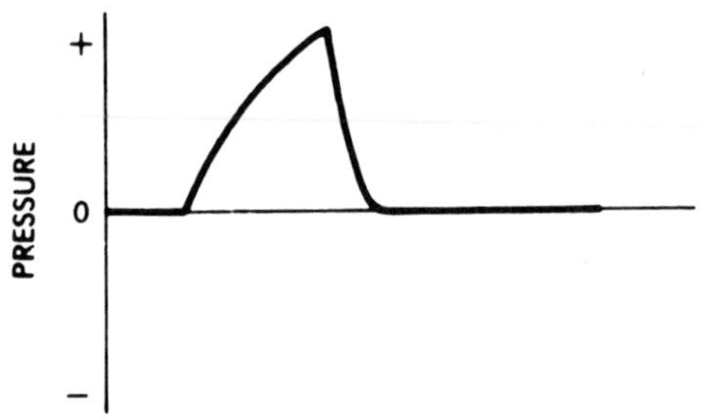

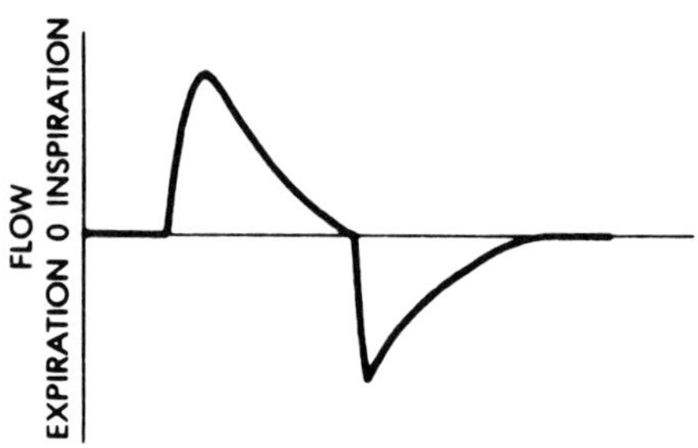

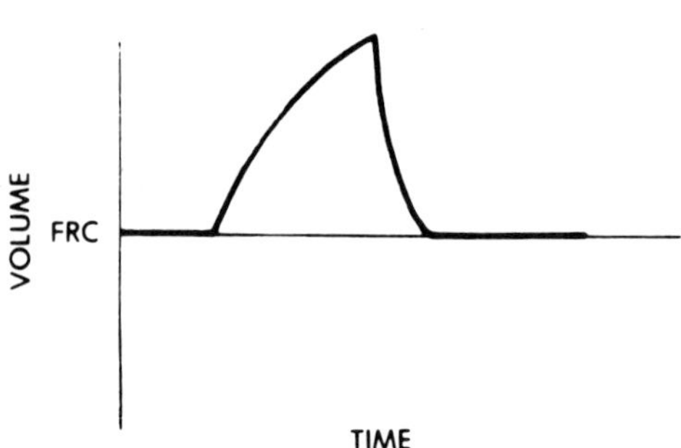

Fig. 2–6. Pressure, flow, and volume waveforms of a ventilator with a low-pressure drive system. Note that flow during inspiration reaches its peak early and then tapers, whereas pressure continues to rise.

Compressor-Driven Bellows

Compressors are commonly used to provide the driving force for double-circuit ventilators. A bellows is usually used for patient gases, and the compressor pressurizes the bellows container to drive it upward, emptying part or all of its contents into the patient circuit (Fig. 2–7). Some compressors or blowers can produce moderate pressures of 100 cm H_2O or more at flow rates exceeding 100 L/min and apply their output directly to the bellows container. An example of such a ventilator is the CCV-2, SIMV unit by Ohio Medical Products.

Other models use compressors that produce pressures of several pounds per square inch gauge (psig) (e.g., 6 to 12 psig), but at flow rates less than 50 L/min. In these systems, a Venturi is used to reduce the maximum pressure and increase the flow from the compressor. Figure 2–7 diagrams such a system and shows the compressor being used to drive the jet of a Venturi while the output of the Venturi drives the bellows. The MA-1 and MA-2 + 2 ventilators from Puritan-Bennett are examples of ventilators using this type of driving system.

Generally, these driving mechanisms produce a relatively square flow pattern until the pressure in the patient circuit increases to within a few centimeters of water pressure of the maximum

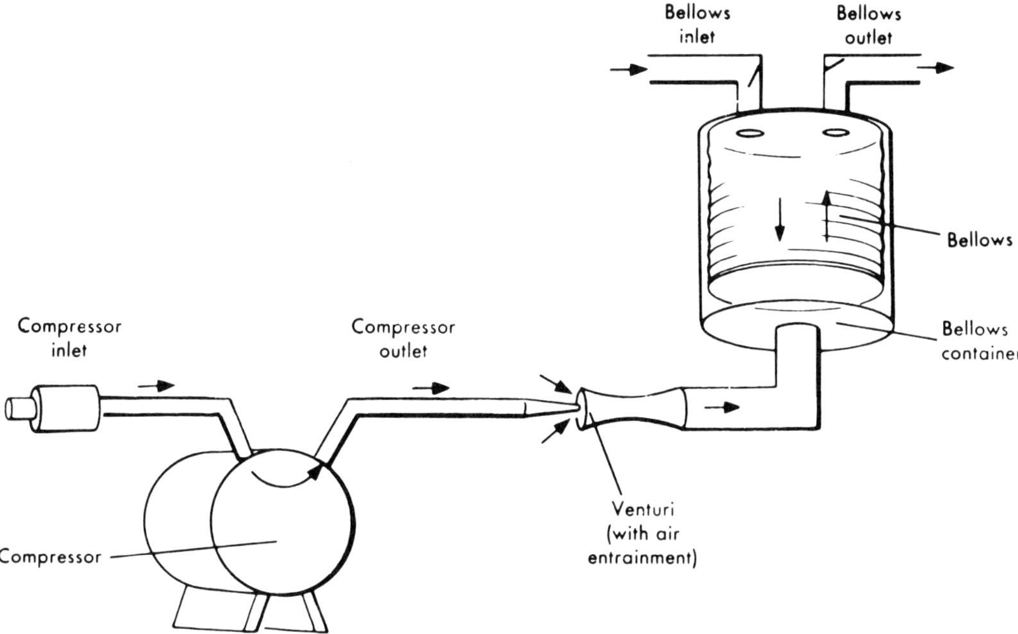

Fig. 2–7. Double-circuit compressor-bellows drive mechanism using a Venturi. The pressure decrement occurring through the Venturi tube increases output from the compressor while additional ambient air is entrained. (From Spearman et al.,[10] with permission.)

driving force, at which time some decrease or tapering of flow occurs.

Initiation of Inspiration

Various mechanisms are available for initiating aspiration in modern mechanical ventilators. The way in which a ventilator is cycled on or "triggered" is a convenient way to categorize the available modes of ventilatory support. These modes vary from complete automatic cycling by the ventilator, through a combination of patient- and ventilator-triggered breaths and spontaneous breathing.

Initiation of the inspiratory phase is often referred to as *cycling,* although this term is also applied to the termination of inspiration and the initiation and termination of expiration as well.[2] We indicate which phase change we are referring to with this term for the remainder of this chapter. The term *triggering* is also synonymous with starting inspiration.

Control Mode (Time-Cycled or Triggered)

Control mode or controlled ventilation is provided when the positive-pressure breaths automatically start by some timing mechanism, regardless, or in the absence, of any patient effort. In this mode, the patient receives a pressurized breath at time intervals determined by the setting of the timing mechanism only. Patients receiving control mode ventilation (CMV) may be totally dependent on the ventilator for support as they are often apneic from either disease processes or drugs, such as neuromuscular blocking agents and sedatives.

A variety of systems are available in modern ventilators to establish a control rate.[1,2] The most common are described here.

Single Rate Control

Some ventilators have an electrical timer system that divides each minute into a set number of breaths. Actually, these timers establish the number of times per minute inspiration *should* begin, whereas some other mechanisms cause inspiration to end.

The controls can be calibrated in breaths per minute (BPM) or in time increments between breaths. In both cases the timer itself is doing the same thing: starting the inspiratory phase at regular intervals. For example, if the timer initiates a mechanical breath every 5 seconds, the control can be calibrated to read "12 BPM" or "5 seconds" of total ventilatory cycle time. The Puritan-Bennett MA-1 and the BEAR-2 ventilators use single rate control knobs which are calibrated in BPM, whereas the Emerson 3-MV uses a single control calibrated in seconds of total time.

Inspiratory and Expiratory Timers

Other ventilators divide the phases of breathing with separate timers. In this case, inspiration is started by one timer and expiration by another. Any change in either of the timers can affect the resulting mechanical rate. As an example, if inspiration lasts 2 seconds and expiration 3 seconds, the total ventilatory cycle time is 5 seconds and the set control rate 12 BPM (60 divided by 5 seconds total). The Emerson 3-PV ventilator uses electrical timers, whereas the Babybird uses pneumatic timers for establishing a control rate.

Independent Expiratory Timer

Another approach to setting an automatic rate for the control mode is the use of an electronic or pneumatic *expiratory* timer. The inspiratory phase begins when this expiratory time ends. The length of inspiration is subject to several factors, such as flow rate and tidal volume or pressure setting; therefore, the rate can be altered not only by the setting of the expiratory timer but also by variables that occur during inspiration. An example of such an electronically controlled system is the Ohio CCV-2, SIMV ventilator, which establishes a control rate based on an expiratory time setting plus tidal volume and flow settings for the inspiratory time. The Bird Mark 7 has a pneumatic timer for the expiratory phase, whereas inspiratory time is controlled by flow and pressure settings. Because the patient's lung condition can influence the flow pattern during the breath and change inspiratory time accordingly, only a maximum expiratory time can be "guaranteed" rather than an actual respiratory rate.

Assist Mode (Patient-Cycled or Triggered)

When a ventilator senses a slight inspiratory effort by the patient and responds by triggering a pressurized breath, assist mode or assisted ventilation is provided. Assist mode ventilation (AMV) implies that the patient's efforts are responsible for the ventilator providing a positive-pressure breath. The number of ventilator breaths occurring per minute is determined solely by the patient's efforts and is quite variable, depending on a variety of factors.

Assist mechanisms can function various ways. Most respond to a change in *pressure* within the patient's tubing circuit. In some ventilators a flexible diaphragm is displaced by the drop in pressure as the patient begins to make an inspiratory effort. If, for example, the diaphragm is moved enough for two electrical contacts to touch, inspiration can be triggered. If the amount of effort required by the patient to trigger inspiration is adjustable, the ventilator is said to have a *sensitivity* or *patient effort* control. If the amount of pressure drop necessary is decreased, the system becomes *more* sensitive, requiring *less* patient effort.

Pressure transducers are also used in some ventilators to provide an assist mode. Here, more sophisticated electronic logic systems are needed to compare a signal on a reference control (e.g., sensitivity) to the signal produced by the pressure transducer in order to trigger an assist breath.

A flow-sensing device can also be used to detect an inspiratory effort. Generally, a slight drop in pressure creates a change in flow. If monitored electronically, the change in flow can also cycle the ventilator on in response to the patient's breathing effort.

Assist mode and sensitivity adjustments are provided by a diaphragm and electrical contact system on the Puritan-Bennett MA-1, whereas a pressure transducer system is used for the Siemens Servo 900B ventilator.[1] A thermistor bead is used with the BEAR-1 to detect the change in flow caused by an inspiratory patient effort.[1]

Assist-Control Mode

An automatic rate mechanism may be combined with an assist mechanism to provide an assist-control mode. In this case the control rate is thought of as the "backup" system and provides the minimum allowable breaths per minute. Should the patient desire to breathe at a rate faster than the control rate, the assist mechanism is triggered. This mode of ventilatory support is very common to modern ventilators, and some cannot be used as strict "controllers" or "assistors" only. Assist-control mode is a convenient way to allow patients to establish their own ventilatory rate in case of respiratory depression or apnea.

Figure 2–8 illustrates the difference between

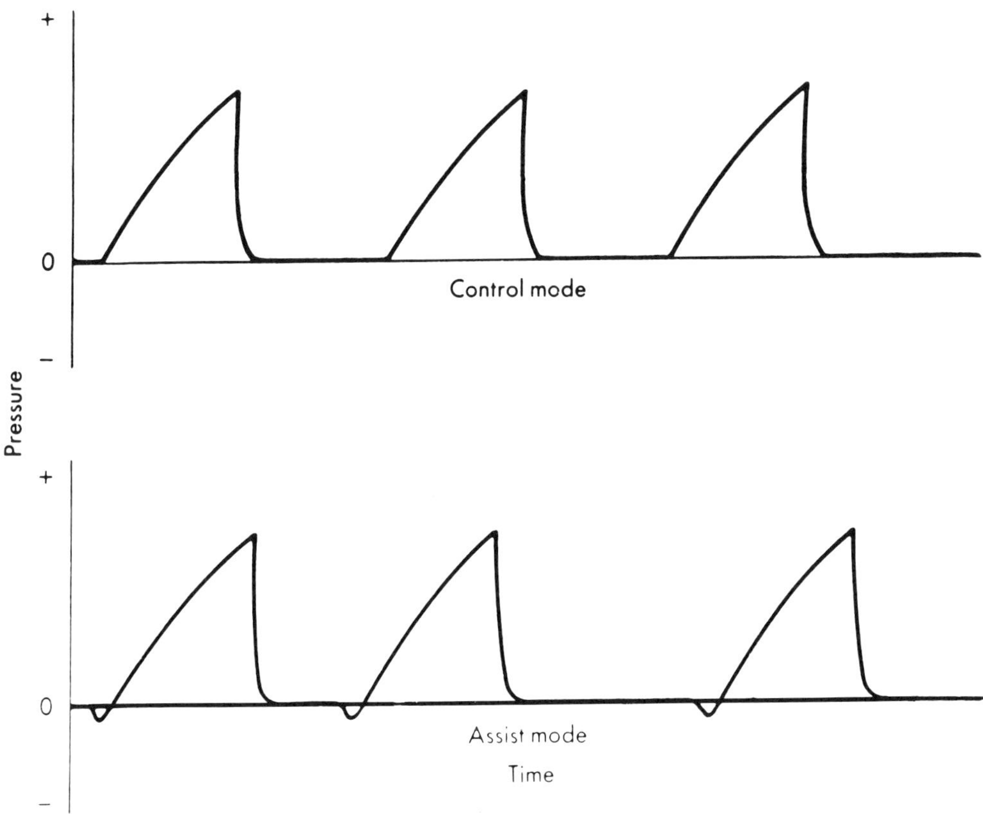

Fig. 2–8. Pressure-time waveforms for control mode and assist mode (IPPV). In this example, the slight "negative" pressure generated by the patient's voluntary inspiratory effort triggers the ventilator during assist mode breathing. (From Spearman et al.,[10] with permission.)

control mode and assist mode in terms of the pressure waveform for each. Pressure is shown on the vertical axis and time on the horizontal axis. Note that for control mode the time intervals between the beginning of one positive-pressure breath and the beginning of the next are quite regular. During assist mode ventilation, a characteristic drop in pressure occurs at the beginning of each breath, indicating that the patient's inspiratory effort triggered or started each breath. The time intervals for the assisted breaths are not as regular as for controlled ones.

Intermittent Mandatory Ventilation

When spontaneous breathing is *combined* with a controlled mechanical rate from a ventilator, the pattern of ventilation is referred to as intermittent mandatory ventilation (IMV).[8–12] The control rate set on the ventilator is provided at preset time intervals, whereas between these breaths the patient inhales from a source of fresh gas at the desired rate and tidal volume. The spontaneous breathing component of IMV infers that the size and number of breaths received are related solely to the patient's ability to inhale spontaneously. The mandatory breaths are those given by the ventilator at regular intervals in a fashion similar to the control mode. Indeed, the primary difference between control mode and IMV is that when a patient attempts to breathe spontaneously between mechanical ventilator breaths in a control mode no fresh gas is available.

IMV allows patients to participate in the ventilation process to varying degrees and may allow them to maintain some of the physiological advantages of spontaneous breathing.[8,13,14] IMV has been used for almost two decades in all age groups as both a primary mode of ventilatory support and a means for weaning patients from the ventilator,[8,12,15–17] although not all patients are candidates for IMV.[18,19]

Most ventilators can be modified easily to supply a source of fresh gas for spontaneous breathing, and many have such a system built in[1,2,20,21] (see Ch. 16).

Physical Principles During Mechanical Inspiration

During conventional mechanical ventilation, certain characteristics of inspiration have been used to classify ventilators. One system, reported by Mushin et al., uses positive pressure.[2] Although few ventilators fit precisely into these categories under all conditions, they are described here for completeness, together with certain clinical implications.

Pressure Generators

Constant-Pressure Generators

When a ventilator applies a relatively constant pressure to the airway throughout inspiration, it is termed a constant-pressure generator. Generally, the mechanisms employed are similar to the low-pressure drive systems previously discussed. Figure 2–9 illustrates theoretical pressure, flow, and volume waveforms for an ideal pressure generator. In each of the examples illustrated, the amount and pattern of applied *pressure* are the same. However, the *flow* pattern and *volume* delivery vary in response to changes in lung or airway characteristics.

Flow is at its highest level at the beginning of inspiration in a pressure generator because the difference in pressure between the ventilator and the patient's lung is greatest at this time. As pressure in the patient's airway increases, the gradient decreases and flow is reduced. If the ventilator and alveolar pressures equilibrate before inspiration ends, flow tapers to zero and the volume delivered is held constant until inspiration is terminated. The tidal volume delivered is a function of the pressure applied, the patient's compliance and airway resistance (Fig. 2–9A).

Figure 2–9B illustrates the effects of decreased lung compliance on flow and volume for the same pressure generator as in Figure 2–9A. Note that flow tapers to zero quickly, and the lung volume is decreased as ventilator and alveolar pressures equilibrate earlier in the cycle.

Figure 2–9C illustrates the effects of increased

airway resistance. Here the flow pattern shows a more gradual taper than in Figure 2–9A, although in the example zero flow is reached before end-inspiration. The flow tapers more slowly because the resistance to flow in the airways impedes the equilibration of alveolar pressure and ventilator pressure. The lung volumes achieved at end-inspiration in Figure 2–9A and 2–9C are the same, indicating that the lung-thorax compliance was the same for both. However, the increased airway resistance in Figure 2–9C caused that volume to be reached later in the breath.

Constant-pressure generators and the low-

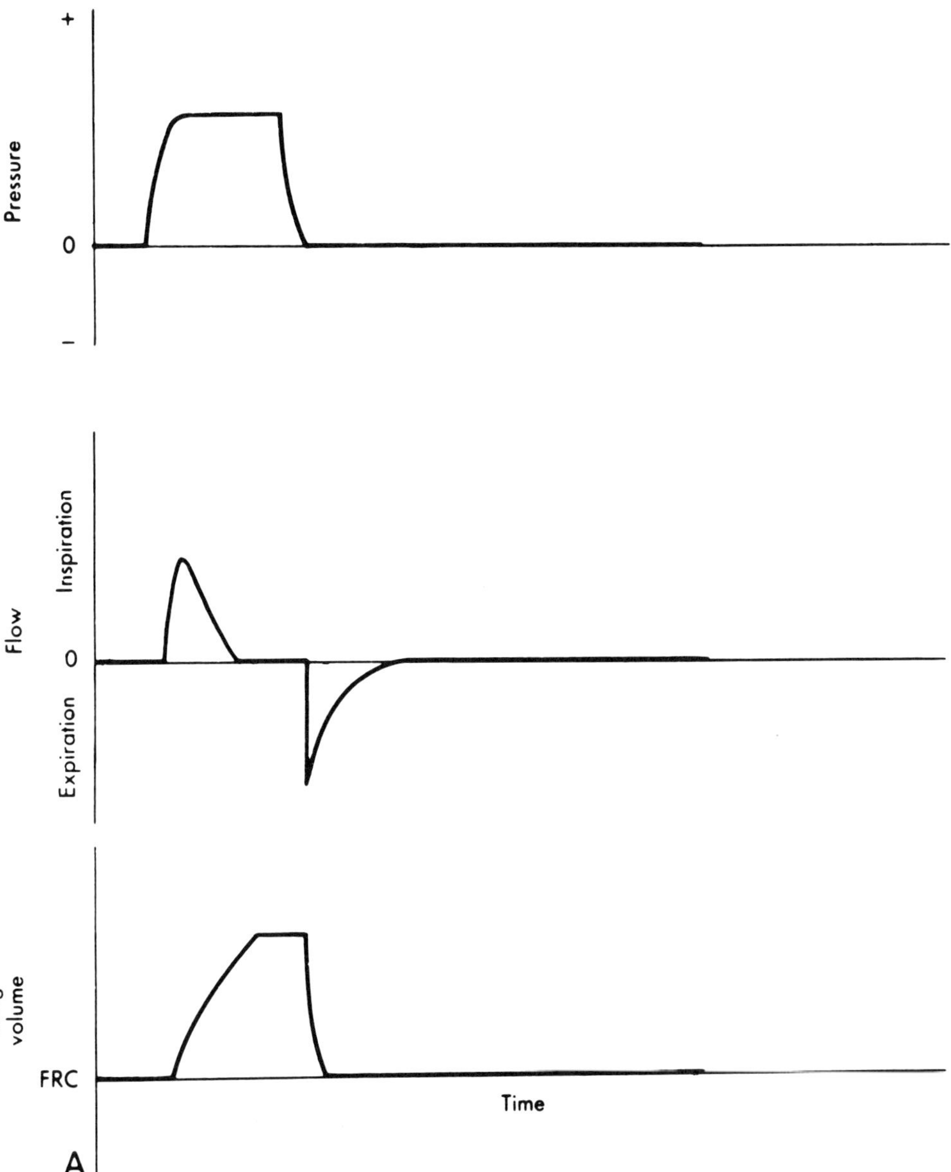

Fig. 2–9. Pressure, flow, and volume waveforms for a constant-pressure generator. **(A)** "Normal" conditions. (*Figure continues*).

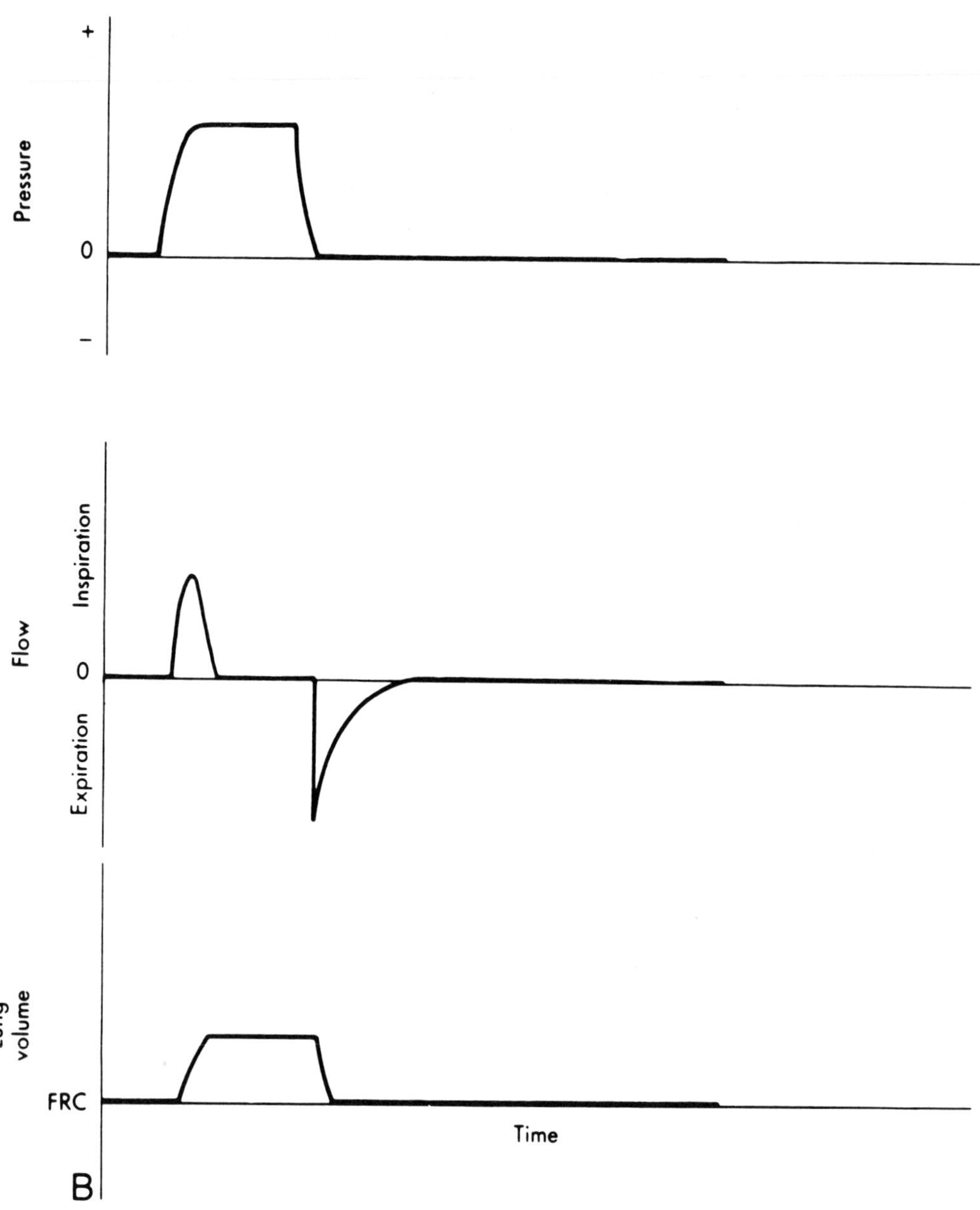

Fig. 2–9 (*Continued*). **(B)** Decreased lung compliance. (*Figure continues*).

pressure driving systems are similar, particularly in the general flow and volume changes that occur with changing patient conditions. A true constant-pressure generator, however, produces the same pressure pattern breath after breath, even when patient conditions vary. A low-pressure drive system may produce the same peak airway pressure each breath (e.g., Puritan-Bennett PR-2), although the pressure pattern or waveform produced can vary substantially. Few pure pressure generators are used in clinical medicine today, although occasionally pediatric ventilators are used so that they produce such a pattern.[1,22–26]

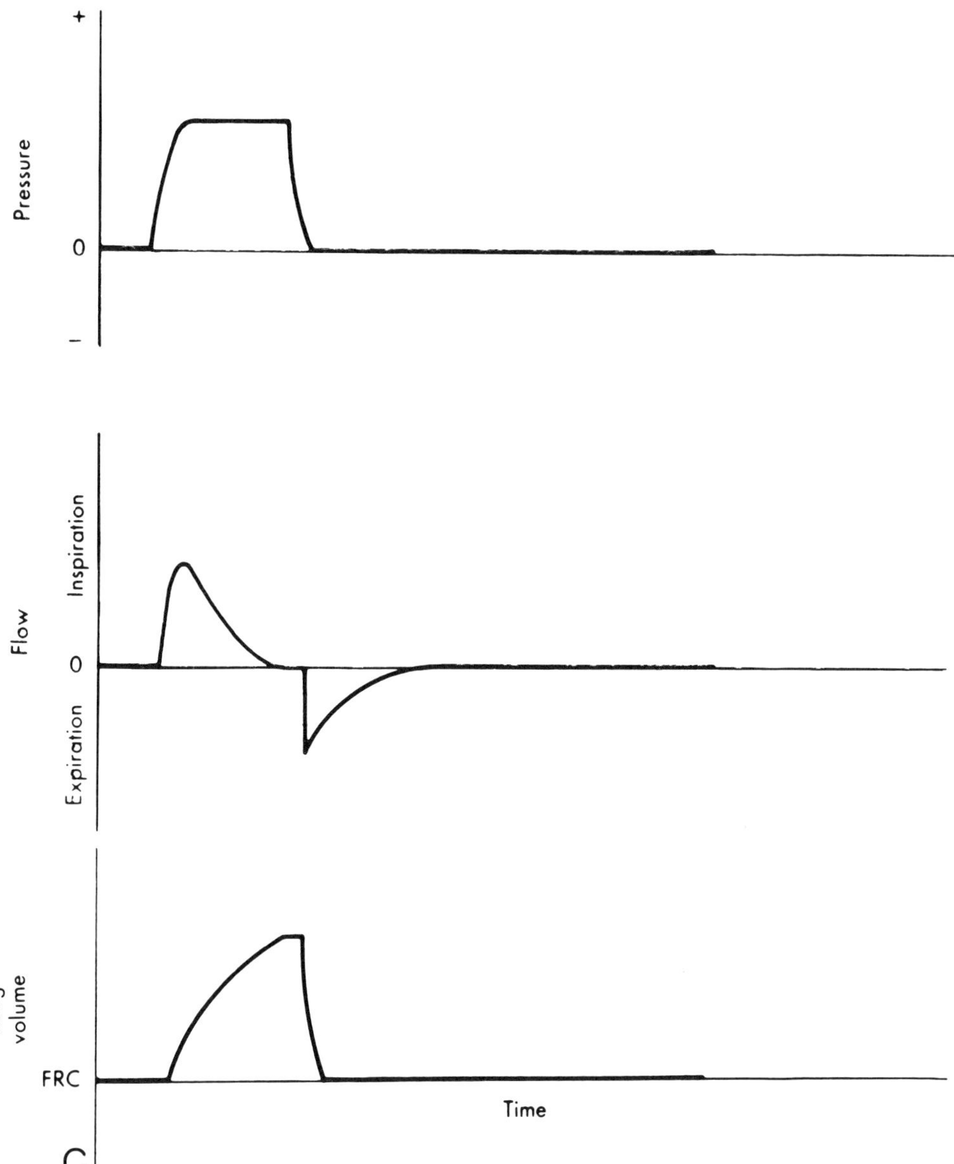

Fig. 2–9 *(Continued)*. **(C)** Increase in airway resistance. A decrease in volume delivery occurs in *B*, whereas in *C* a slowly tapering inspiratory flow is present. (From Spearman et al.,[10] with permission.)

Nonconstant-Pressure Generators

Theoretically, a nonconstant-pressure generator produces a constant *pattern* of pressure from one breath to the next, but the pressure itself is not constant *during* the breath. As an example, the pressure may increase throughout inspiration (nonconstant pressure), but each breath resembles the last in terms of the pressure pattern.[2] Some ventilators approach these operational characteristics, but none can consistently reproduce the same pattern of pressure rise regardless of changing patient conditions; thus none are pure nonconstant-pressure generators.

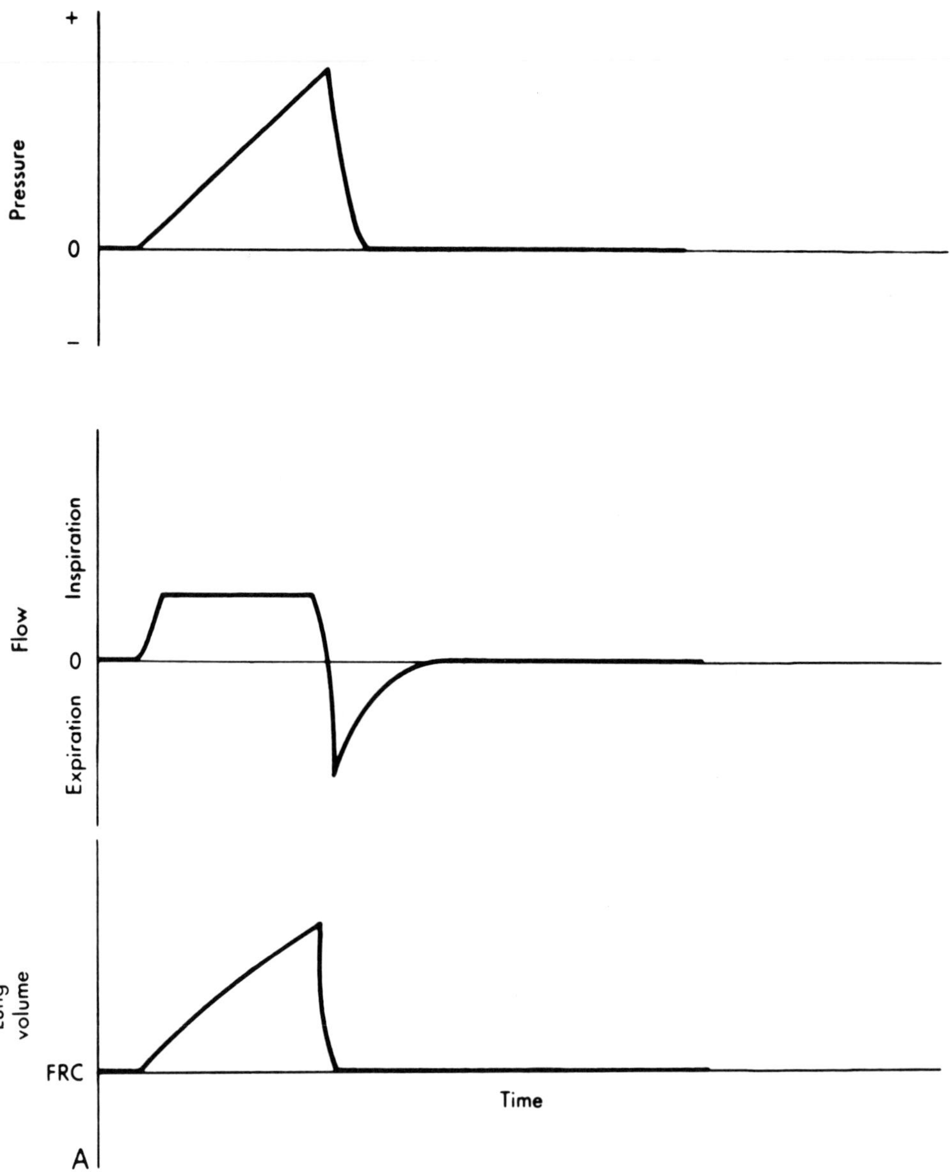

Fig. 2–10. Pressure, flow, and volume waveforms for a constant-flow generator under ''normal'' conditions **(A)** and with decreased compliance. (*Figure continues*).

Flow Generators

Constant-Flow Generators

When a very high pressure is generated within a ventilator, the potential is present for the ventilator to produce a *flow pattern* that is reproducible regardless of changing patient conditions. Such a ventilator is called a *flow generator.*[2] If the actual *flow rate* is the same *during* the breath and the flow *pattern* is the same breath to breath, the ventilator is a constant-flow generator.

Ventilators using high-pressure driving sys-

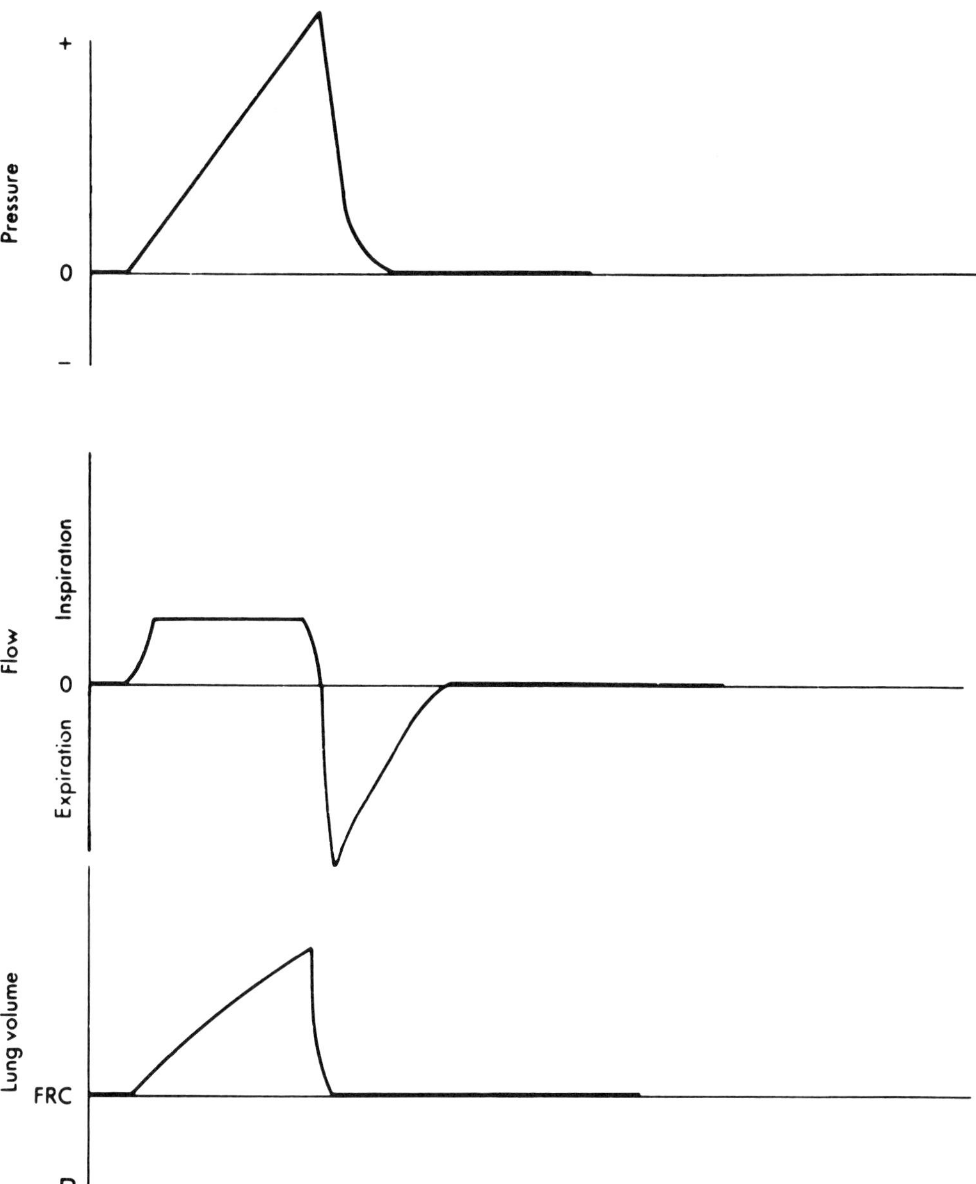

Fig. 2–10 (*Continued*). **(B)** Note that in *B* inspiratory flow remains unchanged whereas inspiratory pressure and expiratory flow increase. Lung volume remains relatively unchanged for the purpose of illustration. (From Spearman et al.,[10] with permission.)

tems with high internal resistance (Fig. 2–5) are constant-flow generators. The driving force is so high that resistance and compliance changes in the ventilator circuit and patient's lungs do not decrease the pressure gradient sufficiently to alter the flow rate during each breath. Figure 2–10 illustrates this point. In Figures 2–10A and 2–10B, inspiratory time is held constant. Note that the flow pattern remains the same, whereas the pressure increases when decreased lung compliance is encountered (Fig. 2–10B). The constant flow pattern during inspiration is commonly referred to as a square wave.

Some ventilators function as constant-flow generators only when inspiratory pressures are relatively low. When high airway pressure is necessary and that pressure approaches the available driving pressure, flow decreases. The Siemens Servo 900 B and Puritan-Bennett MA-1 ventilators have driving pressures equal to or greater than 100 cm H_2O and normally produce a relatively constant flow at typical airway pressures. They are not pure constant-flow generators, as airway pressures close to their driving pressures can be encountered in some clinical situations. The Bourns LS 104–150 piston ventilator and the Monaghan 225/SIMV ventilator are closer to pure constant-flow generators because their driving systems have high force potential.

Nonconstant-Flow Generators

Nonconstant-flow ventilators are exemplified by rotary-driven piston ventilators, producing a sine-wave flow pattern. Because the motor driving the piston can produce a high force, the flow *pattern* produced remains the same in spite of varying patient conditions. Figure 2–11 shows pressure and flow patterns typical of such a ventilator. ''Normal'' conditions are represented by Figure 2–11A, whereas Figures 2–11B and 2–11C illustrate increased airway resistance and decreased compliance, respectively. Although the *pressure* pattern produced is differ-

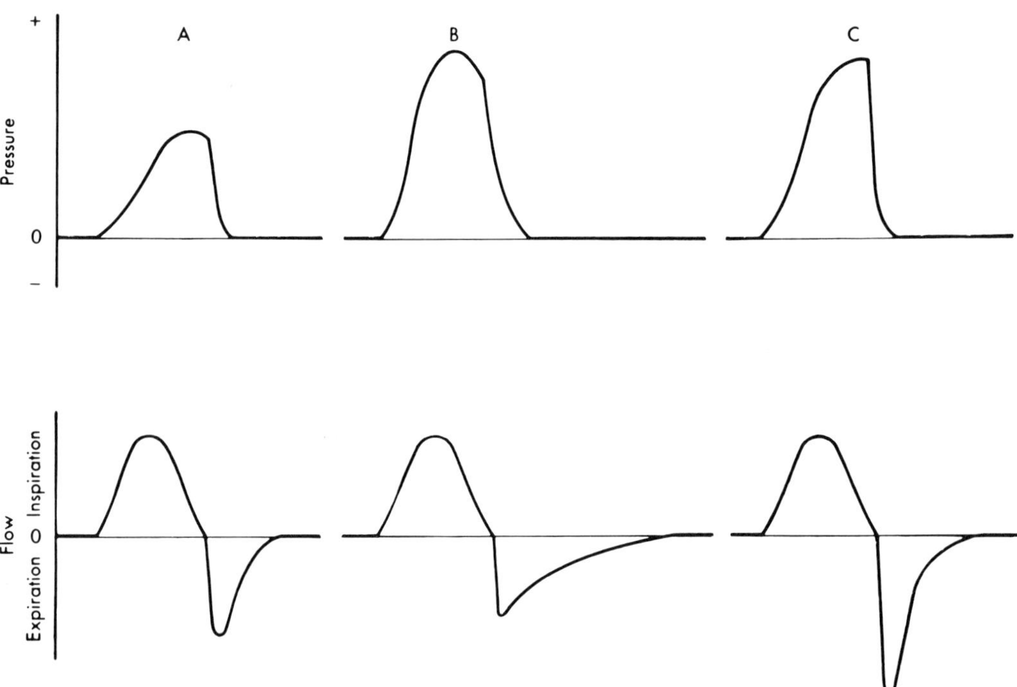

Fig. 2–11. Nonconstant-flow generator (sine-wave type) pressure and flow waveforms. **(A)** ''Normal'' conditions. **(B)** Increased pressure and slow expiratory flow caused by increased airway resistance. **(C)** Increased pressure and expiratory flow caused by a decrease in lung compliance. Note that all inspiratory flow patterns remain the same. (From Spearman et al.,[10] with permission.)

ent for each example, the inspiratory *flow* pattern is the same in all three figures. The Emerson 3-PV and 3-MV ventilators are examples of nonconstant-flow generators.

Ending the Inspiratory Phase

Various terms have been used to indicate the changeover from inspiration to expiration during mechanical ventilation, the most common being *cycle* and *limit*. Neither is fully descriptive, however, because cycle is also used to indicate the changeover from expiration to inspiration, and limit is used to indicate the maximum value for components of the respiratory cycle other than inspiratory time. In this chapter we use the term *cycle* for both the initiation and termination of inspiration, and we distinguish which changeover is occurring. When the term *limit* is used, it refers to a maximal setting or value.

Terminal cycling of the inspiratory phase can be accomplished by *pressure, volume, time, flow,* or a combination of these (see Ch. 15).

Combined Cycling

Many of the ventilators used in critical care units have more than one cycling mechanism available. As an example, a volume-cycled ventilator may use a pressure-cycling feature as a safety backup system. If inspiratory pressure reaches a preselected level before completion of the preselected tidal volume delivery, the pressure-cycling mechanism overrides the volume-cycling one and ends inspiration. This system is employed in the Bennett MA-1 and MA-2 + 2 ventilators.

The BEAR-1 ventilator has a time-cycling mechanism as a secondary backup to its volume-cycling control. The I:E ratio system can end inspiration if it is prolonged beyond one-half the total ventilatory cycle time as set by the rate control.

Inspiratory Limits

As the term *limit* is used here, it infers that some parameter (e.g., pressure or volume) can be set for a maximum allowable value; however, inspiration is not ended or cycled off when that value is reached. As an example, a pressure relief valve can be used to limit pressure during inspiration by allowing the excess gases to vent when the preselected pressure is reached. The pressure is "held" at that level until the breath is volume- or time-cycled off. The Bourns LS 104–150 infant piston ventilator is volume-cycled, yet it has a pressure relief or "pop-off" valve which can limit the pressure during inspiration. Pressure limiting occurs in a similar fashion with Babybird and Babybird-2 ventilators, whereas time is used as the cycling mechanism (see Ch. 15).

Some ventilators are primarily time-cycled but are intended to be used as "volume ventilators." The Servo 900B and 900C ventilators are examples of units that are primarily time-cycled but "attempt" to deliver a consistent volume each breath. If the driving force in these ventilators is inadequate to maintain the necessary flow, volume delivery decreases but inspiratory *time* does not vary. Because this circumstance rarely occurs, these ventilators usually are considered to be volume limited. Regardless of the cycling mechanism used, most ventilators with either tidal volume or minute volume controls available are considered "volume ventilators."

Expiratory Phase Maneuvers

Under normal conditions, expiration is a passive event caused by lung recoil. Expiratory flow is determined by the pressure gradient from the lung to the atmosphere and the resistances to that flow caused by the airways, ventilator tubing, and valving system. Alteration of the expiratory phase has important clinical implications. Three types of expiratory maneuver are described here.

Expiratory Resistance or Retard

Patients with chronic obstructive pulmonary disease (COPD) have been observed to use "pursed lip breathing."[27–29] By so doing, they increase expiratory airway resistance, presumably moving the equal pressure point toward the proximal airway and thereby decreasing air trapping. It is thought that air trapping is relieved by this maneuver, either by its effect on the internal pressure of the flaccid airways or by slowing the respiratory rate.[27,29] Provision of resistance to expiratory air flow during continuous ventilatory support (by decreasing the orifice size through which the patient exhales) mimics this effect. After termination of inspiration, pressure within the airway drops to baseline levels less rapidly when retardation is used than during a typical ventilator breath (Fig. 2–12).

Retardation of expiratory flow can be accomplished by regulating the diameter of the outlet or exhalation valve of the ventilator tubing circuit with an adjustable orifice device or by placing endotracheal tube connectors at the exhalation valve outlet. Some ventilators have an adjustable resistance system (e.g., the Puritan-Bennett MA-1 or the Siemens Servo 900B). The MA-1 control is not calibrated, whereas the Servo 900B adjusts the *maximum* expiratory flow allowed and is calibrated in liters per minute.

All ventilator circuits impose *some* additional resistance to expiratory gas flow compared to normal spontaneous breathing. The amount of resistance is determined primarily by the diameter of the tubing and its connectors, valves, and outlets as well as the length of the tubing. Any continuous flow through the circuit (as occurs with some IMV apparatus) can add additional expiratory resistance as both the continuous flow and the patient's expiratory flow must pass through the same exhalation valve orifice. Excessive intrathoracic pressure can develop during a cough or forced exhalation when the circuit's expiratory resistance is high unless a sensitive pressure relief valve opens abruptly. Intermittent positive-pressure ventilation (IPPV) with added expiratory resistance increases the mean airway and intrathoracic pressures compared to IPPV alone and can *cause* air trapping if the I:E ratio and/or respiratory rate is increased.

Negative End-Expiratory Pressure

Negative end-expiratory pressure (NEEP) applies a subatmospheric pressure to the airway during the expiratory phase. This "negative" pressure is seen at end-expiration (Fig. 2–13). NEEP has been suggested to reduce the mean airway and intrathoracic pressures during positive-pressure mechanical ventilation, thereby augmenting venous return to the right heart.[2]

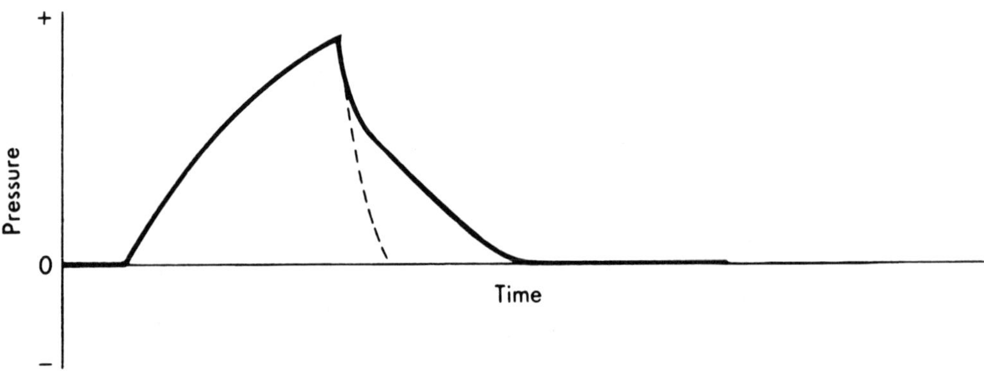

Fig. 2–12. Pressure waveform typical of increased expiratory resistance (retard). Dotted line shows expiratory pattern of system without increased resistance for comparison. (From Spearman et al.,[10] with permission.)

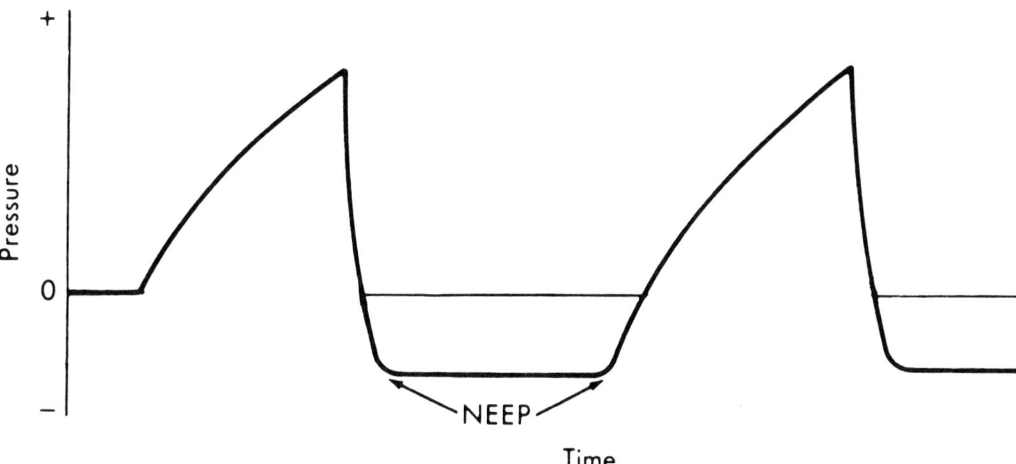

Fig. 2–13. Pressure waveform typical of IPPV with NEEP. (From Spearman et al.,[10] with permission.)

Excessive NEEP can promote airway collapse in both normal and emphysematous patients, and these side effects tend to negate its purported benefits.

Subatmospheric pressure at the airway during exhalation can be generated by entraining air through the exhalation valve from the expiratory side of the ventilator circuit. Typically, a Venturi or similar device is employed.[1] An increase in flow to the jet of the Venturi device is associated with increased entrainment of gas out of the circuit and lowering of airway pressure. Systems for applying NEEP are available for or present in the Bird Mark 8, the Puritan-Bennett MA-1, and the Engström 300 series ventilators.

Positive End-Expiratory Pressure

PEEP maintains a positive airway pressure during expiration. It can be used during both mechanical ventilation and spontaneous breathing. When combined with assist or control modes, it is sometimes called mechanical ventilation with PEEP (MV/PEEP), IPPV/PEEP or continuous positive-pressure ventilation (CPPV).[30–32] When spontaneous breathing uses positive expiratory pressure, various terms are used.[31] Continuous positive-pressure breathing (CPPB) and continuous positive airway pressure (CPAP) describe breathing in which the positive pressures during inspiration and expiration are similar.[28,31,32] (Inspiratory and expiratory pressures fluctuate about the same amount as during spontaneous breathing without a positive-pressure baseline.) When PEEP is applied following a spontaneous peak inspiratory pressure at or below atmospheric pressure, the terms *spontaneous PEEP* (sPEEP) and *expiratory positive airway pressure* (EPAP) have been used.[31,33–36] Mechanical ventilation also can be combined with these spontaneous breathing modes resulting in IMV/CPAP or IMV/sPEEP.[8,10] Pressure waveforms depicting these techniques are illustrated in Figure 2–14.

Expiratory positive pressure can be applied by a variety of devices, some of which are presented here[4,37,38] (see Ch. 15).

Underwater Column

A simple method directs the exhaled gases under water (Fig. 2–15). After bubbling through the water, the gases are vented to the atmosphere. The PEEP level is adjusted by changing the height of the water above the port of gas entry. Raising the water height increases the pressure at and below which further exhalation of gas does not occur. Hence the exhaled volume

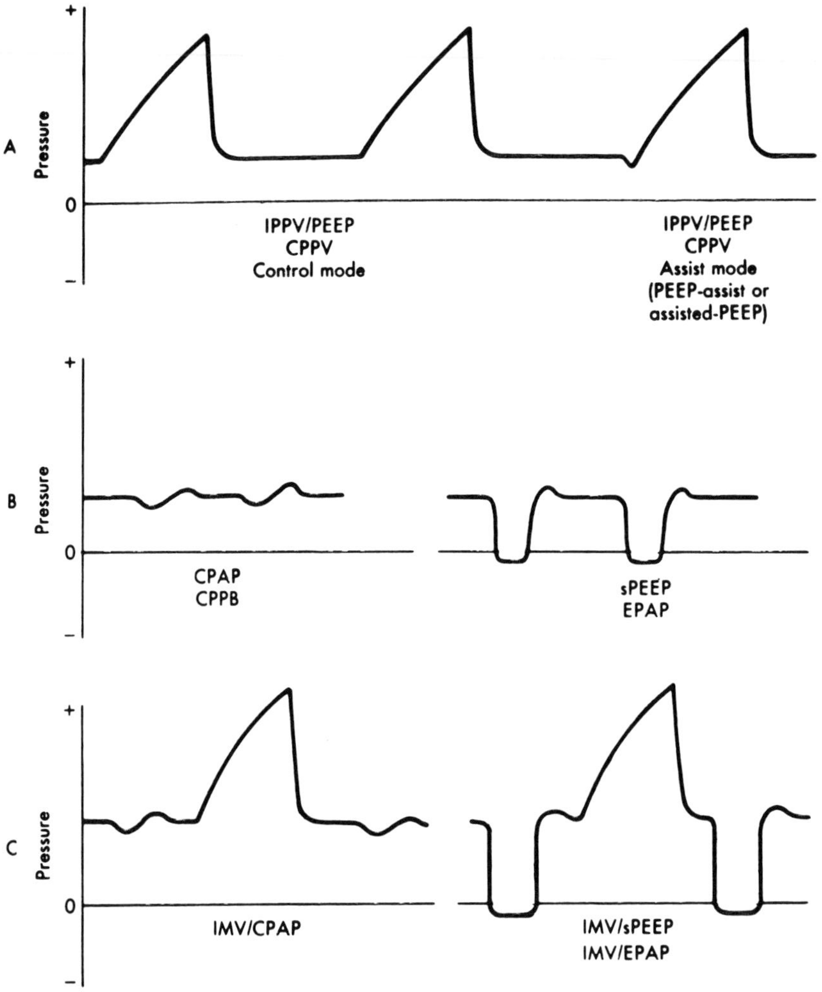

Fig. 2–14. Pressure waveforms and commonly used terminology for various techniques of ventilatory support. PEEP or CPAP is present in each illustration. (From Spearman et al.,[10] with permission.)

decreases, and this gas is "trapped" within the patient circuit and lungs.

If the entry and exit ports on the water column are not restrictive, the PEEP device will have little flow resistance. Therefore, although a positive pressure is present at end-expiration, little or no expiratory flow resistance (or retard) is encountered. If the entry or exit ports are small in diameter, resistance to flow is present and the pressure after a mechanical inspiration takes longer to return to the baseline PEEP level. This flow dependency of airway pressure causes the mean airway pressure to be higher than if the same PEEP level is applied with a resistance-free water column.

Water-Weighted Diaphragm

The J. H. Emerson Co. produces a water column PEEP device which does not require the exhaled gases to bubble through the water (see Ch. 15). Instead, the water is separated from the patient's airway by a flexible dia-

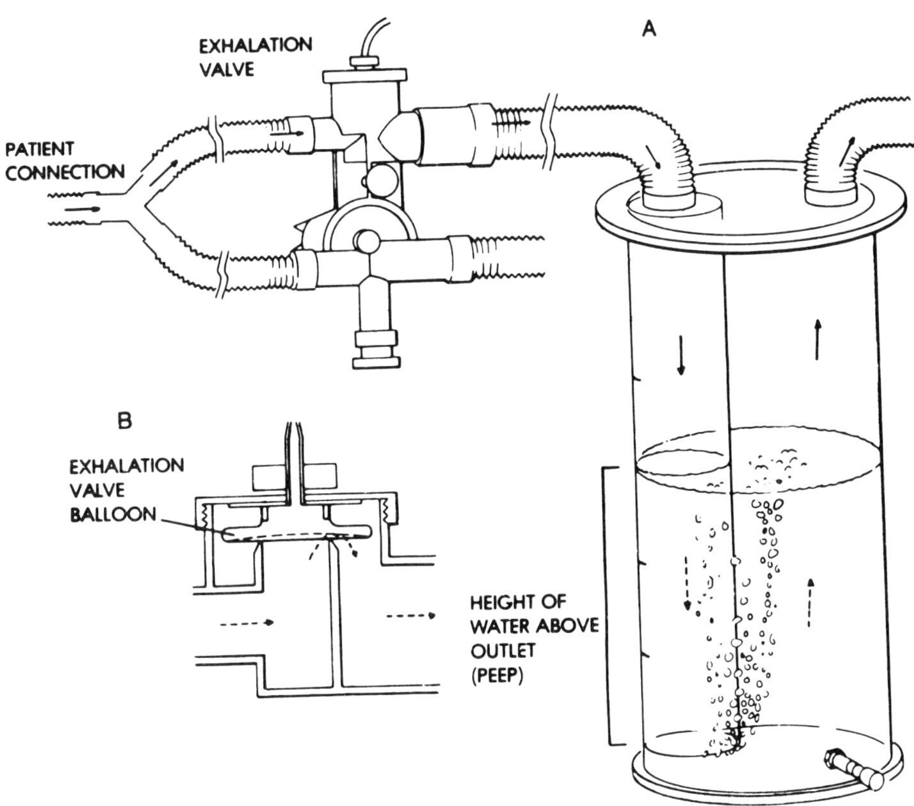

Fig. 2–15. Water column PEEP device. **(A)** Typical ventilator circuit. **(B)** Detail of the exhalation valve balloon. Flexible balloon moves off the seat (dotted lines), allowing exhaled gas to pass on to the water column.

phragm. The diaphragm seat is on the exhalation port which connects to the patient circuit by a large-bore tube. Airway pressure below the diaphragm must be greater than the hydrostatic force exerted by the water column for gas to move the diaphragm off the seat and vent to the atmosphere. When gas and water forces are equal, the diaphragm seals the exhalation port and further exhalation is prevented. The height of the water column regulates the PEEP level.

This device is relatively free of resistance under moderate flow rate conditions. The Emerson 3-PV and 3-MV ventilators apply positive pressure *above* the water level in the valve during mechanical inspiration, forcing the diaphragm to remain seated. Thus the unit functions as a combination exhalation/PEEP valve.

Venturi PEEP Valve

Some ventilators incorporate a Venturi tube to apply PEEP.[1] One method applies the output pressure of the Venturi tube against a one-way valve through which the patient's exhaled air must pass. A high-pressure gas source drives the jet of the Venturi. More pressure applied to the jet results in more pressure exerted against the one-way valve; therefore, more pressure is required to open the valve during exhalation. When the pressure on the patient side of the one way valve exceeds the opposing Venturi pressure, exhaled air moves through the valve and Venturi tube and out through open ports to the atmosphere.

The flow dependence of this type of Venturi

PEEP valve is primarily a function of the one-way valve resistance and the Venturi tube, which is often the narrowest portion of the system. If the one-way valve has a low resistance and the passages for gas flow are relatively wide, the flow-dependent resistance will be low. Two infant ventilators, the Bourns LS 104–150 and BP 200, use this type of Venturi PEEP device.

Spring-Loaded Disk Valve

A spring-loaded valve used for pressure limiting can also be used to create PEEP (Fig. 2–16). An adjustable spring provides tension (force) against a disk which rests on the exhalation port, sealing it from the atmosphere. Expiratory gas pressure opposes the spring tension on the disk. When gas pressure is greater than the spring tension, the disk moves away from its port and the gas vents to the atmosphere. When the gas pressure equals the force of the spring, the disk seals the port and prevents further egress. The PEEP level is raised by compressing the spring, which increases its force on the disk.[38]

Some spring-loaded valves also cause significant expiratory resistance, whereas others offer little resistance to flow.[4,38] The final effect is related primarily to the length of the spring and its movement and the area of the opening for gas flow[4,39] (see Ch. 15).

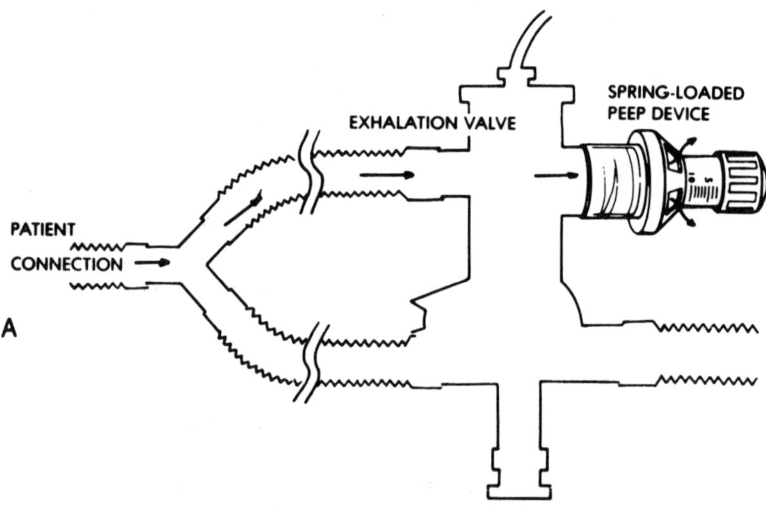

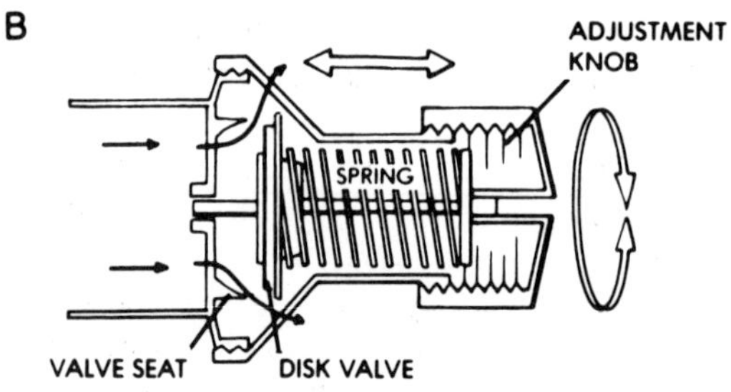

Fig. 2–16. Spring-loaded disk valve. **(A)** Typical ventilator circuit. Arrows shown direction of expiratory flow. **(B)** Detail of spring-loaded valve. See text for description.

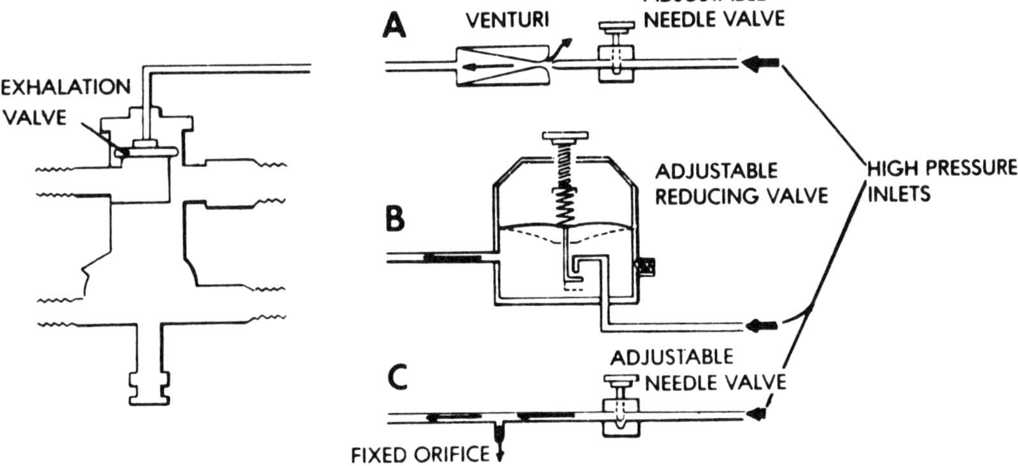

Fig. 2–17. "Trapped" pressure in exhalation valve balloon can be used to generate PEEP in the patient circuit. **(A–C)** Three ways gas pressure within the balloon is controlled. See text for descriptions.

Pressurized Exhalation Balloon Valve

Figure 2–17 shows examples of an exhalation balloon valve PEEP system with different methods of applying pressure within the balloon. In Figure 2–17A a small Venturi applies its output pressure to the balloon. As gas flow to the Venturi jet is increased, balloon pressure also increases. In Figure 2–17B, an adjustable reducing valve applies pressure to the balloon. Greater pressure from the reducing valve results in greater pressure within the balloon. In Figure 2–17C, a system with adjustable flow against a fixed restriction pressurizes the balloon. As flow is increased, a pressure increase results as the resistance of the fixed orifice is increased.

In all three examples, the pressure in the balloon opposes pressure in the patient circuit. Because the area of the balloon applying pressure against the gas outlet is greater than the area below the valve, the pressure within the balloon is less than that within the patient circuit.[38] Pressure in the patient circuit, acting against a smaller area, must exceed the lower pressure in the balloon, which acts on a larger area in order for gas to flow to the atmosphere. These systems can have flow resistance if the opening area for gas flow is small or if the balloon cannot easily deflate.

Systems such as these are the basis of the PEEP mechanisms in several ventilators.[1,2] Venturi pressure applied to an exhalation balloon is used in the BEAR-2 and Puritan-Bennett MA-2 ventilators. The Puritan-Bennett MA-1 has an optional PEEP attachment that uses a reducing valve to apply PEEP.[1] Flow adjustment against a fixed leak to regulate pressure within the exhalation balloon is the mechanism used by the Monaghan 225/SIMV ventilator.[1]

General Characteristics of Ventilation Methods

In our discussion thus far, several methods of ventilatory support have been suggested. This section discusses some general technical and clinical differences for the most common differences for the most common types of positive-pressure ventilation: pressure-cycled, volume-cycled, time-cycled with a volume limit, and time-cycled with a pressure limit.

Pressure-Cycled Ventilation

Pressure-cycled ventilators terminate the inspiratory phase when a preset pressure is reached, regardless of the volume delivered. Therefore, such ventilators are susceptible to changes in compliance and air flow resistance.[3,40,41] As lung compliance decreases or flow resistance increases, they reach their set pressures prematurely and the delivered volume decreases. Under these circumstances, overall hypoventilation may result during control mode ventilation. During assist mode ventilation, patients may respond to the lower tidal volumes by increasing respiratory rate, which increases the I:E ratio and elevates the mean airway pressure.

Raising the peak pressure can restore the tidal volume within the individual ventilator's limitations. However, as compliance and/or resistance to air flow improve, delivered volumes may now increase excessively, leading to hyperventilation and respiratory alkalosis. This potential variation in ventilation makes monitoring of these variables imperative when pressure-cycled ventilation is provided to critically ill patients.

Many patients can be successfully ventilated with pressure-cycled ventilators when adequate supervision and monitoring by a knowledgeable clinician are provided. Patients with normal lungs who receive ventilatory support for short periods postoperatively, patients with relatively stable COPD, and patients weaning from controlled ventilation can be adequately supported by pressure-cycled ventilators with proper management.

Pressure-cycled ventilators can sometimes provide better leak compensation than volume-cycled ventilators.[3] If the leak is not great enough to prevent cycling, these units can provide sufficient volume and flow to "ventilate" both the leak and the patient. In contrast, similar leakage in a volume-preset ventilator decreases the amount of gas received by the patient.[3] Naturally, any such leak should be eliminated, but occasionally this is not possible. Should the leak be large enough to prevent pressure-cycling, a time-cycling mechanism may be needed to terminate inspiration (e.g., Bennett PR-2). Some ventilators (e.g., the Bird Mark 14, the Bird ventilator, and the Bennett PR-2) have special controls which provide additional flow to compensate for the leak.

Generally, pressure-cycled ventilators have peak flows of 80 to 100 L/min and peak pressures of 50 to 60 cm H_2O, and are therefore somewhat limited in their capabilities. Pneumatic oxygen controllers or blenders can be adapted to provide control of delivered oxygen. PEEP and CPAP systems generally can be applied only with special adaptations.[38]

Ventilators using low-pressure drive systems (Venturi or reducing valves described earlier in the chapter) produce a flow pattern that responds to backpressure within the patient system.[42] The decreasing flow rate tends to decrease turbulence, and we have observed repeatedly that specific volumes can be delivered with such ventilators at a lower peak airway pressure in postoperative patients than when the same volume is delivered as a square-wave flow pattern from a volume ventilator.

Most pressure-cycled ventilators (e.g., the Bird Mark series) are pneumatically powered and therefore useful as backup devices to electrically powered volume-cycled or time-cycled ventilators in intensive care units. They are also used for ground and air transport systems, primarily because of their small size and light weight. Such uses require that respiratory therapists, physicians, and nurses be thoroughly familiar with their function and clinical application.

Volume-Cycled Ventilation

Volume-cycled ventilators are the primary types used in critical care units today. Many patients receiving ventilatory support undergo frequent and often rapid changes in lung compliance or airway resistance. Most clinicians believe that volume-cycled ventilators are capable of maintaining more constant ventilation under these circumstances when compared to pressure-cycled ventilators.[3,40,41,43–45] As compliance or resistance worsens, the driving pressure needed to deliver the volume increases automatically. If the pressure reaches a predetermined safety limit, inspiration is terminated by a secondary pressure cycling mechanism or the excess (non-delivered) volume vents to the ambient level through a relief valve, preventing any additional increase of pressure. Modern volume-cycled ventilators are usually capable of high airway pressures (100 to 150 cm H_2O).[1,2]

Volume-cycled ventilators do not deliver constant tidal volumes under all conditions. The inspiratory positive pressure acts on the patient circuit and the ventilator's internal pneumatic system. Gas is compressed by this pressure whereas flexible tubing and other components expand. Thus, part of the preset volume (compressible volume) is lost to the patient because it never reaches the airway.

The volume not received by the patient depends on the pressure generated and the compliance of the system. If the components in which compression occurs are fairly stiff or rigid, the amount of gas compressed is approximately 1 ml/cm H_2O for each liter of available space. If a ventilator has a rigid delivery system of 4 L, 4 ml gas/cm H_2O pressure would be compressed during inspiration. This factor, called the *compressibility factor*, is 4 ml/cm H_2O in this example. If the system is somewhat distensible under pressure, the factor is greater (4.5 or 5 ml/cm H_2O). This value is sometimes termed the *compliance factor* but is generally interchangeable with the compressibility factor.

The significance of the compressed volume during "volume" ventilation depends on a variety of factors, including the preset tidal volume compared with the compressibility factor and the extent of compliance and resistance changes (Fig. 2–18). If the compressibility factor is large

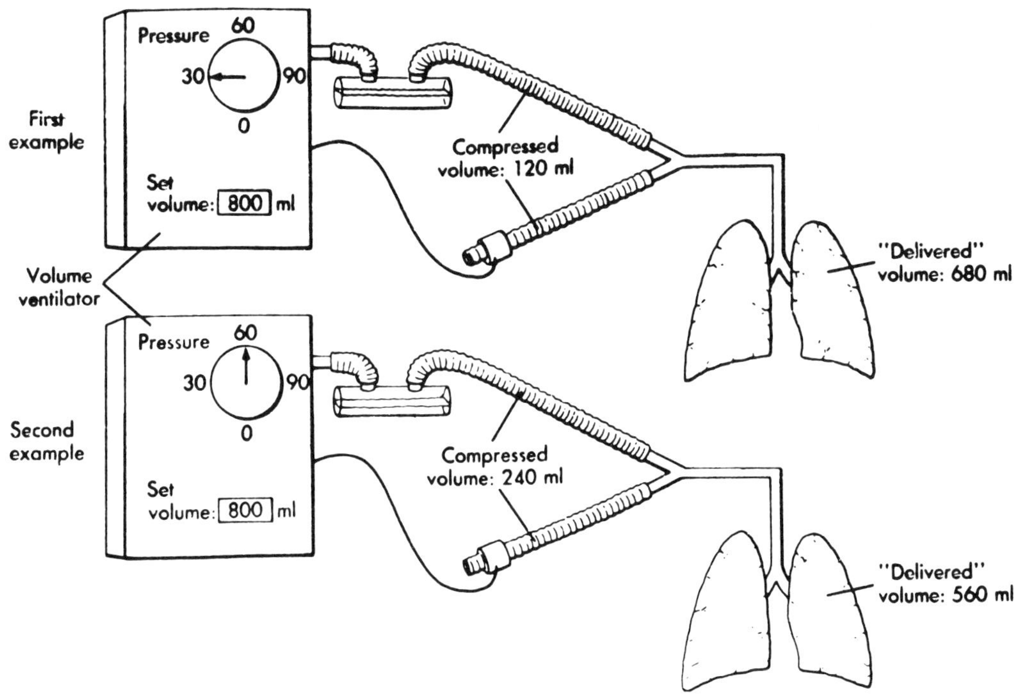

Fig. 2–18. Comparison of tidal volume delivery to a patient when different end-inspiratory pressures occur during volume-cycled ventilation. The first example with a 30-cm H_2O peak pressure results in 680 ml received out of a preset volume of 800 ml. In the second example, a 60-cm H_2O peak pressure results in only 560 ml received. (From Spearman et al.,[10] with permission.)

and small tidal volumes are selected, the ventilator tends to function more like a pressure ventilator in terms of volume delivery. As an example, if the factor is 5 ml/cm H_2O and the tidal volume is 300 ml, this entire amount could be compressed within the system if 60 cm H_2O inflation pressure was applied. The patient would not be ventilated. If end-inspiratory pressure was only 20 cm H_2O, the compressed volume would be one-third the set volume ($5 \times 20 = 100$ ml compressed), whereas a 40-cm H_2O pressure would cause 200 ml of the set volume to be lost, with a resultant substantial reduction of the patient's ventilation. These large decreases in patient-delivered tidal volume are similar to the changes in volume which might be experienced when a pressure-cycled ventilator is used under similar conditions.

The volume in which gas may be compressed is limited primarily to external tubing circuits in some ventilators, whereas others have significant *internal* volume as well.[4,46,47] This fact presents the clinician with a practical problem in volume measurement. Gas collected at a ventilator's exhalation valve is a mixture of that which entered the patient's airway and that compressed primarily in the *external* tubing circuit. (Generally the gas compressed in an internal compartment—bellows or piston cylinder—does not vent through the exhalation valve. Instead, it simply reexpands as that compartment refills immediately after end-inspiration and remains inside the ventilator.)

A simplified ventilator with both internal and external spaces for compressible volumes is illustrated in Fig. 2–19. The set tidal volume, provided by the excursion of the bellows, is 800 ml. Because this bellows begins the inspiratory phase in its full position and empties only part of its volume during the breath, a significant amount of space is available to compress gas within the bellows at end-inspiration. This end-inspiratory internal volume is 2 L, providing a compressibility factor of about 2 ml/cm H_2O. The tubing circuit is the external source of compressible volume and in Figure 2–19 contains 3 L, yielding a compressibility factor of 3 ml/cm H_2O. Thus, a total of 5 ml/cm H_2O is compressed during inspiration and is not delivered to the patient. However, only the 3 ml/cm H_2O compressed in the external circuit is collected with the patient's exhaled gas because the internal system returns to atmospheric pressure as the bellows refills. The one-way valve near the

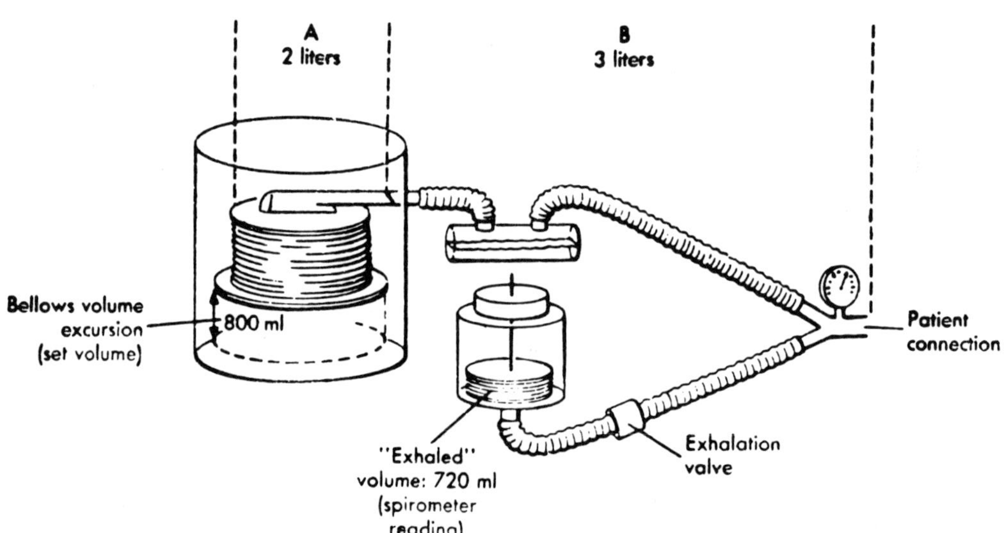

Fig. 2–19. Internal compressed volume **(A)** and tubing circuit compressed volume **(B)** reduce the tidal volume received by a patient during volume-cycled ventilation. Gases compressed internally are not measured on a spirometer. See text for further description of this example. (From Spearman et al.,[10] with permission.)

bellows outlet closes, and the "trapped" gases in the bellows simply reexpand.

If end-inspiratory pressure is 40 cm H_2O, 80 ml is compressed internally (2 × 40), 120 ml is compressed externally (3 × 40), and the patient receives the remaining 600 ml. Only the 120-ml and 600-ml volumes are collected in the spirometer at the exhalation valve, whereas the 80-ml volume remains in the bellows. The spirometer reading is 720 ml, which differs from the set volume of 800 ml. To calculate what portion of the exhaled gas was received by the patient, 3 ml/cm H_2O is subtracted from the *collected* volume recorded by the spirometer. To determine what the patient received compared with the *set* volume of 800 ml, the *total compressibility factor* of 5 ml/cm H_2O is used (800 ml set − 200 ml compressed both internally and externally = 600 ml). Using the *total* factor with the *spirometer* reading *underestimates* the volume received by the patient.

Time-Cycled Ventilation

Time-cycled ventilators end the inspiratory phase once a preset time has passed and manifest relative disregard for airway pressure or volume. However, most time-cycled ventilators are commonly used so that they are also pressure- or volume-limited.

Time-Cycled, Volume-Limited Ventilation

When a time-cycled ventilator is a constant- or nonconstant-flow generator, the volume is also controlled. With a constant-flow generator, the relationship is expressed as

$$\text{Volume (liters)} = \frac{\text{inspiratory time (seconds)} \times \text{flow rate (LPM)}}{60} \quad (1)$$

To use such a ventilator when the desired tidal volume and inspiratory time are known, the necessary flow rate can be found through rearrangement of Eq. (1):

$$\text{Flow rate (LPM) needed} = \frac{\text{desired volume1(liters)}}{\text{inspiratory time (seconds)}} \times 60 \quad (2)$$

Nonconstant-flow generators that are time-cycled produce the same flow *pattern* during the same interval each breath; therefore, a consistent tidal volume results. The most common ventilators of this type are the piston-driven, time-cycled ventilators (e.g., the Emerson 3-PV and 3-MV units). In these devices, the piston stroke establishes the volume, and the rotary drive and inspiratory time setting generate the flow pattern and flow rate, respectively, for that volume. In both examples, inspiration ends after passage of a preselected time interval, even though tidal volume remains constant from one breath to the next. Such ventilators are referred to as time-cycled and volume-limited, and have limitations of volume delivery similar to those described for volume-cycled ventilators. Flow and pressure waveforms for time-cycled, volume-limited ventilators are similar to those shown in Figures 2–10 and 2–11.

Time-Cycled, Pressure-Limited Ventilation

When a pressure relief valve is used to limit the maximum pressure during a time-cycled breath, both flow and volume delivery can vary with changes in the patient's airway resistance and compliance. This pattern is commonly employed with infant ventilators.[1,23,24] In the Babybird-2 and Bear Cub BP-200 ventilators, a flow of gas enters the patient's circuit at all times. Periodically, an expiratory valve is closed and the continuous flow is diverted, under pressure, into the patient's airway. If the pressure limit is reached before inspiratory time is over, some or all of the flow begins to vent through the relief valve, and pressure holds constant for the remainder of the breath.

The volume received by the patient is related primarily to two factors as long as lung pressure equilibrates with the ventilator pressure limit during inspiration: (1) applied pressure, and (2) the patient's lung-thorax compliance. If a peak pressure 30 cm H_2O above PEEP is applied during inspiration and equilibrates with alveolar pressure, then 30 times the patient's compliance equals the volume received. As an example, if the patient's compliance is 1.5 ml/cm H_2O, a 30-cm H_2O pressure results in a tidal volume of 45 ml ($1.5 \times 30 = 45$). Should this compliance value change to 2 ml/cm H_2O, the patient's volume would increase to 60 ml for the same 30-cm H_2O pressure. If the applied pressure does not equilibrate in the alveoli—because of excessive airway resistance, inadequate inspiratory time, or both—the volume may be quite variable.

Examples of time-cycled, pressure-limited ventilation under changing patient conditions are shown in Figure 2–20. In all three examples, sufficient time is allowed for equilibration of

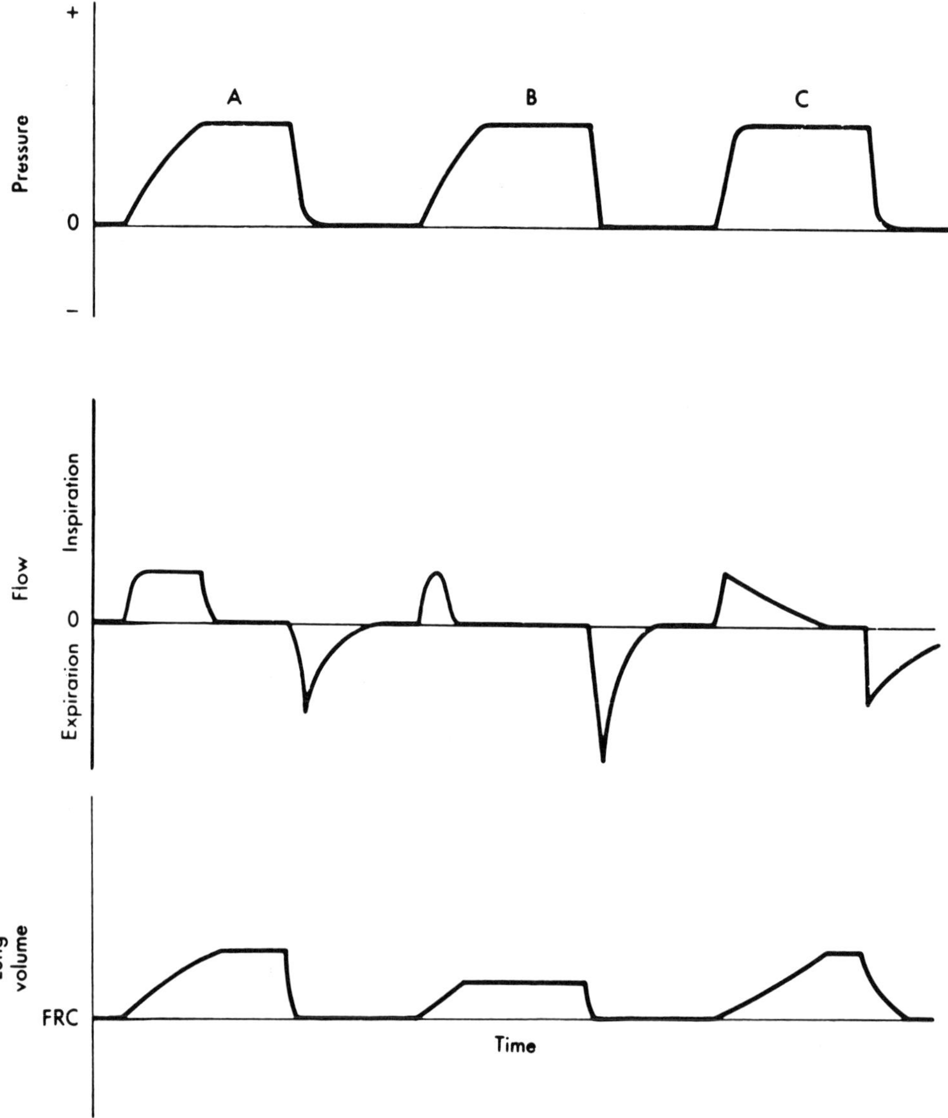

Fig. 2–20. Pressure, flow, and volume waveforms for time-cycled, pressure-limited ventilation during different patient conditions. **(A)** Normal. **(B)** Reduced compliance. **(C)** Increased airway resistance. See text for descriptions. (From Spearman et al.,[10] with permission.)

the applied pressure within the lung. Note that the inspiratory time and pressure limit are the same in each example. The period of zero flow and flattening of the volume curve indicate that pressure in the lung equals the pressure limit applied. Relatively normal conditions are illustrated in Figure 2–20A, whereas a decreased volume delivery results from reduced compliance in Figure 2–20B. The same volume delivery as in Figure 2–20A requires more time in Figure 2–30C because of an increase in airway resistance.

FUNCTIONAL DESIGNS OF OTHER VENTILATOR FEATURES AND SYSTEMS

Air-Oxygen Blending Systems

Most modern ventilators used in critical care can be connected to an oxygen blending system or have one as an integral component part. In general, these systems can be categorized into two types: (1) those requiring both pressurized oxygen and air, and (2) those requiring only pressurized oxygen.

Pressurized Oxygen and Air Blenders

Pressurized oxygen and air blenders generally require inputs from 40 to 50 psig oxygen and air sources. These gas pressures are then either reduced and matched at a lower pressure (e.g., 10 to 12 psig), or the higher of the two pressures is reduced to match the lower pressure (Fig. 2–21). Air and oxygen at equal pressures are then connected to a *proportioning* valve with a single outlet for the blended gases. Because the pressures entering the proportioning valve are equal and the outlet pressure is the same as well, the pressure gradient across this valve is the same for each gas. The *amount* of each

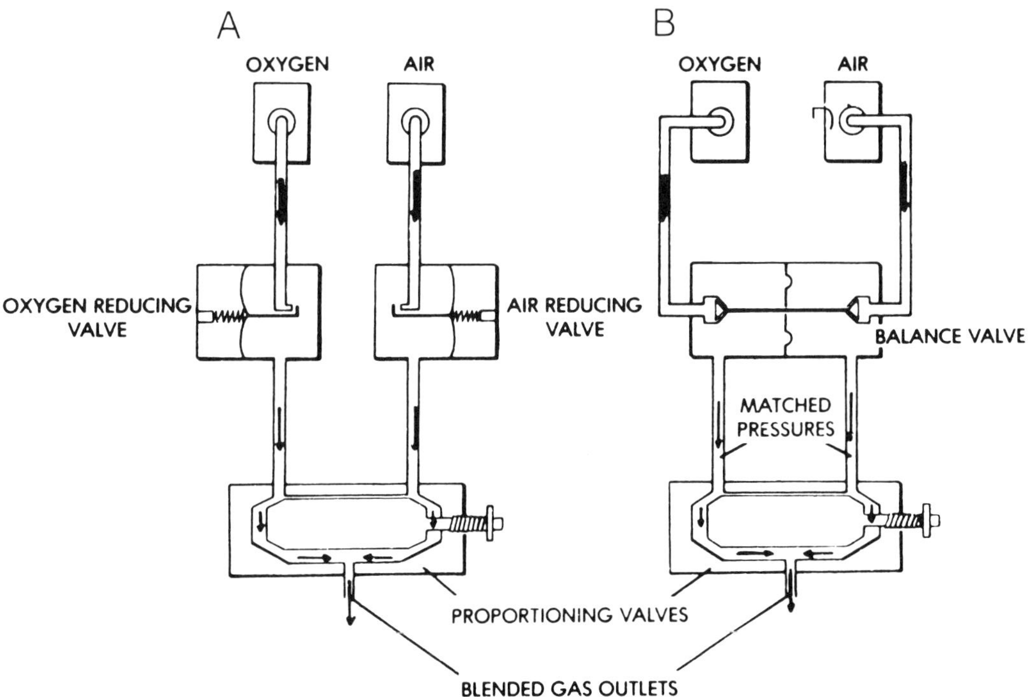

Fig. 2–21. Oxygen blending systems requiring pressurized oxygen and air sources. **(A)** Separate reducing valves set for identical pressures are used to lower oxygen and air pressures proximal to the proportioning valve. **(B)** Both gases are connected to a balance valve, which reduces the higher gas pressure to match the lower pressure proximal to the proportional valve.

gas that passes through the valve is *proportional* to the orifice size for each gas. The valve is constructed so that one side is opened *proportionately* as the other side closes during rotation of the selection knob. When the opening for air is equal to the opening for oxygen (and the pressure gradient across the valve is equal for each gas), the mixture will contain approximately 60 percent oxygen (half the gas is air containing 20.9 percent oxygen and the other half contains 100 percent oxygen). If total occlusion of both sides is possible, concentrations of oxygen from 20.9 percent to 100 percent will be available.

The BEAR-2 and BEAR-CUB ventilators use the system in which compressed air and oxygen are reduced and matched (Fig. 2–21A), whereas the Bird oxygen blender and Puritan-Bennett AO-1 mixer are examples of higher-pressure types which match the higher input pressure to the lower input pressure[1] (Fig. 2–21B).

Pressurized Oxygen Only Blending Systems

Some ventilators require only pressurized oxygen. In these systems oxygen pressure is reduced to nearly atmospheric level. The reduced pressure oxygen and a source of filtered room air for blending then refill the delivery system (Fig. 2–22). A proportioning valve is used to blend air and oxygen. However, the pressure gradient across the valve is from nearly atmospheric pressure for the air and oxygen inlets to a few centimeters of H_2O below atmospheric

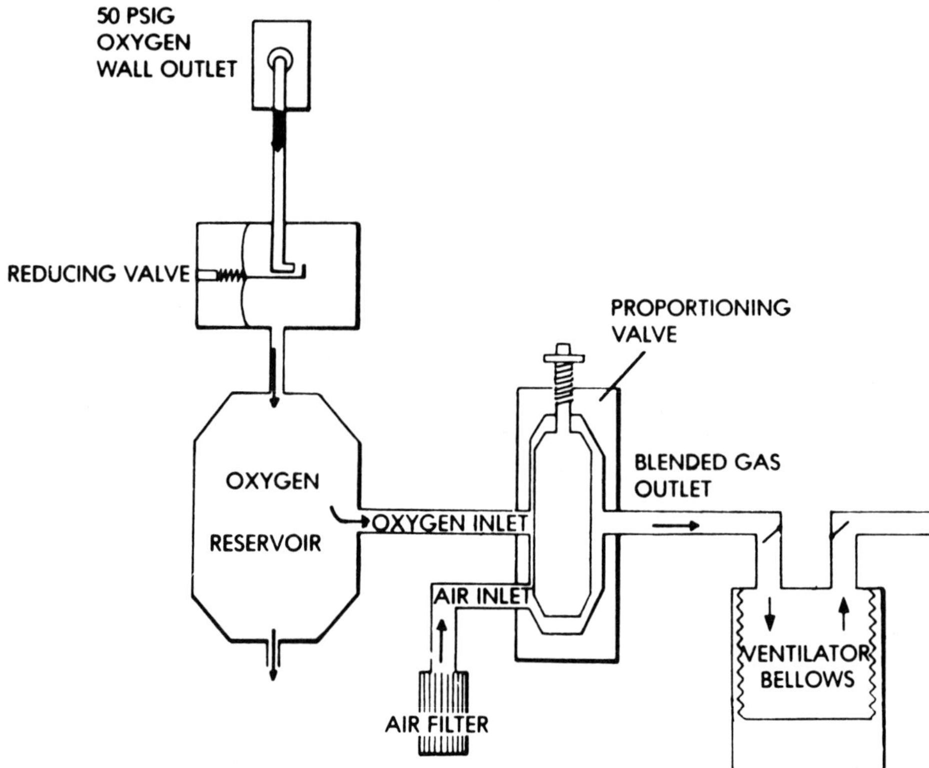

Fig. 2–22. Pressurized oxygen blending system. Oxygen is reduced to near atmospheric pressure in the reservoir. Air and oxygen inlets to the proportioning valve are both at atmospheric pressure. Gas is "pulled" across the valve as the bellows fall during refill.

pressure within the delivery system during its refilling phase. Oxygen blending systems such as these are used in the Puritan-Bennett MA-1 and MA-2 ventilators and the Ohio CCV-2, SIMV ventilator.[1]

Venturi systems using entrainment of room air to mix with 100 percent oxygen have been used; however, these systems are susceptible to backpressure, which causes a decrease in air entrainment and an increase in oxygen concentration.[1,7] If a Venturi system is used to premix oxygen and air in a reservoir system, and the Venturi itself is not exposed to inspiratory positive pressure, reasonably accurate blending can occur. Very early models of the Puritan-Bennett MA-1 used such a system, as did the previously produced Ohio 560.[1]

Various alarms are available for the blenders. Some monitor only pressures within the systems, whereas others use oxygen analyzers to measure oxygen concentration. Some blending systems partially or totally stop supplying gas when one input source fails, whereas others switch entirely over to the remaining gas source regardless of the concentration set on the proportioning valve. Clinicians must be thoroughly familiar with the oxygen system being used so that they can anticipate and respond appropriately in cases of failure.

Humidification Systems

Normally, when the upper airway is intact, inspired air is warmed to near body temperature and is nearly saturated with water vapor by the time it reaches the level of the carina.[48,49] When endotracheal or tracheostomy tubes are used to provide mechanical ventilation, the natural warming and moisturizing functions of the nose, mouth, and trachea are bypassed. Nevertheless, the alveolar air is saturated with water vapor at body temperature even when dry air is inspired. The water deficit of inspired air and the heat needed to warm this air must come from the mucosal surfaces below the artificial airway. Adverse effects of such breathing on mucociliary clearance are well known.[4,14,39,43,45,47]

To avoid this "added burden" on the respiratory tract, heated humidification systems should be used whenever artificial airways are used. In general, they are capable of providing saturated gas over a wide range of temperatures in their simulation of the upper airway functions of heat and moisture control.

The assumption that one must provide gases at 100 percent relative humidity and body temperature (so-called "body humidity") when patients are intubated may be invalid. Some controversy exists concerning the optimal range for humidity and temperature for such patients. Research on anesthetized animals and patients presents conflicting data for lung tissue and surfactant changes, mucous flow, and pulmonary complications at various levels of temperature and humidity.[48–52] When all heat and humidity requirements are supplied externally, natural heat and water vapor losses from the airway are stopped. The clinical significance of this situation is not well understood at present. However, at 50 to 70 percent body humidity mucociliary clearance of secretions is impaired. This function improves when temperatures of 32 to 42°C with 33 mg/L of water vapor are used. Because body humidity equals about 44 mg/L at 37°C, 33 mg/L provides 75 percent body humidity.

Delivered gas for intubated patients should be kept at 80 to 100 percent relative humidity at temperatures of 32 to 37°C (90 to 99°F), and temperature must be monitored closely. Our own clinical experience agrees with that of others for the general use of these guidelines.[4]

Heated Humidifiers

Humidification systems have been evaluated extensively.[1,53,54] Three basic types of heated humidifiers produce water vapor with little or no aerosol: passover or blowby, bubbler or cascade, and wick. Because the bubbler and wick types are the most commonly used, they are described here.

Bubbler and Cascade Humidifiers

In bubbler and cascade humidifiers, gas must pass under and be dispersed through water as relatively small bubbles (Fig. 2–23). This process creates a large surface area for exposure of the gas to the heated water, and evaporation is enhanced. Temperature control is generated by heated rods immersed in the water or a heated plate at the bottom of the humidifier jar. Those using heating rods generally require more agitation of the water for even heating than do the units having a heated plate.

The most commonly used bubbler-style humidifier is the Puritan-Bennett Cascade model. It is produced specifically to provide a relatively low resistance at intermittent high ventilator flow rates. Other examples of bubble humidifiers are the Ohio Heated Humidifier and Chemetron's MICH humidifier system.

Wick-Type Heated Humidifiers

Some humidifiers incorporate a water-absorbing material referred to as a wick. These units are actually ''blowby'' humidifiers because gas flowing through them passes over the water next to the saturated wick, which usually rests against a heated plate (Fig. 2–24).

Several manufacturers produce wick-type heated humidification systems.[1,54] Examples include the Bird Humidifier Model 3000, several models of the Conchatherm/Conchapak systems from Respiratory Care Inc., and the MR500 heated humidifier from Fisher and Paykel Medical, Inc.

Performance Limitations

Most heated humidifiers saturate the gas passing through them if enough heat is applied to the water.[53] In order to deliver the gas near body temperature at the end of a tubing circuit 4 to 6 feet long, it must be heated to a higher temperature before leaving the humidifier. Fig-

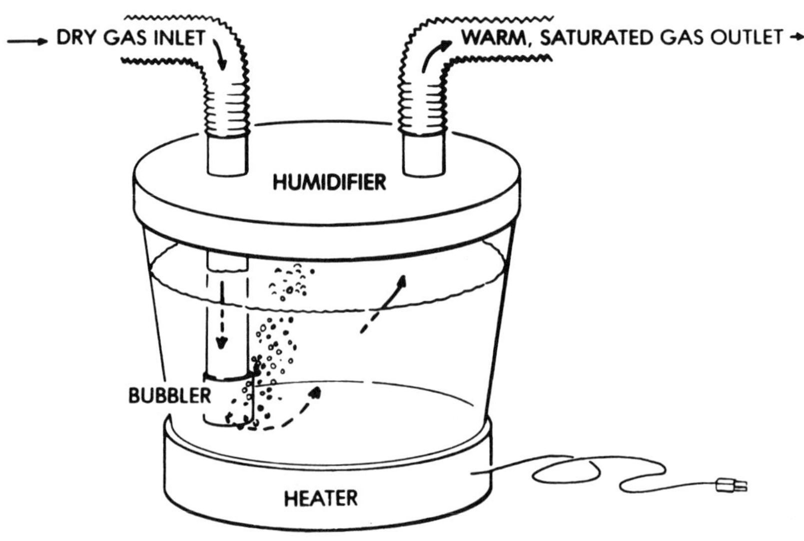

Fig. 2–23. Heated bubbler humidifier. Large-bore tubing, low-resistance bubbling device with high surface area contact between gas and water and heated water provide an efficient ventilator humidification system.

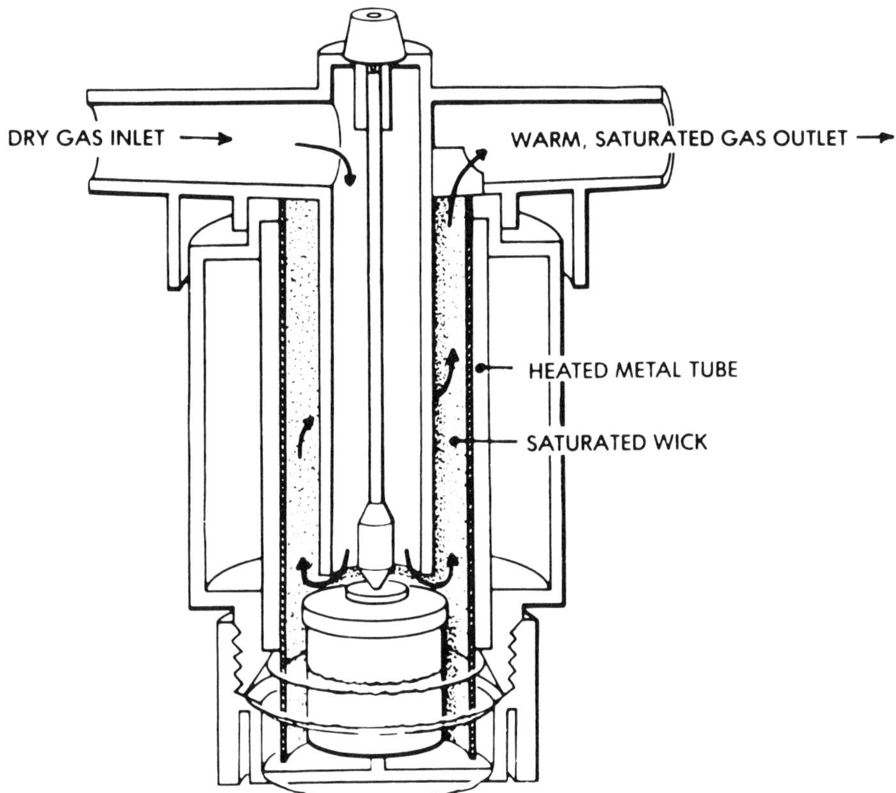

Fig. 2–24. Wick-type humidifier. The saturated wick is warmed by a heated metal tube, and gas passing over the wick gains heat and water vapor.

ure 2–25 illustrates this point. In the example, a high-efficiency humidifier is heated so that its output temperature is 50°C. Saturated air at 50°C contains 84 mg/L water vapor. The room air surrounding the tubing is 22°C, and cooling of the warmed gas occurs as it moves through the tubing to the patient connection. In this example, the temperature at the patient Y connection is 37°C. Because the gas was saturated (100 percent relative humidity) at the humidifier outlet, the temperature drop along the circuit path causes condensation of water vapor to occur, and the absolute humidity decreases from 84 mg/L to 44 mg/L. Nearly one-half the original vapor produced condenses in the tubing circuit as the temperature decreases from 50°C to 37°C. Relative humidity, however, remains at 100 percent (saturated), so the patient is assured of an adequate moisture content of the inspired gas.

The amount of condensation can be reduced significantly by heating the delivery tubing between the humidifier and the patient connection.[55,56] Generally, the humidifier outlet temperature can be within 1 to 2°C of that at the patient connection, so very little condensation occurs.

"Servo-controlling" the humidifier can improve temperature control.[1] When this technique is employed, a probe monitors gas temperature

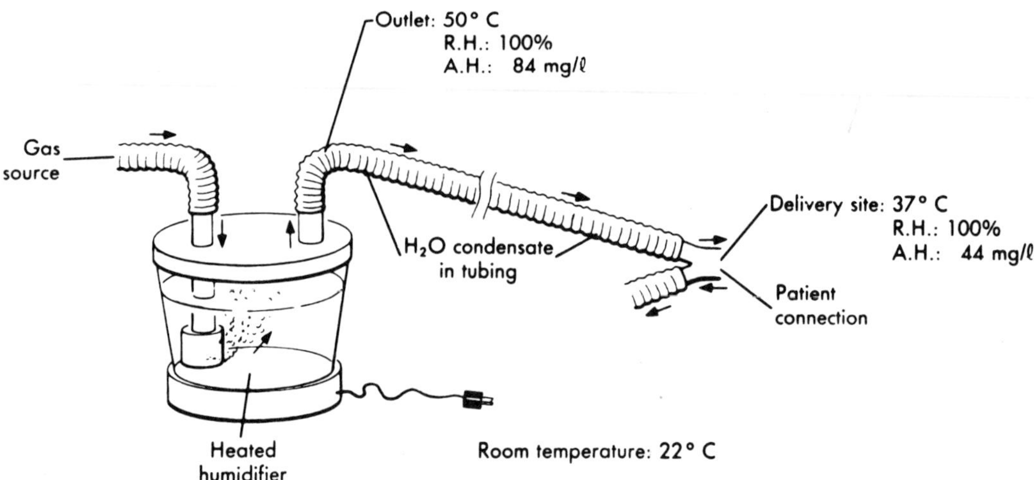

Fig. 2–25. Temperature and humidity changes in the tubing circuit with a heated humidifier. Hot gases saturated with water vapor cool during passage to the patient connection. Condensation occurs, decreasing the absolute humidity (A.H.), whereas the relative humidity (R.H.) stays at 100 percent. Note that in this example almost one-half of the original water vapor condenses in the tubing circuit. (From Spearman et al.,[10] with permission.)

near the patient connection, and water temperature within the humidifier is regulated to maintain the desired gas temperature. These systems tend to compensate for changes in ambient temperature, air currents around the tubing, and bedding insulating the tubing, etc. to ensure a relatively constant gas temperature. If a Servo control is not used, the gas temperature varies with environmental changes, whereas the water temperature remains relatively constant. Examples of Servo-controlled humidifiers include the Puritan-Bennett Cascade II and the Dual Servo MR500.

Thermal mass within a humidifier influences its ability to react quickly to changing gas flow rates or ventilator cycling frequency. As an example, a unit containing 800 to 1,000 ml of water responds to an increased ventilator rate by delivering more heat into the gas. This causes the air temperature breathed by the patient to increase until the ''extra'' heat in the water is dissipated. In some wick humidifiers, the volume of water and hence the thermal mass are very small. These units respond quickly to changing conditions, allowing some wick units to have a shorter ''warmup'' time than some bubblers.[54]

Heat and Moisture Exchangers

Heat and moisture exchangers have been called ''artificial noses'' because they allegedly mimic the heating and humidifying functions of the nose.[43,45,57] They are placed so that they become part of the respiratory dead space or rebreathed volume. During exhalation, saturated gas from the patient condenses some water vapor and gives up some heat to the device. During the subsequent inspiration, the condensed water evaporates and heat is gained from the exchanger, raising the humidity and temperature of the inspired gas toward body levels. A newer design uses a porous material chemically treated to make it hygroscopic and is said to retain more water vapor during the expiratory phase.[58]

Heat and moisture exchangers may provide adequate humidity levels while intubated patients breathe room air or anesthetic gases in semiclosed anesthesia circuits; however, their use in critically ill patients who require mechanical ventilatory support for extended periods needs further study.[57–60] Generally, they provide no more than 50 to 80 percent body humidity when dry gases are breathed, and this level may be inadequate for patients with abnormal clearance of secretions. Condensing units which can provide 80 percent body humidity may prove useful for patients receiving mechanical ventilation whose airways are relatively normal.

Advantages of heat and moisture exchangers include the elimination of condensate in the tubing circuit, reduced compressible volume caused by the absence of a humidifier and water traps, and the avoidance of overheating that can occur with heated humidifiers. Examples of currently available devices are the Servo Humidifier from Siemens-Elema and the Breathaid from Terumo Corp.

Delivery Circuits

Ventilator tubing circuits are varied in their configuration, but most have common features. We first describe a typical system for a volume-cycled ventilator, then compare a general method for modifying the circuit to include IMV.

Standard Ventilator Circuit

Most ventilators use a tubing circuit with the primary components shown in Figure 2–26. The inspiratory side has connecting tubing, a heated humidifier, support manifold, and sometimes a nebulizer and temperature probe. The expiratory limb is comprised of connecting tubing and a gas-powered exhalation valve. A Y-connector connects the inspiratory and expiratory sides to each other and to the patient. Tubing between the Y and the patient is considered *mechanical* dead space because its contents will be rebreathed. Some circuits also have a port for monitoring pressure at the Y as well as bacterial filters, water traps to collect condensate, adaptors for in-line oxygen monitoring, and adjustable relief valves.

During mechanical inspiration the exhalation valve is pressurized at a level equal to or greater than that received by the patient. Because the area under the valve (in the circuit) is smaller than the area within the valve, a surface area

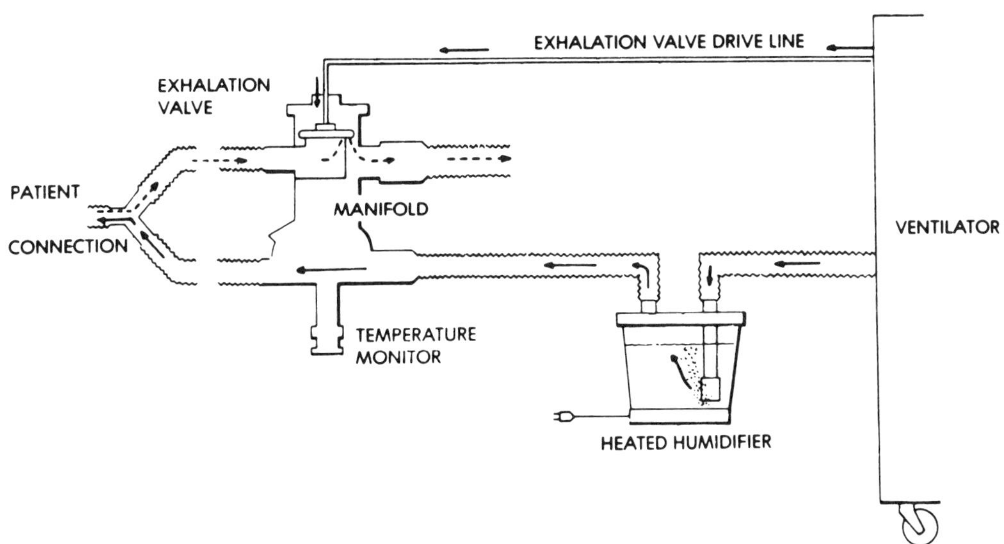

Fig. 2–26. "Typical" volume ventilator circuit. Solid arrows depict inspiratory flow; dashed arrows show expiratory flow.

differential force is established and the valve is held closed.[38] Some ventilators use a predetermined pressure to charge the exhalation valve each breath.[1] During expiration, the valve is depressurized to baseline level (i.e., zero or PEEP), the valve "collapses," and the patient's exhaled gases and those compressed in the tubing circuit vent to the atmosphere.

Other ventilators (e.g., the Servo 900B and Bourns BP-200 models) do not use pneumatically powered exhalation valves. Instead, electronically controlled systems are used and the tubing circuit requires only inspiratory and expiratory large-bore tubes without an expiratory drive line.

IMV Circuit

Since IMV was first popularized for adult ventilation, several modifications to the typical circuit have been suggested.[15,42,48,49,52,57,61] A continuous flow-through system with a reservoir bag is illustated in Figure 2–27. A 3- to 5-L bag is connected to the inspiratory side of the ventilator circuit proximal to the heated humidifier. Continuous gas flow from an oxygen blender enters the bag until it is full, then passes through a one-way valve into the main portion of the patient circuit. Spontaneous breaths are taken from this continuous flow and, if necessary, from the bag.

When the ventilator cycles (mandatory mechanical breath), the one-way valve between the circuit and the bag is closed, preventing the continuous flow from entering the circuit. The valve also prevents the ventilator from "ventilating" the bag instead of the patient. When exhalation begins, the continuous flow moves through the circuit again. During spontaneous breathing, this configuration functions much like a continuous-flow CPAP system.[9,62,63] The spontaneous work of breathing is influenced by the flow through the circuit. Once inspiratory flow exceeds the continuous flow, additional gas must come from the reser-

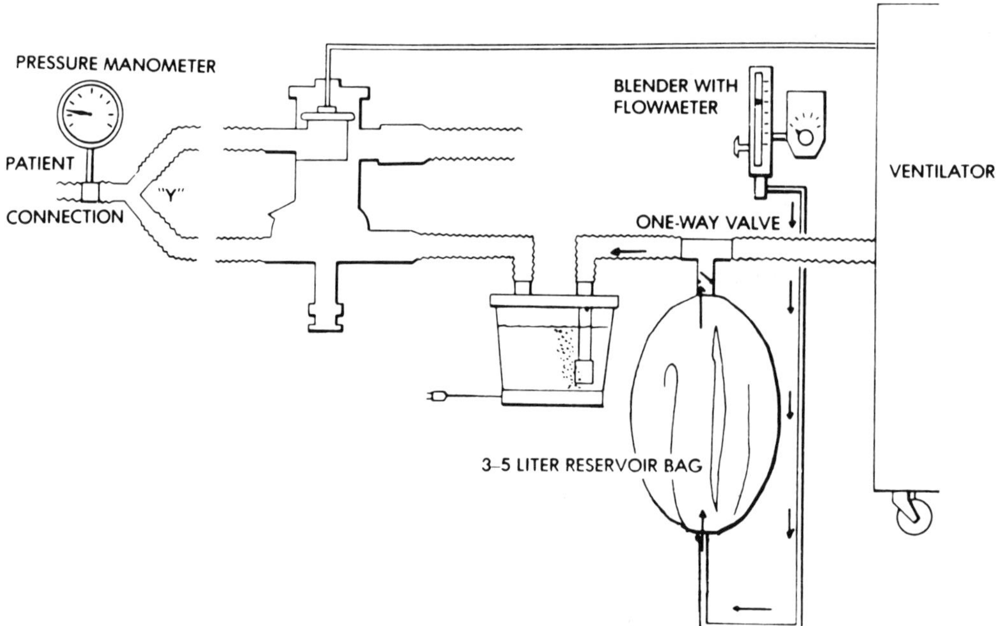

Fig. 2–27. Continuous-flow-through reservoir bag IMV system. Continuous gas flow from the blender fills the bag and flows through the circuit to allow spontaneous breathing. The pressure relief valve on the bag is used to vent excess flow during a mechanical breath. See text for description.

voir bag. If the humidifier is a bubbler or cascade type, the water provides resistance to the patient's breathing. Inspiratory work is least when the continuous flow is higher than the patient's peak inspiratory flow rate (40 to 60 L/min for most patients). Such high flow rates can raise the patient's baseline airway pressure by 2 to 5 cm H_2O, reflecting the circuit's resistance to gas flow. This pressure is sometimes called "inadvertent PEEP" and may be undesirable in some patients.

Another problem is that this high flow must be vented along with the patient's exhaled gas, producing an increase of expiratory resistance or retard. This effect is increased after a mechanical breath from the ventilator. When the ventilator cycles on, the continuous flow is "collected" within the reservoir bag until inspiration ends. As the exhalation valve opens at end-inspiration, the patient's exhaled gases, the continuous flow, and any gases collected in the reservoir bag must all pass through the same exhalation valve, resulting in a substantial increase of expiratory resistance. Some of this resistance can be reduced by a reservoir bag relief valve set for a pressure higher than PEEP but less than the peak pressure during a mechanical breath. In this way the relief valve is closed between mechanical breaths, and flow passes through the circuit as usual. When mechanical inspiration causes the one-way valve to close, the incoming continuous flow causes pressure in the bag to increase until the pressure relief valve opens, venting the extra flow to the atmosphere.

Another problem identified for continuous-flow systems can occur when the ventilator's flow rate is less than the continuous-flow rate.[64] In this case, the one-way valve between the reservoir bag and the circuit remains open, and the tidal volume from the ventilator is increased by the continuous flow. This sequence occurs only if the reservoir bag itself is relatively noncompliant. In our experience, if it can stretch, the pressure in the bag remains lower than that within the circuit, and the one-way valve remains closed during mechanical inspiration.

Lower continuous-flow rates can increase the spontaneous inspiration work, especially if the patient must "pull" gases from the bag through the humidifier's water. If the ventilator pressure manometer is connected to the circuit proximal to the humidifier, it reflects the additional pressure necessary to bubble gas through the water and is several centimeters of water greater than the patient's airway pressure. If a relatively low-resistance humidifier (wick type) is used, the inspiratory work is decreased and the internal pressure manometer reading will be more accurate. A manometer connected at the patient Y best reflects the pressure at the proximal upper airway, regardless of the continuous-flow setting or the type of humidifier used.

A final problem inherent in continuous-flow systems involves the collection of exhaled gases for volume and gas concentration measurements. The continuous flow mixes with the exhaled gases, making such measurements extremely difficult. A pressure differential pneumotachometer placed between the circuit Y and the patient's airway "sees" only inspired and expired gas, and the continuous flow is not measured.[1,47,65] Systems that shunt the continuous flow proximal to a flow sensor so that only inspired and expired gases are monitored have been described.[1,66,67] An additional exhalation valve to isolate the patient's flow so that exhaled gas volumes and concentrations can be monitored has also been used.[67,68]

Because both ventilator-supplied and continuous-flow gas passes through the circuit's heated humidifier, no additional humidification system is needed. Also, only one PEEP device is required because all gas leaves the circuit through a single exhalation valve (unless a special monitoring system is applied). The primary advantage of continuous-flow systems seems to be the relatively low and adjustable work of breathing.[69]

REFERENCES

1. McPherson SP: Respiratory Therapy Equipment. 2nd Ed. CV Mosby, St. Louis, 1981
2. Mushin WW, Rendell-Baker L, Thompson PW, et al: Automatic Ventilation of the Lungs.

3rd Ed. Blackwell Scientific Publications, Oxford, 1980
3. Rattenborg CC, Via-Reque E (eds): Clinical Use of Mechanical Ventilation. Year Book Medical Publishers, Chicago, 1981
4. Sykes MK, McNicol MW, Campbell EJM: Respiratory Failure. Blackwell Scientific Publications, Oxford, 1976
5. Kristensen HS, Neukirch F: Very long term artificial ventilation (28 years). p. 209. In Rattenborg CC, Via-Reque E (eds): Clinical Use of Mechanical Ventilation. Year Book Medical Publishers, Chicago, 1981
6. Smith RK: Respiratory care applications for fluidics. Respir Ther 3:29, 1973
7. Scacci R: Air entrainment masks: jet mixing is how they work; the Bernoulli and Venturi principles are how they don't work. Respir Care 24:298, 1979
8. Kirby RR, Graybar GB (eds): Intermittent mandatory ventilation. Int Anesthesiol Clin 18:1, 1980
9. Smith RA: Respiratory care: mechanical. p. 2177. In Miller RD (ed): Anesthesia. 2nd Ed. Churchill Livingstone, New York, 1986
10. Spearman CB, Sheldon RL, Egan DF: Egan's Fundamentals of Respiratory Therapy. 4th Ed. CV Mosby, St Louis, 1982
11. Kirby RR: Modes of mechanical ventilation. p. 128. In Kacmarek RM, Stoller JK (eds): Current Respiratory Care. B. C. Decker, Toronto, 1988
12. Downs JB, Klein EF, Desautels D, et al: Intermittent mandatory ventilation: a new approach to weaning patients from mechanical ventilators. Chest 64:331, 1973
13. Bynum LJ, Wilson JE, Pierce AK: Comparison of spontaneous and positive pressure breathing in supine normal subjects. J Appl Physiol 40:341, 1976
14. Shapiro BA, Harrison RA, Trout CA: Clinical Application of Respiratory Care. 3rd Ed. Year Book Medical Publishers, Chicago, 1986
15. Venus B, Smith RA, Mathru M: National survey of methods and criteria used for weaning from mechanical ventilation. Crit Care Med 12:530, 1987
16. Kirby RR, Robison EJ, Schulz J, et al: A new pediatric volume ventilator. Anesth Analg 50:533, 1971
17. Lawyer PGP, Nunn JF: Intermittent mandatory ventilation. Anaesthesia 32:138, 1977
18. Fairley HB: Critique of intermittent mandatory ventilation. Int Anesthesiol Clin 18:191, 1980
19. Luce JM, Pierson DJ, Hudson LD: Critical reviews: intermittent mandatory ventilation. Chest 79:678, 1981
20. Desautels DA, Bartlett JL: Methods of administering intermittent mandatory ventilation (IMV). Respir Care 19:187, 1974
21. Spearman CB: Control of inspired oxygen concentration and addition of PEEP or CPAP with the Bourns pediatric ventilator. Respir Care 18:405, 1973
22. Boros SJ: Variations in inspiratory:expiratory ratio and airway pressure wave form during mechanical ventilation: the significance of mean airway pressure. J Pediatr 94:114, 1979
23. Fox WW, Shuttack JG: Positive pressure ventilation: pressure and time-cycled ventilators. p. 101. In Goldsmith JP, Karotkin EH (eds): Assisted Ventilation of the Neonate. WB Saunders, Philadelphia, 1981
24. Harris TR: Physiologic principles. In Goldsmith JP, Karotkin EH (eds): Assisted Ventilation of the Neonate. WB Saunders, Philadelphia, 1981
25. Reynolds EOR: Pressure wave form and ventilator settings for mechanical ventilation in severe hyaline membrane diseases. Int Anesthesiol Clin 12:59, 1974
26. Schacter NE, Lehnert BE, Specht W: Pressure-time relationships of pressure-limited neonatal ventilators. Crit Care Med 11:177, 1983
27. Barach AL: Physiotherapy of advanced disease states. p. 107. In Petty TL (ed): Chronic Obstructive Pulmonary Disease. Marcel Dekker, New York, 1978
28. Barach AL, Bickerman HA, Petty TL: Perspectives in pressure breathing. Respir Care 20:627, 1975
29. Mueller RE, Petty TL, Filley GF: Ventilation and arterial blood gas changes induced by pursed-lip breathing. J Appl Physiol 28:784, 1970
30. Ashbaugh DG, Petty TL: Positive end-expiratory pressure: physiology, indications and contraindications. J Thorac Cardiovasc Surg 65:165, 1973
31. Eross B, Powner D, Grenvik A: Common ventilatory modes: terminology. Int Anesthesiol Clin 18:11, 1980
32. Gregory GA, Kitterman JA, Phibbs RH, et al: Treatment of the idiopathic respiratory distress syndrome with continuous positive airway pressure. N Engl J Med 284:1333, 1971

33. Gillick JS: Spontaneous positive end-expiratory pressure (sPEEP). Anesth Analg 56:627, 1977
34. Greenbaum DM, Millen EJ, Eross B, et al: Continuous positive airway pressure without tracheal intubation in spontaneously breathing patients. Chest 69:615, 1976
35. Schmidt GB, Deepak SP, Bennett T, et al: EPAP without intubation. Crit Care Med 5:297, 1977
36. Sturgeon CL, Douglas ME, Downs JB, et al: PEEP and CPAP cardiopulmonary effects during spontaneous ventilation. Anesth Analg 56:633, 1977
37. Hall JR, Rendleman DC, Downs JB: PEEP devices: flow-dependent increases in airway pressures (abstract). Crit Care Med 6:100, 1978
38. Kacmarek RM, Dimas S, Reynolds J, et al: Technical aspects of positive end-expiratory pressure (PEEP). Parts I, II, and III. Respir Care 27:1478, 1490, 1982
39. Nunn JF: Applied Respiratory Physiology. Butterworth, London, 1987
40. Elam JO, Kerr JH, Janney CD: Performance of ventilators: effects of changes in lung-thorax compliance. Anesthesiology 19:56, 1958
41. Fleming WH, Bowen JC: A comparative evaluation of pressure-limited and volume-limited respirators for prolonged postoperative ventilatory support in combat casualties. Ann Surg 176:49, 1972
42. Edwards WL, Sappenfeld RS: Pressure-cycled ventilators and flow rate control. Anesth Analg 47:77, 1968
43. Bendixen HH, Egbert LD, Hedley-Whyte J, et al: Respiratory Care. CV Mosby, St. Louis, 1965
44. Mapleson WW: The effects of changes of lung characteristics on the functioning of automatic ventilators. Anaesthesia 17:300, 1962
45. Safar P (ed): Respiratory Therapy. FA Davis, Philadelphia, 1965
46. Kirby RR: High frequency positive-pressure ventilation (HFPPV): what role in ventilatory insufficiency? (Editorial.) Anesthesiology 52:109, 1980
47. Osborn JJ: A flow meter for respiratory monitoring. Crit Care Med 6:349, 1978
48. Chalon J, Chandrakant P, Ali M, et al: Humidity and anesthetized patients. Anesthesiology 50:195, 1979
49. Chalon J, Loew DAY, Malebranche J: Effects of dry anesthetic gases on tracheobronchial ciliated epithelium. Anesthesiology 36:338, 1972
50. Forbes AR: Humidification and mucus flow in the intubated trachea. Br J Anaesth 45:874, 1973
51. Forbes AR: Temperature, humidity, and mucus flow in the intubated trachea. Br J Anaesth 46:29, 1974
52. Tsuda T, Noguchi H, Takumi Y, et al: Optimum humidification of air administered to a tracheostomy in dogs. Br J Anaesth 49:965, 1977
53. Klein EF, Shah DA, Modell JH, et al: Performance characteristics of conventional and prototype humidifiers and nebulizers. Chest 64:690, 1973
54. Poulton TJ, Downs JB: Humidification of rapidly flowing gas. Crit Care Med 9:59, 1981
55. Nelson D, McDonald JS: Heated humidification, temperature control, and "rainout" in neonatal ventilation. Respir Ther 7:41, 1977
56. Weigi J: Proximal airway conditions—some theoretical considerations. Respir Ther 6:21, 1976
57. Toremain NG: A heat and moisture exchanger for post-tracheostomy care. An experimental study. Acta Otolaryngol (Stockh) 52:461, 1960
58. Gedeon A, Mebius C: The hygroscopic condenser humidifier: a new device for general use in anesthesia and intensive care. Anaesthesia 34:1043, 1979
59. Walker AKY, Bethune DW: A comparative study of condenser humidifiers. Anaesthesia 31:1086, 1976
60. Weeks DB: Humidification of anesthetic gases with an inexpensive condenser-humidifier in the semiclosed circle. Anesthesiology 51:601, 1974
61. Culpepper J, Snyder J, Pennock B, et al: Effect of PEEP valve resistance on airway pressure and inspiratory work (abstract). Crit Care Med 11:220, 1983
62. Holt TB, Hall MW, Bass JB, et al: Comparison of changes in airway pressure during continuous positive airway pressure (CPAP) between demand valve and continuous flow devices. Respir Care 27:1200, 1982
63. Smith RA, Kirby RR, Gooding JM, et al: Continuous positive airway pressure (CPAP) by face mask. Crit Care Med 8:483, 1980
64. Perel A, Pachys F, Olshwang D, et al: Mechanical inspiratory peak flow as a determinant of tidal volume during IMV and PEEP. Anesthesiology 48:290, 1978
65. Osborn JJ: Monitoring respiratory function. Crit Care Med 2:217, 1974

66. McPherson SP, Glasgow GD, William AA, et al: Methods of administering intermittent mandatory ventilation (IMV). Respir Care 19:187, 1974
67. Weled BJ, Winfrey D, Downs JB: Measuring exhaled volume with continuous positive airway pressure and intermittent mandatory ventilation: techniques and rationale. Chest 76:166, 1979
68. Henry WC, West GA, Wilson RS: An evaluation of a gas collection valve for use in metabolic measurements in high flow CPAP systems. Respir Care 27:282, 1982
69. Gibney RTN, Wilson RS, Pontoppidan H: Comparison of work of breathing on high gas flow and demand valve continuous positive airway pressure systems. Chest 82:692, 1982

3

Microprocessor-Controlled Ventilation Systems and Concepts

Samsun Lampotang

Microprocessors are being used increasingly in ventilators and medical equipment in general. Microprocessor-controlled mechanical ventilators (e.g., Hamilton Veolar and Amadeus, Ohmeda CPU-1, Puritan-Bennett 7200a, Bird 6400 ST, Engström ERICA IV, and Bear 5) represent a clear break from the more traditional, nonmicroprocessor-controlled ventilator designs (e.g., Puritan-Bennett MA-1). Application of microprocessor technology to intensive care and anesthesia ventilators has undoubtedly brought many advantages and desirable features that were previously either unaffordable or impractical, or both. For example, a microprocessor in a ventilator permits monitoring of peak inflation pressure (PIP); mean airway pressure ($\overline{P_{AW}}$); elastic recoil (ERP) and continuous positive airway pressure (CPAP); inspiratory and expiratory flow waveforms and tidal volume (V_T); lung-thorax compliance (C_{LT}); and airway resistance (R_{AW}). These data can be displayed in a user-friendly fashion, allowing the clinician to easily assess patient status. Feature extraction algorithms (see Glossary) can, for example, determine PIP, $\overline{P_{AW}}$, ERP, and CPAP from analysis of the airway pressure waveform. Adjustable alarm levels can be tailored to the patient's ventilatory parameters, and trends can be detected. Closed-loop control systems (see Glossary) can also be implemented. Self-diagnostic capabilities can be provided, as well as helpful error, malfunction, or alarm messages. Essentially, through its computing power, the microprocessor allows "intelligence" to be preprogrammed into the ventilator with the objective of enhancing patient care and safety and helping the clinician do the job efficiently.

In order to understand the capabilities and inherent limitations of microprocessor-controlled ventilators, some familiarity with microprocessors is desirable. The elementary characteristics of microprocessors, along with the relevant concepts and features of microprocessor systems, are presented. Using generic descriptions, general concepts, common to all microprocessor-controlled ventilators, are emphasized rather than the specific characteristics of each ventilator.

MICROPROCESSORS

The microprocessor, also known as a central processing unit (CPU), is the "brain" of a microprocessor-controlled ventilator or, as a more common example, of a personal computer; it is the physical location where computations take place. A microprocessor is a general purpose device mass-produced at low cost and programmed for specific tasks using the appropriate software (see Glossary). For example, the same microprocessor used in an automobile engine control system might be used for controlling a ventilator. Microprocessors in ventilators can also be referred to as microcontrollers or "embedded" controllers. The generic term "microprocessor" is used here for the sake of generality.

Considering its tremendous computing power, the physical size of a microprocessor is surprisingly small. The dimensions of a microprocessor are measured in centimeters, and its weight is only a few grams. Microprocessors cost as little as $2 for an Intel 8088, whereas more powerful units sell for $300. A microprocessor is made of a thin wafer consisting of layers of silicon with miniature electrical circuits etched (integrated) into it (hence the generic name of integrated circuit or silicon chip). Pins on the sides or underside of the microprocessor provide electrical contact to the other components of the microprocessor system. The microprocessor system is defined as a microprocessor and its supporting hardware required for control and operation of the ventilator.

The miniature electrical circuits integrated into the microprocessor enable it to perform arithmetic (addition, subtraction, multiplication, and division), relational, and logical operations, as well as control the operation and the flow of information within the microprocessor system. A relational operation assesses the "truth" of a relational expression such as $x < y$?, $x = y$? or $x > y$? A relational expression can be either "true" or "false." For example, x might be the measured airway pressure and y the high airway pressure alarm limit. If the answer to $x > y$? is "true," a predetermined set of instructions (e.g., sounding an alarm and perhaps aborting the inspiratory phase) is carried out, whereas another set of commands (e.g., do nothing) is performed if the answer is "false."

Logical operations include *NOT, AND,* and *OR* and operate on the result of relational expressions. Logical operations have the same meaning as their counterparts in the English language. For example, *NOT true* is false and *NOT false* is true. The *AND* function operates on two relational expressions and requires that both expressions be true for the result to be true; *true AND true* is true; *true AND false* is false. The *OR* function requires that at least one of the two relational expressions is true for the result to be true; *true OR false* is true and *false OR false* is false. With these deceptively simple building blocks—the fundamental elements of computer language—very powerful sets of instructions (programs referred to as software) are written to make the ventilator perform specific tasks, which impart to a microprocessor the appearance of "intelligence."

Simplified flow diagrams depicting ventilator software routines are used to illustrate these concepts. An example of a generic routine for controlling the operation of a microprocessor-controlled ventilator is illustrated in Figure 3–1. Software routines that check that airway pressure is within preselected alarm limits are also used (Fig. 3–2). Another software routine is the calculation of delivered tidal volume (Fig. 3–3). Routines or algorithms, such as those portrayed in Figures 3–2 and 3–3, are employed to calculate a host of other ventilatory parameters, including exhaled tidal volume, exhaled minute volume, CLT, and RAW.

BITS AND BYTES

A *bit* is an element that can have only one of two possible states, "1" or "0," "ON" or "OFF," "true" or "false," at any given time. For example, a two-way switch (like a light switch) can be considered a bit with the ON position corresponding to 1 and the OFF to 0. The voltage on an electrical wire or across a capacitor (see Glossary) can also be considered a bit if 1 is defined as a voltage between +3 and +5 V and 0 as a voltage between 0 and +0.5 V, and if the voltage is not allowed to reside outside these two ranges. This scheme is known as transistor logic (TTL) and is precisely how a bit is implemented on most microprocessor systems.

With only one bit, two combinations are pos-

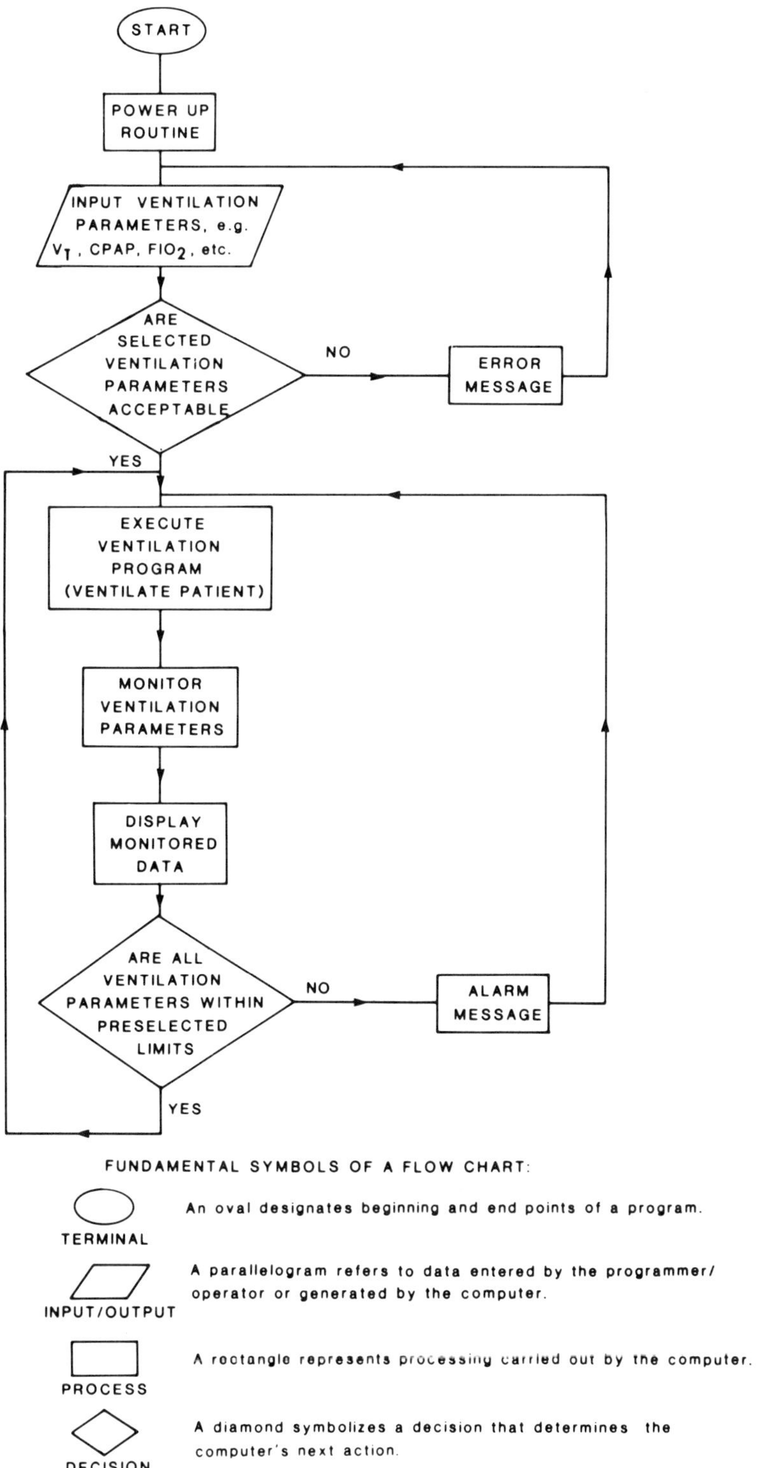

Fig. 3–1. Flowchart of a generic ventilation control program for a microprocessor-controlled ventilation.

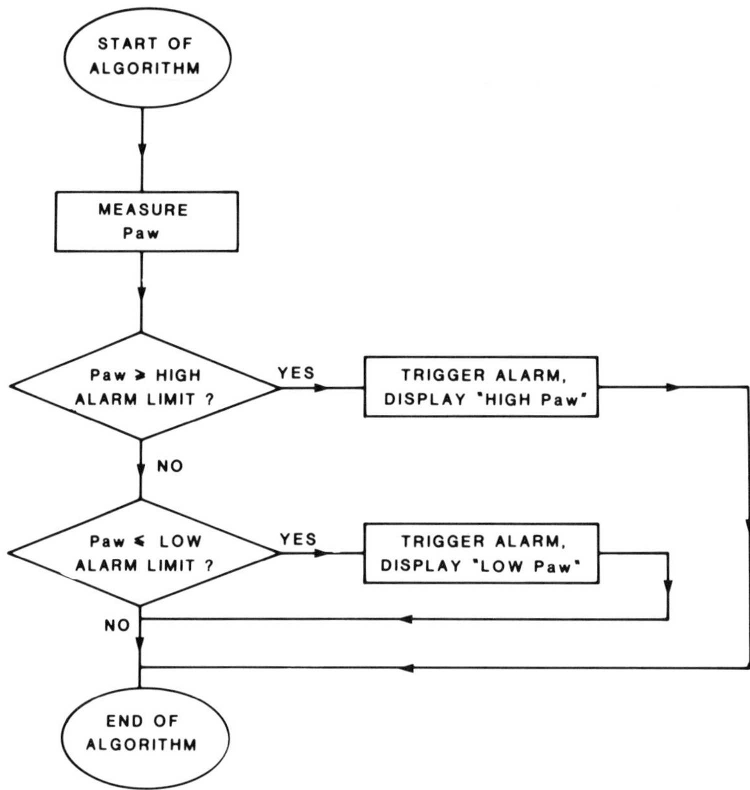

Fig. 3–2. Algorithm to check that the airway pressure (PAW) is within a specified range selected by the clinician. If the measured PAW is in violation of the preselected alarm limits, audible and visual alarms are activated.

sible. With 2 bits, 4 combinations are possible; with 3 bits, 8 combinations, and so on. Each additional bit doubles the amount of combinations possible (Table 3–1). In fact, the number of unique combinations or bit patterns possible with *n* bits is 2 to the power of *n*. A byte is defined as 8 bits and permits the representation of 256 (2^8) states or combinations. By assigning a specific meaning to each unique combination or bit pattern, a code is created for communicating data: the American Standard Code for Information Interchange (ASCII) code for encoding characters and numbers. For example, the ASCII codes for A, a, and 3 are 01000001, 01100001, and 00110011, respectively. Data encoded in the form of a bit pattern are called digital data. The number of bits determines the number of unique combinations possible, and hence the range of integer values that can be represented. For example with 8 bits, the range of integer values would be 0 to 255.

Microprocessors differ in their capabilities. Some can handle 8 bits, while others can process 16 bits or 32 bits at a time; hence the name 8-bit, 16-bit and 32-bit microprocessors. Microprocessors that can process a larger number of bits simultaneously can access a larger memory and a larger range of integer values.

CLOCK FREQUENCY

An important characteristic of a microprocessor system is the clock frequency, also known as clock cycle or clock speed. Typically, an excited quartz crystal, similar to that used in a digital watch, provides pulses at frequencies in the megahertz (MHz), or one million pulses

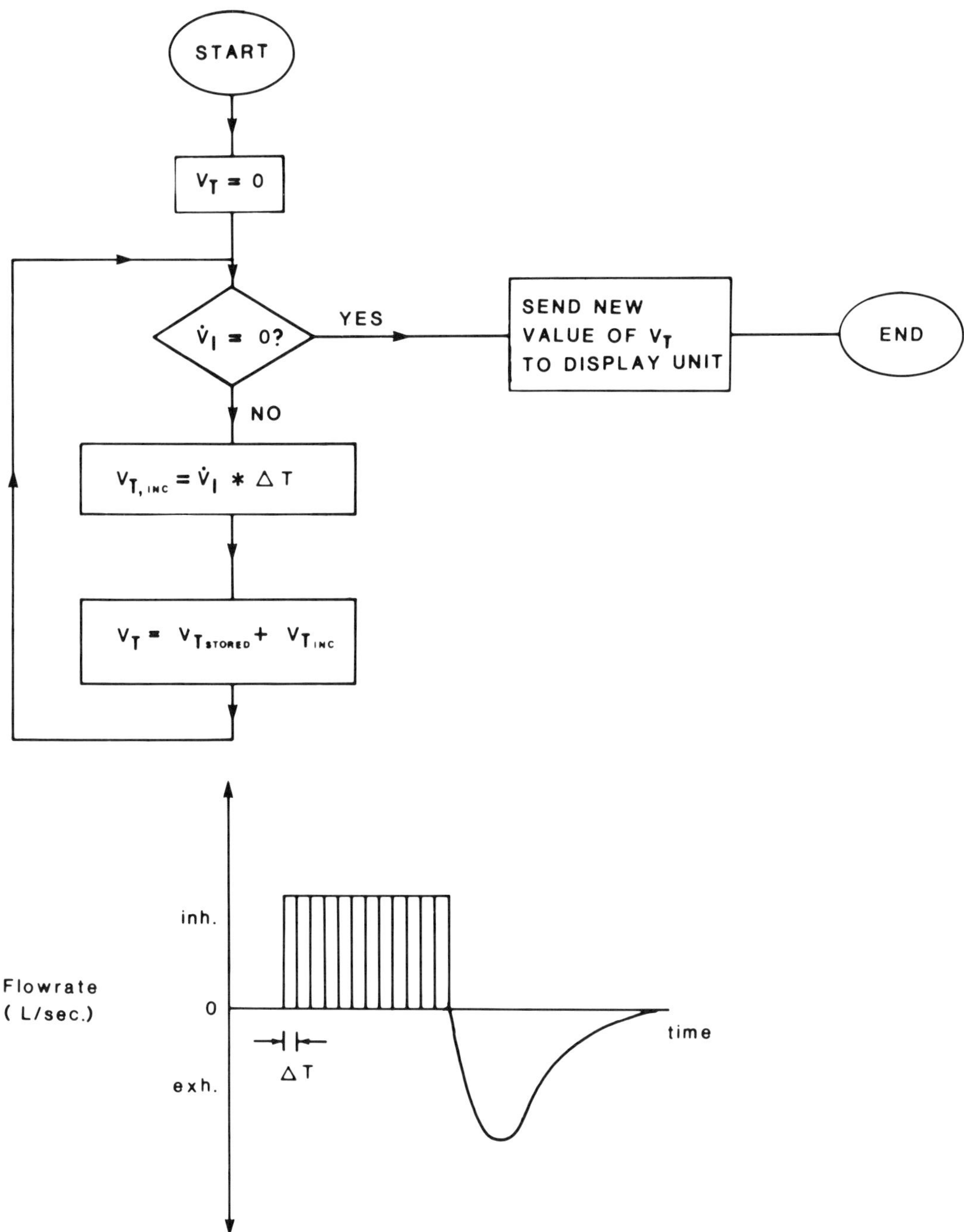

Fig. 3–3. Example of an algorithm to calculate tidal volume (VT) from inspiratory flow rate ($\dot{V}$I) during mechanical inhalation. At the onset of mechanical inhalation, VT is reset to zero (VT = 0). The inspiratory flow waveform is sampled at regular time intervals (ΔT), and $\dot{V}$I is assumed constant during each time interval. The incremental change in tidal volume (VT, inc) is cumulatively added to the stored tidal volume (VT, stored) during each pass through the loop. VT is the integration of $\dot{V}$I with respect to time, during inhalation. When $\dot{V}$I stops (end of mechanical inhalation; $\dot{V}$I = 0), the loop is exited and the updated value of VT is displayed.

Table 3–1. Unique Combinations (Bit Patterns) as a Function of Number of Bits Available

Bits Available	Combinations (bit patterns)				No. of unique combinations[a]
1	0	1			$2^1 = 2$
2	00	01			$2^2 = 4$
	10	11			
3	000	001	010	011	$2^3 = 9$
	100	101	110	111	

[a] The base number refers to the two possible states of a bit (i.e., 1 or 0) while the exponent refers to the number of bits available.

per second, range that synchronize the operations of a microprocessor system, and hence the ventilator. During each clock cycle, the microprocessor can execute one operation.

A clock cycle is in the order of microseconds, a time span below the temporal resolution of humans, so that the microprocessor appears to perform operations instantaneously and simultaneously. In actuality, the microprocessor processes instructions serially, that is, one after the other. At any point in time, the microprocessor is performing only one operation, but at phenomenal speed, so that thousands of operations can be performed per second. For example, every second, a microprocessor acquires data from the ventilator's flow and pressure transducers, checks whether any alarm limits have been violated by comparing the measured values with the limits entered by the operator, manipulates and displays old and new data, and controls the overall operation of the ventilator.

MEMORY

To display intelligence, humans require memory. Similarly, memory is essential for the operation of microprocessor-controlled ventilators. For example, a trend for PIP over a given time period could be displayed. A trend can only be displayed if a ventilator can "remember" previous PIP values by storing them in memory. Memory provides a convenient place to store data for later retrieval when the data are not currently being used by the microprocessor. Memory typically consists of memory locations (cells), each with a unique address (see Glossary).

Random access memory (RAM) and read-only memory (ROM) are two types of memory found in both microprocessor-controlled ventilators and computers. The flow of data between RAM and the microprocessor is two-way. The microprocessor can write data into RAM for storage and can also retrieve data by reading from the memory locations of interest. When new data are placed into a memory cell, old data stored in that cell are written over and lost.

RAM is volatile; that is, when electrical power is switched off, all stored data are lost. Therefore, RAM would be unsuitable for storing a ventilator control program for two reasons: (1) a ventilator control program stored in RAM would be lost when power is turned off; even when the supply of electrical power is reestablished, the ventilator would not function because the control program would be permanently lost; and (2) since it is possible to write into RAM, parts of the program could accidentally be written over and deleted, resulting in ventilator malfunction.

ROM, also known as permanent memory, solves the aforementioned problems of RAM. ROM is nonvolatile and, as the name implies, data cannot be written into ROM but can only be read from it. The ventilator control program is written into ROM at the factory and cannot accidentally be written over during ventilator operation. Data transfer is unidirectional, flowing only from ROM to the microprocessor. Therefore, a ventilator control program stored in ROM is not lost when electrical power is discontinued, and cannot be accidentally deleted or written over. ROM chips are not general purpose, but application specific. Such specificity makes ROM economical only if a large number of identical ROM chips are required. For smaller volume applications, programmable ROM (PROM) is generally used. PROM chips are general purpose chips and are rendered specific to the application by permanently programming ("burning") the desired software into them.

PROM has the disadvantage, especially during the prototype stage of a ventilator, that if small changes have to be made to the ventilator control program (e.g., to increase the time duration or pitch of the alarm tone), the existing PROM chip cannot be altered, and a new PROM chip must be programmed. Erasable PROM (EPROM) is ideal for this situation. As the name implies, a program in EPROM can be erased and the improved software programmed into the same EPROM.

The ventilator control program can be stored in any of the above mentioned types of ROM. Since the ventilator control program (software) is totally self-contained in the ROM-type module, an upgrade simply consists of replacing the old ROM-type device with a new chip containing the improved software. The relative ease of software alteration, without expensive hardware changes, allows ventilator manufacturers to be more responsive to design suggestions and requests from clinicians.

When new modalities of ventilation are introduced, they may be implemented by altering the software, via a ROM-type chip change, and adding the necessary hardware to the ventilator. Some ventilators allocate space and keypads on the control panel for future retrofits and upgrades; thus protecting the clinicians' investment from premature obsolescence.

MICROPROCESSOR SYSTEM

In a microprocessor system, data are transferred via the data bus (Fig. 3–4). A data bus consists of a set of parallel wires that carry data in the form of bit patterns. The address bus is used to indicate which component of the microprocessor system needs to be accessed. For that purpose, each of the input and output ports and each memory location are identified by the unique address assigned to it. The control bus provides timing signals and coded instructions that coordinate the operation of the system and dictates the kind of operation to be performed. For example, if data need to be read from memory, the desired memory location is addressed via the address bus. Then the control bus sends instructions that data are to be read from that memory location, and stored data are transferred via the data bus to the microprocessor (Fig. 3–4).

The microprocessor system communicates and interacts with the outside world via the input and output ports. Digital input and output (I/O) of the microprocessor system are of two types: serial and parallel. In serial output, the 8 bits in a byte are transferred serially, one at a time over the same wire; for example, an RS 232 is a popular serial communication standard or interface. A serial I/O port is mainly characterized by its baud rate—the number of bits that can be transferred per second. In parallel output, all 8 bits in a byte are transferred simultaneously, each bit on a separate wire, such as the Centronics interface, a popular scheme for printers. Consequently, parallel I/O provides faster data transfer than does serial I/O at the expense of a larger number of wires, which is impractical for long-distance data transmission.

DIGITAL AND ANALOG SIGNALS

The concepts of digital and analog signals are essential in understanding the operation of microprocessor-controlled ventilators. A microprocessor processes only digital signals (i.e., data in the form of bits). However, the real world is an analog world. Commonly encountered physical variables, such as flow rate, pressure, and voltage, are analog in nature; that is, they have an infinite range of values. In an analog signal, an infinite number of values exists between the two values because any interval between two numbers can always be divided into even smaller intervals ad infinitum. In other words, there is no restriction on the value that an analog signal may assume.

By contrast, with digital data the number of bits determines the number of combinations possible. If 8 bits are used to represent digital information, then only 256 (2^8) combinations are possible. Since each combination can be assigned to represent a unique value, only 256

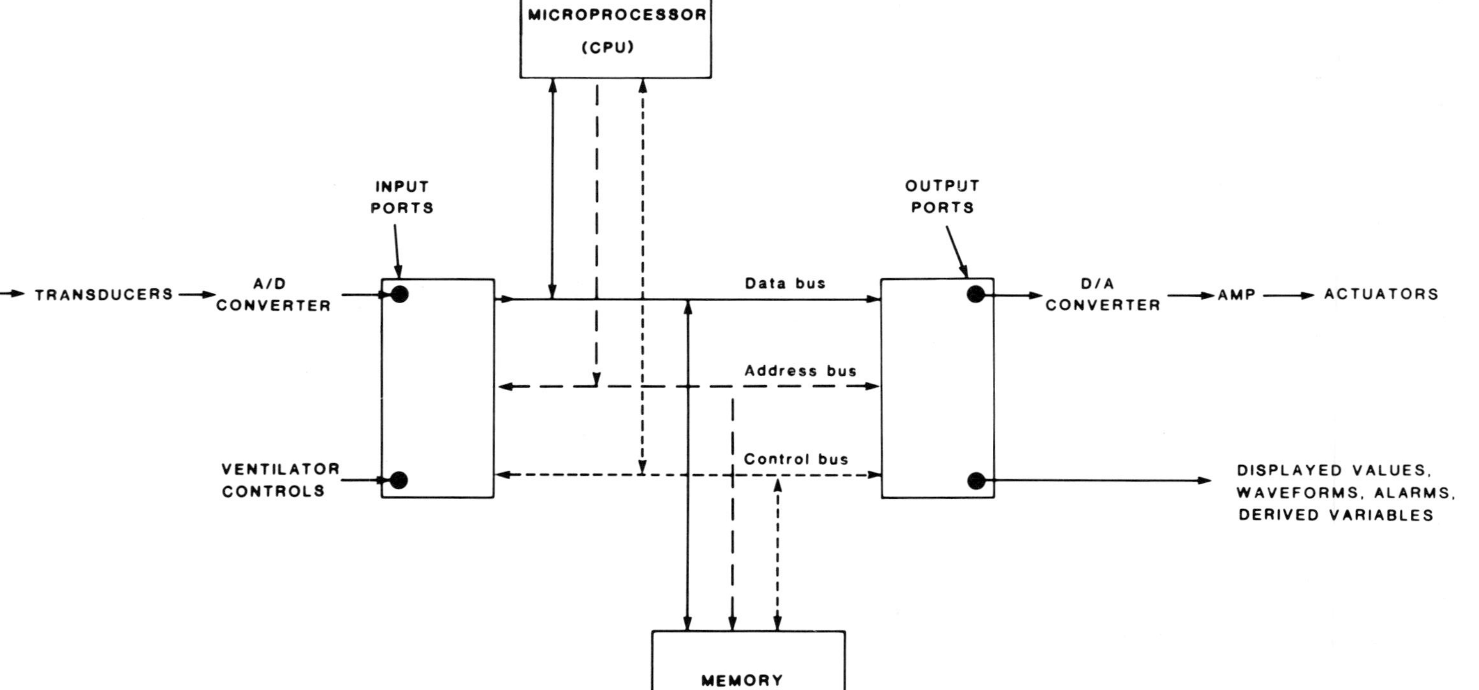

Fig. 3–4. Diagrammatic representation of a microprocessor system in a mechanical ventilator. Arrows indicate the direction in which data and/or instructions can flow. The transducers measure variables such as pressure and flow rate, which are inputs to the system. An analog-to-digital (A/D) converter transforms the analog voltages from the transducers into digital data. These data are then placed onto the data bus so that they can be routed to any of the subsystems connected to the data bus (i.e., memory, microprocessor, or output port). The address bus is used by the microprocessor to indicate which component it wants to access. The control bus is used to send instructions so that the appropriate operation is performed in the correct sequence. The actuators are the inspiratory flow valve and the exhalation valve, which are under the control of the microprocessor.

specific values can be encoded. Therefore, an 8-bit digital signal having a range of 0 to 1 V can only have 256 values represented within that range. If the values are equally spaced, the voltages that can be represented will be 0, 1/256, 2/256, . . . , 254/256, 255/256 V, and the resolution (see Glossary) is 1/256 V.

CONTINUOUS-TIME AND DISCRETE-TIME

Time in the real world is continuous. Any time interval, however small, can be subdivided into an infinite number of even smaller time intervals. In a continuous-time signal, the signal has a value at each of the infinite number points in time. Signals in the real world (e.g., flow rate, pressure, FIO_2) are predominantly continuous-time and analog (e.g., the airway pressure signal using an aneroid manometer).

In a discrete-time system, time can only be represented at specific or discrete points. A discrete-time signal has a value only at each discrete point in time. For example, a continuous-time signal sampled at a rate of 1 Hz (1 sample per second) becomes a discrete-time signal, since the signal only has a value at the sampling time and nothing is known about the signal during the 1-second interval between sampling times.

ANALOG-TO-DIGITAL CONVERTERS

Since a microprocessor in a microprocessor-controlled ventilator works only with digital signals, analog and continuous-time signals must be transformed into equivalent digital and discrete-time signals by an analog-to-digital converter (A/D converter). The A/D converter samples a continuous-time analog signal at a given sampling frequency or rate and converts the resulting signal to a discrete-time digital signal that the microprocessor can process (Fig. 3–5).

The resolution of an A/D converter is an important characteristic and is a function of the input range and the number of bits used to represent the digital values. The more bits used in an A/D converter, the finer the resolution becomes. Too coarse a resolution might introduce inaccuracies in data acquisition, since the A/D converter approximates the actual value of the signal to the closest value that can be represented. The resolution of an A/D converter affects the accuracy of a transducer. For example, a flowmeter might have a range of 0 to 100 L/min and an accuracy of 0.1 L/min. If the A/D converter is an 8-bit design, 256 (2^8) values can be represented. Therefore, the resolution of the digital flowmeter signal will be 100/256 L/min, approximately 0.4 L/min, which is less than the accuracy of the transducer. Consequently, the original accuracy of the transducer is effectively degraded to 0.4 L/min. Using an A/D converter with 12 bits ($12^2 = 4{,}096$) will increase the resolution to 100/4,096 = 0.025 L/min, conserving the original accuracy of the transducer.

In general, the A/D converters in a microprocessor-controlled ventilator will have sufficient sampling frequency and resolution for routine clinical applications. The ease of experimental data collection with microprocessor-controlled ventilators makes such ventilators potentially useful research tools. In research applications, however, sampling rate and resolution can become limiting factors especially when high-precision measurements of fleeting phenomena, such as pressure transients caused by a demand valve opening, are attempted. If the sampling frequency of the A/D converter is too low, the transient phenomenon might not be captured. For low-amplitude phenomena, an A/D converter with a coarse resolution might not be able to capture the event. Before using a microprocessor-controlled ventilator as a research tool, the researcher should check the resolution and sampling rate of its A/D converter(s) to determine whether the experimental requirements are met. If that is not the case, higher-precision instruments, such as pneumotachographs and electronic transducers, should be used.

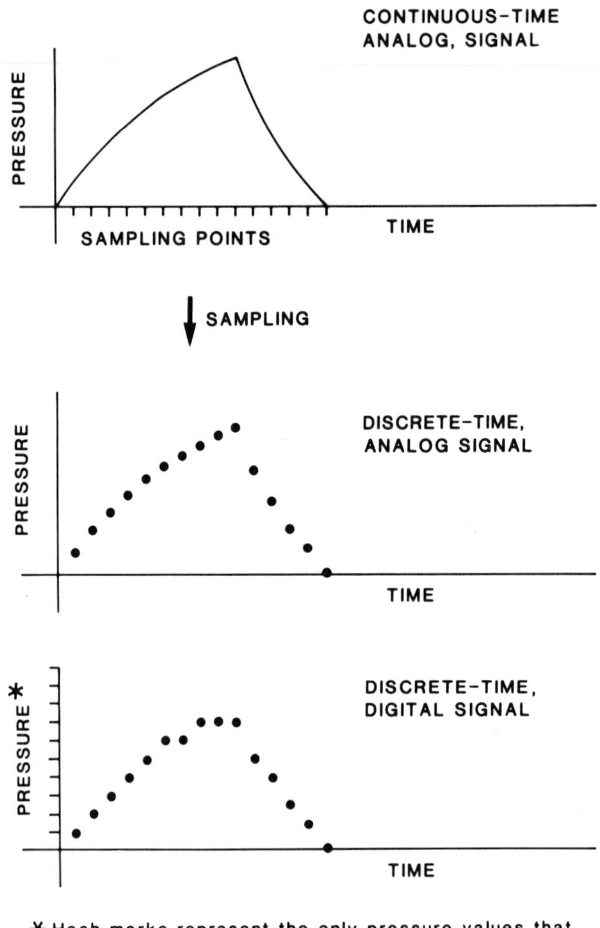

Fig. 3–5. Conversion of a continuous-time analog signal to a discrete-time digital signal is diagrammed. The sampling process captures the value of a given variable (e.g., pressure at a specific sampling instant). The analog-to-digital (A/D) converter can only represent a limited amount of discrete numbers per unit time.

DIGITAL-TO-ANALOG CONVERTERS

The digital data from a microprocessor are meaningless to the outside world. Therefore, a digital-to-analog converter (D/A converter) is required to transform discrete-time digital signals into a continuous-time analog voltage. A D/A converter functions in a manner opposite that of an A/D converter. The power output of a D/A converter is usually too low to drive an actuator (see Glossary), for example, the ventilator's inspiratory flow valve. An amplifier interposed between the D/A converter and the actuator is used to amplify the output from the D/A converter to the required level (Fig. 3–4).

MEASURED AND DERIVED VARIABLES

Most transducers convert a physical variable, such as airway pressure to an analog voltage. With a linear transducer, the output voltage is proportional to the magnitude of the variable, within the range of operation of the transducer. It is important to differentiate between measured variables and derived variables. Measured variables are parameters, such as airway pressure and inspiratory flow rate, which can be measured directly by pressure and flow transducers, respectively. Measured variables are inputs to a microprocessor system. Derived variables are computed from measured variables and are outputs of a microprocessor system. For example, airway resistance is derived from measured variables, that is, change in airway pressure divided by inspiratory flow rate. Another example is lung-thorax compliance derived from two measured variables, that is, change in volume divided by change in airway pressure. Since a microprocessor has computational ability, derived variables are readily calculated if the required measured variables are available.

REAL TIME

The term *real time* is often used in connection with microprocessor-controlled ventilators. Real time means that a signal is processed as fast as it is being physically generated and that the processed results are immediately made available (e.g., a real-time display of exhaled tidal volume). Real-time monitoring of airway pressure, flow, and volume is provided with some microprocessor-controlled ventilators. These data may then be used to calculate derived variables such as CLT, RAW, and work of breathing.

CONTROL SYSTEMS AND CONCEPTS

Control systems are used whenever a variable or ventilator parameter needs to be controlled in a prescribed way. Control systems can be either open loop or closed loop. Open-loop control systems do not use feedback and are generally time cycled. Feedback is the process by which the output of a system is measured and fed back to be used as part of the input of the system. An example of an open-loop control system is the MA-1 volume-cycled ventilator; the ventilator cycles off when a preselected VT has been ejected from the ventilator. There is no feedback of the output (delivered VT) to the ventilator control mechanism. Closed-loop control systems use feedback and are therefore also called feedback control systems. A closed-loop control system (Fig. 3–6) uses the difference (error) between the reference input and the measured output to drive the controlled system toward the desired output. A digital closed-loop control system requires A/D and D/A converters as well as a microprocessor. For example, Figure 3–6 is a representation of a closed-loop digital control system for delivering a constant inspiratory flow rate during mechanical inhalation, irrespective of changes in PIP.

The reference input to a closed-loop control system can be either constant or time varying. A constant input is used for VT delivery for example, since the desired VT is a constant and does not change over the course of an inspiratory cycle. Time-varying inputs provide a changing reference input over time and are used, for example, to shape the inspiratory flow waveform to sinusoidal, square, accelerating, and decelerating patterns over one inspiratory cycle. The output (inspiratory flow rate) is compared with the time-varying reference input, and the actuator (e.g., a proportional flow control valve) delivering the inspiratory flow rate is accordingly modulated to make the output track the reference input.

It should be noted that a closed-loop control system usually consists of components arranged in series as part of a loop. For example, in the closed-loop control system depicted in Figure 3–6, the microprocessor, the D/A converter, the amplifier, the inspiratory flow valve, and the flow transducer are arranged in a cascade. There is a cause-and-effect relationship linking the components in series in the sense that the output of the upstream component (e.g., the inspiratory flow valve) is the input to the component immediately downstream (flow transducer). The effect of an input at the top of the

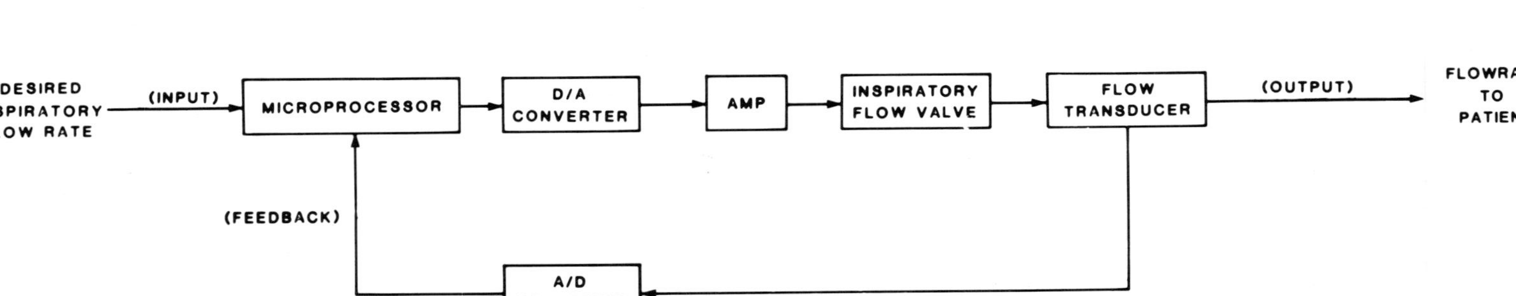

Fig. 3–6. Representation of a digital closed-loop control system for inspiratory flow rate during mechanical inhalation. Input is the preselected inspiratory flow rate. Output is the flow rate of gas to the patient and is measured by a flow transducer. The analog voltage from the flow transducer is converted to digital data by an analog-to-digital (A/D) converter. In the microprocessor, the difference between the input and the measured output is computed and used to evaluate how much the inspiratory flow valve should be opened or closed. The instructions from the microprocessor to the inspiratory flow valve are digital and have to be transformed into analog signals by a digital-to-analog (D/A) converter. Since the analog output from the D/A converter is too low to drive the inspiratory flow valve, an amplifier is usually placed between these two components.

series trickles down the cascade and is eventually felt at the bottom of the series. Each component has its characteristic response time and influences the overall response time of the whole system. There are many definitions of response time; in essence, response time is a measure of the time that a system takes to react or respond to an input or instruction. For example, if an initially closed inspiratory flow valve is instructed to deliver a flow rate of 60 L/min, the elapsed time between the instruction and flow rate actually reaching 60 L/min might be, for example, 20 msec. This value is the response time.

A microprocessor cannot speed up the response time of the mechanical or electromechanical components in a microprocessor-controlled ventilator. The microprocessor can only provide the ability to acquire measured data, compute derived variables from measured data, make decisions, and initiate actions based on these computations at very high speed. However, if a component of the system has a longer response time relative to the other components, the response time of the whole system will be dominated by that slow-acting component, no matter how fast the computing speed of the microprocessor. In other words, the response time of the system is only as fast as that of the slowest component in the system.

Data collected by other contributors to this book (M. J. Banner, P. Blanch, D. A. Desautels) seem to indicate that, contrary to the manufacturers' claims, microprocessor-controlled ventilators do not maintain the preselected inspiratory flow rate when faced with increased PIP. Inspiratory flow rate, hence V_T delivery to the patient, are reduced when PIP increases, with several microprocessor-controlled ventilators. There are many possible reasons for this observation. For example, if the response time of the components (e.g., the inspiratory flow valve) in the closed-loop control system for constant V_T delivery is too slow, the control system will not be able to respond fast enough to compensate for the effects of increased PIP. Another possibility is the location in the breathing circuit of the sensor used for feedback.

FEATURES TO LOOK FOR IN MICROPROCESSOR-CONTROLLED VENTILATORS

When choosing a microprocessor-controlled ventilator, several factors should be considered. For example, what happens in case of power failure? Is there automatic battery backup of essential monitors and alarms? Can manual breaths be given in case of electrical power failure? Are there redundant analog devices, such as the float in an oxygen flowmeter that continues to function in the absence of electrical power? The ability to upgrade is a desirable fearure. Has extra room been allocated on the ventilator's control panel for possible future additions of keypads and control knobs? Is the design of the ventilator modular in nature? A modular design facilitates troubleshooting and maintenance.

Ease of patient data collection is another factor to consider. Compatibility with existing data collection systems, and specifically with the ubiquitous IBM-PC microcomputer, should be investigated. Are there easily accessible digital and analog outputs on the ventilator? What is the voltage range of the analog output? What type of interface is used for the digital signal and what is the range? If a hard copy of the patient trends is required, is there a parallel port at the back of the ventilator, and what type of interface is used? Are there provisions for automatic record-keeping and downloading of information into the hospital information system (HIS) computer?

The location of the pressure and flow transducers in the ventilator's breathing circuit affects the validity of airway pressure, flow, and V_T measurements. For example, if the flow transducer for measuring exhaled flow and V_T is located between the Y piece and the endotracheal tube (e.g., Hamilton Veolar and Amadeus ventilators), V_T measurements will be more accurate than with a ventilator in which the flow transducer is located distal to the exhalation valve. (See *Accuracy of Displayed Exhaled Tidal Volume,* Ch. 15.) Questions regarding self-diagnostic capabilities in case of malfunction should be raised. Is an automatic maintenance reminder displayed after a predetermined number of operating hours?

The consumer/clinician should establish whether the manufacturer's claims about the performance characteristics (pressure, flow rate, and volume delivery) of the microprocessor-controlled ventilator have been supported by independent research. For example, during mechanical inhalation, does the inspiratory flow rate, and thus the V_T remain constant when PIP increases? If a closed-loop control system for inspiratory flow rate is employed (Fig. 3–6), inspiratory flow rate and V_T should theoretically remain fairly constant, even if PIP increases.

Questions concerning the characteristics of system components used in the data acquisition system should be broached. For example, what are the operating characteristics of the A/D converters, and what is the accuracy of the pressure and flow transducers in the system?

THE FUTURE

With the advent of cheaper and more powerful microprocessors and memory, expert systems can be installed in microprocessor-controlled ventilators that will suggest possible therapies to the clinician. Microprocessor-controlled ventilators have the essential features of a computer (CPU, I/O, and memory) so that these ventilators can literally be considered a microcomputer and a ventilator contained in the same box. Therefore, existing and future computer technology could be extended to microprocessor-controlled ventilators. A microprocessor-controlled ventilator with a video terminal, a keyboard, and a modem can be used to communicate with a central computer that might be the HIS computer or a regional or national database computer. A patient's medical history and any past complications could be identified by the expert system and brought to the clinician's attention.

A concept that may be possible using microprocessor technology is employing the partial pressure of end-tidal CO_2 ($PetCO_2$) and arterial oxygen saturation (pulse oximetry) as feedback data in a closed-loop ventilation system. As $PetCO_2$ and oxygen saturation vary from the clinically acceptable values, the ventilator would automatically adjust its rate, V_T, F_IO_2, CPAP, and other factors accordingly. A caveat, using $PetCO_2$ as feedback data in a closed-loop ventilation system, is that patients with acute and chronic respiratory failure may have $PetCO_2$ values of 20 mmHg lower than the arterial PCO_2 (normal arterial to end-tidal PCO_2 difference is approximately 5 mmHg). Thus, reliance on $PetCO_2$ as feedback data in a closed-loop ventilation system may be fraught with inappropriate ventilator settings for some patients.

The possible applications of microprocessors in mechanical ventilators are many; it is the responsibility of the clinician to be discerning and recognize the useful from the gimmicky. Microprocessors are not a panacea and should be used wisely if they are not to become marketing gadgets.

BIBLIOGRAPHY

Bear Medical Systems Bear-5 ventilator instruction manual. Part number 50000–10700. Bear Medical Systems, Riverside, CA

Hamilton Veolar Operator's Manual: Part number 610131. Hamilton Medical, Reno, NE

Kamen EW: Introduction to Signals and Systems. Macmillan, New York, 1987

Kuo BC: Digital Control Systems. Holt, Rinehart, New York, 1980

Money SA: Microprocessors in Instrumentation and Control. McGraw-Hill, New York, 1986

Norton P: Inside the IBM PC. Prentice-Hall, Englewood Cliffs, NJ, 1986

Ogata K: Modern Control Engineering. Prentice-Hall, Englewood Cliffs, NJ, 1970

Puritan-Bennett 7200 Series Microprocessor Ventilator Operator's Manual: Part number 20500A. Puritan Bennett Corporation, Kansas City, KS, 1986

Siemens Servo Ventilator 900C Operating Manual. 3rd Ed. Solna, Sweden, 1984

Spearman CB, Sanders HG: The new generation of mechanical ventilators. Conference Proceedings. Respir Care 32:403, 1987

Thompson JD: Computerized control of mechanical ventilation: closing the loop. Respir Care 32:440, 1987

GLOSSARY

Actuator: a generic term for a device that performs an action. For example, a flow-control valve that controls inspiratory flow rate.

A/D converter: Analog-to-digital converter; a device to transform an analog signal to a digital signal.

Address: a unique number assigned to each input/output (I/O) port and memory location that allows the microprocessor to specify which location it wants to access.

Algorithm: a set of instructions designed to perform a specific function, for example, extracting features such as CPAP and PIP from an airway pressure waveform.

Analog: refers to a signal that can have an infinite number of values.

ASCII: American Standard Code for Information Interchange. A convention for encoding letters and numbers in the form of 8-bit patterns.

Baud rate: the number of bits that can be transmitted per second on a serial communication line.

Bit pattern: a combination of 0 and 1 that is used to encode digital information.

Capacitor: a device for storing electrical charge.

Centronics: a parallel input/output interface standard.

Closed loop: refers to a control system in which the output state is used to determine the control action; also known as feedback control system.

CPU: central processing unit (e.g., a microprocessor); the device with which computations and overall supervision of the system are performed.

D/A converter: digital-to-analog converter; an electronic device for transforming analog signals to digital signals.

Database: an information bank designed to permit fast retrieval of information.

Digital: refers to data encoded in the form of binary digit (bit) patterns.

DRAM: dynamic random access memory; a form of memory storage that requires dynamic update of the data in storage; uses capacitors.

EEPROM: electrically erasable programmable read-only memory; a ROM-type device similar to an EPROM, except that erasure is done electrically rather than with ultraviolet light.

Expert system: a form of artificial intelligence that codifies the knowledge and expertise of an acknowledged expert in a given field into a software program.

EPROM: erasable programmable read-only memory; a general-purpose form of ROM that is erasable with high-intensity ultraviolet light.

Feature extraction: the process of obtaining data from analyzing the shape, level, and/or trend of data and waveforms.

Feedback: the process of measuring the state of the output and comparing it with the reference input to determine the appropriate control action.

Hardware: the physical components that make up a microprocessor system: CPU chip, RAM, EPROM, and data bus.

Interface: a mechanism, convention, or protocol that enables two separate systems to communicate with each other, that is, to be interfaced.

I/O: abbreviation for the input/output of data in a computer system.

Keypad: a device for entering data into the microprocessor-controlled ventilator.

Memory: the location in a microprocessor system where digitally encoded data are stored.

Microprocessor: also known as a CPU; the location at which computations and supervision of the system are performed.

Modem: abbreviation for MOdulator/DEModulator—at the transmitting end, a modem modulates digital data into sound frequencies transmitted over a phone line. At the receiving end, another modem demodulates the sound frequencies back into digital data.

Modularity: an approach to system design that emphasizes each subsystem as a self-contained module.

Open loop: refers to a control system in which the state of the output is not measured or used for control purposes.

Parallel I/O: a form of input/output whereby the bits in a bit pattern are transferred simultaneously, with each bit transferred over a separate line.

"Pot": an abbreviation for potentiometer (e.g., a standard rotating-type control knob is attached to a "pot.")

Potentiometer: an electromechanical device that converts displacement (rotary or linear) into a change in electrical resistance.

PROM: programmable read-only memory; a general-purpose form of ROM that is programmable but not erasable.

RAM: random access memory (also known as read and write memory or temporary memory); memory used for storing temporary data that can be retrieved later.

Real-time: pertaining to the ability of a microprocessor system to process data at least as fast as that information is physically generated, without significant delay.

Resolution: the smallest interval between two points on a scale (e.g., time, length, sound) below which they are undistinguishable and appear to be one single point.

Response time: a measure of how fast a system or component takes to react to an instruction.

ROM: read-only memory; its main characteristics are that it is nonvolatile and data cannot be written into ROM but can only be read from it.

RS232: a serial input/output interface standard.

Serial I/O: a form of input/output in which the bits in a bit pattern are transferred one at a time, that is, in a serial fashion, over the same wire.

Software: the set of instructions and data stored in a program designed to perform a specific task, for example, software to control a ventilator.

SRAM: static random-access memory; a form of memory that does not require dynamic update of data and is faster than dynamic random-access memory (DRAM); uses transistors.

4

Ventilator Performance Evaluation

David A. Desautels

The purchase of mechanical ventilators should be a rational, objective, and calculating decision. Diligent control of costs can limit skyrocketing expenditures. Consumers (patients), patient's families, respiratory therapists, nurses, and physicians must be the driving force behind ventilator pricing. Decisions regarding the type and function of ventilators should be made unemotionally, without bias, and with special regard to the type of patient to be ventilated and the quality of support services needed. As an example, the most expensive and elaborate ventilator is not essential in a chronic care unit where complications are minimal; a quality product that provides only the necessary ventilation modes is required. Ventilators that meet and remain within their specifications with reasonable use and without premature breakdowns are needed.

One of the purposes of this chapter is to aid those who purchase ventilators to evaluate them by objective criteria. Such a purchase should be approached like that of any expensive automobile. Economic virtues, recommendations, flexibility, and need should be investigated. The possibility that the device in question might someday be used for a friend, loved one, or oneself should be considered. Personal inspection of ventilators that are already owned, on trial, or anticipated for purchase is essential and should not be limited only to those ventilators one is familiar with.

PERFORMANCE EVALUATION FORMS

A program that permits an objective and comprehensive evaluation of any ventilator should include forms based on classification and specifications by which similarities, differences, and results of bench testing and subjective evaluations can be recorded. Even a picture of the front panel and a schematic diagram of the various ventilators may be useful. The forms should be comprehensive yet succinct. Too much detail makes forms cumbersome and discourages thoroughness.

Various performance evaluation forms are presented in this chapter to assist in obtaining the most comprehensive and objective analysis possible (Figs. 4-1 to 4-6). Such forms help a prospective purchaser or user compare ventilators objectively. Although some forms may seem irrelevant (e.g., the classification form), all are essential for good decision-making.

As additional ventilators are evaluated for purchase, the forms can be accumulated so that, eventually, a complete file of objective and unsolicited information is available with which to make practical and realistic decisions, to keep

VENTILATOR CLASSIFICATION ANALYSIS MODEL ____________________

(Check if available)

I. Ventilator power variables	
A. Pressure differential	
1. Subambient pressure	
2. Positive pressure	
B. Power source	
1. Electrical	
a. Mechanical	
b. Electronic	
2. Gas	
a. Pnuematic	
b. Fluidic	
3. Mixed	
C. Gas transmission	
1. Direct	
2. Indirect	
D. Internal mechanism	
1. Eccentric wheel piston	
2. Direct drive piston	
3. Solenoid/gate valve	
4. Venturi (injector)	
5. Compressor	
6. Bellows/bag	
7. High pressure gas	
8. Spring	
9. Weight	
II. Ventilator phase variables	
A. Inspiratory phase	
1. Normal generators	
a. Constant pressure	
b. Nonconstant pressure	
c. Constant fow	
d. Nonconstant flow	
2. Modification	
a. Pressure	
1.Inspiratory hold	
b. Flow wave	
1. Square	
2. Sinusoidal	
3. Decelerating	
4. Accelerating	
B. Change from inspiratory to expiratory	
1.Classic method	
a. Time cycled	
b. Pressure cycled	
c. Volume cycled	
B. Change from inspiratory to expiratory (cont.)	
d. Flow cycled	
e. Mixed cycle	
2. Limits	
a. Pressure	
b. Volume	
c. Mixed	
C. Expiratory phase	
1. Classic method - generators	
a. Constant pressure	
b. Nonconstant pressure	
c. Constant flow	
d. Nonconstant flow	
2. Modified method	
a. Distending pressure	
b. Ambient pressure	
c. Retard	
D. Change from expiratory to inspiratory	
1. Classic method	
a. Time cycled	
b. Pressure cycled	
c. Volume cycled	
d. Mixed cycled	
2. Traditional	
a. Control	
b. Assist	
c. Assist/control	
d. Intermittent mandatory ventilation	
e. Synchronized intermitt. ventilation	
f. Mandatory minute ventilation	
g. Pressure support	
h. Airway pressure release ventilation	
III. High frequency ventilation ventilation	
A. High frequency positive pressure ventilation	
B. High frequency oscillation	
C. High frequency jet ventilation	

Fig. 4-1. Form to evaluate a ventilator by its classification.

VENTILATOR SPECIFICATIONS - I

Manufacturer ______________________

Model ______________________

Cost ______________________

	Capability		Alarm/Monitor				
	Minimum	Maximum	Low	High	Type	Delay	Comment
Inspiration							
Rate (breath/min)							
Volume (ml)							
Flow rate (L/min)							
Pressure limit (cm H_2O)							
Time (sec)							
Effort (sensitivity) (cm H_2O)							
Hold (sec)							
Oxygen (%)							
Demand flow (L/min)							
Safety pressure limit (cm H_2O)							
Expiration							
Volume (ml)							
Time (sec)							
Positive end-expiratory pressure and continuous positive airway pressure (cm H_2O)							
Retard (L/min)							
Ratio of inspiration to expiration							
Ratio							
Inverse							
Sigh							
Rate (breath/hour)							
Volume (ml)							
Pressure limit (cm H_2O)							
Multiples							
Humidity							
Temperature (°C)							
Volume (ml)							

Fig. 4-2. Form to evaluate a ventilator by its specifications.

ventilators within their specifications, to pass inspections, and to become oriented to new products.

VENTILATOR CLASSIFICATION

The New World Dictionary defines a ventilator as, "a thing that ventilates; especially any opening or device used to bring in fresh air and drive out foul air." The American College of Chest Physicians describes a ventilator as, "a device designed to augment or replace the patient's spontaneous ventilation." A ventilator is different from a respirator which is defined by the New World Dictionary as: "1. A contrivance such as gauze worn over the mouth, or mouth and nose to prevent the inhalation of harmful substances, to warm the air breathed,

VENTILATOR SPECIFICATIONS - II — Model ______

Manufacturer ______ — Cost ______

(Check if available or fill in correct number)

	OPTIONALS		WAVEFORM	
	Power switch		Constant	
	Lamp test		Decelerating	
	Delay selector		Accelerating	
	Alarm reset		Sinusoidal	
	Alarm volume		POWER	
	Single breath trigger		Electric	
	Oxygen pressure gauge		MISCELLANEOUS	
	Air pressure gauge		Apneic period (sec)	
	Elapse timer		Humidifier volume (ml)	
	Minute volume counter		CURRENT LEAKAGE (UV)	
	MODE SELECTOR		ELECTRIC CONSUMPTION (watt)	
	Control		GAS CONSUMPTION (L/min)	
	Assist		MINUTE VOLUME	
	Assist/Control		Rate × tidal volume	
	Intermittent mandatory ventilation		Flow × inspiration time × expiration time	
	Synchronized intermittent mandatory ventilation		Flow × inspiration time × I :E ratio	
	Pressure support ventilation		PHYSICAL DIMENSIONS	
	Mandatory minute ventilation		Size	
	Airway pressure release ventilation		Weight	
	Continuous positive airway pressure			
	Compressible volume (ml/cm H_2O)			
	Resistance (cm H_2O/L/sec)			

Fig. 4-3. Form to evaluate a ventilator by its specifications—does not require testing at minimum and maximum settings.

etc. 2. An apparatus for giving artificial respiration. 3. A gas mask.'' The proper term, *ventilator,* is used throughout this chapter.

Proper classification cannot be summed up by a simple phrase such as ''a volume ventilator.'' Although such a description may have been meaningful during the 1960s when intermittent positive-pressure breathing (IPPB) was in vogue, it has little use at present. The sophistication in ventilators of the 1980s and 1990s dictates a more elaborate method of classification (Fig. 4-1).

Power Variables

Ventilators are first characterized according to power variables, subdivided as follows: (1) pressure differential, (2) power source, (3) mechanism of transmission, (4) internal mechanisms.[1,2] Pressure differential has been limited in use since the early 1960s, primarily due to the advent of positive-pressure ventilation; however, many iron lungs and chest cuirasses, which belong in the subambient pressure category, are still available.

The power source is divided into electrical and gas components, each with further subdivisions: electronic or mechanical and fluidic or pneumatic, respectively. Many ventilators use several power sources. Examples include the Emerson ventilator, which has some electronic components but is basically a mechanical device, and the Puritan-Bennett MA-1 ventilator, which has some mechanical components but is primarily electronic. Similar overlap also occurs with fluidic and pneumatic ventilators.

VENTILATOR CONTROLS ORIENTATION
(Check if available)

I. Minute volume delivery		C. Environment controls	
A. Flow and time controls		1. Oxygen concentration	
1. Flow rate		2. Humidification: heater	
2. Time		3. Nebulizer	
a. Rate		D. Sigh controls	
b. Inspiratory time		1. Rate	
c. Expiratory time		2. Volume	
d. Inspiratory:expiratory ratio		3. Pressure	
B. Volume and time controls		4. Multiple sigh	
1. Volume		III. Expiratory modification controls	
a. Minute volume		A. Flow	
b. Tidal volume		1. Retard	
2. Time		2. Expiratory flow gradient	
a. Rate		B. Pressure	
b. Inspiratory time		1. Subambient pressure	
c. Expiratory time		2. Distending pressure	
d. Inspiratory:expiratory ratio		IV. Alarms	
II. Delivery modification controls		A. Minute volume	
A. Initiation		1. Power failure	
1. Manual trigger		2. High pressure	
2. Sensitivity		3. Low pressure	
a. Pressure sensitivity		4. High volume	
b. Volume sensitivity		5. Low volume	
B. Inspiratory modification controls		6. Long expiration	
1. Inspiratory hold		7. Short expiration	
2. Flow pattern		B. Supplemental alarms	
a. Biphasic flow		1. Oxygen concentration	
b. Flow taper		2. Distending pressure	

Fig. 4-4. Form for orientation to ventilator control knobs.

Subjective Checklist for Ventilator Evaluation

(1 = poor, 2 = fair, 3 = average, 4 = good, 5 = excellent)

	Weight	1	2	3	4	5	Total
Ease of operation							
Durability							
Flexibility							
Cost							
Monitor/Alarms							
Dependability							
Simplicity							
Esthetics							

Fig. 4-5. Form for the subjective evaluation of ventilators.

Checklist for Inspection by the Joint Commission for the Accreditation of Hospitals

REQUIREMENTS FOR EACH VENTILATOR	A	B	C	D	E
Policy and procedure					
Assembly and operation instructions					
Objectives of use					
Orientation documents					
Continuing education documents					
Entry level knowledge documentation					
Quality assurance program					
Preventative maintenance program					
Specifications on file					
Component calibration records					
Pressure monitoring available					
Oxygen monitoring available					
Temperature monitoring available					
PIN index and diameter index safety system					
Infection control measures					
Cleaning and sterilizing procedures					
Adverse reaction criteria					
Equipment change requirements					
Instructions for discharged patients					
GENERAL REQUIREMENTS					
Samples of forms					
Records of equipment changes					
Prescription record on patient's chart					
Record of new piping installation testing					
Documentation of goals and objectives on patient's chart					
Efficacy of treatment on patient's chart					
Drugs and reagents in date					
Drug refrigerator documented at 40°C					
Documentation of long–term oxygen use					

Fig. 4-6. Checklist with which to prepare ventilators for inspection by the Joint Commission on Hospital Accreditation.

The mechanism of transmission describes how gas is delivered to the patient. If the power source is the medium by which gas is transmitted to the patient, direct transmission is involved; if not, the gas is transmitted indirectly. Examples of direct-transmission ventilators include the Emerson 3-PV and Babybird, whereas the Puritan-Bennett MA-1 and Engström Erica IV ventilators represent indirect transmission types.

A ventilator also can be categorized according to the internal mechanism by which it operates. Here, the emphasis is on the mechanical components responsible for ventilator function. Many are similar from one ventilator to another, whereas others are unique. Some ventilators operate by more than one basic mechanism. Primary mechanisms include eccentric wheel pistons, direct-drive pistons, solenoid/gate valves, Venturis, compressors, bellows/bags, high-pressure gas, springs, and weights. The drive mechanisms are directly responsible for the type of inspiratory flow waveform developed during mechanical inhalation. As an example, an eccentric wheel piston develops a sine wave inspiratory flow pattern, whereas a solenoid gate valve produces a square or constant inspiratory flow waveform.

Phase Variables

Mushin's classic description[1,2] remains the prototype of classification systems. He divided the ventilatory cycle into four components: (1) the inspiratory phase, (2) the change from inspiratory to expiratory phase, (3) the expiratory phase, and (4) the change from expiratory to inspiratory phase. To begin inspiration, a positive-pressure ventilator must have an internal pressure different from (higher than) that of the lung, that is, pressure differential. Important factors include the volume of gas to be delivered, the rate at which gas must flow, the airway pressure required to move gas, and the alveolar pressure that results once gas has been delivered.[1–11]

Inspiratory Phase

The inspiratory phase (perhaps the most frequently misunderstood category) is dependent on either pressure or flow generators.[1,2,5]

Constant-Pressure Generator

A constant-pressure generator develops a low source pressure and maintains a low pressure gradient. Pure constant-pressure generators equilibrate with the patient's alveolar pressure within several time constants. A time constant τ is the time required for completion of 63 percent of the exponentially changing function when the total time for the function change is unlimited. The percentage of equilibrium value obtained in each time constant is related to the reciprocal of the natural log *e:*

$$\tau = \frac{1}{\log^e} \tag{1}$$

$$\begin{aligned} \frac{1}{2.718} &= 0.3679;\ 1.0 - 0.3679 \\ &= 0.63 \text{ (one time constant)} \\ (0.3679)^2 &= 0.1354;\ 1.0 - 0.1354 \\ &= 0.865 \text{ (two time constants)} \\ (0.3679)^3 &= 0.4971;\ 1.0 - 0.04971 \\ &= 0.95 \text{ (three time constants)} \end{aligned}$$

In the ventilator/patient system, the rate of change of pressure and volume depends on the product of total resistance and total compliance. If the resistance was 10 cm H_2O/L/sec and the compliance was 0.05 L/cm H_2O, the time constant is 0.5 seconds. This means that in 0.5 seconds, 63 percent of the equilibrium pressure and volume will be delivered; in 1.0 second, 86.5 percent; in 1.5 seconds, 95 percent; and so forth. Thus, the ventilator inspiratory phase progresses toward equilibrium at an exponential rate so that, in the first time constant, 63 percent of the equilibrium is attained; in the second, 86.5 percent; in the third, 95 percent; and so forth.

A theoretical pure constant-pressure generator is represented by an inverted bellows connected to a lung. If a weight that generates exactly the pressure required for proper lung excursion is placed on the bellows, gravity pulls the weight down and gas flows into the lung. However, perfect equilibrium is never attained, only approximated. After a specific period of time, even though equilibrium may be only 99.996 percent complete, the expiratory phase begins.

Examples of dynamic curves for constant pressure generators demonstrate the exponential function of these ventilators. Volume (V) delivered to the lung relative to the volume attained at equilibrium may be determined at any time constant (Fig. 4-7). The volume to be delivered at equilibrium is equal to the product of generated pressure (P) and system compliance (C):

$$\text{V (liters)} = \text{P (cm } H_2O) \times \text{C(L/cm } H_2O) \tag{2}$$

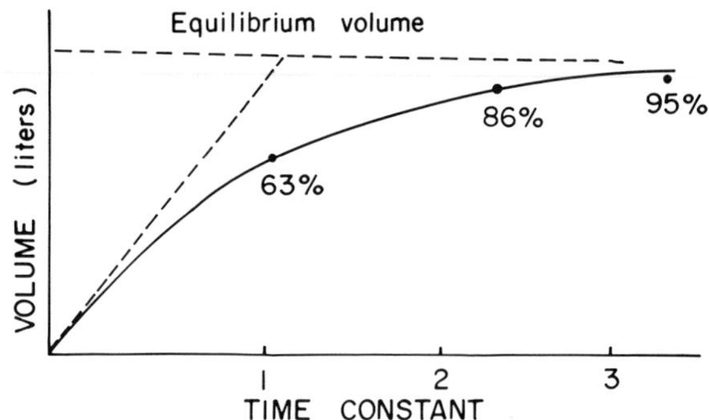

Fig. 4-7. Dynamic volume curve during mechanical ventilation with a constant-pressure generator.

For example, if 0.8 L is the equilibrium volume, in one time constant, 63 percent of that volume (or 0.0504 L) is delivered; in two time constants, 86 percent of that volume (or 0.688 L) is delivered, and so on.

Inspiratory flow rate ($\dot{V}_I$) (Fig. 4-8) is determined relative to the initial flow rate capability of the constant-pressure generator, which is equal to pressure (P) divided by the system's resistance (R):

$$\dot{V}_I = \frac{P}{R(\text{patient} + \text{ventilator})} \quad (3)$$
$$= \frac{\text{cm } H_20}{\text{cm } H_2O/\text{L/second}}$$
$$= \text{L/sec}$$

Therefore, if the pressure generated is 20 cm H_2O and the resistance of the system (patient and ventilator) is 30 cm H_2O/L/sec, the initial flow rate delivered into the lung occurs over a period of 0.67 L/sec. In the first time constant, the inspiratory flow rate diminishes to 37 percent of the initial value (1 − 0.63) (or 0.2479 L/sec); in two time constants, to 13.5 percent (1 − 0.865) (or 0.0905 L/sec), and so forth.

Alveolar pressure (P_A) (Fig. 4-9), relative to the pressure attained at equilibrium, may also be determined at any time constant. The alveolar pressure at equilibrium should equal that of the constant-pressure generator. This value is equal to the volume at equilibrium divided by the compliance (C) of the system:

$$P_A = \frac{V}{C(\text{patient} + \text{ventilator})} \quad (4)$$
$$= \frac{L}{\text{L/cm } H_2O}$$
$$= \text{cm } H_2O$$

As with volume, if the equilibrium pressure is 20 cm H_2O, in the first time constant, P_A is 63 percent (or 12.6 cm H_2O); in two time constants, P_A is 86.5 percent (or 17.3 cm H_2O) of the equilibrium pressure.

As gas flows, mouth (or oral) pressure (P_M)

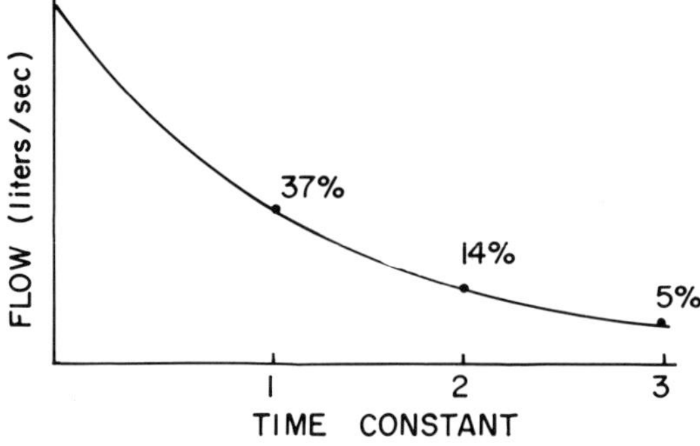

Fig. 4-8. Dynamic flow curve during mechanical ventilation with a constant-pressure generator.

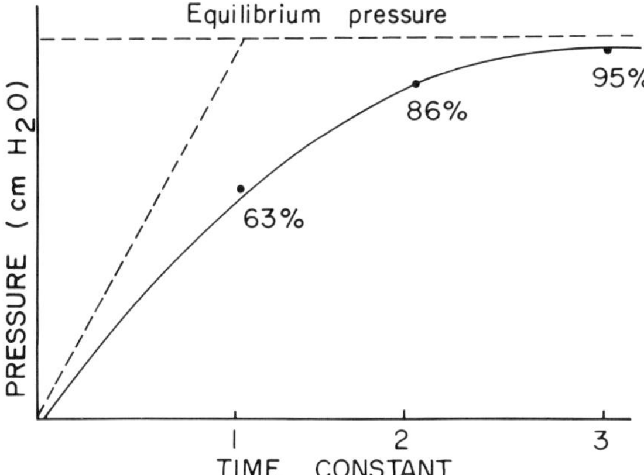

Fig. 4-9. Dynamic alveolar pressure curve during mechanical ventilation with a constant-pressure generator.

(Fig. 4-10) exceeds alveolar pressure by the ratio of the patient's resistance to the system's total resistance:

$$P_M = \frac{\text{R(patient)}}{\text{R(patient + ventilator)}} \times P \qquad (5)$$

$$= \frac{\text{cm } H_2O\text{/L/second (patient)}}{\text{cm } H_2O\text{/L/sec (patient + ventilator)}} \times \text{cm } H_2O$$

$$= \text{cm } H_2O$$

In this case, the instantaneous pressure must first be determined. The time constants are then applied to the difference between instantaneous pressure and equilibrium pressure. For example, if the ratio of the patient's resistance to the total resistance is 75 percent, 75 percent of the generated pressure is registered instantaneously on the pressure gauge before any gas flow occurs. If this value is 15 cm H_2O (75 percent of 20 cm H_2O, the first time constant relation of 63 percent is applied to the difference between equilibrium pressure and instantaneous pressure (20 − 15). Thus, in the first time constant the oral pressure is 18.15 cm H_2O (15 + 3.15). In actual fact, few constant-pressure ventilators are in use today.

Nonconstant-Pressure Generator

In the nonconstant-pressure generator, ventilator pressure, instead of remaining constant, is allowed to vary. It is the same at any designated point during each mechanical inhalation

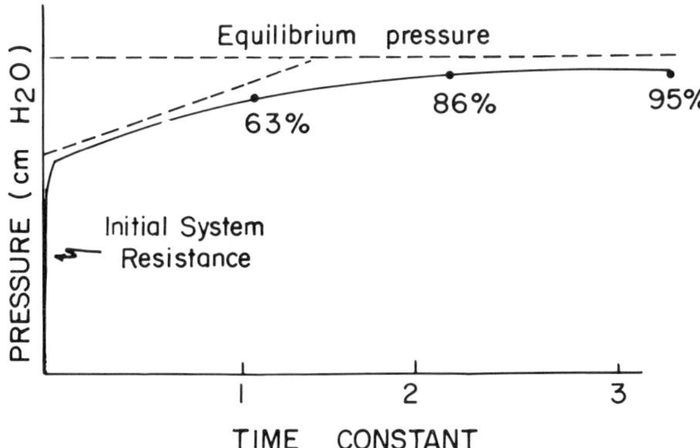

Fig. 4-10. Dynamic oral pressure curve during mechanical ventilation with a constant-pressure generator.

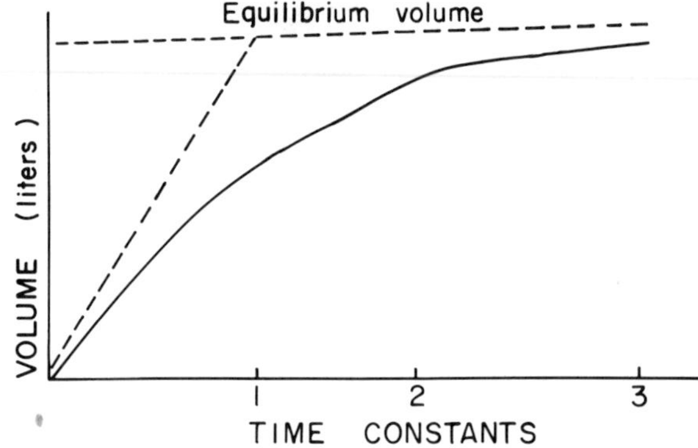

Fig. 4-11. Dynamic volume curve during mechanical ventilation with a nonconstant-pressure generator.

but is affected by the patient's lung-thorax compliance (CLT) and airway resistance. Equilibrium with the patient is developed within specific time constants, as with a constant-pressure generator, although each time constant is determined trigonometrically rather than arithmetically.

Dynamic curves for nonconstant-pressure generators (Figs. 4-11 to 4-14) follow the same principles as those for constant-pressure generators except that with nonconstant-pressure, the curves may not be exponential and may vary at each time constant.

Constant-Flow Generator

A ventilator that is a constant-flow generator theoretically is not influenced by changes in patient CLT and airway resistance because the ventilator driving pressure is at least ten times greater than that required for normal lung expansion. The pressure gradient is so large that time constants are measured in minutes rather than seconds, and inspiratory time is measured in seconds rather than time-constant increments.

Most constant-flow generators have high internal resistance as a safety feature. The neces-

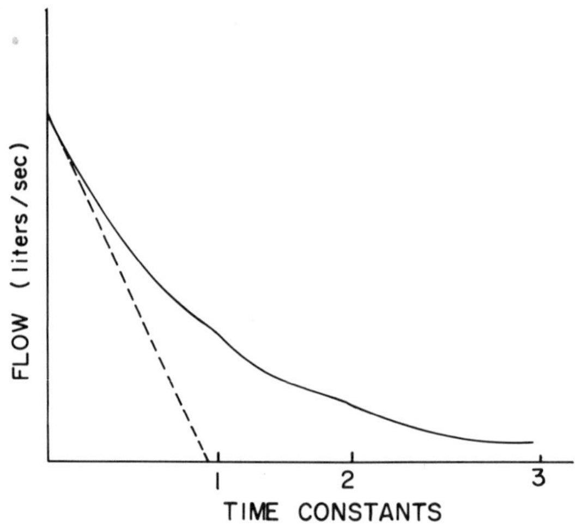

Fig. 4-12. Dynamic flow curve during mechanical ventilation with a nonconstant-pressure generator.

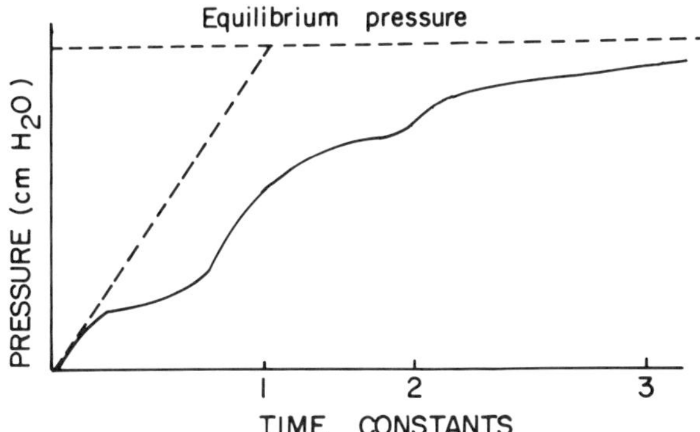

Fig. 4-13. Dynamic alveolar pressure curve during mechanical ventilation with a nonconstant-pressure generator.

sity of this feature can be readily understood if a pure constant-flow generator, represented by a cylinder of compressed gas at 2,200 psig, is examined. If this gas source is connected to a patient's airway and a solenoid valve is placed between the cylinder and the patient, a pure constant flow generator results. When the solenoid valve is opened for a fraction of a second, the patient's resistance and compliance have little effect on gas flow. However, in the absence of an internal reducing regulator, the patient is exposed to a high risk of injury.

Constant flow through the ventilator can be mistaken for that induced by a constant flow generator; however, there is a distinction, as in the Babybird ventilator. A constant-flow generator applies only to the mechanical inspiratory phase, whereas constant flow through a ventilator applies to both inspiratory and expiratory phases.

The volume (Fig. 4-15) of gas flowing to the lung is determined by the inspiratory flow rate and elapsed time (t):

$$\begin{aligned} V &= \dot{V}_I \text{ (L/sec)} \times t\text{(sec)} \\ &= L \end{aligned} \tag{6}$$

Because the internal resistance of the system is so great, most constant-flow generators have a time constant greater than 6 minutes, making such a value of little practical or clinical significance. Therefore, elapsed time (inspiratory time) is determined in seconds. If the constant inspiratory flow rate is 1.0 L/sec (60 L/min) and the inspiratory time is 1 second, the volume

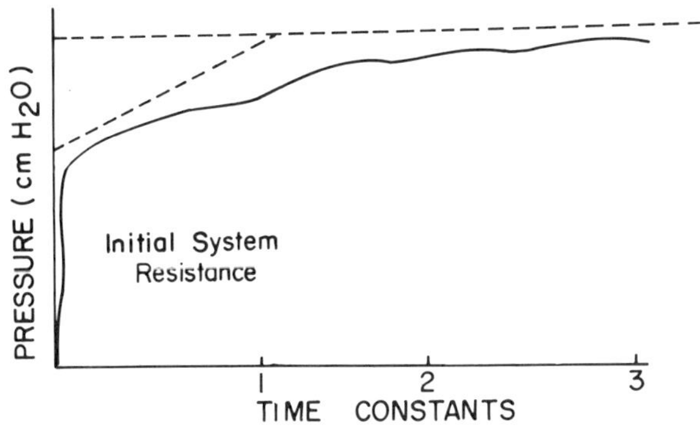

Fig. 4-14. Dynamic oral pressure curve during mechanical ventilation with a nonconstant-pressure generator.

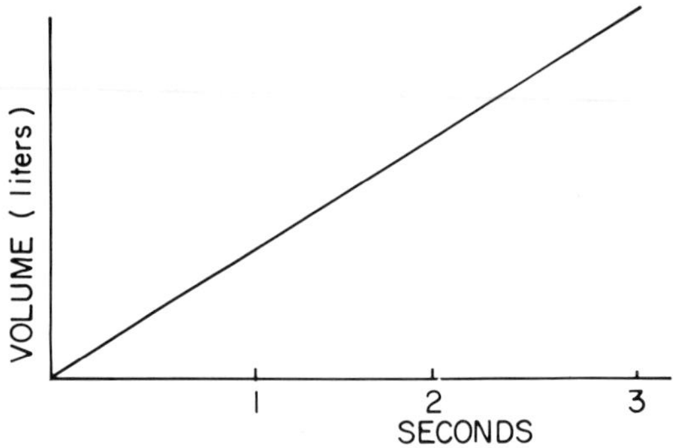

Fig. 4-15. Dynamic volume curve during mechanical ventilation with a constant-flow generator.

delivered is 1 L in spite of resistance and compliance factors of the patient, because of the high pressure differential.

Gas-flow rate (Fig. 4-16) into the lung, as implied, proceeds at a constant rate. It is equal to the generating pressure (PG) divided by the resistance (R) of the system:

$$\dot{V}_I = \frac{P_G}{R} = \frac{\text{cm } H_2O}{\text{cm } H_2O/\text{L/sec}} = \text{L/sec} \quad (7)$$

If P_G = 4,000 cm H_2O and R = 8,000 cm H_2O/L/sec, $\dot{V}_I$ = 0.5 L/sec.

Alveolar pressure (Fig. 4-17) is calculated as the ratio of the inspiratory flow rate to the compliance of the system:

$$P_A = \frac{\dot{V}_I}{C} = \frac{\text{L/sec}}{\text{L/cm } H_2O} = \text{cm } H_2O/\text{sec} \quad (8)$$

Note that this value varies as a function of time. If during mechanical inhalation the constant flow rate is 0.5 L/sec and the compliance of the system is 0.05 L/cm H_2O, the alveolar pressure increases at 10 cm H_2O/sec.

Mouth or oral pressure (Fig. 4-18) exceeds alveolar pressure during gas flow; therefore, a differential pressure equal to the product of the

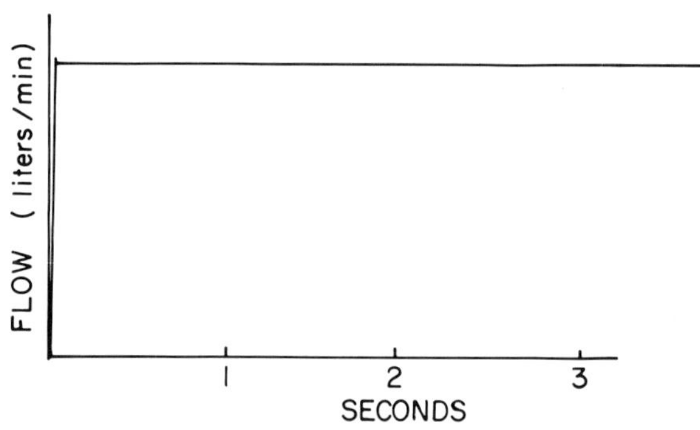

Fig. 4-16. Dynamic flow curve during mechanical ventilation with a constant-flow generator.

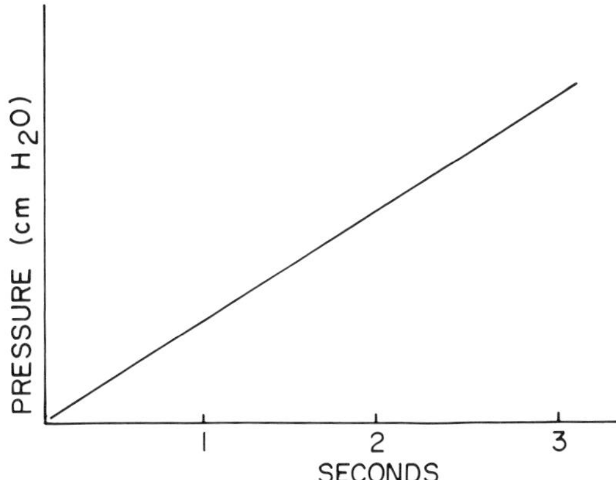

Fig. 4-17. Dynamic alveolar pressure curve during mechanical ventilation with a constant-flow generator.

patient's airway resistance and the flow rate must be added to the alveolar pressure:

$$\begin{aligned} P_M &= P_A + (\text{airway resistance} \times \dot{V}_I) \quad (9) \\ &= \text{cm } H_2O + (\text{cm } H_2O/L/sec \times L/sec) \\ &= \text{cm } H_2O \end{aligned}$$

If the alveolar pressure in the first second is 10 cm H_2O) and the differential pressure is 2.5 cm H_2O (resistance of patient = 5 cm $H_2O/L/sec$ and inspiratory flow rate = 0.5 L/sec), the P_M in the first second is 12.5 cm H_2O.

Nonconstant-Flow Generators

Ventilators of the nonconstant-flow generator-type generate sine wave flow patterns during mechanical inhalation. The pressure gradient, similar to that of constant-flow generators, is so large that ideally, the delivered flow rate is not influenced by the patient's C_{LT} or airway resistance. Examples of dynamic function curves during mechanical ventilation with nonconstant-flow generators are shown in Figures 4-19 to 4-22.

The reader should be aware that "pure" constant-flow generators and constant-pressure generators are theoretical constructs in the clinical setting. To the extent that a ventilator's functional characteristics approach one or the other of these categories more closely, it is classified accordingly.

End-Inspiratory Pause

An end-inspiratory pause (EIP), or hold, is incorporated into many ventilators. Some venti-

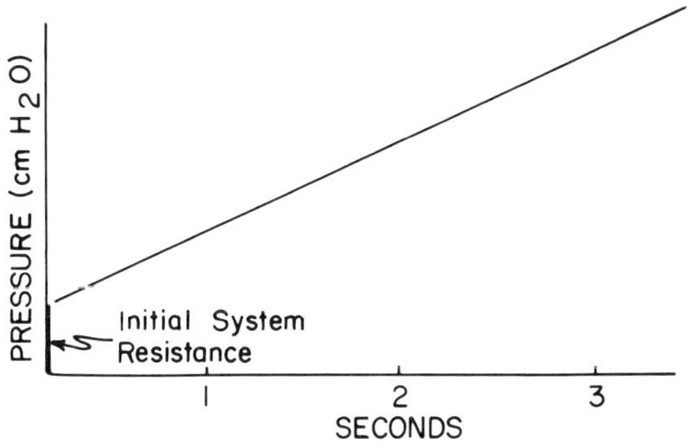

Fig. 4-18. Dynamic oral pressure curve during mechanical ventilation with a constant-flow generator.

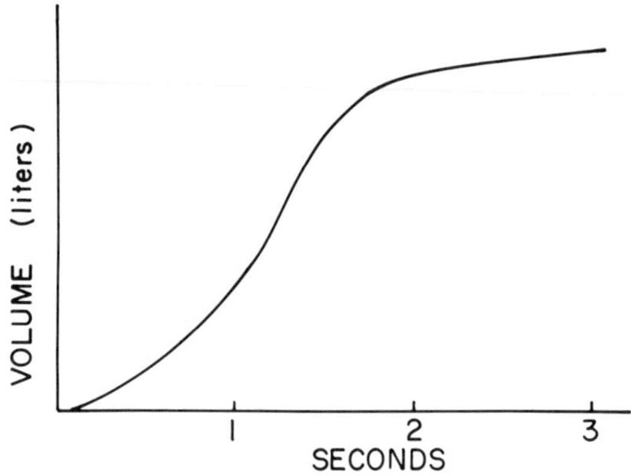

Fig. 4-19. Dynamic volume curve during mechanical ventilation with a nonconstant-flow generator.

lators hold pressure in the lung for a set period, whereas volume in others is maintained at a constant level. Finally, additional gas flow may be provided after the normal tidal delivery during the EIP period.

Inspiratory Flow Waveform

The advent of microprocessor-controlled ventilators has allowed various types of inspiratory flow waveforms to be delivered during mechanical inhalation. Constant flow generators provide a constant or a square inspiratory flow waveform by setting a constant inspiratory flow rate for a designated inspiratory time. Patient resistance and/or compliance do not alter the shape of the inspiratory flow waveform; therefore, a square wave is delivered. Constant-pressure generators do respond to patient resistance and compliance, delivering a decelerating inspiratory flow waveform. Microprocessor-controlled, nonconstant-flow ventilators are able to vary the inspiratory flow waveform, producing a sine wave flow profile. The ability to alter the pressure differential during mechanical inhalation allows microprocessor-controlled, nonconstant-flow ventilators to deliver decelerating or accelerating inspiratory flow waveforms as well. Patient resistance or compliance will not alter these waveforms due to the high-pressure differential provided.

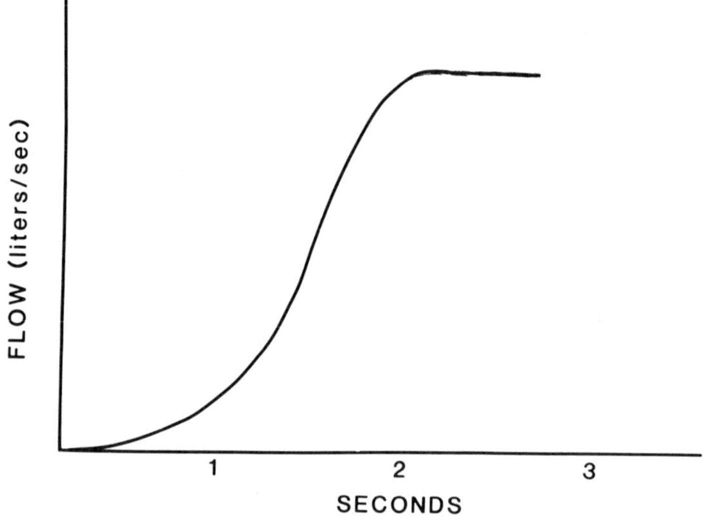

Fig. 4-20. Dynamic flow curve during mechanical ventilation with a nonconstant-flow generator.

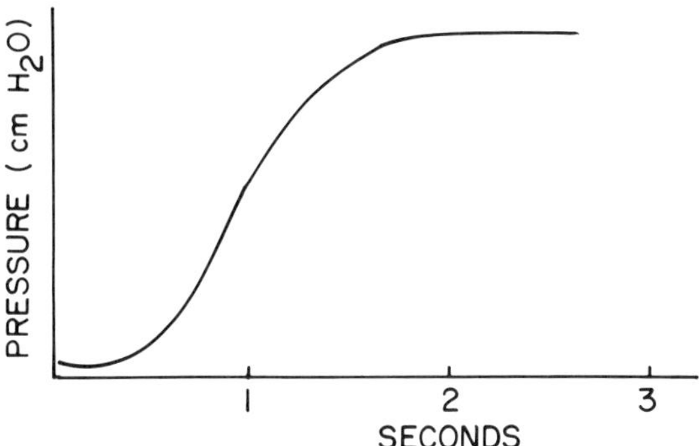

Fig. 4-21. Dynamic alveolar pressure curve during mechanical ventilation with a nonconstant-flow generator.

Inhalation to Exhalation Phase

Elam et al.[4] classified ventilators as volume-limited and pressure-variable or pressure-limited and volume-variable, a system that was generally accepted until Mapleson[6] introduced the concepts of time, pressure, volume, and flow cycling. This method of classification has survived to the present despite the proposal of other systems (e.g., that of Hunter[12,13]), which classed ventilators as pressure preset and volume preset.

An important distinction should be made between *cycling* and *limiting*. Cycling refers to termination, whereas limiting implies restriction. Thus, pressure-cycled is completely different from pressure-limited. If a ventilator is pressure-cycled, it cycles to the exhalation phase, once the designated pressure is reached. By contrast, a pressure-limited ventilator reaches and holds its designated pressure without cycling to the exhalation phase. Ventilators may be pressure- or volume-limited, but they cannot be time-limited; if time is limited and that time elapses, an exhalation must result. Such a ventilator is actually time-cycled.

Exhalation Phase

The same classification used for the inhalation phase can also be applied to the exhalation phase. However, such a classification is limited in that exhalation is most dependent on the functional characteristics of exhalation valves, which are widely variable. A more practical approach is to consider what therapeutic regimens are employed during exhalation (distending pressure, subambient pressure, retardation). Distending pressure, otherwise known as

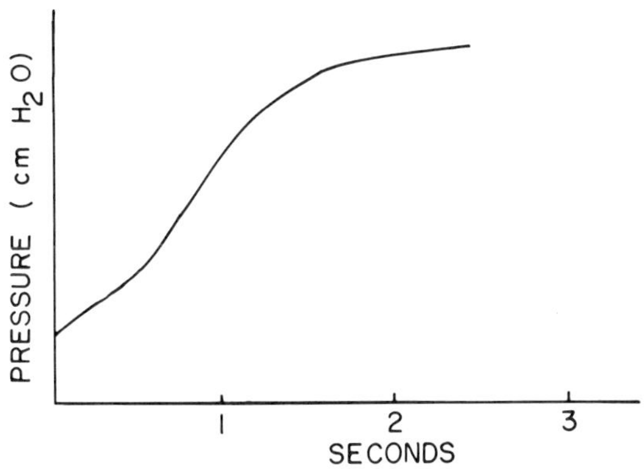

Fig. 4-22. Dynamic oral pressure curve during mechanical ventilation with a nonconstant-flow generator.

continuous positive airway pressure (CPAP), is positive pressure maintained throughout the spontaneous inhalation and exhalation phases. Subambient or negative pressure refers to airway pressure that is less than zero and may be used to reduce resistance of the breathing circuit (e.g., Babybird ventilator). Retardation of flow rate and volume from the lungs during exhalation is regulated by venting exhalation through a valve with a restricted orifice.

Exhalation to Inhalation Phase

Mapleson[6] classified this phase as similar to the change from inhalation to exhalation phase, that is, that phases are cycled by time, pressure, volume, the patient, or a combination thereof. More useful, perhaps, is that of Holaday and Rattenborg,[14] which describes assistors, controllers, and assist-controllers to which may be added intermittent mandatory ventilation (IMV), synchronized intermittent mandatory ventilation (SIMV), mandatory minute ventilation (MMV), high-frequency jet ventilation (HFJV), pressure-support ventilation (PSV), and airway pressure release ventilation (APRV).

Assisted (patient-triggered) ventilation is regulated by the patient's spontaneous breathing effort, which initiates a positive-pressure breath response from the ventilator. Controlled ventilation is machine-initiated (time-cycled on) at a designated rate. With assistor-controllers, the assist mode is dominant unless the patient fails to trigger the ventilator within a specified period of time; in the latter event, the control mode dominates. IMV is a combination of controlled and spontaneous ventilation, whereas SIMV represents a combination of assisted and spontaneous ventilation. MMV allows the ventilator to mandate a specific minute volume. Should the patient attain the prescribed minute ventilation through spontaneous ventilation, the ventilator adjusts itself to decrease mandated breaths. This modification allows the ventilator to control part of the weaning process and is available on the Engström Erica, Hamilton Veolar, Ohmeda CPU-1, and Bear 5 ventilators. HFJV is similar to controlled mechanical ventilation; however, the breathing frequency is much faster (e.g., 100 breaths/min) and the peak inflation pressures are lower.

Newer microprocessor-controlled ventilators (e.g., Puritan-Bennett 7200a, Hamilton Veolar) include PSV that operate in conjunction with their demand-flow systems. In the PSV mode, the ventilator is patient-triggered ON, to a preselected positive-pressure limit. As long as the patient's inspiratory effort is maintained, the preselected airway pressure stays constant with a variable flow of gas from the ventilator. Inspiration cycles OFF when the patient's inspiratory demand decreases to a preselected percentage of the peak mechanical inspiratory flow rate. The ventilator is thus flow-cycled in the PSV mode, following which passive exhalation occurs. The airway pressure, flow, and lung volume changes during PSV are more akin to assisted intermittent positive-pressure ventilation (IPPV) than to spontaneous breathing with CPAP.

Airway pressure release ventilation (APRV) is a unique mode of ventilatory support that provides alveolar ventilation by intermittently *decreasing* airway pressure from a preselected level of CPAP to either ambient pressure or a lower level of CPAP. As pressure is released from a higher to a lower level, a change in airway pressure (Δ PAW) results. Tidal volume (Vt) with APRV is equal to the product of PAW and CLT.

Airway Pressure Curves

For descriptive purposes, the PAW tracing may be divided into four components[14a]: (1) *baseline* (end-expiratory), the pressure level from which all respiratory maneuvers are accomplished; (2) *assist-effort pressure,* the pressure level the patient must generate in order to initiate a mechanical inhalation; (3) *peak inflation pressure* (PIP), the maximum airway pressure during a mechanical ventilator breath; and (4) *spontaneous inspiratory effort,* the airway pressure measured during a spontaneous inhalation. The values in all four levels represent gauge pressure in absolute numbers, and not deviations above and below the baseline.

Putting the entire sequence together, one is able to describe any respiratory pressure curve by an abbreviation and a set of numbers (Fig. 4-23), such as *SIMV 10/8/30/7*. In this example, SIMV is characterized by a baseline pressure of CPAP of 10 cm H_2O, and PAW drops to 8 cm H_2O during patient-triggering of the mechanical ventilator. A PIP of 30 cm H_2O is generated by the ventilator, and a baseline pressure is then maintained until a spontaneous breath occurs, during which time the PAW drops below the baseline level of CPAP to 7 cm H_2O. When a numerical value is not applicable for a given measurement, a blank or an asterisk is used. For example, the assist and spontaneous inspiratory effort pressures would not be applicable during controlled mechanical ventilation with Positive end-expiratory pressure (PEEP) and might be described in this way: *CMV-PEEP 10/*/30/**. In this instance, the baseline pressure is 10 cm H_2O, and a PIP of 30 cm H_2O is generated during delivery of the VT by the mechanical ventilator. Since neither assisted nor spontaneous breaths are accomplished by the patient, these categories are designed by a blank or an asterisk.

The proposed nomenclature not only describes the ventilatory mode, but also allows a more detailed description of the fluctuations in airway pressure that are created during ventilatory assistance. Adopting such a system of terminology would do much to eliminate the confusion that exists during communication between practitioners of respiratory care.

SPECIFICATIONS

Specifications pertain to ventilator controls without regard to ventilator classification. The specifications listed in the operating manual should not be considered constant for any ventilator; a ventilator that has been in use for even a brief time requires calibration to ensure specific levels of performance. The majority of pertinent information with which to evaluate specifications is shown in Figures 4-1 to 4-4. This information is not listed by priority, nor is all of it necessary to evaluate a ventilator satisfactorily.

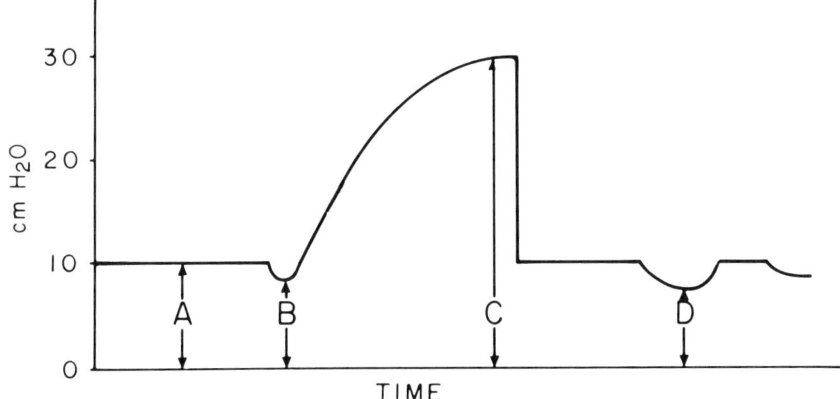

Fig. 4-23. Nomenclature for describing airway pressure curves. Four major components are shown. **(A)** Baseline (end-expiratory) pressure. **(B)** Assist effort. **(C)** Peak inflation pressure. **(D)** Spontaneous inspiratory effort. The pressure values for these components are used in a shorthand system to describe any ventilatory pattern. For example, the above pressure tracing represents a patient breathing with synchronized IMV and CPAP (10 cm H_2O). Using this nomenclature to describe the ventilatory pattern, the values A, B, C, and D, would be 10/8/30/7, respectively. (See text for details.)

Controls

The range (minimum to maximum) of each control is indicated in the manufacturer's operating manual, or is measured by specific monitors or gauges. Although some controls are not applicable to every ventilator, controls available should be evaluated to make comparison easier. If the range of a control is not given in the proper unit of measure, the necessary conversion should be made. For example, the pressure limit may be stated in millimeters of mercury (mmHg), but centimeters of water (cm H_2O), through common usage, is appropriate for most ventilators. Although often not listed in the manufacturer's specifications, inspiratory time is very helpful when making comparisons. Should specifications for certain parameters not be available from the manufacturer, the following suggestions may help in assessing the requisite values.

Rate. Values can be determined best by counting the number of breaths per minute as the machine cycles at the lowest and highest settings.

Volume. A pneumotachograph or a respirometer may be used with volume at minimum and maximum values. It is advisable to make several measurements at the minimum setting, which tends to fluctuate the most. If only minute volume is indicated, this value is divided by the number of breaths counted. Alternately, tidal volume VT can be calculated from the inspiratory flow rate and inspiratory time[15] [Eq. (6)]:

$$\begin{aligned} V_T &= 0.5 \text{ L/sec} \times 1 \text{ sec} \\ &= 0.5 \text{ L} \end{aligned} \tag{9}$$

Flow Rate. To measure flow rate exactly requires expensive flowmeters or a pneumotachograph. A rough approximation can be made from VT and inspiratory time:

$$\dot{V} = \frac{V_T}{\text{inspiratory time}} \tag{10}$$

$$\begin{aligned} \dot{V}_I &= \frac{0.5 \text{ L}}{1 \text{ sec}} \\ &= 0.5 \text{ L/sec (30 L/min)} \end{aligned}$$

Pressure Limit. The pressure-limit value should be measured at minimum and maximum settings. The maximum deflection of the pressure gauge should not be assumed to be the pressure limit. Generally, the needle oscillates and moves back toward the true reading because of a damping effect.

Inspiratory and Expiratory Times. Inspiratory (Ti) and expiratory times (Te) are difficult to determine without expensive measuring devices. However, an approximate value can be determined easily:

$$Ti = \frac{V_T \text{ (L)}}{\dot{V} \text{ (L/sec)*}} \tag{11}$$

For example,

$$\begin{aligned} Ti &= \frac{0.5 \text{ L}}{0.5 \text{ L/sec}} \\ &= 1 \text{ sec} \end{aligned}$$

In addition, T_i and T_e can be determined if the rate and the ratio of inhalation to exhalation (I:E) are known. Calculation at a rate of 16 breaths/min with an I:E ratio of 1:2 follow:

$$\begin{aligned} \text{Respiratory cycle time} &= \frac{60 \text{ sec/min}}{16 \text{ breaths/min}} \\ &= 3.75 \text{ sec/breath} \end{aligned}$$

$$\begin{aligned} \text{Fractional units of respiratory cycle} &= \frac{\text{respiratory cycle time}}{\text{I + E}} \\ &= \frac{3.75 \text{ sec/breath}}{1 + 2} = \frac{3.75}{3} \\ \text{Inspiratory time} &= 1 \text{ fractional unit} \\ &= 1.25 \text{ second} \end{aligned}$$

$$\begin{aligned} \text{Expiratory time} &= 2 \text{ fractional units} \\ &= 2.50 \text{ seconds} \end{aligned}$$

Inspiratory Effort. The inspiratory effort can be measured by placing a T connector in the breathing circuit, and measuring the deflection of a pressure gauge during inhalation with the airway occluded.

---

* Assuming a constant inspiratory flow rate.

Inspiratory Hold. Similar to the measurement of inspiratory effort, a T connector may be placed in the breathing circuit to observe the level and duration of an inspiratory "plateau."

Oxygen Concentration. An oxygen analyzer should be placed in the ventilator breathing circuit to monitor the minimum and maximum concentrations of oxygen.

Demand Flow. During spontaneous inhalation with CPAP, a pneumotachograph or similar device is essential in determining maximum flow rate from the system. Efforts to obtain flow rates greater than the capacity of the system do not increase the flow rate further.

Positive End-Expiratory Pressure/Continuous Positive Airway Pressure. To measure PEEP and CPAP, a T connector is inserted into the breathing circuit with a length of tubing connected to a pressure manometer. This measurement should always be made at the Y piece (patient/ventilator interface).

Retard. Retardation of exhaled flow, volume, and pressure from the lungs are measured in liters per minute (L/min) for exhaled flow rate, in milliliters (ml) for lung volume, and in centimeters of water (cm H_2O) for PAW. A pneumotachograph or respirometer and an PAW transducer are required to obtain these measurements.

I:E Ratio. An accurate assessment of the I:E ratio requires measurement of pressure with a transducer on a strip-chart recorder at a predetermined speed. Once the graph is recorded, measurement of the time of each phase from the chart speed is a simple matter to those familiar with graph tracings.

Other Factors. Each control on the ventilator also may have as a minimal requirement a corresponding alarm/monitor, the range of which should be listed. Thus, alarms for power failure, high and low pressures, high and low volumes, and long or short inspiratory and expiratory times may be necessary. Additional alarms that detect failure to maintain oxygen concentration and CPAP are desirable. The type of alarm (audible, visual, or both) should be characterized. The alarm delay, or that period of time that elapses before the alarm is activated, should be recorded. Alarm systems for ventilators have undergone rapid development during the past few years, almost to the point that some ventilators are overloaded and basic functions tend to be overlooked.

Of major importance in evaluating ventilator performance is the peak flow rate at designated PIP. Pressure relief pop-off valves with known pressure limits are helpful for measuring the ability of the ventilator to work against significant backpressure. If the valves are placed at the patient Y piece and the ventilator cycled, an in-line flowrater indicates the flow-rate capabilities against the generated backpressure. Often a ventilator that functions well during demonstration under ideal conditions, fails in a clinical setting when significant backpressure (PIP) is present.

A specification sheet should be a composite reflection of the major categories and components of most ventilators and should serve as a guide that can be adjusted as necessary for ventilator comparison. A detailed schematic diagram of the internal mechanisms of a ventilator should be included in ventilator performance evaluation and can be obtained from the ventilator manufacturer. A knowledge of schematic diagrams can lead to an in-depth understanding of ventilators. To clarify the functions available on a ventilator a diagram of the front panel and controls of the ventilator should be obtained. Such diagrams are available from the manufacturer or may be found in this and other texts.[1,2,16–19]

SUBJECTIVE EVALUATION

The subjective evaluation has no rules; the ventilator should be upgraded according to one's feelings about anything from color, control panel layout, operation, ease of operation, ease of understanding, and so forth (Fig. 4-5). However, the prospective purchaser should be fair and not make decisions based on past experience or because a salesperson may present the product poorly.

BENCH TEST EVALUATION

A bench test evaluation should be included in the ventilator performance evaluation program. Although a great deal can be learned from publications, manufacturer's information, and ventilator trials, until the ventilator actually has been tested under varied conditions, a complete understanding of its advantages, disadvantages, and best application cannot be obtained. An operational bench test includes a lung analogue to simulate physiologic variables (e.g., compliance, resistance, and air leaks) and instruments with which to measure the ventilator variables (e.g., flow rate, time, pressure, and volume). The measuring instruments need not be expensive and elaborate; simple tools are often better than expensive devices. For example, measurement of resistance can be expensive or—with a water-filled U tube, flowmeter, some tubing and a flowrater—inexpensive.

Lung analogues have long presented a perplexing problem to physiologists. Considering the multitude of complex factors that influence the human lung, it is hardly surprising that our ability to mimic the lung and its function is less than satisfactory. From using beer barrels to expensive wedge-type lung analogues experts have tried to simulate natural lung functions during mechanical ventilation, although mechanical ventilation is anything but natural. Publication of the American National Standards for Breathing Machines for Medical Use, ANSI standards Z79.7, in January 1976 brought some order out of the previously existing chaos.[20] Without these standards, physicians and respiratory therapists would be faced with an extremely difficult job of product evaluation and comparison.

Once a bench test has been established, it may also be used for teaching and testing new techniques. Flow, pressure, and volume curves can be demonstrated under a wide range of ventilator settings, and elaborate lung analogues can be useful in demonstrating: (1) how volume remains static or changes as a patient's compliance and resistance are altered; (2) how gas can be trapped at some settings when the ventilator is not functioning properly; (3) what happens during an inspiratory plateau; (4) how a particular CPAP system operates; and (5) a multitude of other concepts that require direct observation for complete understanding.

PURPOSES OF AN EVALUATION PROGRAM

Ventilator Operation

How a ventilator is adjusted depends on the needs of the patient. If a patient requires a respiratory rate of 30 breaths/min, the ventilator should provide that rate. A patient should never be made to breathe inappropriately because the ventilator cannot provide the appropriate rate. A variety of ventilatory modes should be available to meet ordinary and unusual requirements.

Additional mechanisms can modify or initiate mechanical breathing, including sensitivity control, which determines the spontaneous effort required to initiate a breath, and manual buttons, which generate an inflation when they are pushed.

Once the mode has been selected, a frequency must be chosen. Some ventilators use inspiratory and expiratory time controls rather than rate controls, per se. The expiratory and inspiratory times determine the rate, the minute volume, or both. The expiratory time is extended to decrease the number of breaths/min. This extension can also be used to permit more spontaneous respiration with IMV and SIMV. Miscellaneous controls that modify frequency include sigh rate, multiple sigh breaths, I:E ratio, and safety time-limit controls. An inspiratory hold modifies frequency by prolonging the inspiratory time through maintenance of either pressure or volume in the lung at the end of the inspiratory phase.

Although most critical care ventilators are generally referred to as volume ventilators (even though they often are not volume-cycled), pressure ultimately limits their capabilities. Pressure limit is determined by the operator; however, the pressure limit does not cycle the ventilator into the expiratory phase. The pressure setting on constant-pressure generators, is the end point of ventilator function. If the pressure attained by the ventilator is in equilibrium with the alveoli within six time constants, the ventilator is classified as a constant-pressure generator, such as the Gill 1 ventilator or Siemens 900B ventilator (when minute volume is high and the working pressure control is set at a low level).

Gas-flow rate in a ventilator system occurs because of a pressure gradient. Hence, pressure and flow are intrinsically related and interdependent. The settings for flow rate and inspiratory time generate a specific VT into the breathing circuit in time-cycled ventilators. Some ventilators use an inspiratory flow-tapering mechanism to produce a decelerating inspiratory flow waveform. Just as inspiratory flow rate can be modified, so also can the expiratory flow rate. An expiratory flow gradient (negative pressure) may be used to eliminate inadvertent PEEP or an expiratory retard valve employed to decrease flow rate and prevent air trapping.

Distending pressure controls maintain positive pressure during either the exhalation phase of the ventilator or throughout the entire respiratory cycle when the patient breathes spontaneously (i.e., CPAP). A threshold resistor expiratory pressure valve that maintains expiratory airway pressure at a preselected value is preferable (e.g., Emerson water column valve). An ideal threshold resistor maintains a constant airway pressure irrespective of the gas-flow rate directed through the valve. A flow resistor (restricted orifice) expiratory pressure valve, which increases or decreases airway pressure as flow rate increases or decreases, respectively, is sometimes employed. The latter exerts expiratory flow retardation as well as PEEP/CPAP, whereas a threshold resistor has minimal flow retardation.

Ventilator Malfunction

Caution must be exercised when dealing with ventilators that malfunction. Initially, the extent of the malfunction must be assessed. If the malfunction can be easily pinpointed and corrected and does not jeopardize the patient's well-being, the clinician can proceed with corrective actions. However, if any doubt exists regarding the origin or extent of the malfunction or the means to correct it, the ventilator must be disconnected from the patient immediately and alternative manual or mechanical ventilation provided. A troubleshooting algorithm is useful and is usually available in the instruction manual which comes with the ventilator. If a significant problem is documented which is intrinsic to the ventilator, it should be detailed sufficiently for publication or forwarded to an organization such as the ECRI, Inc., which publishes hazard bulletins and investigates problems of more than passing interest to medical consumers (see Ch. 16).

Ventilator Comparison

To gain a perspective on available ventilators, one should first thoroughly evaluate those ventilators at hand. To understand a ventilator's capabilities and limitations, the investigator should employ it under clinical and laboratory settings. One difficulty with this approach is that familiarity may mask objectivity. The use of forms similar to those presented earlier in this chapter are helpful in cataloging information and maintaining a neutral outlook. The forms which in all likelihood are of greatest use pertain to classification specifications. Probable clinical applications should be considered, particularly when flow rates and pressure-limit capabilities are important determinants of function. Specification forms help to remove some subjective aspects of decision-making; if they are properly used and weighed appropriately for each criterion for each ventilator, many dilemmas of decision-making are obviated.

If possible, once a particular "make and model" of ventilator is chosen, several "samples" should be tested. Surprising differences in performance in apparently identical machines may be detected. Ventilators, like automobiles, require periodic calibration and tune-ups. In fact, the Joint Commission on Accreditation of Hospitals (JCAH) requires calibration of ventilators to manufacturer's specifications at intervals designated by the manufacturer (usually annually, but quarterly is preferable).

When comparing ventilators, one should initially compare the base or stripped models before considering optional accessories. If options are necessary to make products comparable, the additional cost should be considered in the final evaluation.

Often, ventilators are modified by the user to achieve some perceived advantage in performance. In such instances, changes must be well thought out. Should the integrity of the ventilator be affected in a way not approved by the manufacturer, the user becomes liable for any mishaps and the ventilator warranty is invalidated. After major alterations, animal studies are appropriate before the ventilator is applied clinically.

Ventilator Purchase

Ventilators to be considered for purchase should be submitted to an in-hospital trial and performance evaluation. New or trial equipment must be introduced cautiously to clinical use. Although manufacturers have used engineering prototypes, animal experiments, and clinical trials in the development of their product, the ventilator is new to the prospective buyer and staff. Proper orientation must be given to all personnel who will be required to operate the device before it is used for patient care. Untrained persons should not use the ventilator under any circumstances. When in-service education is provided, the personnel signatures, date of training, and lecturer should be documented and filed.

Should a given hospital or teaching institution be involved with clinical trials or research protocols for ventilator development, such protocols normally are approved by the hospital's Institutional Review Board (IRB). If the ventilator is a prototype developed after May 28, 1976, its use falls under the Food and Drug Administration regulations concerning all new class 3 medical devices.[21,22] A thorough cost analysis helps and should be established when ventilator purchases are considered. In addition to depreciation, each of the items in Table 4-1 must be taken into account to arrive at a true estimate of dollar outlay.

Table 4.1. Analysis of Ventilator True Cost

Ventilator
Breathing circuit
Sterilization
Repair
Preventative maintenance
Quality assurance
Additional monitoring
Replacement
Operation
Interest on money borrowed to purchase the ventilator

Justification for purchase of very expensive ventilators may be difficult when one deals with health care administrators who are striving to reduce costs. Once a ventilator is chosen, data should be presented, if possible, to show that it can provide the best medical care for the fewest dollars. Later, the decision to purchase should be evaluated objectively to determine if prepurchase considerations have actually been verified.

JOINT COMMISSION ON ACCREDITATION OF HOSPITALS INSPECTION

A performance verification program should be instituted to comply with JCAH standards[23] and should include the records, preventive maintenance, and quality control for each ventilator in use, as well as documentation of employment, orientation and continuing education program of persons using the ventilators.

A checklist to help with JCAH inspections is provided in Fig. 4-6. This checklist, complied from several JCAH documents and other support materials, should be used for each ventilator. Also, policies and procedures related to each type of ventilator in the department, should be formulated and written, as well as for orientation, in-service, and continuing education.[24] Records of attendance at continuing education programs should be kept in each personnel file, together with an outline of the lecture, signatures of the lecturers, and persons attending. A separate schedule of lectures should also be maintained.

Many quality-assurance programs can be built around each ventilator. These should contain criteria for evaluation, a detailed survey or collection of data, results, follow-up, and indication of the corrective actions that may be taken. Each ventilator must have a repair and preventive maintenance record that contains the instructions, specifications, and manufacturer's suggested maintenance schedule. This requirement applies also to all ventilator components as well as the gases used.

For proper documentation, all ventilator therapy must be recorded on the patient's chart, including diagnosis; goals and objectives of care; prescriptions; type, frequency, and duration of any treatment; type, dose, and diluent of medication; oxygen concentration; patient's vital signs at regular intervals; and results of therapy. All these data must be accompanied by the initials of the responsible person.

Additional policies and procedures that should be available pertain to documents to substantiate the competence of any respiratory therapist on staff, tests on all newly installed gas piping systems, routine checks on existing systems, and compliance of ventilator systems with PIN index or DISS safety systems. Policies of infection control, which should address requirements and methods for ventilator equipment changes, cleaning, and sterilization should also be maintained. Further documentation should substantiate the actions to be taken in the event of complications—how the complication is identified and how it should be corrected.

REFERENCES

1. Mushin WW, Rendell-Baker L, Thompson PW, et al: Automatic Ventilation of the Lungs. 1st Ed. Blackwell, London, 1959
2. Mushin WW, Rendell-Baker L, Thompson PW, et al: Automatic Ventilation of the Lungs. 3rd Ed. Blackwell, London, 1980
3. Baker AB, Babington PCB, Colliss JE, et al: Effects of varying inspiratory flow waveform and time in intermittent positive pressure ventilation. Br J Anaesth 49:1207, 1977
4. Elam JO, Kerr JH, Janney CD: Performance of ventilators: effects of changes in lung-thorax compliance. Anesthesiology 19:56, 1958
5. Jansson L, Jonson B: A theoretical study on flow patterns of ventilators. Scand J Respir Dis 52:237, 1972
6. Mapleson WW: The effect of changes of lung characteristics on the functioning of automatic ventilators. Anaesthesia 17:300, 1962
7. Nunn JF: Applied Respiratory Physiology. Butterworth, Boston, 1977
8. Peslin RL: The physical properties of ventilators in the inspiratory phases. Anesthesiology 30:3, 1969
9. Robbins LS, Crocker D, Smith RM: Tidal volume losses of volume-limited ventilators. Anesth Analg 46:428, 1967
10. Simbruner G, Gregory GA: Performance of neonatal ventilators: the effects of changes in resistance and compliance. Crit Care Med 9:509, 1981
11. Sullivan M, Saklad M, Demers R: Relationships between ventilator waveform and tidal-volume distribution. Respir Care 22:386, 1977
12. Hunter AR: The classification of respirators. Anaesthesia 16:231, 1961
13. Perry D: A simplified diagram for understanding the operation of volume-preset ventilators. Respir Care 22:42, 1977
14. Holaday DA, Rattenborg CC: Automatic lung ventilators. Anesthesiology 23:413, 1962

14a. Desautels DA, Sanderson RR, Klein EF: A unified approach to pulmonary ventilation terminology. Respir Care 23:42, 1978

15. Slonin NB, Hamilton LH: Respiratory Physiology. 2nd Ed. CV Mosby, St. Louis, 1971
16. Burton GB, Gee GN, Hodgkin JE: Respiratory Care. 1st Ed. JB Lippincott, Philadelphia, 1977
17. Egan D: Fundamentals of Respiratory Therapy. 2nd Ed. CV Mosby, St. Louis, 1973
18. Heironimus TW, Bogeaut RA: Mechanical Artificial Ventilation. 3rd Ed. Charles C Thomas, Springfield IL, 1977
19. Young JA, Crocker O: Inhalation Therapy. 2nd Ed. Year Book Medical Publishers, Chicago, 1976
20. American National Standards Institute: American National Standard for Breathing Machines

for Medical Use. ANSI 279.7–1976, January 26, 1976

21. United States Department of Health and Human Services: Investigational Device Exemption Regulation. Food & Drug Administration, Washington DC, July 1980
22. United States Department of Health and Human Services: Guidelines for the Arrangement and Content of a Premarket Approval Application. DHHS, Washington, DC, November, 1980
23. Accreditation Manual for Hospitals: Joint Commission of Accreditation of Hospitals, 1984
24. Hunsinger DL, Maurizi JJ, Lisnerski KS, et al: Respiratory Technology. 2nd Ed. Reston Publishing, Reston, VA, 1976

5

Physiologic Principles of Conventional Mechanical Ventilation

Scott Norwood

Respiratory support of critically ill patients has evolved from controlled mechanical ventilation (CMV) during the 1960s to a variety of techniques, including intermittent and synchronized intermittent mandatory ventilation (IMV/SIMV), assisted (patient-triggered) ventilation (AV), pressure-support ventilation (PSV), and various forms of high-frequency ventilation (HFV). Although each of these techniques is somewhat different, all are forms of positive-pressure ventilation (PPV). When used with or without positive end-expiratory pressure (PEEP) or continuous positive airway pressure (CPAP), these therapeutic techniques produce complex cardiopulmonary and extrathoracic organ interactions that may prove either beneficial or detrimental to oxygen delivery and end-organ function. Clinicians should understand these effects, because some forms of ventilation may prove more detrimental than therapeutic under certain conditions. The clinician who understands these physiologic effects will be able to choose the form of support that is most beneficial, considering the underlying disease process.

The purpose of this chapter is to present both the beneficial and detrimental physiologic effects of conventional PPV and PEEP/CPAP. HFV and airway pressure release ventilation (APRV) are discussed elsewhere in the book and are not subjects for this chapter (see Chs. 6, 7, and 15).

DEFINITIONS AND TERMINOLOGY

Conventional PPV is defined as any technique that incorporates a commercially available ventilator to improve either oxygenation or ventilation, or both with oxygen-enriched air. These goals are accomplished by the generation of increased airway pressure as the tidal volume (V_T) is delivered. PEEP and CPAP may also be used.

Mechanical ventilatory modes are classified according to the method by which the mechanical V_T, and the pressure/flow characteristics of the generated waveform are produced (see Chs. 6 and 15). Previously, discussions of pressure-cycled versus volume-cycled mechanical ventilation reflected differences in ventilator performance rather than the techniques of support. Early pressure-cycled ventilators generated 30 to 40 cm H_2O inspiratory pressure, as a result of which an adequate V_T could not be delivered to patients with severely decreased lung-thorax compliance (C_{LT}). They also were compliance variable, that is, if the patient resisted inflation, airway pressure rapidly increased, and the inspiratory phase was terminated prematurely before a sufficient VT was delivered.

By contrast, early volume-cycled ventilators could generate high peak inspiratory pressure (PIP) so that an adequate tidal volume usually could be maintained, even if compliance were markedly reduced. The change from inspiration to expiration occurred not at a fixed inspiratory pressure, but only after the desired VT was delivered. However, most volume-cycled (and time-cycled) ventilators have pressure-limiting safety devices built into the circuit. If a preselected maximal PIP is exceeded, the inspiratory cycle is aborted. Therefore, modern ventilators ultimately are pressure limited, regardless of their primary cycling mechanism.

VENTILATOR MODES

A variety of techniques have been advocated for optimal ventilator support. Each has its advocates, but none has clearly demonstrated superiority. Controlled mechanical ventilation, AV,[1,2] IMV/SIMV,[3–7] PSV,[8–10] and pressure-contolled ventilation (PCV) are most popular today. The relative merits of some of the newer techniques have been debated,[11–13] and their effects are undergoing careful evaluation. Their potential clinical application is described in detail in Chapters 6 and 9.

CARDIOPULMONARY INTERACTIONS

Numerous cardiopulmonary interactions are in effect during both spontaneous ventilation (SV) and PPV. They have variable effects on oxygen delivery, as summarized in this section. A more detailed analysis is presented later in the chapter.

During PPV, changes in pressure, flow, volume, and inspiratory time can be altered to minimize or completely eliminate spontaneous respiratory muscle work.[14] This potentially useful effect must be weighed against possibly adverse side effects. Such risk/benefit analysis should be individualized, depending on the patient's underlying cardiopulmonary status and the primary disease process.

Lung volume is related directly to the transpulmonary pressure (PL), which represents the difference between airway pressure (PAW) and intrapleural pressure (Ppl) (Fig. 5-1). Thus,

$$P_L = P_{AW} - Ppl \qquad (1)$$

During SV, when Ppl decreases (becomes more negative) as a result of respiratory muscle contraction, the thorax expands. Airway pressure may decrease slightly with SV but returns to baseline at end-inspiration.

During PPV, lung volume also increases. However, this change results from an increase in PAW, rather than from a decrease in Ppl. As PAW becomes positive, so does Ppl, although to a lesser degree. This basic difference in the

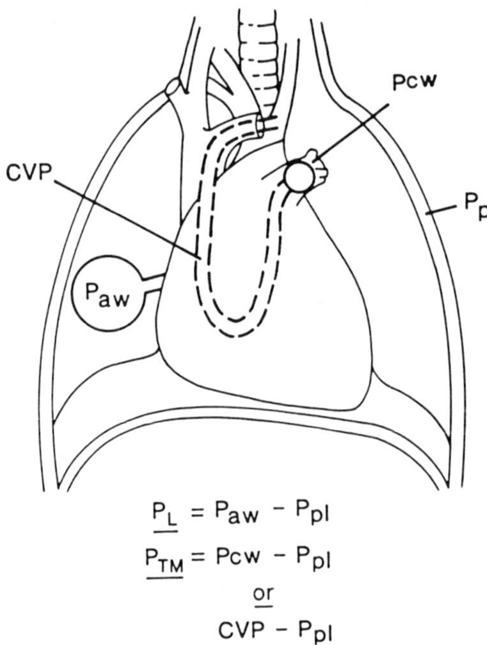

Fig. 5-1. Relationship among transpulmonary pressure (PL), airway pressure (PAW), and pleural pressure (Ppl). Note that the effective cardiac filling pressure, or transmural pressure (PTM) is also influenced by Ppl. Therefore, PAW or measured cardiac filling pressures [wedge pressure (PCWP) or central venous pressure (CVP)] are more accurate if referenced to Ppl. (From Boysen and McGough,[14] with permission.)

mechanism by which the same end point of increased lung volume occurs is responsible for most of the physiologic differences between SV and PPV.

Because SV decreases Ppl, venous return to the right side of the heart is enhanced. The opposite effect results from PPV; this diminution in venous return becomes more clinically significant in patients who are hypovolemic. Conversely, SV may inhibit ventricular systole by decreasing the pressure surrounding the heart.[15] Under certain conditions, left ventricular (LV) function is enhanced by PPV, decreasing afterload. This LV assist mechanism is more pronounced when myocardial contractility is compromised, and adequate preload is ensured by enhanced venous return.[16]

When lung volume is increased significantly, both SV and PPV increase right ventricular (RV) afterload, but the effect is generally more pronounced with PPV. As a result, an intravascular volume appropriate for SV, with or without PEEP/CPAP, often proves inadequate when PAW is increased with PPV. Conversely, the appropriate intravascular volume status when PAW is high may prove excessive at lower PAW or during SV.[16]

Optimal distribution of ventilation and perfusion ($\dot{V}/\dot{Q}$) is generally better during SV.[17] However, the work of breathing necessary to provide the same level of ventilation is always greater during SV than during CMV, regardless of the degree of respiratory dysfunction.[16,18]

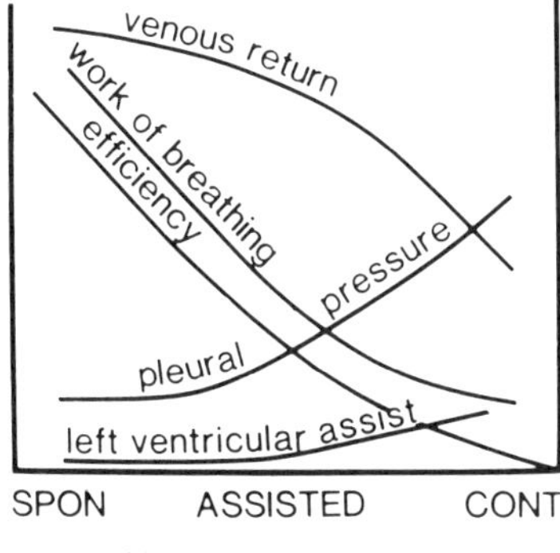

Fig. 5-2. Graphic presentation of the spectrum from spontaneous to controlled mechanical ventilation. SPON, spontaneous; CONT, controlled. (From Snyder et al.,[16] with permission.

Thus, the principal advantages of PPV (to decrease the work of breathing and improve alveolar recruitment by increasing PL)[16] must be weighed against the advantages of SV (improved venous return, less cardiac compromise, and better $\dot{V}/\dot{Q}$ relationships). Careful assessment and reassessment of each patient's ventilatory needs for the existing clinical condition usually provide the basis for a logical integration of PPV with SV, so that the advantages of both can be realized (Fig. 5-2).

PULMONARY EFFECTS OF CONVENTIONAL MECHANICAL VENTILATION

Observations in both normal and uniformly damaged lungs have shown that techniques designed to improve gas exchange may actually exacerbate the underlying disease process. Comparisons between conventional PPV and HFV suggest that cyclic stretching of the lung may induce structural damage.[19,20] However, lung compliance decreases within 2 hours during normal constant VT ventilation without PEEP.[21,22] Oxygenation and compliance both improve when PAW is increased, presumably because of improved alveolar recruitment. These findings, combined with the early observation that the dead space to tidal volume ratio (VD/VT) was increased by CMV, led to the common practice of delivering larger mechanical VT (12 to 15 ml/kg) than those associated with spontaneous breathing (5 to 7 ml/kg).

Large volume mechanical ventilation is accompanied by increased surfactant turnover, increased surface tension, and decreased lung compliance. Increased surface tension predisposes to alveolar collapse, which is more pronounced in normal lung units.[16] The result is decreased interstitial fluid pressure (PIF), which can lead to increased transudation of fluid from extra-alveolar vessels and the development of pulmonary edema[16] (Fig. 5-3). The application

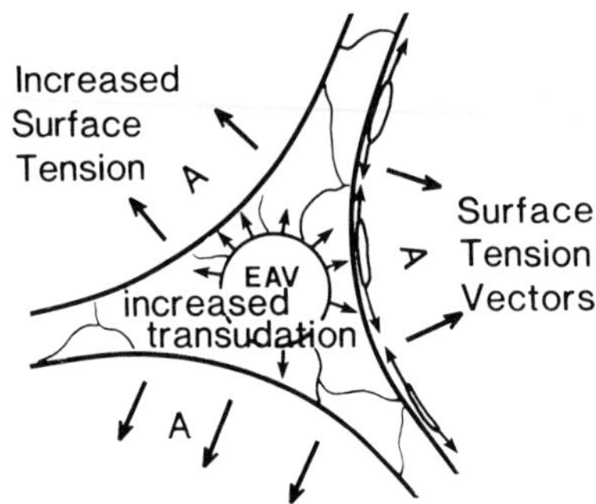

Fig. 5-3. As surface tension increases from surfactant loss, alveoli begin to collapse, pulling the walls of the interstitium apart and lowering interstitial fluid pressure. This alteration promotes increased fluid transudation from the extra-alveolar vessels (EAV). A, alveolus. (From Snyder et al.,[16] with permission.)

of up to 10 cm H_2O PEEP may improve the balance between surfactant generation and loss when large tidal volumes are used.[23]

Alveolar overexpansion with large VT or excessive PEEP may also produce adverse effects on PIF relationships. As lung volume increases above the normal functional residual capacity (FRC), the interstitial space enlarges, with a resultant decrease in PIF. Extra-alveolar vessels are thereby increased in volume, promoting fluid transudation into the interstitial space[24] (Fig. 5-4). This phenomenon can occur with either SV or PPV. The resulting low PIF may explain the sudden appearance of pulmonary edema after atelectatic lung reexpansion.[25] Thus, large VT and high inflation pressure, which are used to counteract the decreased CLT and increased VD/VT, often have an adverse effect on normal alveoli.

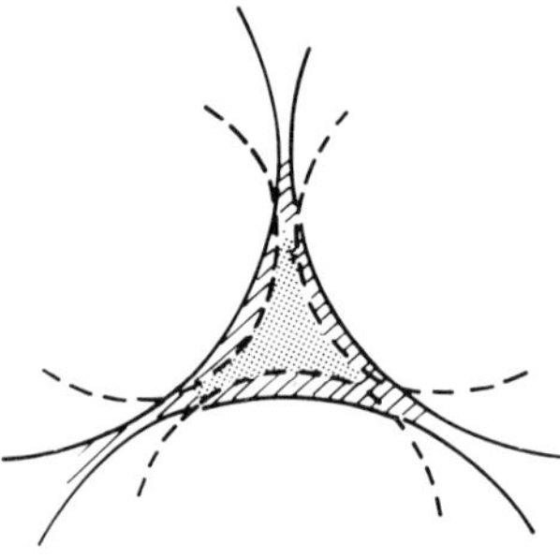

Fig. 5-4. Overinflation of the lung causes enlargement of the interstitial space as the alveoli enlarge. This results in decreased interstitial fluid pressure, which may cause increased fluid transudation into the interstitial space. This occurs with both SV and PPV. (From Snyder et al.,[16] with permission.)

Some investigators believe that a large VT repeatedly delivered over a prolonged period produces structural damage to the lung parenchyma.[20] This hypothesis is supported indirectly by the observation that mechanically ventilated patients with adult respiratory distress syndrome (ARDS) frequently develop further diffuse alveolar damage or bronchopulmonary dysplasia (BPD.[26] The avoidance of cyclic inflation, when possible, may help resolve such lesions.[27] HFV combined with PEEP is thought to be beneficial in this regard,[20] although a recent study showed no difference in the incidence of BPD in infants ventilated with high-frequency oscillation compared with a similar group treated conventionally.[28]

Snyder and Froese[20] postulated that it is not the lungs as a whole that are important, but rather the regional differences in expansion due to variable compliance, airway resistance (RAW), and Ppl. Since volume is distributed preferentially to those areas of greatest compliance and least resistance, normal alveoli become overdistended during peak inflation. The functional loss of one-third of the lung parenchyma results in a 50 percent increase in ventilation to the remainder. If a VT of 15 ml/kg is delivered overall, the effect is a VT of 22.5 ml/kg to the uninvolved lung segments, a volume that is 4.5 times normal spontaneous VT. Altered $\dot{V}/\dot{Q}$ relationships, increased VD/VT, and increased $PaCO_2$ are predictable. Yet the usual treatment for increased $PaCO_2$ is to increase the number and volume of positive-pressure breaths, which may worsen the structural damage. An inexperienced clinician often falls into this vicious cycle without realizing it is occurring. The same phenomenon may be seen in patients who receive too much PEEP or CPAP. Although seemingly paradoxical, the correct intervention in such cases is to reduce the level of support.

RESISTANCE AND COMPLIANCE

Airway resistance and CLT depend on the delivered VT and can be altered by varying inspiratory flow rate ($\dot{V}_I$) and the inspiratory time (TI). These relationships are defined in the following equations:

$$V_T = \dot{V} \times T_I \quad (2)$$

$$C_{LT} = V/P \quad (3)$$

where V is change in volume, and P is change in pressure (PIP − PEEP).

$$R_{AW} = P/\dot{V}_I \quad (4)$$

where P = PIP − EIP (end-inspiratory pressure)

The EIP is a static pressure measured at the end of inspiration following occlusion of the expiratory limb of the ventilator circuit (Fig. 5-5).

During PPV, the PIP results from the sum of elastic, flow restrictive, and, less importantly, inertial properties of the lungs and chest wall.[29] Total pulmonary resistance is due primarily to RAW, with less than 10 percent contributed by tissue flow resistance.[28] The magnitude of airflow resistance depends on whether flow is laminar (pressure α $\dot{V}_I$) or turbulent (pressure α $\dot{V}_I^2$). Usually, both laminar and turbulent flow are present in different parts of the airway. Airway radius also is a major determinant of resistance. When flow is laminar, RAW α 1/radius^4, but with turbulent flow, RAW α 1/radius.[5] Airway caliber may be decreased (RAW increased) by intraluminal obstruction (secretions, blood, edema, inflammation) or an increase in airway smooth muscle tone (asthma).[14] When PPV is used to overcome reduced CLT or increased RAW, the PIP and mean PAW, with their inherent undesirable effects, increase.[14] The problem may be compounded by the use of small bore endotracheal tubes[30] (Fig. 5-6).

Expiration usually occurs passively by the elastic recoil of the lungs and chest wall during both SV and PPV. However, increased RAW prolongs the expiratory time, while a low CLT shortens it. The ventilator rate must be decreased and/or the inspiratory to expiratory (I:E) time ratios must be adjusted to allow adequate time

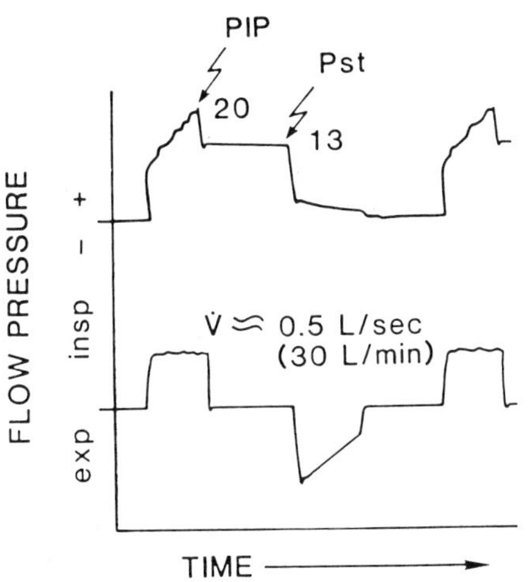

Fig. 5-5. Pressure, flow, and volume are all related and are essential for determination of airway resistance (RAW) and lung-thorax compliance (CLT). The peak inspiratory pressure (PIP) relates to RAW, while the static airway pressure (PST) with the lung expanded is used to calculate both RAW and CLT. (From Boysen and McGough,[14] with permission.)

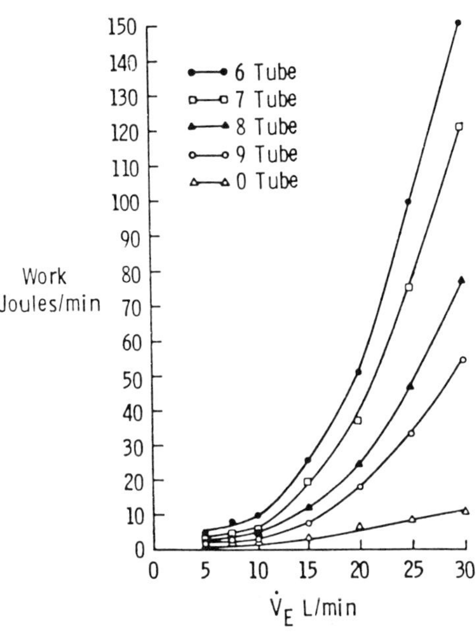

Fig. 5-6. Relationship between increasing minute ventilation ($\dot{V}_E$) and imposed work of breathing by various sized endotracheal tubes. (From Shapiro et al.,[30] with permission.)

for expiration and to prevent air trapping[14] (see section on auto-PEEP).

Time Constants

Inspiratory flow rate, CLT, and to a lesser extent, the V̇I pattern (waveform) control the distribution of alveolar gas. A brief discussion of time constants is essential to an understanding of those relationships (see also Ch. 3). A time constant denotes the time required for a lung unit to reach (1) its final volume at an initial constantly held flow rate, or (2) 63 percent of its final volume with a constantly applied pressure. An exponential decrease in flow rate occurs as volume increases.[29] The value for a time constant is quantitated by multiplying resistance and compliance:

$$T = R_{AW} \times C_{LT} \qquad (5)$$

Consider 1 L of gas delivered at 30 L/min with a PIP (P_1) equal to 40 cm H_2O and EIP (P_2) equal to 35 cm H_2O. If PEEP equals 5 cm H_2O, the following relationships hold:

$$R_{AW} = \frac{(40 - 35)\text{ cm } H_2O}{30\text{ L/min}} = \frac{5\text{ cm } H_2O}{0.5\text{ L/sec}} = 10\text{ cm } H_2O\text{/L/sec}$$

$$C_{LT} = \frac{1\text{ L}}{35 - 5\text{ cm } H_2O} = \frac{1\text{ L}}{30\text{ cm } H_2O} = 0.033\text{ L/cm } H_2O$$

$$T = 10\text{ cm}H_2O\text{/L/sec} \times 0.033\text{ L/cm}H_2O = 0.33\text{ sec}$$

In supine, spontaneously breathing patients, the posterior (dependent) portion of the diaphragm has a much greater excursion than does the anterior (nondependent) portion (Fig. 5-7). Thus, an increased percentage of the VT is delivered to the dependent lung regions. The majority of pulmonary blood flow also is dependent, and V̇/Q̇ relationships are well matched.

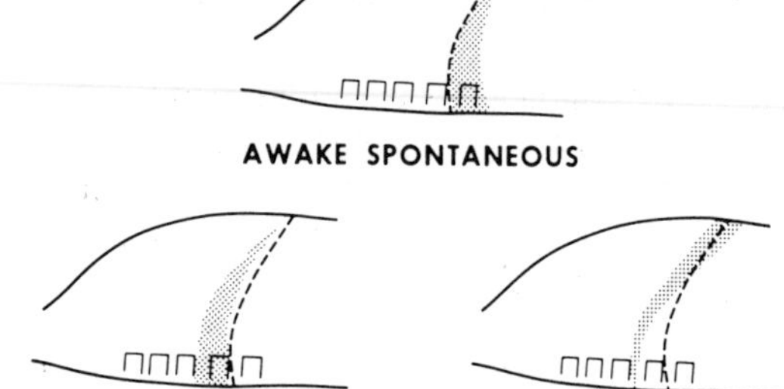

Fig. 5-7. Diaphragm movement during spontaneous (SV) and positive-pressure ventilation (PPV) in supine individuals. Broken line corresponds to baseline FRC. Shaded area corresponds to diaphragmatic movement during SV and PPV. The FRC is less with SV during anesthesia and with PPV and muscle paralysis. (From Froese and Bryan,[17] with permission.)

When the diaphragm is paralyzed or otherwise noncontractile, and PPV is employed, the dependent portion moves very little, even with a large, mechanically generated VT. Movement is greatest in the nondependent region where opposing abdominal pressure is least (Fig. 5-7). This phenomenon is similar to that which occurs when an inflated excised lung is placed under water; most of the volume is displaced to the nondependent areas in which the opposing hydrostatic pressure is least.[17] Neither PEEP nor increased VT can restore the diaphragm (and lungs) to the normal FRC present with SV. An increase in VD/VT is a necessary result of PPV because of overdistention of the nondependent lung regions. Maintenance of SV whenever possible offsets some of this abnormality.[17]

Areas with high RAW are slower to fill and may be incompletely expanded compared with the overdistention of other less resistant lung units. Inspiratory flow and TI are more important than are the compliance factors with respect to the distribution of ventilation.[14,29] If TI is increased to approach the longest time constants in regions with the poorest ventilation, inspired gas can be more evenly distributed to both the fast filling and slow filling lung units, with a resultant improvement of improved $\dot{V}/\dot{Q}$ matching.

Flow Patterns

Although various flow patterns have been advocated to improve ventilation, few data support the superiority of one waveform compared with another in most patients. Nevertheless, in my experience, a deceleration pattern (Fig. 5-8) appears to be beneficial when Tɪ must be prolonged to improve filling of lung units with longer time constants.[14]

PULMONARY BLOOD FLOW

During both SV and PPV, pulmonary blood flow is greater to dependent portions of the lungs in both the upright and supine positions. With PPV, this relationship is disadvantageous since, as outlined previously, most ventilation in the supine position is nondependent. The resulting maldistribution of ventilation produces a nondependent increase of $\dot{V}/\dot{Q}$ and a dependent decrease. Neither PEEP nor increased Vᴛ returns the diaphragm to its normal position with SV.[17] This inherent inefficiency of gas exchange may reduce PaO_2 (increased shunt, $\dot{Q}s/\dot{Q}t$) and may increase $PaCO_2$ (increased Vᴅ/Vᴛ).[16]

Pressure effects on pulmonary blood flow have been studied primarily with PEEP or CPAP rather than with PPV, although it is logical to assume that any therapy that increases alveolar pressure and volume will produce similar results. Two basic effects have been demonstrated: (1) at high lung volume, increased alveolar pressure compresses alveolar vessels; as a result, upstream extra-alveolar vessels develop in-

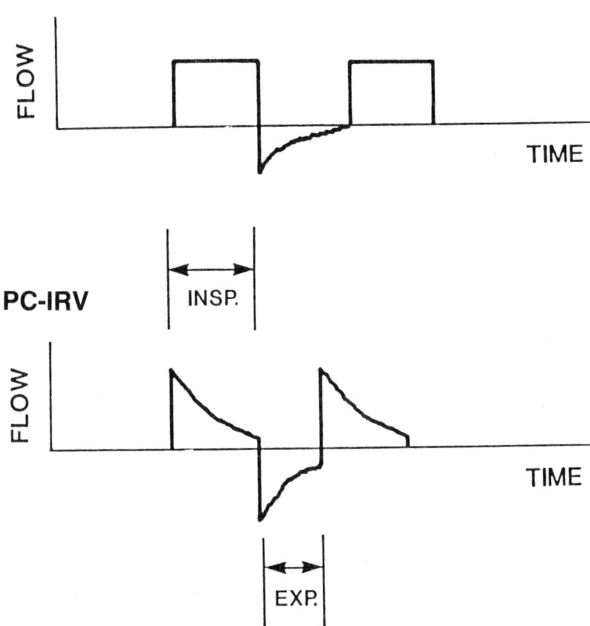

Fig. 5-8. Differences in flow-time curves between pressure-controlled inverse-ratio ventilation (PC-IRV) and conventional volume controlled, normal-ratio ventilation (top diagram). Note the decelerating flow-pattern with PC-IRV, which, in combination with a square-wave pressure delivery and prolonged inspiration, improves the ventilation of slow-filling alveoli with longer time constants. The result is improved oxygenation and ventilation at lower peak pressures and PEEP without an increase of minute ventilation. (From Tharatt et al.,[63] with permission.)

creased pressure and vascular resistance;[16] and (2) spontaneous ventilation decreases Ppl, thereby increasing venous return and pulmonary microvascular pressure.[16]

Using in vivo photomicrography, Nieman and Brendenberg[31] showed that increased positive airway pressure reduced pulmonary capillary flow ($\dot{Q}c$) by 25 percent, even after the effects on cardiac output had been corrected. When alveolar pressure exceeds the alveolar capillary perfusion pressure, $\dot{Q}c$ decreases due to direct compression and collapse of the vessels. However, when alveolar pressure exceeds the extra-alveolar vessels perfusion pressure, blood flow remains about the same.[31] As the lungs expand, radial traction applied to these vessels pulls outward on their walls, keeping them open and maintaining blood flow.[32,33] In dogs treated with 20 cm H_2O PEEP and injected with radionucleotide microspheres, a two- to threefold decrease in total pulmonary blood flow was demonstrated, together with augmentation of the usual vertical gradient of blood flow (decreased flow to nondependent lung units) and a shift of blood flow to the lung periphery.[34]

A final effect of PPV and PEEP/CPAP, the clinical relevance of which is unknown, is a decrease in bronchial blood flow.[33] The bronchial circulation is derived from aortic tributaries. Blood empties distally into a dual venous system of bronchial veins, one portion of which empties back into the right atrium, while another anastomoses with the pulmonary circulation and enters the left atrium via the pulmonary veins.

A 70 to 85 percent decrease in bronchial blood flow is seen in dogs treated with PEEP.[35] A preferential increase in blood return to the left atrium with low-level pressure (less than 10 cm H_2O) and to the right atrium with high-level pressure (greater than 10 cm H_2O) also has been described.[36] Since bronchial blood flow represents a small percentage of total pulmonary blood flow, these changes may be of no consequence. However, bronchial blood flow may be important in lung repair process following the ARDS if extensive pulmonary thrombosis precludes adequate nutrient flow to the lungs.[37]

WORK OF BREATHING

The work of breathing (WOB) may be defined mathematically by the following expression:

$$W = \int PV \qquad (6)$$

In addition to this definition of mechanical work, the WOB can also be characterized by the oxygen cost of breathing in ml O_2/L ventilation.[38] However, measurement of oxygen consumption by the respiratory muscles alone is not possible.

Respiratory muscle work is determined by (1) the required oxygen consumption ($\dot{V}O_2$) and carbon dioxide production ($\dot{V}CO_2$) (i.e., the amount of gas exchange needed), (2) the mechanical efficiency of the thoracic cage, (3) the mechanical properties of the lungs, and (4) the degree of $\dot{V}/\dot{Q}$ matching (i.e., the efficiency of the lungs in exchanging gas).[39] In normal human subjects breathing spontaneously, the oxygen cost of breathing at rest is about 1 to 4 percent of the entire body's $\dot{V}O_2$,[40] or about 0.35 to 1.0 ml/L of ventilation.[38,41] During exercise with ventilation of 70 L/min, only about 10 to 15 percent of the entire $\dot{V}O_2$ in normal subjects is used by the respiratory muscles. This value may be as high as 35 to 40 percent in patients with chronic obstructive pulmonary disease (COPD).[42] The mechanical WOB in obesity or COPD is 2.6 to 3.0 times the normal resting value.[38] Such observations have led some clinicians to downplay the importance of an increased WOB during respiratory failure in patients with previously normal pulmonary function, while others potentially overemphasize WOB in COPD patients with acute exacerbations. The magnitude and clinical relevance of the WOB is difficult to ascertain, since the evaluation of muscle function at the bedside is problematic.[43]

As with other skeletal muscles, respiratory muscles can be either ''strength'' conditioned or ''endurance'' conditioned. Strength conditioning develops more sarcomeres per unit area of muscle and is achieved with high pressure, low volume WOB.[43] Endurance conditioning develops increased mitochondrial density and therefore more fatigue-resistant fibers, best achieved with low pressure, high volume WOB.[43]

Since optimal pressure/volume WOB changes are not well defined, a controversy exists concerning whether patients with respiratory failure should rest completely by totally removing all WOB or be allowed to breath at whatever level they are capable (and therefore prevent muscle atrophy), as long as minute ventilation is adequate, as evidenced by a normal $PaCO_2$. Complete muscle rest can lead to atrophy in 72 to 96 hours.[44] Changes in the imposed WOB, or the amount of work added to the intrinsic (lung and chest wall) WOB due to artificial airways, ventilatory circuitry, and types of ventilators used,[38] has further fueled this controversy.

Positive-Pressure Ventilation

Inspiratory Work

The work required for SV is influenced by the impedance (resistance and compliance) to chest inflation, and the depth, rate, and shape of the inspiratory pressure waveform.[38] Gherini et al.[45] determined that to minimize the WOB in patients receiving CPAP, airway pressure must be maintained at a near constant level throughout the entire respiratory cycle. If airway pressure decreases during inspiration, added inspiratory WOB is imposed [Eq. (6)]. Conversely, if PAW rises above the level of PEEP or CPAP during expiration, additional expiratory work is imposed.[45]

Airway pressure changes can be minimized by reducing the resistance and the reactance of the circuit components.[46] Continuous-flow CPAP systems provide a constant high flow of fresh gas during spontaneous ventilation. Demand flow systems, which were developed to conserve gas, deliver fresh gas only in response to spontaneous inspiration and a reduction of the circuit pressure. If demand flow CPAP systems require a significant decrease in airway pressure to operate the valve in the CPAP mode, increased WOB, as evidenced by increased $\dot{V}O_2$ and $\dot{V}CO_2$, may result when compared to continuous flow systems.[47] Other studies[48–51] have produced similar results, leading to the recommendation that demand valves should respond to pressure decrements no greater than 2 cm H_2O and opening delays less than 0.15 seconds.[52]

Ventilator manometers sometimes measure internal machine pressure and often underestimate the reduction in pressure required to open the demand valve. Accurate measurements may be determined by placing a catheter attached to an aneroid manometer within or adjacent to the endotracheal tube.[53]

In any breathing circuit, the inspiratory pressure is determined by the flow rate of fresh gas and the resistance of the circuit [Eq. (4)]. Most continuous flow systems incorporate a reservoir bag so that fresh gas inflow can be reduced below peak inspiratory flow rates. However, a high gas-flow rate ensures that the reservoir bag volume varies minimally with spontaneous breathing. Accordingly, WOB is reduced, since circuit pressure changes are minimized. Some increase in circuit resistance can result from turbulence associated with high flow, but this effect is usually minimal.[54] If gas flow from the system is greater than the patient's demand, and the reservoir bag remains distended even at peak inspiration, the decrease in airway pressure, and therefore the WOB, is minimal with spontaneous ventilation.

Modern ventilators have improved demand valve systems, and some incorporate a pressure support mode so that the imposed WOB is significantly reduced (75 to 100 percent increases down to 2 to 50 percent increases compared with normal breathing)[55] (see also Ch. 15). All tested ventilators exhibit the highest inspiratory WOB at 0 PEEP/CPAP. Accordingly, when spontaneous breathing is desirable, a small amount of CPAP (up to 5 cm H_20) should be provided.[55] At appropriate levels, CPAP improves lung mechanics in patients recovering from acute respiratory failure by reducing total pulmonary power, defined as the rate of change of the WOB during inspiration, while simultaneously improving 0_2 and $C0_2$ exchange.[51]

The effects of endotracheal tube diameter and length on WOB have been mentioned earlier.[30] At constant laminar flow, endotracheal tube resistance increases in direct proportion to the length and inversely to the fourth power of the radius (i.e., a 50 percent reduction in radius increases resistance 16-fold). With turbulent flow, resistance varies inversely to the fifth power of the radius. Katz and Marks[51] showed that WOB through a T-piece was approximately twice the normal value in healthy volunteers whose tracheas were not intubated. Breathing through a properly designed CPAP circuit required 59 percent less work than breathing through a T-piece prior to extubation. Thus, some of the imposed WOB due to the artificial airway may be offset by using CPAP up to the time of extubation. Pressure support ventilation can also eliminate the imposed WOB from small endotracheal tubes and poorly designed demand valve CPAP circuits, which may be as much as 54 to 240 percent above normal.[55]

Expiratory Work

During PPV, the expiratory airway pressure is controlled primarily by the exhalation valve. A significant increase in expiratory work may be induced by some commercially available devices. When high-resistance exhalation valves are combined with high-resistance demand valves, overall WOB can be increased to intolerable levels. Expiratory ''loading'' also leads to dyspnea.[37]

Exhalation valves are classified as either variable pressure-flow resistors or threshold resistors.[56] When flow resistor valves are used, the level of PEEP/CPAP is directly proportional to the product of the gas flow through the orifice of the expiratory pressure valve and the resistance of the valve.

$$P \propto R\dot{V} \tag{7}$$

Such valves are associated with a significant reduction of airway pressure during inspiration if a continuous gas-flow IMV or CPAP circuit is used (gas is diverted from the valve to the patient), causing WOB to increase.[57] [Eq. (6)].

With threshold resistors, the PEEP/CPAP level is determined by the force applied to the surface area of the valve:

$$P \propto F/SA \tag{8}$$

In general, threshold resistors decrease the imposed WOB compared with variable pressure-flow resistors, since the pressure generated is independent of flow. Thus, during spontaneous breathing, significant changes in airway pressure do not result from inspiratory and expiratory flow changes.[56] As a general rule, if increased WOB is a concern, threshold valves with low resistance to flow should be used to apply CPAP/PEEP.

INVERSE-RATIO VENTILATION

During the early development of PPV, exhaustive studies of airway pressure curves and their relationships to inspiration and expiration were performed in normal individuals.[14] On the basis of these studies, I:E ratios of 1:1, 1:2, and 1:3 were considered optimal. At higher I:E ratios (e.g., 2:1, 3:1), airway pressure did not return to ambient pressure during expiration, resulting in no obvious respiratory advantage but producing significant deterioration of cardiac output.

Inverse ratio ventilation (IRV) gained popularity initially in the management of neonates with the idiopathic respiratory distress syndrome (IRDS), and several studies have reported improvements in oxygenation with lower peak airway pressures using I:E ratios as high as 4:1.[58–60] It has also been applied in adults, although experience here, until recently, was limited.[61,62] Currently, interest in IRV has been renewed with respect to its use in combination with pressure-controlled ventilation (PC-

IRV).[63] Pressure-controlled ventilation provides essentially the same flow wave characteristics as pressure support ventilation, but in a time-cycled on/off mode rather than a patient-triggered mechanism.[14] Neuromuscular blockade and heavy sedation are often necessary in order to avoid patient discomfort and/or prevent "fighting" against the ventilator.[64] This requirement is reminiscent of earlier experience with conventional CMV.

The proposed advantage of PC-IRV is that adequate oxygenation and ventilation can be achieved at lower PEEP and PIP.[63] The physiologic mechanism by which PC-IRV improves alveolar ventilation without changing minute ventilation is unclear but is clinically evident by the frequent decreases in $PaCO_2$ that have been noted. Indeed, this effect may be more useful clinically than is the maintenance of oxygenation at a somewhat lower PEEP and PIP. One theory suggests that PC-IRV increases mean airway pressure which improves oxygenation,[58,65] but this mechanism has not been substantiated in laboratory studies.[66] A more likely explanation is an increase in PL. Functional residual capacity is improved with PC-IRV just as with PEEP, but this effect probably is due to the decreased expiratory time which prevents full expiration (auto-PEEP).[62] Others believe the improved oxygenation results from increased alveolar recruitment, stabilization, and improved gas diffusion.[64]

Alterations in the pressure and flow wave form characteristics may also be instrumental in the improvement of oxygenation and ventilation. Sustained inflation with a constant (square wave) pressure combined with a rapidly decelerating inspiratory flow (Fig. 5-8) appear to be superior in terms of increasing PaO_2 compared with volume-controlled ventilation with a constant inspiratory flow at similar I:E ratios.[67]

Improved ventilation probably results from increased duration of the inspiratory phase, allowing areas with longer time constants to receive greater flow than would otherwise occur with conventional volume-controlled ventilation and the usual I:E ratios.[62]

PRESSURE SUPPORT VENTILATION

Pressure support ventilation was developed partially because of concerns that standard mechanical ventilation may not be optimal for patient comfort or muscle reconditioning during weaning.[68] Proponents of PSV believe that the potential disadvantages of volume-controlled IMV and AV are clinically significant in certain patients and lead to exacerbation of respiratory muscle dysfunction.

Many of the responsible factors have been discussed. They include intermittent and irregular respiratory muscle loads, with high diaphragm tensions resulting from the increased impedance imposed by the underlying lung disease, poorly designed ventilator circuits or demand valves, and the endotracheal tube. This "qualitative" respiratory work defect cannot be improved simply by increasing the IMV rate.[69] With PSV, muscle exercise generally is more regular, and the diaphragm tension characteristics of each ventilator-assisted breath resemble those seen with normal breathing. Thus, WOB is improved not only quantitatively, but also qualitatively.

Patient-triggered PSV is associated with a rapid, almost immediate, rise in airway pressure to a predetermined limit, accompanied by a decelerating flow rate (Fig. 5-8). Tidal volume is variable, depending on the patient's inspiratory effort.[14] The most important physiological aspect of PSV may be its ability to better match the patient's inspiratory flow demands, thereby minimizing respiratory muscle effort as compared with other forms of mechanical ventilation.[70,71]

McIntyre[68] reported a constantly lower spontaneous ventilatory rate and increased comfort with PSV compared with IMV in patients with acute and chronic respiratory problems. These effects are believed to be caused by an altered central nervous system (CNS) ventilatory pattern in response to changes in arterial blood gas (ABG) partial pressures and the mechanical work of breathing. The ventilatory frequency and tidal volume pattern associated with PSV is postulated to supply the necessary alveolar ventilation with the minimum respiratory muscle energy expenditure. As the level of PSV is increased, muscle work should decrease and V_T increase. The optimal ventilatory pattern thus becomes progressively slower and deeper.[68]

POSITIVE END-EXPIRATORY PRESSURE

Positive end-expiratory pressure is a general term designating an increase of airway pressure to achieve a greater expiratory lung volume.[72] Other terms, such as CPAP, expiratory positive airway pressure (EPAP), and continuous distending airway pressure (CDAP), represent special technical applications of PEEP.

Improvement of gas delivery to poorly ventilated, but well-perfused alveoli (areas of low $\dot{V}/\dot{Q}$, and to areas with complete alveolar collapse are the goals of PEEP therapy. Supplemental oxygen may improve hypoxemia but does nothing to reverse the pathophysiologic alterations leading to poor $\dot{V}/\dot{Q}$ matching. Furthermore, a high fraction of inspired oxygen (F_{IO_2}) will depress ciliary and macrophage function, enhance adherence of bacteria to the lower respiratory tract epithelium, and promote fibrogenesis.[73] By maintaining lung volume above the critical closing level, PEEP is thought to lower oxygen requirements, thereby reducing the risk of oxygen toxicity, and also to prevent early deterioration of pulmonary function from absorption atelectasis.[74]

Although the terms are frequently interchanged in the clinical setting, PEEP and CPAP are not synonymous. The latter is a form of PEEP, although all PEEP systems do not deliver CPAP. With some applications of PEEP, airway pressure falls to atmospheric or subatmospheric levels during inspiration[56]; by contrast, CPAP maintains airway pressure above atmospheric throughout the entire respiratory cycle (Fig. 5-9). For purposes of the following discussion, CPAP refers to continuous positive pressure thoughout inspiration and expiration, and PEEP denotes pressure which is positive during expiration only, returning to atmospheric or subatmospheric levels with spontaneous inspiration.

Both interventions improve oxygenation by increasing FRC. Schlobohm et al.[75] evaluated 18 patients with mild to moderate acute respiratory failure and compared CPAP and PEEP levels of +5 and +10 cm H_2O. The PaO_2 and FRC improved more with CPAP than with PEEP. In addition, the P_L at CPAP +10 cm H_2O increased more with PEEP +10 cm H_2O at end-expiration and was correlated with a higher FRC. This difference is postulated to occur from changes in the mechanical properties of either the lung or the chest wall, or a combination of both. Since lung compliance curves were no different with CPAP or PEEP, Schlobohm

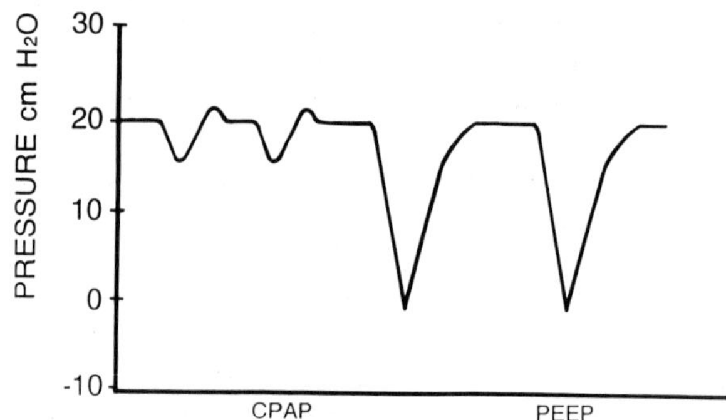

Fig. 5-9. Difference between positive end-expiratory pressure (PEEP) and continuous positive airway pressure (CPAP). Note that with CPAP, airway pressure remains positive during the entire breathing cycle but falls to zero or below during inspiration with PEEP. CPAP is a form of PEEP, but not all PEEP systems deliver CPAP.

and co-workers believed that increased chest wall elastic recoil occurred with CPAP (i.e., a tendency for greater chest wall expansion). By contrast, PEEP, by allowing airway pressure to return to zero or below, may increase expiratory muscle tone (and work), thereby increasing the tendency for alveolar collapse.

Because of the viscoelastic properties of both the lungs and chest wall, improvements in lung volume at constant pressure are time dependent. They are also related to the initial FRC. When the FRC is normal, further increase with positive airway pressure results in hyperinflation, a decrease in lung compliance, increased elastic WOB, and poor gas exchange.[51] Thus, CPAP should be used preferentially in patients whose lung volume is reduced and in whom a return to a normal FRC is desirable. Improvement usually is more pronounced in the supine rather than upright positions.

Gherini et al.[76] studied the effects of CPAP and PEEP on the WOB in 10 healthy volunteers. A linear increase in mean total WOB/min (116 percent) and total WOB/L (121 percent) occurred with PEEP up to 20 cm H_2O. With CPAP, total work/min decreased from baseline by 45 percent at +10 cm H_2O and did not increase any further with +15 to +20 cm H_2O CPAP. Expiratory WOB seems to increase the most at zero CPAP, especially if poorly designed exhalation valves and demand valves are used.[77] Thus, CPAP improves and maintains FRC and reduces the WOB when compared with spontaneous breathing with other conventional forms of PEEP that allow airway pressure to return to ambient levels during inspiration.[78]

Beneficial Pulmonary Effects

Mechanisms of improved oxygenation with PEEP/CPAP include (1) maintenance of alveolar patency throughout the respiratory cycle (which improves FRC); (2) recruitment of new (collapsed) alveoli; (3) favorable effects on the volume and distribution of pulmonary extravascular lung water; and (4) improved $\dot{V}/\dot{Q}$ matching.[33]

Distention of already patent alveoli, which prevents expiratory collapse, and recruitment of closed alveoli, both contribute to the improved FRC associated with PEEP, along with distention of small and moderate sized proximal conducting airways.[79,80] Studies in explanted lungs[81] suggest that PEEP/CPAP expand atelectatic lung by promoting airflow through collateral air channels (pores of Kohn).

Normally, multiple forces govern the egress of water from the pulmonary alveolar and extra-alveolar capillaries to the interstitium.[82] Since the alveolar-capillary membrane is permeable to water, the hydrostatic pressure gradient tends to promote fluid movement out of the capillaries into the interstitium. This hydrostatic pressure gradient is partially balanced by a gradient in the oncotic pressures between the plasma (blood) and the interstitial fluid.[83] Decreased interstitial protein concentration, increased interstitial pressures, and increased lymphatic flow normally prevent pulmonary edema.[69] With PEEP, the transvascular fluid flux may increase, decrease, or remain constant depending on the pressure transmitted to the alveolar and extra-alveolar vessels.[33] Regional differences of extravascular lung water (EVLW) accumulations are in part dependent on the level of PEEP reflected in those areas.

Most animal and human studies suggest that EVLW either increases or remains constant with PEEP but that it is redistributed away from the primary gas exchange areas (i.e., peribronchial/perivascular space). Shunt decreases as a result of improved $\dot{V}/\dot{Q}$ relationships and increased alveolar recruitment. Vascular derecruitment has been postulated as a possible cause for the improved $\dot{Q}_{sp}/\dot{Q}_t$. This theory emphasizes that shunt may be reduced because of decreased blood flow to areas of poor ventilation associated with a lower cardiac output. However, most patients seem to improve because of a direct effect on alveolar recruitment, since PaO_2 usually increases when cardiac output is held constant.[33]

The effect of PEEP on $\dot{V}/\dot{Q}$ abnormalities is variable. Low levels of PEEP (less than 10 cm H_2O) decrease shunt and abolish low $\dot{V}/\dot{Q}$ areas but may increase dead space when the initial shunt is less than 0.4. With severe shunting (over 0.4), low level PEEP also reduces the shunt, but dead space increases only at levels above 15 cm H_2O. In humans the change in dead space is much more variable and unpredictable.[33]

Adverse Pulmonary Effects

A number of changes have been attributed to PEEP. However, similar alterations result from PPV, and separating the effects of one from the other is difficult when they are applied simultaneously. Developmental bronchiolectasis (dilatation of the terminal bronchioles) has been reported in patients treated with PEEP for long periods.[84] Although this probably is a reversible phenomenon,[85,86] it may contribute to the frequent increase of dead space and elevated $PaCO_2$ in later stages of therapy. Acute increases in $PaCO_2$ also can result from overdistention of relatively normal lung areas. This change often is seen in patients with localized lung disease (e.g., lobar pneumonia) or in patients with relatively few damaged alveoli in relationship to healthy alveoli.

Another possible adverse effect is the stretched-pore phenomenon, postulated to occur in both animals[87] and humans[88] and thought to be a mechanism responsible for the apparent increase in lung water associated with PEEP. Increased pulmonary vascular permeability also has been demonstrated with large volume mechanical ventilation.[89] It presumably occurs because of hyperinflation and stretching of intercellular junctions when the delivered volume approaches total lung capacity.[90] Such changes also are more likely to occur in normal alveoli.

Miscellaneous Applications

The addition of 3 to 5 cm H_2O PEEP/CPAP is believed by some to substitute for the effect of the glottic-laryngeal apparatus that is eliminated by translaryngeal intubation or tracheotomy.[91] Extubation at zero PEEP often is accompanied by improvement in FRC and gas exchange, suggesting that glottic function is important in the restoration of lung volume if the FRC is reduced during a period of tracheal intubation.

Pain and immobilization lead to a series of events altering lung and chest wall mechanics, which eventually increase WOB and may affect gas exchange profoundly following chest or abdominal surgery. Typically, V_T decreases and spontaneous respiratory rate increases. This fast, shallow breathing pattern results in decreased alveolar ventilation unless minute ventilation increases to maintain adequate gas exchange. Alveolar collapse ensues owing to a lack of periodic hyperinflation, resulting in decreased compliance, further hindering gas exchange and increases WOB. Most affected are the dependent lung regions in which gas exchange normally is greatest, further compounding the problem.[39]

These restrictive lung changes following elective abdominal surgery are reversed by PEEP/CPAP. Lindner showed that 12 cm H_2O CPAP administered to patients for 1 hour immediately following tracheal extubation, followed by 3 hours daily for the first 5 days, resulted in major improvements in vital capacity when compared to patients receiving no CPAP.[92] The decrease in expiratory reserve volume due to restricted diaphragm function (from surgery) was aborted by CPAP administered over 2-hour intervals during the first 3 postoperative days following upper abdominal surgery and was accompanied by more rapid normalization of FRC and decreased atelectasis.[93] Anderes et al.[94] prevented decreases in FRC if 5 cm H_2O CPAP were administered for 3 hours following extubation.

Auto-PEEP

Auto-PEEP usually results from insufficient expiratory time.[95] This phenomenon is also referred to as gas trapping, occult PEEP, intrinsic PEEP, endogenous PEEP, and inadvertent PEEP.[96] It most commonly occurs during PPV in patients with airflow obstruction and a prolongation of exhalation. If the ventilator expiratory phase is too short, progressive air trapping and an increase in alveolar pressure develop. Auto-PEEP is potentially dangerous because the increased pressure is not reflected by the usual proximal airway pressure measurements. Only when the exhalation port is occluded at the precise moment the next ventilator breath should be delivered, will the presence of auto-PEEP be revealed, a technique which is difficult in the best of circumstances, and not possible with many newer ventilator designs.

Auto-PEEP should be suspected if any of the following problems develop: (1) unexplained hypotension or other forms of hemodynamic compromise; (2) falsely elevated/artifactual pulmonary artery occlusion pressure (PAOP); (3) evidence of increased work of breathing when ventilators with demand valves are used. Since a reduction of airway pressure is necessary to open the valve, WOB will be increased if the distal airway pressure prior to inspiration is higher than the preset proximal airway pressure set on the ventilator; and (4) unexplained barotrauma. This problem can be decreased or avoided by reducing the ventilator rate to the minimum level that maintains adequate minute ventilation, and increasing the inspiratory gas flow rate, which allows more time for expiration.[96]

EFFECTS OF POSITIVE PRESSURE VENTILATION AND PEEP/CPAP ON ORGAN FUNCTION

Heart

Support of cardiac function is often necessary in patients with respiratory failure who require mechanical ventilation. Adjustment and "fine-tuning" of the physiologic determinants of cardiac output (CO) insure that the potentially adverse cardiac effects of PPV do not hinder oxygen delivery to the peripheral tissues. Since oxygen delivery is dependent on both arterial oxygen content (CaO_2) and CO, an understanding of how mechanical ventilation affects cardiac function is essential. Pinsky[97] described the heart as a pressure chamber within another pressure chamber, the thorax. Changes in Ppl, pulmonary vascular resistance (PVR), and capacitance, systemic vascular resistance (SVR), and LV preload can significantly affect CO and oxygen delivery.[97]

The Fick equation describes the relationship between CO, $\dot{V}O_2$, CaO_2, and mixed venous oxygen content ($C\bar{v}O_2$).[1]

$$CO = \frac{\dot{V}O_2}{CaO_2 - C\bar{v}O_2} \tag{9}$$

In the relatively short period of time required to measure cardiac output by thermodilution techniques, and to obtain arterial and mixed venous blood, $\dot{V}0_2$ remains relatively constant.[98] Thus, an increased arterial-venous oxygen content difference [$C(a\text{-}\bar{v})O_2$] usually reflects a decrease in $C\bar{v}O_2$, mixed venous oxygen partial pressure ($P\bar{v}O_2$), and saturation ($S\bar{v}O_2$). A decreased $P\bar{v}O_2$ and $S\bar{v}O_2$ suggest that the cardiac output is inadequate for the existing level of $\dot{V}O_2$.[99] These changes usually occur before other clinical signs of cardiovascular dysfunction develop. Hence, the monitoring of $S\bar{v}O_2$ may be useful to provide early warning of cardiovascular deterioration.[100,101]

Cardiac Output

Cardiac output is the product of stroke volume and heart rate. Three major factors influence stroke volume: preload, afterload, and contractility. The interaction of these factors and their effects on muscle work were first described by Frank[102] and later emphasized by Starling and co-workers.[103]

Preload

Preload defines the relationship between end-diastolic fiber length and work performed by the contracting cardiac muscle.[104] Starling's law of the heart states that "the energy of contraction, however measured, is a function of the length of the muscle prior to contraction."[105] Ventricular muscle fiber length is proportional to end-diastolic volume, which in turn is proportional to end-diastolic pressure. A measurement of PAOP provides a reasonable approximation of LV end-diastolic and left atrial pressures in many clinical settings.[106] Right ventricular (RV) preload is assessed clinically by right atrial or central venous pressure (CVP) measurements, which approximate RV end-diastolic pressure. Although useful, wedge pressure and CVP measurements do not always reflect volume status accurately.

Afterload

Afterload is defined as the "load" that the cardiac muscle is asked to move when it contracts,[104] or more specifically, the ventricular wall tension that is required to eject a given stroke volume.[107] Two primary factors influence ventricular afterload: SVR and the ventricular radius.

$$SVR = \frac{MAP - CVP}{CO} \times 79.9 \qquad (10)$$

where MAP is mean arterial pressure (normal SVR = 900 – 1,200 dynes/cm/sec^{-5}).

Ventricular radius and ventricular wall tension having the following relationship:

$$\text{Wall tension} \approx \frac{\text{distending pressure} \times \text{radius}^n}{\text{wall thickness}} \qquad (11)$$

As the ventricular radius increases, wall tension must increase exponentially to produce the same amount of work at a constant preload and wall thickness.[108]

When preload and contractility remain constant, increased afterload results in decreased muscle shortening with contraction, that is, a less efficient ventricle.[109] The presystolic ejection period (PEP), defined as the interval between closure of the mitral valve and opening of the aortic valve, is the time when wall tension increases prior to stroke volume ejection. Increased afterload prolongs the PEP. This period of isovolemic contraction markedly increases myocardial oxygen consumption ($M\dot{V}O_2$), a detrimental effect in patients with coronary artery disease and limited myocardial blood flow.

Contractility

The rate of generation of crosslinkings between actin and myosin determines the state of contractility[110] and controls stroke volume when preload and afterload are constant. This process is related intimately to the quantity of available ionized calcium and the level of norepinephrine, the intrinsic cardiac adrenergic transmitter.

Studies correlating ventricular-pressure changes over time (dp/dt), PEP, and LV ejection time (LVET) are useful to evaluate contractility during cardiac catheterization. Unfortunately, no readily available studies permit quantitation of contractility in the intensive care setting. Therapeutically induced augmentation of contractility is empiric. Improved CO and oxygen delivery at constant preload and afterload are often used to gauge the appropriate endpoint.

Heart Rate

If stroke volume remains constant, CO increases in linear fashion up to a heart rate of approximately 150/min. Rate is determined primarily by a balance between the parasympathetic nervous system cholinergic receptors in the sinoatrial node (decreased rate) and the sympathetic nervous system's stimulation of β-adrenergic receptors (increased rate).

Cardiac output in younger individuals with normal function generally is rate-dependent. In acutely ill patients, the benefits of improving CO by increasing heart rate must be weighed against the detrimental increases in $M\dot{V}O_2$, especially in those patients with coronary artery disease.

Although the four determinants of CO can be measured separately, and for purposes of discussion are distinct, they are clinically interdependent. A change in one may effect an increase or decrease in one or more of the other three factors. For instance, augmentation of preload by fluid administration increases end-diastolic volume and myocardial muscle fiber length. Depending on LV compliance, the ventricular radius may increase significantly, with a resultant increment of wall tension, or afterload. This afterload increase often proves detrimental, offsetting the advantage of increased preload on the ultimate balance of CO, oxygen delivery, and $M\dot{V}O_2$. Inotropic agents used to improve contractility are deleterious if an increased heart rate limits ventricular filling, reduces stroke volume, and increases $M\dot{V}O_2$ significantly. Therapeutic interventions should be followed by appropriate assessment of the physiological determinants of CO and oxygen delivery to determine whether the desired benefits actually are achieved.

Adverse Effects

Patients with respiratory failure treated with mechanical ventilation and PEEP may require an augmentation of cardiac function to achieve therapeutic endpoints. However, determination of these endpoints may be difficult. The PAOP clinically is used to assess the adequacy of end-diastolic volume and changes in ventricular preload. On occasion failure to understand ventricular pressure-volume relationships may result in erroneous conclusions and inappropriate therapy.[111] Such errors can prove catastrophic in patients who require high level mechanical ventilation and/or PEEP/CPAP for respiratory failure.[112]

An appreciation of the role of ventricular compliance is essential. Studies by Glantz and Parmley[113] and Grossman and McLaurin[114] demonstrated a fall in ventricular compliance at higher filling pressures. When filling pressure is low, large increases in LV end-diastolic volume may be reflected by minimal changes in end-diastolic pressure. Conversely, large PAOP changes often result from small changes in the volume of noncompliant ventricles. Compliance is altered by a number of therapeutic interventions. It is increased in various cardiomyopathies, but is reduced by myocardial ischemia or infarction and by overdistention of the lungs by PPV, PEEP, or CPAP.

An understanding of the relationship between pressure, volume, and compliance is crucial in order to interpret the PAOP. Trends in intravascular volume status reflected by the PAOP usually are meaningful if the pressure-volume relationships are considered when the data are analyzed. Therapy should be directed toward physiologic improvement rather than "optimization of the numbers" in every case.

Cardiac output depression is a potential problem with any mode of therapy that increases airway pressure. The principal effects of positive airway pressure on oxygen transport occurs by means of changes in CO and pulmonary venous admixture. Decreased CO has been attributed to a reduction of venous return to the heart,[115,116] cardiac fossa compression,[117,118] increased PVR,[119–121] myocardial depressant agents released into the circulation,[122] reflex mediated depression of ventricular function by pulmonary baroreceptor stimulation,[123,124] and hypocarbia.[125]

Although any or all of these factors may be detrimental, changes in Ppl transmitted to the mediastinal contents (heart and great vessels) with resulting alterations of venous return and ventricular function seem to be the primary culprits. Lower levels of PPV and, therefore, lower Ppl combined with spontaneous breathing usually are associated with improved cardiac output. One study of 20 patients following coronary artery bypass surgery[126] showed that a change from CMV to IMV had salutary effects on hemodynamic performance in these patients with normal LV reserve function. In those patients with poor LV function, a decrease in the number of positive-pressure breaths was associated with deterioration of cardiac function; however, the changes were reversed with low levels of PEEP. The investigators postulated that the adverse effects resulted from increased RV afterload which altered the geometry of the already dysfunctional left ventricle. They also felt that the subatmospheric Ppl during spontaneous breathing with IMV in the absence of PEEP may have affected LV function adversely by increasing transmural pressure and, therefore, afterload.[112]

Similarly Nikki et al.[127] showed that a combination of low level IMV (4 breaths/min) and PEEP (10 cm H_2O) produced the best results in terms of reduced pulmonary venous admixture, no adverse effect on cardiac function, and improved oxygen delivery in nine patients with acute myocardial infarction and respiratory failure. Thus, a decrease of achieved Ppl, achieved by ventilatory techniques that do not significantly increase mean airway pressure ($P\overline{AW}$), assures the best overall level of cardiac function.

Decreased lung compliance may, under certain clinical circumstances, have a protective effect against the adverse cardiac consequences of PPV. According to this view, less airway pressure is transmitted to the heart and great vessels, and venous return is better maintained. At least one laboratory study, however, does not support the presumption that low lung compliance blunts the hemodynamic consequences of increased airway pressure,[128] although this concept is still prevalent.

Acute RV dysfunction associated with respiratory failure or its treatment may impair LV stroke volume. The right ventricle traditionally has been regarded as a more or less passive conduit for blood flow to the pulmonary vascular bed and the left side of the heart.[129] Alterations of normal RV function, however, can diminish LV stroke work, reduce CO, and ultimately diminish oxygen delivery to the systemic circulation. Those factors that determine LV output (preload, afterload, contractility, and heart rate) also influence the right ventricle. Any decrease of RV preload or contractility, or increases of RV afterload, may have a negative influence on LV performances. Increases in RV end-diastolic pressure and volume generally increases RV stroke work. However, Vlahakes et al.[130] showed that this response may be limited in the right ventricle because of insufficient coronary blood flow, a situation most critical in patients with coronary artery disease. Right ventricular afterload is determined primarily by the interaction of the PVR[129] and ventricular wall tension (Laplace's Law).[131]

A number of investigators have documented an increased mortality when acute respiratory failure is associated with pulmonary artery hypertension.[132,133] However, pulmonary hypertension is not a constant clinical finding,[134] and its importance as a singular risk factor is difficult to establish. Nevertheless, any increase in RV afterload (i.e., pulmonary hypertension) can cause RV dilation, increased RV pressure, leftward (posterior) shift of the interventricular septum, decreased LV compliance and end-diastolic volume, and, ultimately, decreased LV stroke volume and CO.[112]

This septal shift is due in part to the pericardium, which restricts right ventricular expansion. Septal shift is minimized in animal models when the pericardium is removed.[135] Sibbald et al.[136] showed that pulmonary hypertension in patients with ARDS decreases RV ejection fraction and increases RV end-diastolic volume. Increasing RV preload will improve RV stroke volume and maintain LV preload, if no factors limit contractility (i.e., coronary insufficiency). Intravascular volume expansion may be successful if right ventricular contractility is diminished, for example, by myocardial contusion,[137] or if afterload is increased by a mean pulmonary artery pressure above 40 mmHg.[138] Severe pulmonary hypertension appears to decrease RV contractility because of myocardial ischemia resulting from increased RV wall tension and duration of the PEP.[129]

Beneficial Effects

When cardiac function is normal, increased Ppl is generally associated with decreased cardiac output for the reasons described in the previous sections. There is, however, a subgroup of patients in which increased airway pressure and PPV may improve cardiac function. This improvement is dependent on adequate LV filling, decreased LV afterload, and possibly improved coronary artery perfusion resulting from increased mean aortic pressure.[139] Such effects are most pronounced and clinically more evident in patients with severe LV dysfunction. Cardiac pressure and volume changes associated with SV and PPV are complex and/or mediated by the forces determining RV and LV interactions, direct pressure on the heart, and changes in systemic and pulmonary venous return.[140]

When reduced cardiac function is associated with elevated LV filling pressures, an increase of Ppl associated with increased airway pressure may augment CO despite a relative decrease in LV preload.[139] Such insensitivity to decreasing preload is seen only in the most severely damaged and dilated left ventricles exemplified by a depressed cardiac function curve.[141] With less severe impairment, augmentation of cardiac function with increased airway pressure is achieved only with optimization of preload and is least beneficial when preload is reduced.[139]

Increased LV stroke work and CO following the application of positive airway pressure is also attributed to decreased LV afterload, which follows an increase in the pressure gradient between the intrathoracic and extrathoracic vascular beds.[142] Transmural LV pressure (defined as the LV pressure minus Ppl) more accurately reflects LV afterload than does systolic aortic pressure alone.[143] Large negative pressure swings which may accompany SV at ambient pressure will decrease Ppl, thereby increasing LV transmural pressure and afterload.[143] Treating such patients with intermittent PPV or low levels of CPAP aborts these pressure fluctuations, decreases afterload, and improves cardiac efficiency, if the venous return is not simultaneously decreased or if RV function is not impaired by increased PVR.[143]

These salutary effects on LV function have been attributed both to PPV[139,142,143] and to CPAP.[140,141,144] The common denominator for success with both forms of therapy is similar to the beneficial effect seen with vasodilator therapy: decreased afterload with optimization of preload (or without compromising preload). Hence, the subgroup of critically ill patients with moderate to severe LV dysfunction benefits from increased airway pressure, which improves rather than decreases cardiac function.

Extrathoracic Organs

The majority of extrathoracic organ effects related to PPV result from impaired cardiac function. Selected factors of importance should be understood regarding specific organ systems.

Central Nervous System

The detrimental effects of PPV[145] and PEEP[146] on intracranial and cerebral perfusion pressure (CPP) have been extensively reported. Earlier studies involved patients with normal pulmonary function. Subsequently, despite moderate reluctance on the part of many clinicians, PEEP was successfully (and safely) used in head-injured patients.[147,148]

The relationship between positive airway pressure and intracranial pressure (ICP) is dependent on both lung compliance and intracerebral elastance. Cerebral blood flow and its relation to ICP is regulated by a "Starling resistor" between the sagittal sinus and the cerebral veins.[149] As intrathoracic pressure increases, lung distention and increased right atrial pressure decrease venous return from the head. Superior vena caval and sagittal venous pressures can increase up to a "waterfall" pressure without adversely increasing ICP or cerebral blood flow. However, once this pressure is exceeded, a direct relationship exists between superior vena caval, sagittal sinus, and cerebral venous pressures.[149]

Apuzzo et al.[150] studied the effects of PEEP in 25 patients who sustained severe head injury with and without associated pulmonary injury. Patients with increased intracerebral elastance (or decreased intracerebral compliance) were identified by at least a 2 mmHg/ml increase in ICP when a given volume of air was injected intracranially (the volume/pressure response test).[150] Patients were then treated with 10 cm

H_2O PEEP, and the ICP responses again measured. A significant increase in ICP was defined as twice baseline or greater than 13 mmHg. Only 4 of 25 patients had responded with ICP above 13 mmHg, while 21 patients had ICP less than 13 mmHg.

Of importance is the fact that minimal pulmonary impairment was present in this group of patients. Therefore, PEEP may have been inappropriate under these clinical conditions. Whether patients with increased or normal intracerebral elastance and significant decreases in pulmonary compliance would react similarly cannot be ascertained from this study. My clinical experience and that of others[151,152] suggests that PEEP or CPAP applied in the appropriate clinical setting does not adversely affect ICP. Decreased lung compliance associated with acute respiratory failure appears to prevent transmural conductance of airway pressure to the right atrium and the consequent increase of ICP. If high levels of PPV or PEEP/CPAP are needed, ICP monitoring is strongly recommended.

Liver

Increased airway pressure can impair hepatic function, but does not appear to affect hepatic perfusion redistribution directly. Manny and colleagues[153] showed that decreased hepatic, splenic, and bronchial blood flow was secondary to the reduction of CO. Bonnet et al.[154] determined that hepatic plasma flow correlated directly with CO and remained a constant fraction of CO with increasing levels of PPV and PEEP. Thus, adverse hepatic effects appear to be avoided by preventing deterioration of CO.

Kidneys

While the effects of positive airway pressure on hepatic blood flow are relatively straightforward, renal effects are multifactorial. The differences in SV and PPV are more pronounced in the kidneys than perhaps any other extrathoracic organ. Renal function also has received the most study, because the combination of respiratory and renal failure carries such a high mortality in critical care units.

Early experimental investigations demonstrated that PPV decreased urine flow in both man and experimental animals, while negative pressure breathing increased it.[155] These changes in urine flow were postulated to result from different levels in activity of stretch receptors in the walls of the atria and great vessels of the thorax, which regulated antidiuretic hormone (ADH) activity and/or were associated with the control of renal hemodynamic function.[156,157]

Unanesthetized subjects responded to negative pressure breathing (no change in respiratory rate) with as much as a 10-fold increase in urine output but no difference in urine pH and total sodium or potassium excretion.[158] In other words, with negative pressure breathing, free water excretion increased, possibly as a result of decreased ADH activity. Later the effects of PPV, CPAP, and SV on ADH levels and free water clearance were evaluated. Hemmer et al.[159] demonstrated that ADH increased at least 100 percent and free water clearance decreased during continuous and intermittent PPV compared to SV, alone or in combination with CPAP, in patients with flail chest injuries.

Other studies have questioned the increased airway pressure effect on ADH secretion. Payen et al.[160] stated that earlier studies failed to demonstrate parallel changes in free water clearance and serum ADH when PEEP was used. These workers suggested that PEEP simply induced a decrease in CO and renal blood flow (RBF), provoking a reflex stimulation of the renin-angiotensin system but no effect on ADH.[160]

Positive airway pressure does alter renal hemodynamic function. Some effects presumably result from direct depression of cardiac output and RBF.[161–163] Actual improvement in renal function with positive airway pressure has been noted as well.[164] The frequently observed increase in urinary sodium retention during PPV may be explained by redistribution of RBF from cortical to medullary regions.[164,165]

Data also suggest that a decrease of atrial natriuretic factor (ANF) results from positive airway pressure and is responsible for the reduction of urine output.[166] This 28-amino acid peptide is released from granules located in the atrial cardiocytes in direct response to atrial distention or pressure elevation.[167,168] This substance has multiple biologic and physiologic actions whose concerted effect is to lower cardiac filling pressure. At pharmacological doses (up to 100 μg), ANF causes as much as a fourfold increase in urinary sodium excretion and a twofold increase in urinary volume.[169] The natriuretic and diuretic response is short-acting, returning to baseline in about 45 minutes.[169] These effects are predominantly due to a significant increase in the glomerular filtration rate.[170] Aldosterone release also is inhibited by ANF, with a resultant producing profound inhibition of vascular contraction and decrease in the vascular effects of norepinephrine and angiotension II.[170]

Inariba[171] measured ANF levels in mechanically ventilated patients with acute respiratory failure. Three minutes after cessation of PPV, ANF increased from 32.5 to 85.7 pg/ml, with a resulting increase in urine volume and sodium concentration. The measured levels dropped precipitously at 15 minutes and returned to normal 45 minutes later.[171]

Thus the effects of positive airway pressure on renal function are complex. Decreases in CO, alterations in ADH secretion, changes in the renin-angiotensin system, redistribution of cortical/medullary blood flow, and variations in the secretion of ANF all play a role, the end result of which is a significant reduction of urine volume and urinary sodium.

SUMMARY

Understanding of the relationship among cardiopulmonary physiology, extrathoracic organ function, and mechanical ventilation is increasingly important for the treatment of pulmonary abnormalities. Most forms of mechanical ventilation find broad application, while others may be beneficial to only a selected few patients.

Observations of patients with normal pulmonary function cannot be applied broadly to those with acute respiratory failure or chronic lung disease but may aid in understanding many of the adverse effects of PPV and PEEP/CPAP. The range of pulmonary abnormalities that must be treated clinically is much more complex and variable than that which is developed in animal models.

Management of critically ill patients with respiratory failure necessitates a rational and educated integration of the physiologic observations of healthy and diseased lungs. Patients often have components of both, and therapy directed toward improving diseased lung function may adversely affect normal lung. Recognition of the physiologic principles of PPV and PEEP/CPAP should prevent one from branding a form of therapy as useless, when in reality it was only inappropriately applied.

REFERENCES

1. Llewellyn MA, Swyer PR: Assisted and controlled ventilation in the newborn period: effect on oxygenation. Br J Anaesth 43:926, 1971
2. Marini JJ, Rodriguez RM, Capps JS, et al: The inspiratory work of breathing during assisted mechanical ventilation (Abstract). Crit Care Med 13:310, 1985
3. Downs JB, Klein EF, Desautels DA, et al: Intermittent mandatory ventilation: a new approach to weaning patients from mechanical ventilation. Chest 64:331, 1973
4. Mathru M, Rao TLK, Venus B: Ventilator-induced barotrauma in controlled mechanical ventilation versus intermittent mandatory ventilation. Crit Care Med 11:359, 1983
5. Peterson GW, Baier H: Incidence of pulmonary barotrauma in a medical ICU. Crit Care Med 11:67, 1983
6. Kumar A, Pontoppidan H, Falke K: Pulmonary barotrauma during mechanical ventilation. Crit Care Med 1:188, 1973
7. Heenan TJ, Downs JB, Douglas ME, et al: Intermittent mandatory ventilation: is synchronization important? Chest 77:598, 1980
8. MacIntyre NR: Pressure support ventilation.

Effects on ventilatory reflexes and ventilatory-muscle workloads. Respir Care 32:447, 1987

9. Brochaul L, Harf A, Lorino H, et al: Optimal level of pressure support (PS) in patients with unsuccessful weaning from mechanical ventilation. Am Rev Respir Dis (Abstract) 135:A-51, 1987
10. Brochaul L, Harf A, Lorino H, Lemaire F: Pressure support decreases work of breathing and oxygen consumption during weaning from mechanical ventilation. Am Rev Respir Dis (Abstract) 135:A-51, 1987
11. Banner MJ, Kirby RR: Similarities between pressure support ventilation and intermittent positive-pressure ventilation. Crit Care Med 13:997, 1985
12. Prakesh O, Meij S: Cardiopulmonary response to inspiratory pressure support during spontaneous ventilation versus conventional ventilation. Chest 88:403, 1985
13. Mathru M, Rao TLK, El-Etr AA, et al: Hemodynamic response to changes in ventilatory patterns in patients with normal and poor left ventricular reserve. Crit Care Med 10:613, 1982
14. Boysen PG, McGough PG: Pressure-control and pressure-support ventilation: flow patterns, inspiratory time, and gas distribution. Respir Care 33:126, 1988
15. Summer WR, Permutt S, Sagawa K, et al: Effects of spontaneous respiration on canine left ventricular function. Circ Res 45:719, 1979
16. Snyder JV, Carroll GC, Schuster DP, et al: Mechanical ventilation: physiology and application. Curr Prob Surg 21:40, 1984
17. Froese AD, Bryan AC: Effects of anesthesia and paralysis on diaphragmatic mechanics in man. Anesthesiology 41:242, 1974
18. Op't Holt TB: Work of breathing and other aspects of patient interaction with PEEP devices and systems. Respir Care 33:444, 1988
19. Hamilton PP, Onayemi A, Smyth JA, et al: Comparison of conventional and high frequency ventilation: oxygenation and lung pathology. J Appl Physiol 55:131, 1983
20. Snyder JV, Froese A: Respiratory lung. p. 358. In Snyder JV, Pinsky MR (eds): Oxygen Transport in the Critically Ill. Year Book Medical Publishers, Chicago, 1987
21. Ferris BG, Pollard DS: Effect of deep and quiet breathing on pulmonary compliance in man. J Clin Invest 39:143, 1960
22. Bendixen HH, Hedley-White J, Chir B, et al: Impaired oxygenation in surgical patients during general anesthesia with controlled ventilation. N Engl J Med 269:991, 1963
23. Webb H, Tierney D: Experimental pulmonary edema due to intermittent positive pressure ventilation with high inflation pressures: protection by positive end-expiratory pressure. Am Rev Respir Dis 110:556, 1974
24. Inoue H, Inoue C, Hildebrandt J: Vascular and airway pressures, and interstitial edema, affect peribronchial fluid pressure. J Appl Physiol 48:177, 1980
25. Marland AM, Glauser FL: Hemodynamic and pulmonary edema protein measurements in a case of re-expansion pulmonary edema. Chest 81:250, 1982
26. Churg A, Golden J, Fligiel S, et al: Bronchopulmonary dysplasia in the adult. Am Rev Respir Dis 127:117, 1983
27. Gattitoni L, Pesenti A, Pellizola A, et al: Extracorporeal carbon dioxide removal in acute respiratory failure. Ann Chir Gynaecol 71 (suppl):77, 1982
28. HIFI Study Group: High-frequency oscillatory ventilation compared with conventional mechanical ventilation in the treatment of respiratory failure in preterm infants. N Engl J Med 320:88, 1989
29. Hillman DR: Physiological aspects of intermittent positive pressure ventilation. Anaesth Intens Care 14:226, 1986
30. Shapiro M, Wilson RK, Casar G, et al: Work of breathing through different sized endotracheal tubes. Crit Care Med 14:1028, 1986
31. Nieman GF, Bredenberg C: Pulmonary microvascular perfusion during positive end-expiratory pressure (PEEP). Respir Care 33:93, 1988
32. Fung YC, Sobin SS, Tremer H, et al: Patency and compliance of pulmonary veins when airway pressure exceeds venous pressure. J Appl Physiol 54:1538, 1983
33. Stoller JK: Respiratory effects of positive end-expiratory pressure. Respir Care 33:454, 1988
34. Hedenstierna G, White FC, Wagner PD: Spatial distribution of pulmonary blood flow in the dog with PEEP ventilation. J Appl Physiol 47:938, 1979
35. Cassidy SS, Haynes MS: The effects of ventilation with positive end-expiratory pressure on the bronchial circulation. Respir Physiol 66: 269, 1986
36. Baile EM, Albert RK, Kirk W, et al: Positive

end-expiratory pressure decreases bronchial blood flow in the dog. J Appl Physiol 56:1289, 1984

37. Albert RK: Non-respiratory effects of positive end-expiratory pressure. Respir Care 33:464, 1988
38. Marini JJ: The role of the inspiratory circuit in the work of breathing during mechanical ventilation. Respir Care 32:419, 1987
39. Peters RM: Work of breathing and abnormal mechanics. Surg Clin North Am 54:955, 1974
40. Otis AB: The work of breathing. Physiol Rev 34:449, 1954
41. Campbell EJM, Westlake EK, Cherniak RM: The oxygen consumption and efficiency of the respiratory muscles of young male subjects. Clin Sci 18:55, 1959
42. Levison H, Cherniack RM: Ventilatory cost of exercise in chronic obstructive pulmonary disease. J Appl Physiol 25:21, 1968
43. Leith DE, Bradley M: Ventilatory muscle strength and endurance training. J Appl Physiol 41:508, 1976
44. Braun NMT, Faulkner J, Hughes RL, et al: When should respiratory muscles be exercised? Chest 84:76, 1983
45. Gherini S, Peters R, Virgilio R: Mechanical work on the lungs and work of breathing with positive end-expiratory pressure and continuous positive airway pressure. Chest 76:251, 1979
46. Hillman DR, Finucane KE: Continuous positive airway pressure: a system to minimize respiratory work. Crit Care Med 13:38, 1985
47. Henry WC, West GA, Wilson RS: A comparison of the oxygen cost of breathing between a continuous flow CPAP system and a demand-flow CPAP system. Respir Care 28:1273, 1983
48. Gibney RTW, Wilson RS, Pontoppidan H: Comparison of work of breathing on high gas flow and demand valve continuous positive airway pressure systems. Chest 82:692, 1982
49. Op't Holt TB, Hall MW, Ban JB, et al: Comparison of changes in airway pressure between demand valve and continuous flow devices. Respir Care 27:1200, 1982
50. Poulton TJ, Downs JB: Humidification of rapidly flowing gas. Crit Care Med 9:59, 1981
51. Katz JA, Marks JD: Inspiratory work with and without continuous positive airway pressure in patients with acute respiratory failure. Anesthesiology 63:598, 1985
52. Cox D, Niblett DJ: Studies on continuous positive airway systems. Br J Anaesth 56:905, 1984
53. Christopher KL, Neff JA, Bowman JI, et al: Demand and continuous-flow intermittent mandatory ventilation systems. Chest 87:625, 1985
54. Hillman DR, Finucane KE: Continuous positive airway pressure with minimal work of breathing. Chest 91:796, 1987
55. Fiastro JF, Habib MP, Quan SF: Pressure support compensation for inspiratory work due to endotracheal tubes and demand continuous positive airway pressure. Chest 93:499, 1988
56. Gammage GW: Airway pressure support. p. 543. In Kirby RR, Taylor RW (eds): Respiratory Failure. Year Book Medical Publishers, Chicago, 1986
57. Banner MJ, Downs JB, Kirby RR, et al: Effects of expiratory flow resistance on inspiratory work of breathing. Chest 93:795, 1988
58. Boros SJ: Variations in inspiratory:expiratory ratio and airway pressure wave form during mechanical ventilation: the significance of mean airway pressure. J Pediatr 94:114, 1979
59. Reynolds EOR: Effect of alterations in mechanical ventilator settings on pulmonary gas exchange in hyaline membrane disease. Arch Dis Child 46:159, 1971
60. Spahr RC, Klein AM, Brown DR, et al: Hyaline membrane disease. A controlled study of inspiratory to expiratory ratio and its management by ventilator. Am J Dis Child 134:373, 1980
61. Ravizza AG, Carugo D, Cerchiari EL, et al: Inverse ratio and conventional ventilation: comparison of the respiratory effects. Anesthesiology 59:A523, 1983 (abst)
62. Cole AGH, Weller SF, Sykes MK: Inverse ratio ventilation compared with PEEP in adult respiratory failure. Intensive Care Med 10:227, 1984
63. Tharatt RS, Allen RP, Albertson TE: Pressure controlled inverse ratio ventilation in severe adult respiratory failure. Chest 94:755, 1988
64. Gurevitch MJ, Van Dyke J, Young ES, et al: Improved oxygenation and lower peak airway pressure in severe adult respiratory distress syndrome. Treatment with inverse ratio ventilation. Chest 89:211, 1986
65. Duncan SR, Rizk NW, Raffin TA: Inverse ratio ventilation. PEEP in disguise? Chest 92:390, 1987
66. Berman LS, Downs JB, Van Eeden A, et al: Inspiration:expiration ratio. Is mean airway pressure the difference? Crit Care Med 9:775, 1981

67. Lachmann B, Danzmann E, Haendly B, et al: Ventilator settings and gas exchange in respiratory distress syndrome. p. 143. In Prakash O (ed): Applied Physiology in Clinical Respiratory Care. Martinus Nijhoff, Boston, 1982
68. MacIntyre NR: Respiratory function during pressure support ventilation. Chest 89:677, 1986
69. MacIntyre NR: Weaning from mechanical ventilatory support: volume-assisting intermittent breaths versus pressure-supporting every breath. Respir Care 33:121, 1988
70. Marini JJ, Capps JS, Culver BH: The inspiratory work of breathing during assisted mechanical ventilation. Chest 87:612, 1985
71. Marini JJ, Rodriguez MR, Lamb VJ: The inspiratory workload of patient-initiated mechanical ventilation. Am Rev Respir Dis 134:902, 1986
72. Spearman CB: Positive end-expiratory pressure: terminology and technical aspects of PEEP devices and systems. Respir Care 33:434, 1988
73. Rinaldo JE, Rogers RM: Adult respiratory distress syndrome. N Engl J Med 306:900, 1982
74. Downs JB, Douglas ME: Applied physiology and respiratory care. p. III (E)2. In Shoemaker WC (ed): Critical Care State of the Art. Vol 3. Society of Critical Care Medicine, Anaheim, CA, 1982
75. Schlobohm RM, Falltrick RT, Quan SF, et al: Lung volumes, mechanism, and oxygenation during spontaneous positive-pressure ventilation: the advantage of CPAP over EPAP. Anesthesiology 55:416, 1981
76. Gherini S, Peters RM, Virgilio RW: Mechanical work on the lungs and work of breathing with positive end-expiratory pressure and continuous positive airway pressure. Chest 76:251, 1979
77. Capps JS, Ritz R, Pierson DJ: An evaluation, in four ventilators, of characteristics that affect work of breathing. Respir Care 32:1017, 1987
78. Zebrowski M, Geer R: Low flow continuous positive airway pressure with a modified fresh gas reservoir. Crit Care Med 9:106, 1981
79. Barach AL, Swenson PC: Effect of breathing bases under positive pressure on lumens of small and medium-sized bronchi. Arch Intern Med 63:946, 1979
80. Dueck R, Wagner PD, West JB: Effects of positive end-expiratory pressure on gas exchange in dogs with normal and edematous lungs. Anesthesiology 47:359, 1977
81. Anderson JB, Qvist J, Kann T: Recruiting collapsed lung through collateral channels with PEEP. Scand J Respir Dis 60:260, 1979
82. Staub NC: Pulmonary edema. Physiol Rev 54:678, 1974
83. Taylor AE: Capillary fluid filtration: Starling forces and lymph flow. Circ Res 49:557, 1981
84. Slavin G, Nunn JF, Crow J, et al: Bronchiolectasis—a complication of artificial ventilation. Br Med J 285:931, 1982
85. Navaratnarajah M, Nunn JF, Lyons D, et al: Bronchiolectasis caused by positive end-expiratory pressure. Crit Care Med 12:1036, 1984
86. Ingebar DH, Matthay RA: Pulmonary sequelae and lung repair in survivors of the adult respiratory distress syndrome. Crit Care Clin 2:629, 1986
87. Rizk NW, Luce JM, Hoeffel JM, et al: Site of deposition and factors affecting clearance of aerosolized solute from canine dogs. J Appl Physiol 56:723, 1984
88. Marks JD, Luce JM, Lazar NM, et al: Effect of increases in lung volume on clearance of aerosolized solute from human lungs. J Appl Physiol 59:1242, 1985
89. Parker JC, Townsley MI, Rippe B, et al: Increased microvascular permeability in dog lungs due to high peak airway pressures. J Appl Physiol 57:1809, 1984
90. Kim KJ, Crandall ED: Effects of lung inflation on alveolar epithelial solute and water transport properties. J Appl Physiol 52:1498, 1982
91. Smith RA: Physiologic PEEP. Respir Care 33:620, 1988
92. Lindner KH, Lotz P, Alnefield FW: Continuous positive airway pressure effect on functional residual capacity, vital capacity, and its subdivisions. Chest 92:66, 1987
93. Stock CM, Downs JB, Gauer PK, et al: Prevention of postoperative pulmonary complications with CPAP, incentive spirometry, and conservative therapy. Chest 87:151, 1985
94. Anderes C, Anderes U, Gasser D, et al: Postoperative spontaneous breathing with CPAP to normalize late postoperative oxygenation. Intensive Care Med 6:15, 1979
95. Pepe PE, Marini JJ: Occult positive end-expiratory pressure in mechanically ventilated patients with airflow obstruction, the auto-PEEP effect. Am Rev Respir Dis 126:166, 1982
96. Benson MS, Pierson DJ: Auto-PEEP during mechanical ventilation of adults. Respir Care 33:557, 1988

97. Pinsky MR: The hemodynamic effects of artificial ventilation. p. 319. In Snyder JV, Pinsky MR (eds): Oxygen Transport in the Critically Ill. Year Book Medical Publishers, Chicago, 1987
98. Giovannini I, Boldrini G, Sgonga G, et al: Quantification of the determinants of arterial hypoxemia in critically ill patients. Crit Care Med 11:644, 1983
99. Shapiro BA, Harrison RA, Walton JR: Clinical Application of Blood Gases. Year Book Medical Publishers, Chicago, 1982
100. Norwood SH, Nelson LD: Continuous monitoring of mixed venous oxygen saturation during aortofemoral bypass grafting. Am Surg 52:114, 1986
101. Schweiss JF: Continuous Measurement of Blood Oxygen Saturation in the High Risk Patient. Beach International, San Diego, 1983
102. Frank O: Die grundform des arteriellen pulses. Z Biol 37:483, 1898
103. Patterson SW, Pipper H, Starling EH: The regulation of the heart beat. J Physiol (Lond.) 48:465, 1914
104. Ayres SM: Ventricular function. p. I (C)1. In Shoemaker WC, Thompson WL (eds): Critical Care: State of the Art. Vol. 1. Society of Critical Care Medicine, Fullerton, CA, 1980
105. Starling EH: The Linacre Lecture on the Law of the Heart. (Presented at Cambridge in 1915.) Longmans, Green, London, 1918
106. Sibbald WH, Calvin J, Driedger AA: Right and left ventricular preload, and diastolic ventricular compliance: implications of therapy in critically ill patients. p. III (F)2. In Shoemaker WC, Thompson WL (eds): Critical Care: State of the Art. Vol. 3. Society of Critical Care Medicine, Fullerton, CA, 1982
107. Glass DD: Cardiovascular drugs. In Civetta JM (ed): Intensive Care Therapeutics. Appleton-Century Crofts, E. Norwalk, CT, 1980
108. Sonnenblick EH, Ross J, Braunwald E: Oxygen consumption of the heart: newer concepts of its multifactorial determination. Am J Cardiol 22:238, 1968
109. Sonnenblick EH: Determinants of active state in heart muscle: force, velocity, instantaneous muscle length, time. Fed Proc 24:1396, 1965
110. Norwood SH, Civetta JM: Ventilatory support in patients with ARDS. Surg Clin North Am 65:895, 1985
111. Calvin JE, Driedger AA, Sibbald WJ: Does the pulmonary capillary wedge pressure predict left ventricular preload in critically ill patients? Crit Care Med 9:437, 1981
112. Jardin F, Farcot JC, Boisante L, et al: Influence of positive end-expiratory pressure on left ventricular performance. N Engl J Med 304:387, 1981
113. Glantz SA, Parmley WW: Factors which affect diastolic presure volume curve. Circ Res 42:171, 1978
114. Grossman W, McLaurin LP: Diastolic properties of the left ventricle. Ann Intern Med 84:316, 1976
115. Kumar A, Falke KJ, Geffin B, et al: Continuous positive-pressure ventilation in acute respiratory failure: effects on hemodynamics and lung function. N Engl J Med 283:1430, 1970
116. Qvist J, Pontoppidan H, Wilson RS, et al: Hemodynamic responses to mechanical ventilation with PEEP: the effect of hypervolemia. Anesthesiology 42:45, 1976
117. Lloud TC Jr: Respiratory system compliance as seen from the cardiac fossa. J Appl Physiol 53:57, 1982
118. Freeman GL, LeSinter MM: Determinants of intrapericardial pressure in dogs. J Appl Physiol 60:758, 1986
119. Cassidy SS, Robertson CH, Pierce AK, et al: Cardiovascular effects of positive end-expiratory pressure in dogs. J Appl Physiol 44:743, 1978
120. Fewell JE, Abendschein DR, Carlson CJ, et al: Mechanism of deceased right and left ventricular end-diastolic volume during continuous positive-pressure ventilation in dogs. Circ Res 47:467, 1980
121. Manny J, Patten MT, Liebman PR, et al: The association of lung distention, PEEP, and biventricular failure. Ann Surg 187:151, 1987
122. Utsonomiya T, Krausz MM, Dunham B, et al: Depression of myocardial ATPase activity by plasma obtained during positive end-expiratory pressure. Surgery 91:322, 1982
123. Shepherd JT: The lungs as receptor sites for cardiovascular regulation. Circulation 63:1, 1981
124. Cassidy SS, Echenbacher WL, Johnson RL: Reflex cardiovascular depression during unilateral lung hyperinflation in the dog. J Clin Invest 64:620, 1979
125. Morgan BL, Crawford EW, Hornbein TF, et

al: Hemodynamic effects of changes in arterial carbon dioxide tension during intermittent positive pressure ventilation. Anesthesiology 28: 866, 1967

126. Mathru M, Rao TLK, El-Etr AA, et al: Hemodynamic response to changes in ventilatory patterns in patients with normal and poor left ventricular function. Crit Care Med 10:423, 1982
127. Nikki P, Räsänen J, Tahvanainen J, et al: Ventilatory pattern in respiratory failure arising from acute myocardial infarction. Crit Care Med 10:75, 1982
128. Venus B, Cohen LE, Smith RA: Hemodynamic and intrathoracic pressure transmission during controlled mechanical ventilation and positive end-expiratory pressure in normal and low compliant lungs. Crit Care Med 16:686, 1988
129. Sibbald SJ, Driedger AA: Right ventricular function in acute disease states: pathophysiologic considerations. Crit Care Med 11:339, 1983
130. Vlahakes GJ, Turley K, Hoffman JI: The pathophysiology of failure in acute right ventricular hypertension: hemodynamic and biochemical correlations. Circulation 63:87, 1981
131. Weber KT, Janicki JS, Shroffs AS, et al: Contractile mechanics and interaction of the right and left ventricles. Am J Cardiol 47:686, 1981
132. Sibbald WJ, Patterson NA, Holliday RL, et al: Pulmonary hypertension in sepsis: measurement of the pulmonary arterial diastolic-pulmonary wedge gradient and the influence of passive and active factors. Chest 73:583, 1978
133. Zapol W, Snyder MT: Pulmonary hypertension in severe acute respiratory failure. N Engl J Med 296:476, 1977
134. Gallagher TJ, Civetta JM: Normal pulmonary vascular resistance during acute respiratory insufficiency. Crit Care Med 9:647, 1981
135. Goldstein JA, Vlahakes GJ, Verrier ED, et al: The role of right ventricular systolic dysfunction and elevated intrapericardial pressures in the genesis of low output in experimental right ventricular infarction. Circulation 65:513, 1982
136. Sibbald WJ, Driedger AA, Pong H: Biventricular function in human ARDS: assessment by increasing afterload with the cold pressor test (CPT) (Abstract). Ann R Coll Phys Surg Can 15:282, 1982
137. Sutherland G, Calvi J, Driedger AA, et al: Anatomical and cardiopulmonary responses to trauma with associated blunt chest injury. J Trauma 27:1, 1981
138. McIntyre K, Sasahara AA: Determinants of right ventricular function and hemodynamics after pulmonary embolism. Chest 65:534, 1974
139. Pinsky MR, Matuschak GM, Klain M: Determinants of cardiac augmentation by elevations in intrathoracic pressure. J Appl Physiol 58:1189, 1985
140. Räsänen J, Vaisanen IT, Heikkila J, et al: Acute myocardial infarction complicated by respiratory failure. The effects of mechanical ventilation. Chest 85:21, 1984
141. Räsänen J, Vaisanen IT, Heikkila J, et al: Acute myocardial infarction complicated by left ventricular dysfunction and respiratory failure. Chest 87:158, 1985
142. Robotham JL, Cherry D, Mitzner W, et al: A reevaluation of the hemodynamic consequences of intermittent positive pressure ventilation. Crit Care Med 11:783, 1983
143. Pinsky MR, Summer WR: Cardiac augmentation by phasic high intrathoracic pressure support in man. Chest 84:370, 1983
144. Alderman EL: Effect of intrathoracic pressure on left ventricular performance. N Engl J Med 301:453, 1979
145. Raley RA, Schlobohm RM, Pitts LH, et al: Mechanical hyperventilation in patients with head trauma potentiates the ICP response in $PaCO_2$ (Abstract). Anesthesiology 57:A90, 1982
146. Aidinis SJ, Lafferty J, Shapiro HM: Intracranial responses to PEEP. Anesthesiology 45:275, 1976
147. Cooper KR, Boswell PA, Choi SC: Safe use of PEEP in patients with severe head injury. J Neurosurg 63:552, 1985
148. Frost EA: Effects of positive end-expiratory pressure on intracranial pressure and compliance in brain-injured patients. J Neurosurg 47:195, 1977
149. Luce JM, Husby JS, Kirk W, et al: A Starling resistor regulates cerebral venous outflow in dogs. J Appl Physiol 53:1496, 1982
150. Apuzzo MLJ, Weiss MH, Petersons V, et al: Effect of positive end-expiratory pressure ventilation on intracranial pressure in man. J Neurosurg 46:227, 1977
151. Huseby JS, Pavlin EG, Butler J: Effect of positive end-expiratory pressure on intracranial pressure in dogs. J Appl Physiol 44:25, 1978

152. Burchid KJ, Steege TD, Wyler AR: Intracranial pressure changes in brain-injured patients requiring positive end-expiratory pressure ventilation. J Neurosurg 8:443, 1981
153. Manny J, Justice R, Hechtmann HB: Abnormalities in organ blood flow during positive end-expiratory pressure ventilation. Crit Care Med 15:106, 1987
154. Bonnet F, Richard C, Glaser P, et al: Changes in hepatic flow induced by continuous positive pressure ventilation in critically ill patients. Crit Care Med 10:703, 1982
155. Murdaugh HV, Sieker HO, Manfred F: Effect of altered intrathoracic pressure on renal hemodynamics, electrolyte excretion, and water clearance. J Clin Invest 38:834, 1959
156. Henry JP, Gauer OH, Reeves JL: Evidence of the atrial location of receptors influencing urine flow. Circ Res 4:85, 1956
157. Van Dyke HB: The regulation of water excretion by the neurohypophysis. Bull NY Acad Med 29:24, 1953
158. Gauer OH, Henry JP, Sieker HO, et al: The effect of negative pressure breathing on urine flow. J Clin Invest 33:287, 1954
159. Hemmer M, Viquerat CE, Suter PM, et al: Urinary antidiuretic hormone excretion during mechanical ventilation and weaning in man. Anesthesiology 52:395, 1980
160. Payen DM, Farge D, Beloucif S, et al: No involvement of antidiuretic hormone in acute antidiuresis during PEEP ventilation in humans. Anesthesiology 66:17, 1987
161. Gammanpila S, Bevan DR, Bhuda R: Effect of positive and negative expiratory pressure on renal function. Br J Anaesth 49:199, 1977
162. Jarnberg PO, DeVillota ED, Eklund J, et al: Effects of positive end-expiratory pressure on renal function. Acta Anaesth Scand 22:508, 1978
163. Gabriele G, Rosenfield CR, Fixler DE, et al: Continuous airway pressure breathing with the head-box in the newborn lamb: effects on regional blood flow. Pediatrics 59:858, 1977
164. Manny J, Justice R, Hechtman HB: Abnormalities in organ blood flow and its distribution during positive end-expiratory pressure. Surgery 85:425, 1979
165. Hall SV, Johnson EE, Hedley-Whyte J: Renal hemodynamics and function with continuous positive pressure ventilation in dogs. Anesthesiology 41:452, 1974
166. Leitner C, Frass M, Pacher R, et al: Mechanical ventilation with positive end-expiratory pressure decreases release of alpha-atrial natriuretic peptide. Crit Care Med 15:484, 1987
167. Atlas SA: Atrial natriuretic factor: A new hormone of cardiac origin. Rec Prog Horm Res 42:207, 1986
168. Needleman P, Greenwald JE: Atriopeptin: A cardiac hormone intimately involved in fluid, electrolyte, and blood pressure hemostasis. N Engl J Med 314:828, 1986
169. Trippodo NL, Cole FE, Macphee AA, et al: Biologic mechanisms of atrial natriuretic factor. J Lab Clin Med 109:112, 1987
170. Genest J, Cantin M: Atrial natriuretic factor. Circulation 75:I118, 1987
171. Inariba H, Kohno M, Matsuura T, et al: Circulating atrial natriuretic peptides during weaning from mechanical ventilation. Chest 91:797, 1987

6

Modes of Mechanical Ventilatory Support

Jukka Räsänen
John B. Downs

PHYSIOLOGIC PRINCIPLES OF MECHANICAL VENTILATION

Mechanical ventilatory support entails enhancement of alveolar ventilation using apparatus external to the body's ventilatory pump. According to this definition, stimulation of the phrenic nerves to effect diaphragmatic contraction and change in lung volume is not a form of mechanical ventilatory support because ventilatory work is still done by the patient. Neither does this definition include extracorporeal CO_2 removal, which replaces rather than enhances alveolar ventilation. We include in this discussion most of the techniques that have been widely used clinically for ventilatory support. High-frequency ventilation (HFV) and pressure-support ventilation (PSV) are discussed in detail in Chapters 5, 9, and 15 and, therefore, are mentioned only briefly here.

Pressure Gradients

All clinically used methods of artificial ventilation depend on a change in transpulmonary pressure, the differential between the alveolar pressure (PA) and the pleural pressure (Ppl), to effect alteration in lung volume. Transpulmonary pressure can be altered either by raising or lowering Ppl or by increasing or decreasing PA. Intrapleural pressure can be altered by applying positive or negative pressure to the thoracic cage. Change in PA is accomplished by changing pressure in the proximal airway. Decreases in extrathoracic pressure and increases or decreases in airway pressure (PAW) are used clinically to administer mechanical ventilatory support.

The response of lung volume to a given change in transpulmonary pressure is affected by the compliance of the lung and by the amount of time allowed for lung inflation or deflation. The extent to which manipulations of extrathoracic pressure or PAW will alter transpulmonary pressure depends on the effect that these maneuvers have on Ppl. Transmission of pressure into the pleural space depends on both lung compliance and chest wall compliance. Furthermore, in the event that the exposure of the pulmonary system to a transpulmonary pressure gradient is limited in time, the length of this exposure will also influence the resulting change in lung volume. The effects of inspiratory and expiratory time are related to the time constant (the product of compliance and resistance) of the respiratory system (see Ch. 4) Therefore, an increase in airway resistance (RAW) or lung-thorax compliance (CLT) will retard complete inflation or deflation of the lungs, while a decrease in either variable allows lung volume to change more rapidly.

Adverse side effects of mechanical ventilatory support affect both the respiratory and the cardiovascular systems. Positive-pressure lung inflation can cause structural pulmonary damage if alveoli are overdistended by excessive pressure. In addition to outright tissue destruction, hyperinflation of lung units on the one hand and alveolar collapse on the other may result in functional pulmonary impairment by destabilizing ventilation/perfusion ($\dot{V}/\dot{Q}$) relationships. Finally, inappropriately high or low Ppl can adversely affect right and left ventricular function or peripheral circulatory performance, depending on the initial hemodynamic status of the patient.

Healthy lungs in a patient with normal cardiorespiratory function can be mechanically ventilated with relative ease and safety using a variety of techniques. However, severe and often inhomogeneous alterations in pulmonary compliance and resistance in patients with acute or chronic pulmonary disease complicate respiratory support and increase the susceptibility of the cardiorespiratory system to the adverse effects of therapy. Since its inception, an intensive search has been conducted to find the ideal technique of ventilatory support. As a result, a confusing array of techniques has been introduced rapidly into clinical use. The clinical research to validate these methods lags seriously behind.

EVOLUTION OF MECHANICAL VENTILATION

Iron Lung and Cuirass Ventilators

Interest in mechanical ventilation developed from attempts to resuscitate victims of drowning during the late seventeenth century. Tracheal cannulation and positive-pressure lung inflation were suggested as means of ventilatory assistance during the late seventeenth and the early eighteenth centuries. However, the first ventilators that were developed for human use in the middle of the nineteenth century did not deliver positive-pressure ventilation. Instead, they operated by creating a subambient pressure around the body. These "iron lung" or cabinet ventilators enclosed the patient's entire body, leaving only the head exposed to ambient air (see Ch. 1, Fig. 1-11). The opening around the neck provided an airtight seal, allowing subambient pressure to be generated in the chamber.

Iron lungs were associated with a variety of problems. The patients suffered from lack of nursing care, neck sores, venous engorgement of the head and face, and the adverse psychological effects of being partially (and often permanently) enclosed. However, they provided, for the first time, life-saving long-term support to patients with ventilatory failure.

By the end of the nineteenth century, a simplified version of the iron lung, the cuirass ventilator, was developed (see Ch. 1, Fig. 1-13). It also effected subambient extrathoracic pressure but covered only the patient's chest and/or abdomen. It gained popularity because it allowed easier access to the patient than did iron lungs and was more economical and portable. The negative pressure required by the cuirass ventilator for a given tidal volume (V_T) was larger compared with the negative pressure required by the iron lung, but the obvious advantages for many patients outweighed the lesser ventilatory efficiency.

Positive-Pressure Ventilation

Tracheal intubation and positive-pressure lung inflation were adopted as adjuncts of thoracic surgery during the first decade of the twentieth century. However, these techniques were not commonly employed until the 1950s. The final breakthrough of mechanical ventilatory support outside the operating room was triggered by the experience gained from the 1952 epidemic of poliomyelitis in Copenhagen, Denmark. Thereafter, positive-pressure ventilation spread rapidly into various clinical applications in critical care units and pulmonary medicine.

Mechanical ventilators available before the 1970s were capable only of ventilator-triggered (controlled) or patient-triggered (assisted) positive-pressure ventilation. Weaning from ventilatory support was accomplished by simple disconnection of the patient from the ventilator circuit. However, during the late 1930s, Barach et al.[1] discovered that continuous positive airway pressure (CPAP) without mechanical ventilation could be used to alleviate ventilatory insufficiency and arterial hypoxemia in patients with respiratory failure of variable etiology. These findings were validated later by Frumin et al.[2] and Ashbaugh et al.[3] in adults and by Gregory et al.[4] in neonates by 1970. Subsequently, Kirby et al.[5] and Downs et al.[6] introduced the first adjustable ventilatory support modality—intermittent mandatory ventilation (IMV)—which made it possible to administer mechanical ventilation in a graded fashion. These developments established the essential philosophy of modern fractional respiratory support: independent application of CPAP, supplemental oxygen, and mechanical ventilation to match the particular pathophysiologic derangements of individual patients.

Four techniques of ventilatory support have been introduced since the initial description of IMV. Attempts to attenuate interference with cardiovascular measurements produced by pulmonary inflation in animal experiments led to the development of HFV by Sjöstrand[7] in 1967. During the ensueing 20 years, various methods of high-frequency, low V_T, mechanical ventilatory support have been the topic of a large number of scientific experimental and clinical reports. However, the full role of these modalities in clinical respiratory therapy remains to be established.

Mandatory minute ventilation (MMV) was described by Hewlett et al.[8] in 1977 as a means to provide on-demand partial ventilatory support for patients recovering from anesthesia. Pressure support ventilation was described by Norlander[9] in 1982 as a method to improve the V_T of spontaneously initiated breaths, so that they would be recognized more readily during MMV. Later, PSV was reassessed as an independent mode of partial ventilatory support.

The latest addition to the spectrum of ventilatory techniques—airway pressure-release ventilation (APRV)—introduced by Downs and Stock[10] in 1987, is the only ventilatory mode that is based on intermittent decrease of lung volume (V_L) and P_{AW}. It currently is undergoing experimental and clinical testing and is not yet in wide clinical use.

The popularity of mechanical ventilation, rapid progress in technology, and economic incentives have led to the design of ever more complex ventilators with various functions, many of which are of unproven clinical significance. Gas flow, pressure, and cycling frequency can be manipulated rapidly in endless combinations. New ventilators incorporate most ventilatory modalities, even though little scientific validation of their efficacy is available. At the same time, there is growing concern that the key to improving the prognosis of patients with respiratory failure may not lie in the development of more advanced techniques of mechanical ventilation, but rather by other means, such as extracorporeal support and pharmacologic interventions. Mechanical ventilation, accordingly, is being forced into an era of critical evaluation.

TRADITIONAL VENTILATOR CLASSIFICATION

Mechanical ventilatory support has been characterized largely by the historical sequence and popularity of the individual techniques and their modifications. Understanding of the development of positive-pressure ventilation was enhanced greatly by the work of Mushin et al.[11] These investigators divided available mechanical ventilators on the basis of four key factors (Table 6-1). The criteria included whether (1) flow or pressure was held most constant during inspiration; (2) V_T was limited by flow, pressure, or volume; (3) the mechanism responsible for cycling the ventilator from expiration to inspiration was sensitive to flow, pressure, volume, or time; and (4) inspiration was triggered by the patient or by the ventilator. This classification still provides the simplest method for understanding the operation of a given ventilatory modality; it is applicable even to the newest

Table 6-1. Mechanical Ventilator Classification

Gas delivery
Flow generators
Pressure generators
Tidal volume delivery
Flow cycled
Pressure cycled
Volume cycled
Changeover from expiration to inspiration
Flow cycled
Pressure cycled
Volume cycled
Time cycled
Changeover from inspiration to expiration
Patient-triggered (assisted)
Ventilator-triggered (controlled)

(From Mushin et al.,[11] with permission.)

Table 6-2. Independent Classes of Ventilatory Support

1. Decreased intrapleural pressure
2. Increased airway pressure (VT > VD)
   - IMV
   - MMV
   - PSV
3. Increased airway pressure (VT ≤ VD)
   - HFV
4. Decreased airway pressure
   - APRV

positive-pressure ventilators. However, in order to cover those ventilatory techniques that do not rely on the generation of positive airway pressure and to look at ventilatory support from the point of view of the patient, a more basic physiologic approach is used here. This classification divides the various methods of mechanical ventilatory support into groups based on two physiologic events involved in the generation of mechanical VT: (1) how transpulmonary pressure is altered, and (2) whether the principal factor in alveolar ventilation involves conventional mass gas movement.

Transpulmonary pressure can be altered by changing Ppl or PAW. Mass movement of gas is assumed to be principally responsible for CO_2 elimination when the volume of the mechanical breath is greater than the average dead-space volume (VD) of the respiratory system. In addition, other mechanisms are proposed when VT is equal to or less than VD. Hence, there are four groups of mechanical ventilatory support for currently available techniques of mechanical ventilation (Table 6-2).

The iron lung is a typical example of a group 1 ventilator, which generates a subambient Ppl. All techniques that produce positive-pressure lung inflation at a rate approaching the normal spontaneous respiratory frequency, such as IMV and PSV, belong to group 2. Various methods of HFV, which generally use smaller VT, fall into group 3, while group 4 currently includes only APRV.

Further analysis of the methods within these groups suggests that each is technically unique and capable of providing full or partial alveolar ventilation. Therefore, among the most widely used group 2 methods, only three separate entities can be distinguished: IMV, MMV, and PSV. Conventional controlled mechanical ventilation (CMV) and IMV differ in the level of ventilatory support but use the same basic technique. Intermittent mandatory ventilation, MMV, and PSV, however, are completely different techniques with respect to the interfacing of spontaneous breathing and mechanical ventilation. This grouping of ventilatory modalities should help the clinician to recognize similarities between allegedly different methods and to anticipate the variability in physiologic response between truly different techniques.

TOTAL AND PARTIAL VENTILATORY SUPPORT

Rationale for Partial Ventilatory Support

Ventilator therapy varies widely. Most clinicians use a technique that allows the administration of variable levels of ventilatory support. Partial ventilatory support has been seen historically as an independent technique, leading to controversy regarding the merits of, for example, CMV and IMV. A more fruitful approach, and the one used here, is to view partial ventilatory support as a necessary technical feature of any useful ventilatory modality.

Mechanical ventilatory support in patients with acute respiratory failure must be viewed as symptomatic treatment of alveolar hypoventilation or increased respiratory work. It does not correct any of the pathophysiologic derangements responsible for the development of respiratory failure, even though it can eliminate respiratory acidosis and excessive work of breathing.

Adverse Effects of CMV

Total control of ventilation has not been shown to provide any advantage compared with a level of partial ventilatory support that adequately reduces respiratory work and augments alveolar ventilation. This is true even for patients with heart failure, who theoretically would be most likely to benefit from a high level of positive-pressure mechanical ventilation because of the functional characteristics of their circulation.[12] In contrast, several claims have been made regarding the advantages of partial ventilatory support.

To control ventilation the patient's intrinsic respiratory drive must be extinguished or the patient's neuromuscular transmission interrupted to abolish spontaneous breathing. The former method requires a level of mechanical ventilation that will lower arterial CO_2 tension below the apneic threshold. The apneic threshold can be increased with sedatives allowing control of ventilation at normocarbic levels. However, sedation deep enough to induce apnea with normocarbia is likely to have significant cardiovascular adverse effects and is therefore seldom advisable. Prolonged neuromuscular blockade subjects the patient to hazards associated with the loss of muscle tone and the prolonged recovery of normal neuromuscular function and to a potentially catastrophic event if a circuit disconnection occurs.

For these reasons, induction of respiratory alkalosis is frequently employed to obtain mechanical control of respiration. However, respiratory alkalosis is associated with decreased cardiac output, cerebral vasoconstriction, increased tissue oxygen consumption, and bronchospasm, all of which are potentially hazardous to a critically ill patient.[13] Studies of IMV have shown that a patient who is allowed to perform spontaneous breathing usually will adjust the arterial pH to normal.[14,15] Therefore, partial ventilatory support frequently obviates the need for deep sedation, muscle paralysis, and induced respiratory alkalosis.

Radiographic studies have demonstrated striking differences in the distribution of pulmonary airflow during positive-pressure ventilation and spontaneous breathing.[16] Mechanical positive-pressure breaths delivered to a supine subject direct inspiratory gas flow primarily to anterior (nondependent) lung regions, away from the dependent areas of maximal pulmonary blood flow (Fig. 6-1). This maldistribution cre-

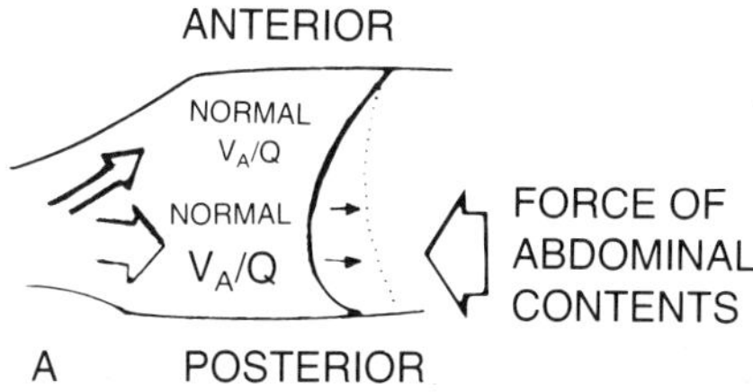

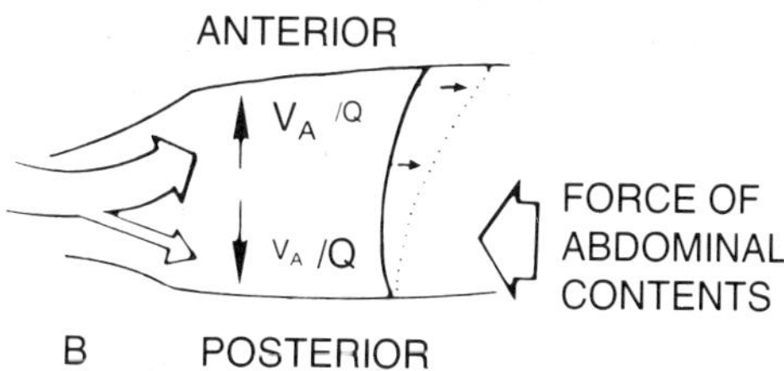

Fig. 6-1. (A) Spontaneous breathing in the supine position is associated with greater posterior diaphragmatic and lung movement. Accordingly, $\dot{V}/\dot{Q}$ relationships here are more closely matched. Less ventilation and perfusion are present anteriorly. **(B)** When the diaphragm does not contract and the patient is manually or mechanically ventilated, most ventilation is anterior (high $\dot{V}/\dot{Q}$), while most perfusion remains (low $\dot{V}/\dot{Q}$) posterior. The result is a potentially significant alteration in normal overall $\dot{V}/\dot{Q}$.

ates $\dot{V}/\dot{Q}$ mismatching and increases the V_D/V_T ratio.[17] As a result, the total minute ventilation required to effect sufficient CO_2 removal will increase, necessitating an increasing level of mechanical ventilatory support.

Advantages of Spontaneous Breathing

During spontaneous breathing, the posterior diaphragm generates greater contractility and movement. Thus, spontaneous ventilation is directed preferentially to the well-perfused dependent lung regions, ensuring optimum $\dot{V}/\dot{Q}$ matching, minimal wasted ventilation, and maximal efficiency of arterial blood oxygenation[18] (Fig. 6-1).

Long periods of CMV have been noted to cause disuse atrophy and discoordination of respiratory muscles.[19] Asynchrony and weakness of these muscle groups may cause considerable problems when weaning to spontaneous breathing is attempted after prolonged ventilator therapy. A method of ventilatory support that allows spontaneous breathing throughout the treatment period tends to maintain respiratory muscle strength and coordination as compared with total control of ventilation. However, muscle strength may be diminished by excessive respiratory work that leads to respiratory muscle fatigue.[20] Therefore, an adequate level of ventilatory support must be assured throughout the period of ventilatory assistance.

When mechanical ventilatory support is effected using methods that increase P_{AW} and Ppl, venous blood return to the heart diminishes.[21] The ensuing decrease in right and left ventricular preload usually causes a decrease in stroke volume in normovolemic or hypovolemic patients. Significant augmentation of intravascular volume and inotropic support may be necessary to counteract the circulatory depression induced by increased Ppl. The adverse hemodynamic effects of positive-pressure ventilation can be minimized by the use of an adequate level of partial ventilator support, allowing some spontaneous breathing activity to persist[22] (Fig. 6-2). Spontaneous breathing produces a decrease in Ppl that augments venous return and cardiac output. An intermittent decrease in Ppl (APRV) may reduce or obviate the need for blood volume and inotropic support measures, and allows the application of appropriate levels of CPAP to correct any aberrant pulmonary mechanical function.

Partial ventilatory support in patients with left heart failure has been criticized because a periodic fall in Ppl increases left ventricular afterload. Furthermore, the failing ventricle may not benefit from increased venous return, because the chamber already is maximally dilated in end-diastole. Adequate ventilatory support and CPAP are critically important in cardiogenic respiratory failure.[23,24] However, studies comparing CMV and IMV in patients with acute myocardial infarction and heart failure have shown that total mechanical control of ventilation is not indicated and that it commonly produces a decrease in cardiac output.[12,24]

The generally accepted relationship between mechanical ventilatory support and cardiovascular function may undergo a change with the introduction of APRV. This method augments alveolar ventilation by producing a decrease in P_{AW} and Ppl (Fig. 6-3). Thus, an increase in ventilatory support with APRV actually decreases mean Ppl. Experimental evidence indicates that APRV can assure mechanical control of respiration without any impairment in the circulatory performance of spontaneously breathing, normovolemic dogs.[25]

The popularity of positive-pressure ventilation has led to increased concern over the possible structural damage that may result from periodic high-pressure lung inflation. A critical factor associated with pulmonary barotrauma is the peak lung volume during a mechanical breath. Therefore, the chances of developing pulmonary parenchymal damage are maximized when ventilation is controlled with large positive-pressure ventilation. Modalities that reduce the peak transpulmonary pressure and lung volume of a mechanical breath, or the frequency of such breaths, should lower the incidence of pulmonary barotrauma.

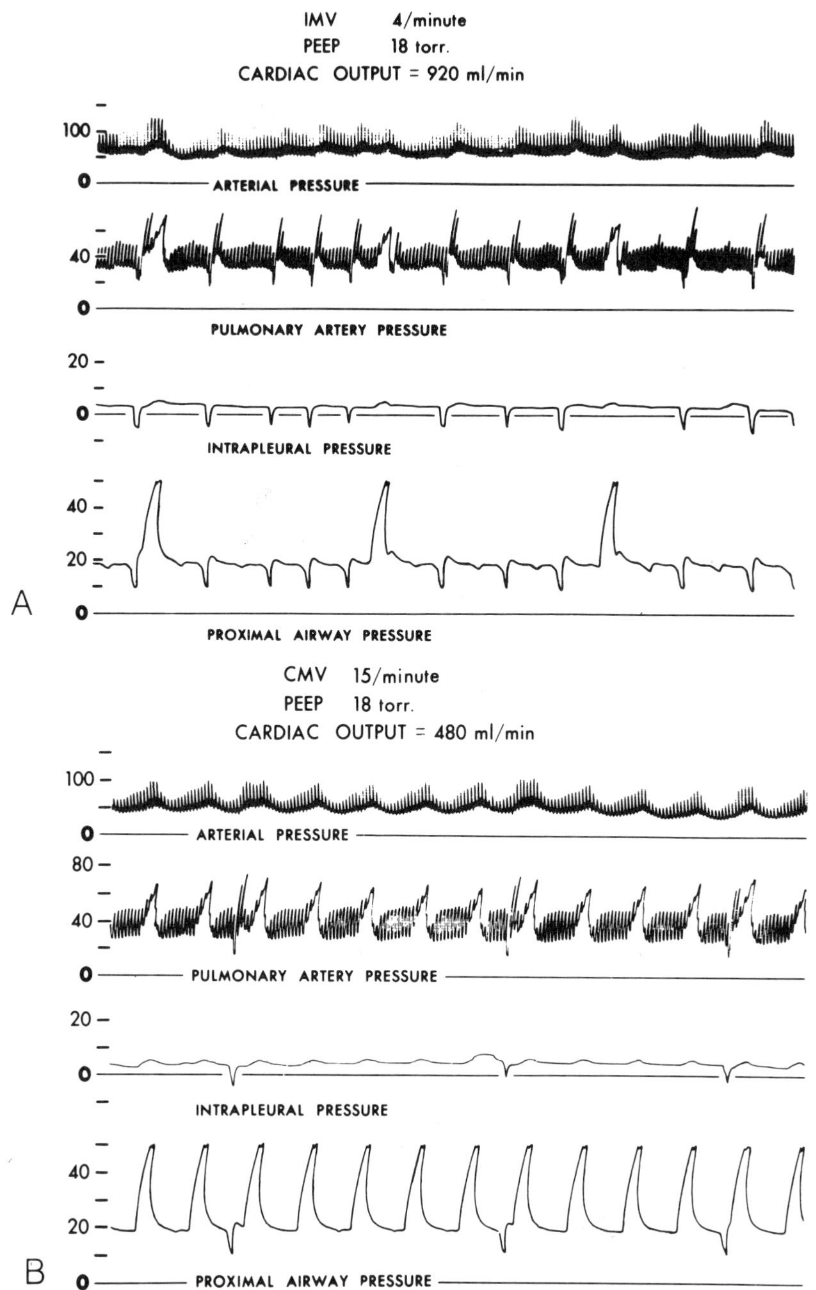

Fig. 6-2. Because of the maintenance of spontaneous ventilation with fewer high-pressure mechanical cycles, IMV **(A)** is associated with less cardiovascular depression than is CMV **(B).** (From Brunner,[73] with permission.)

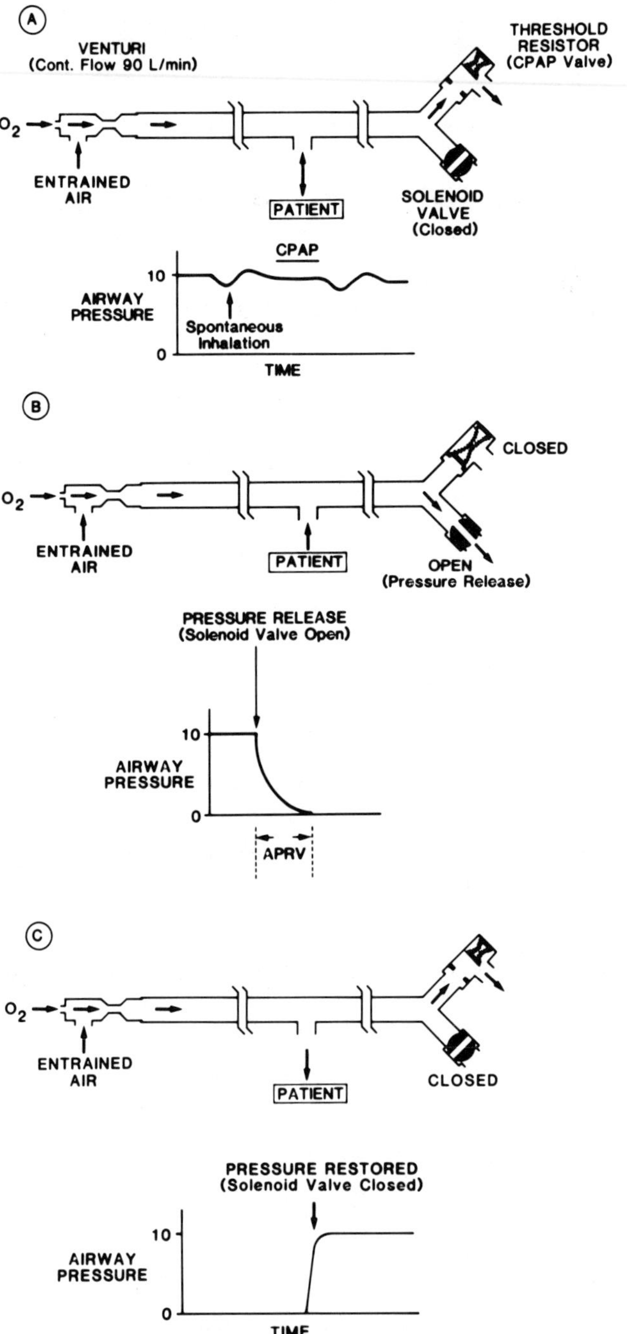

Fig. 6-3. Airway pressure-release ventilation (APRV). **(A)** High continuous gas flow against a closed solenoid valve results in continuous positive airway pressure (CPAP) determined by the threshold resistor. **(B)** Opening of the solenoid valve for a specific time interval results in an immediate decrease in airway pressure (PAW). A large exhalation occurs. **(C)** Closure of the solenoid valve allows immediate restitution of PAW back to the preselected CPAP. The highest pressure level is determined by the CPAP valve. (Courtesy of M.J. Banner, Ph.D.)

This concept is substantiated by clinical studies implicating peak PAW as the clinically measured variable that has the strongest association with pulmonary barotrauma.[26] Partial ventilatory support with IMV reduces the incidence of barotrauma in adults, and cardiopulmonary support with extracorporeal membrane oxygenation (ECMO) decreases the risk of bronchopulmonary dysplasia in neonates with respiratory failure.[27,28] Avoidance of pulmonary barotrauma mandates the lowest level of positive-pressure assistance compatible with adequate ventilation and acceptable respiratory work. Ventilatory techniques that operate with low peak PAW, such as APRV, should prove advantageous.

Partial ventilatory support requires a breathing circuit that allows the patient to breathe and to maintain control of the spontaneous VT. Such integration of patient and ventilator is likely to result in better patient comfort with little need for sedation and none for muscle paralysis. Preservation of spontaneous breathing improves the safety of therapy by decreasing the probability of severe respiratory compromise should the patient become disconnected from the ventilator.

A major advantage of partial ventilatory support is the ability to meet changing requirements by gradually adjusting the level of ventilatory support. This therapeutic flexibility is particularly important when the patient is ready for ventilator weaning. A surprising controversy still prevails regarding the weaning of patients from mechanical ventilation.[29–31] Some clinicians have claimed that partial ventilatory support with IMV does not offer any weaning advantage and prolongs ventilator therapy unnecessarily.[31] It would be inappropriate, although probably not dangerous, to apply a gradual weaning technique routinely to patients who have been mechanically ventilated during general anesthesia. However, sudden discontinuation of ventilatory support of a patient who is recovering from cardiogenic respiratory failure with borderline left ventricular function[24] would be highly inappropriate and extremely dangerous. Therefore, the ability to adjust the level of mechanical ventilation in relation to spontaneous breathing is an essential technique of modern ventilatory support.

INTERFACING BETWEEN SPONTANEOUS AND MECHANICAL VENTILATION

Several techniques have been devised to combine spontaneous breathing and mechanical ventilation during partial ventilatory support. Some do little more than add to the cost of the equipment; others promote clinically significant practical differences.

Nonsynchronized Partial Support

The simplest technical interfacing allows unrestricted spontaneous breathing and delivers the mechanical breaths irrespective of the spontaneous respiratory cycle phase. It is the rule during HFV and is common to APRV (Fig. 6-3) and IMV (Figs. 6-4 and 6-5B). The advantages of nonsynchronized, partial ventilatory support relate to mechanical simplicity. No feedback loop between the patient and ventilator controls means lower cost and increased equipment reliability. The potential disadvantages are patient discomfort associated with asynchronous mechanical lung inflation and pulmonary hyperinflation when the mechanical breath occurs at the end of spontaneous inspiration. Criticism of nonsynchronized partial ventilatory support remains largely theoretical, however, and no data indicate that lack of synchronization between mechanical ventilation and spontaneous breathing presents a hazard or clinically significant discomfort to the adult patient.

Synchronized Partial Support

The most common technique of partial ventilatory support uses patient-triggered mechanical ventilation. An airway pressure sensor detects a reduction in PAW when the patient attempts

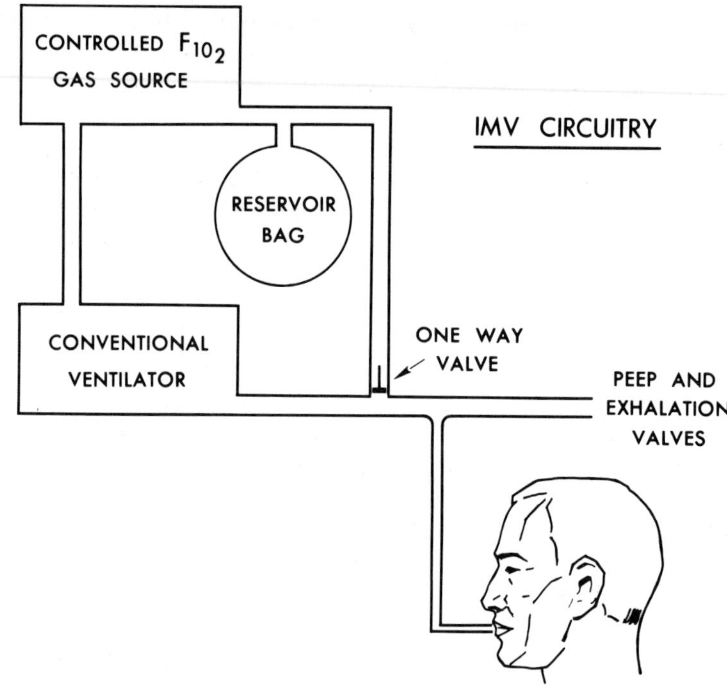

Fig. 6-4. Prototype intermittent mandatory ventilation (IMV) circuit that allows unrestricted spontaneous breathing from the reservoir bag between ventilator-generated mechanical breaths.

to breathe. The impulse is transmitted to the ventilator, which initiates a mechanical breath in response to the pressure change (Fig. 6-5A). Synchronized breaths may be delivered with a set frequency—synchronized intermittent mandatory ventilation (SIMV)—even though the patient's spontaneous respiratory rate may vary (Fig. 6-5C). Spontaneous breaths in excess of the set mechanical rate are unassisted. Breath-to-breath partial ventilatory support with variable intensity is also possible with PSV. In contrast, assisted ventilation (AV) is a form of breath-to-breath partial ventilatory support in which the degree of mechanical assistance cannot be varied externally (Fig. 6-5A).

Successful synchronization of mechanical breaths to spontaneous respiratory effort depends on the sophistication of the sensing mechanism. If the triggering sensitivity is too low, the patient must make a strong inspiratory effort before the ventilator provides gas flow. If the sensitivity is too high, the ventilator may cycle in response to extraneous oscillations in PAW (movement, cardiac impulse). The delay from the start of the triggering deflection until sufficient gas flow is achieved may be long enough to result in a large negative deflection in PAW increased work of breathing, and considerable discomfort. Synchronization is essential in breath-to-breath assist techniques. Comparisons between nonsynchronized (IMV) and synchronized (SIMV) and partial ventilatory support reveal no advantage to synchronization.[32,33]

On-demand mechanical ventilation represents yet another method of interfacing spontaneous and mechanical ventilation. This coupling is unique to MMV.[8] The ventilator is set to respond by administering a mechanical breath or by increasing breath-to-breath ventilatory assistance whenever spontaneous minute ventilation falls short of a minimum, preset level. At other times it remains inactive, and the patient breathes entirely spontaneously. If the patient makes no respiratory efforts, the ventilator will deliver CMV with a minute ventilation equal to the set minimum level. A recently introduced modi-

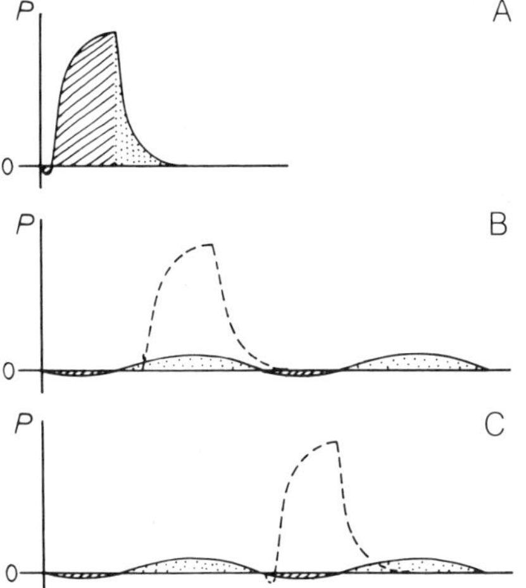

Fig. 6-5. Comparison of airway pressure tracings with three modes of mechanical ventilation. **(A)** Assisted ventilation: A small "negative"-pressure deflection associated with spontaneous inspiration triggers the ventilator and a positive-pressure breath is delivered. **(B)** Intermittent mandatory ventilation: A positive-pressure breath is delivered by the ventilator at a preselected rate independent of the patient's spontaneous effort (asynchronously). **(C)** Synchronized intermittent mandatory volume: The ventilator tidal volume is delivered in response to the negative-pressure deflection of the patient's spontaneous effort (synchronously). Between mechanical cycles, spontaneous breathing occurs as with IMV. (From Eross et al.,[74] with permission.)

fication of this technique increases breath-to-breath ventilatory assistance when the patient's spontaneous respiratory rate exceeds a preselected maximum value.[34] The clinical applicability of these concepts is discussed later.

INDICATIONS FOR TOTAL AND PARTIAL VENTILATORY SUPPORT

The choice between total and partial ventilatory support is determined on an individual basis. Under most circumstances we favor partial ventilatory support for the reasons outlined earlier. However, in some clinical situations, total ventilatory support is appropriate.

The level of ventilatory support should be set according to the patient's ability to breathe spontaneously. A patient with depressed or absent respiratory drive or a patient with impaired neuromuscular respiratory function may be able to perform little or no spontaneous respiratory work without developing respiratory acidemia. Controlled ventilation is entirely appropriate in such a case.

Sometimes extrapulmonary factors necessitate control of respiration. Deliberate hyperventilation may be required to decrease elevated intracranial pressure or to alleviate pulmonary hypertension in the neonate, even when the patient's ventilatory status and pulmonary gas exchange are unimpaired. In these cases, an appropriate level of ventilation is easily achieved because the respiratory mechanics are normal.

Most patients who receive ventilatory support require augmentation of alveolar ventilation to decrease the work of breathing associated with acute or chronic lung disease. Ventilatory support should be adjustable from 0 to 100 percent. The appropriate level administered at different stages of the disease process will be determined by analysis of $PaCO_2$ and pH and by observing clinical signs of respiratory work.

Since $\dot{V}/\dot{Q}$ and gas exchange relationships during mechanical ventilation are often altered unfavorably, mechanical techniques will induce some inatrogenic increase to the amount of support required on the basis of the patient's lung function.[17,18] The same holds true also with respect to respiratory work. No currently marketed ventilator has an ideal flow capability and circuit resistance that allow patients to maintain spontaneous breaths without added work of breathing. Some ventilator circuits are so poorly designed that anything less than total ventilatory support subjects patients to an intolerable increase of respiratory work.[35] Appropriate use of partial ventilatory support with these ventilators is not possible, unless compensatory mechanisms such as AV are activated simultaneously.

Circulatory status influences the choice of therapy. Patients with acute myocardial ischemia and cardiogenic pulmonary edema initially should receive a high level of ventilatory support. Performance of a dilated, afterload-sensitive, failing left ventricle is not likely to be further impaired by elevated PAW and Ppl.[36] A decrease in myocardial ischemia resulting from the alleviation of respiratory work may make left ventricular failure more readily responsive to medical therapy. Accurate evaluation of the circulatory status is essential, because in other conditions, such as pericardial tamponade, the initiation of CMV may bring about sudden and severe cardiovascular collapse.

Finally, some ventilatory support techniques are not compatible with spontaneous respiration because of poor patient tolerance or difficulties with the interfacing spontaneous and mechanical ventilation. The unphysiologic timing of inspiration and expiration during reverse inspiratory to expiratory (I:E) ratio ventilation—inverse ratio ventilation (IRV)—frequently cannot be tolerated and necessitates abolition of spontaneous breathing. Differential (independent) lung ventilation presents such a difficult task of patient-ventilator interfacing that deep sedation, muscle paralysis, and control of ventilation are commonly used.

MECHANICAL VENTILATION BY DECREASED EXTRATHORACIC PRESSURE

The logical first approach to maintaining or augmenting alveolar ventilation in the mid–nineteenth century was to emulate the decrease in Ppl that generates gas movement into the lungs during spontaneous breathing. Unfortunately, this technique required cumbersome apparatus, provided poor control of VT and was fraught with nursing problems caused by limited patient access. Therefore, more effective, albeit less physiologic, ventilatory techniques eventually were developed. During the period of rapidly growing popularity of positive-pressure ventilators, few clinicians anticipated that negative-pressure ventilation would still have a place in respiratory care during the late 1980s. However, reports describing its successful use in various clinical situations are increasing.

Description

The iron lung is used for most negative-pressure ventilation. The tank accommodates the patient's lower body and chest up to the neck, leaving the head outside (see Ch. 1, Fig. 1-11). A neck opening provides an airtight seal enabling a suction device (piston) to generate intermittent subambient pressure that retracts the chest wall outward and the diaphragm downward. An increase in transpulmonary pressure and VT results from the decrease of Ppl. Upon termination of the suction phase, pressure in the tank becomes ambient, allowing passive exhalation to occur.

The cuirass ventilator consists of a rigid cylindrical shell placed around the patient's chest and abdomen, leaving a space anteriorly (see Ch. 1, Fig. 1-13). A vacuum can be generated within the shell, or it may be covered with a nylon or plastic ''coat'' that produces an airtight seal around the shell and chest wall.

Iron lungs perform adequately in many patients; exceptions are those with severe chest wall deformities and/or markedly reduced CLT. Cuirass ventilators usually need to be custom-fitted for optimum performance, and they generally produce less efficient alveolar ventilation. Patients can breathe spontaneously throughout the negative-pressure ventilatory cycle; the mechanical and spontaneous breaths are not synchronized.

Decreased Ppl can also be used in sustained rather than intermittent fashion, to increase the functional residual capacity (FRC) in patients with acute respiratory failure. Restoration of VT results in a decrease of spontaneous respiratory work and improvement in gas exchange in a manner identical to CPAP but without tracheal intubation, mask application, and so forth.

Documentation

Curran[37] and Braun et al.[38] reported stabilization or improvement in the respiratory function of patients with progressive neuromuscular disease when night-time, negative-pressure ventilation was instituted. A significant improvement in ventilatory function was observed by Cropp and DiMarco[39] in a randomized study of negative-pressure ventilation administered for 3 days, 3 to 6 hours daily, to patients with chronic obstructive pulmonary disease (COPD). Splaingard et al.[40] reported 20 years of experience with home negative-pressure ventilation in 40 patients who had neuromuscular disease. The ventilator appeared to be safe, economical, and reliable, with mechanical problems occurring less than once yearly per patient.

Negative-pressure ventilation recently has generated interest as a means of postoperative ventilatory support and weaning. Favorable results were reported in 10 patients with COPD who failed conventional weaning from mechanical ventilation.[41] Early extubation in such patients, with resumption of normal sleeping pattern, speech, and alimentation, may avoid some of the pulmonary and cardiovascular complications of prolonged tracheal intubation and positive-pressure ventilatory support.

Several reports describing the use of sustained negative extrathoracic pressure therapy were published during the early 1970s in neonates,[42] children,[43] and adults.[44] Despite the obvious efficacy of such therapy, its usefulness is limited by the associated problems with nursing care and the availability and acceptance of the CPAP mask.

Advantages

The primary use for negative-pressure ventilation is night-time respiratory muscle rest for patients with COPD or neuromuscular disorders. Quality of life is improved since alveolar ventilation can be augmented and symptoms of chronic hypoventilation alleviated without tracheal intubation or tracheotomy. The patient is able to speak, drink, sleep, and eat normally; complications associated with endotracheal or tracheostomy tubes are avoided. Since the mechanical ventilatory cycle is associated with a decrease in Ppl, cardiovascular impairment is unlikely to occur in patients with normal circulatory function.

Hazards

A patent airway is a prerequisite of negative-pressure ventilation. If the airway is open, the VT depends on lung and chest wall compliance, the level of subambient pressure around the chest wall, the duration and sequencing of pressure changes, and the space available for the chest and abdominal wall to expand. Tidal volume cannot be adjusted accurately and has a definite upper limit. Time required for the subambient pressure to develop does not allow large increases in ventilator rate to compensate for the low VT. Negative-pressure ventilation requires bulky apparatus and is relatively inefficient. Limitations in nursing care for patients who do not tolerate opening of the cabinet even for short periods of time have been mentioned. Psychological problems related to long-term confinement are often problematic.

Current Status

Negative-pressure ventilation has a place in modern respiratory therapy. It may be a favored alternative to tracheotomy and positive-pressure ventilation in patients who need intermittent ventilatory assistance to alleviate COPD. Its use in postoperative respiratory support or the treatment of acute respiratory failure will be minimal.

VENTILATION BY INCREASED AIRWAY PRESSURE (VT > VD)

Conventional positive-pressure ventilation includes any ventilatory support technique that increases PAW and generates a VT greater than the volume of the patient's respiratory dead space. Three separate ventilatory techniques fall into this category: IMV, MMV, and PSV (Table 6-2). The clinically important differences between them relate to the method by which mechanical ventilation is interfaced with spontaneous breathing. However, when used to deliver a high level of mechanical ventilation, they are remarkably similar. The major difference is that PSV cannot be used for controlled ventilation because each breath is initiated by spontaneous patient effort. Only IMV and MMV are discussed in this chapter; for a detailed presentation of PSV, the reader is referred to Chapters 5, 9, and 15.

Assisted ventilation and IRV frequently are presented as separate ventilatory modalities. With regard to tidal volume ($V_T > V_D$), they are classified as conventional. However, in contrast to IMV, MMV, and PSV, neither can be used to cover the full range of ventilatory support. Therefore, they are not separate ventilatory support techniques in the broad sense we have described. For historical reasons only, they are discussed as separate entities.

Generation of Tidal Volume

To initiate a conventional positive-pressure breath, a mechanical ventilator predominantly regulates either flow or pressure. The flow or pressure may be constant throughout inspiration, or it may vary. A second variable limits inspiration to a given pressure, volume, or flow, while a third cycles the ventilator from inspiration to expiration using pressure, volume, time, or flow as the determinant (Table 6-1).

Little or no solid data support the view that any flow or pressure profile used to generate a positive-pressure breath is clearly superior in routine clinical use. However, Al-Saady and Bennett[45] reported a significant improvement in lung mechanics when a decelerating rather than a constant inspiratory flow pattern was employed. Setting an inspiratory pressure limit for constant-flow neonatial ventilators probably is useful to protect the lungs from barotrauma caused by inadvertently high peak pressures.

Cycling mechanisms have been emphasized when comparing the operational characteristics of various mechanical ventilators. However, none of the available inspiratory to expiratory cycling mechanisms assures constant V_T if the C_{LT} varies sufficiently. Of more practical importance than the principles of operation are the absolute capabilities of ventilator to generate flow and pressure, the maximum flow available for spontaneous inspiration, and the resistance that the patient must overcome to breathe spontaneously through the ventilator circuit at low levels of ventilatory support.[46]

Intermittent Mandatory Ventilation

Description

Intermittent mandatory ventilation delivers conventional positive-pressure ventilation at a fixed mechanical rate, while (in theory) allowing unrestricted, unassisted spontaneous breathing to occur between mechanical cycles (Figs. 6-4, and 6-5B). Mandatory mechanical breaths may or may not be synchronized to spontaneous breathing (IMV and SIMV). The technique sets no restrictions with respect to the generation, limiting, or cycling of the mechanical breaths. Any level of mechanical support from 0 to 100 percent may be delivered with IMV. Control of ventilation is achieved by increasing the frequency and/or V_T of the mandatory breaths, until the $PaCO_2$ is lowered below the apneic threshold, and the patient's spontaneous respiratory efforts cease. Weaning from IMV is accomplished by gradually lowering the mandatory rate. The technique can be employed simultaneously with ambient, positive, or subambient expiratory airway pressure.

During SIMV, the mechanical breaths are triggered by the patient, if spontaneous respiratory efforts are present within a time period suitable for the selected ventilator rate. Should the ventilator not sense spontaneous ventilatory

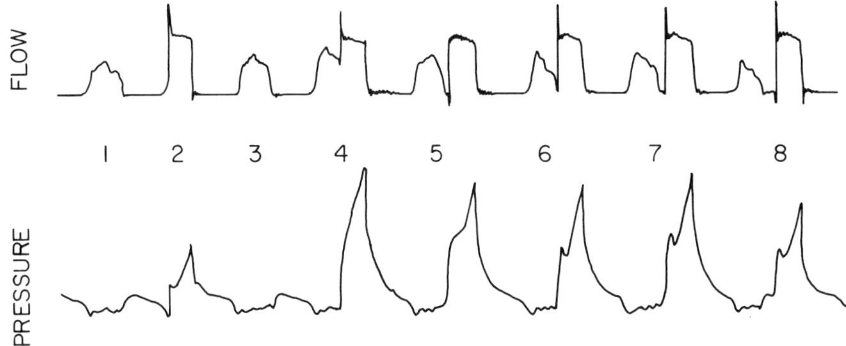

Fig. 6-6. Potential problems of breath stacking with IMV. Breath 1 is spontaneous; breath 2 is a ventilator-delivered IMV. Breath 3 is spontaneous. In breaths 4–7, the IMV cycles are delivered before the patient's spontaneous exhalations are complete. A much higher airway pressure results. With breath 8, the "normal" relationship begins to be reestablished. (From Graybar & Smith,[75] with permission.)

efforts at the appropriate time, it will deliver nonsynchronized mandatory breaths according to the set IMV rate.

Synchronization was designed to avoid "stacking" of mechanical and spontaneous breaths[47] (Fig. 6-6). A ventilator breath occurring at the end of a spontaneous inspiration was thought to predispose to high PAW and Ppl, with a resultant increased risk of barotrauma and cardiovascular compromise. However, Hasten et al.[32] found no difference in cardiopulmonary function of 35 patients in a randomized comparison of IMV and SIMV. These workers noted that patients appeared to synchronize their breathing to the mechanical ventilator rate during IMV and, therefore, benefited little from ventilator-engineered synchronization.

Heenan et al.[33] found no physiologic difference between IMV and SIMV in an experimental study in which the two techniques were applied with or without CPAP, before and after near-drowning. Although peak and mean airway pressures were an average of 2 mmHg higher than IMV, no difference was found in Ppl. Presumably, a "stacked" IMV breath started at a lower level of Ppl than did a triggered SIMV breath. Therefore, improved cardiovascular function did not result from synchronization. The reported difference in airway pressure probably is not large enough to alter the incidence of barotrauma significantly. Synchronization of IMV breaths appears to be an unnecessary technical feature that makes ventilators more complex, more costly, and more likely to malfunction.

Documentation

Intermittent mandatory ventilation initially was described as a method of providing mechanical ventilatory support to infants.[5,48] Later, the successful use of IMV in six adult patients who had failed weaning by conventional T-piece trials was described.[6] A further report of three cases presented evidence for the applicability of IMV in weaning patients with COPD.[49] In 1974, Downs et al.[50] published a study that compared IMV and controlled mechanical ventilation in weaning 24 patients with respiratory failure of variable etiology. This report indicated that weaning could be accomplished more rapidly and with more normal acid-base status using IMV. Furthermore, IMV did not seem to affect arterial blood oxygenation adversely or to produce increased oxygen consumption in these patients. This study has been roundly criticized, particularly with respect to the claim that the period of weaning could be shortened, by IMV.[30,31]

Although IMV was introduced for weaning, it rapidly became the standard technique of long-term ventilator support in many institutions. This development was directed primarily by clinical experience and by the lack of alternative techniques that provided adjustable partial-through-total ventilatory support. Comparisons between IMV and CMV have been made with respect to pulmonary function, cardiovascular performance, and oxygen cost of breathing.[12,51,52] However, as we have suggested, such comparisons really address the effects of different levels of the same type of ventilatory support, and thus cannot be used to validate or refute IMV in general. Studies comparing IMV and AV are similarly irrelevant, because the results depend on the level of ventilatory support arbitrarily selected for IMV in counter-distinction to the fixed support with AV. No controlled studies compare the outcome of ventilator therapy with IMV and alternative methods, such as PSV, MMV, or APRV.

Advantages

Intermittent mandatory ventilation is the most accurately documented ventilator mode currently in use. Mechanical tidal volume delivery is predictable and influenced by a limited number of physiologic variables that are accessible for evaluation using clinical observation and simple measurements. As a result, the beneficial and adverse physiologic effects of different levels of IMV can be predicted with considerable accuracy.

The relative amount of mechanical ventilation (0 to 100 percent) in conjunction with the patient's spontaneous rate and tidal volume maintain normal $PaCO_2$ and pHa. Spontaneous respiratory activity can be observed and analyzed while the prescribed level of mechanical support is applied. A continuous clinical evaluation of the patient's respiratory status and accurate assessment of the effects of other therapy on the mechanisms of breathing is easily achieved. During HFV and PSV, the actual level of ventilatory assistance is difficult to ascertain, and the patient's spontaneous ventilation can be observed only by turning off the ventilator. The circuitry required for IMV is inexpensive, simple to build, and easy to maintain, because it does not require complex synchronization and regulating devices.

Hazards

The major drawback to IMV is that not all spontaneous breaths are assisted. As a result, the characteristics of the breathing circuit and expertise of the physician are increasingly important. If the ventilator circuit has high flow resistance, low flow capability, or a poorly functioning demand valve, the resulting spontaneous inspiratory work may be sufficiently high to preclude effective spontaneous breathing.[35] Such a ventilator should not be used for IMV, but only to provide total ventilatory support.

Similarly, if patients are not given proper therapy to improve their pulmonary mechanics, the intrinsic respiratory work may be too high to permit unassisted spontaneous breathing. Reports of increased oxygen consumption and deterioration of circulatory function during IMV can be traced frequently to inadequate equipment design or inappropriate use of CPAP.[24,52] However, despite optimization of ventilator circuit characteristics and intrinsic respiratory mechanical function, the spontaneous work of breathing remains unacceptably high and necessitates total ventilatory support for some patients. Whether breath-to-breath support with PSV will allow a reduction of ventilatory assistance in these cases is unknown.

The method of tidal volume delivery constitutes a hazard common to all conventional forms of ventilatory support. A relatively large VT is added to an FRC which, ideally, has been restored to near-normal with CPAP. Consequently, the peak PAW is high (often excessively so) and subjects the patient to an increased risk of barotrauma and adverse circulatory side effects when increased ventilatory support is required. This problem was not solved by the introduction of HFV. Whether APRV will circumvent it remains to be seen.

The absolute amount of ventilatory support is fixed for a given IMV rate. The ventilator is not sensitive to increases in the total amount of ventilatory work associated with changes in lung mechanics, metabolic rate, or nutrition. Some compensation for increased ventilatory requirement is provided by methods such as PSV that provide breath-to-breath support. Mechanical ventilation with PSV increases if the patient triggers the ventilator more frequently in response to an increase in CO_2 production or decrease in lung compliance.[53] However, this compensation may not occur if airway resistance increases, because the latter usually causes a decrease in respiratory rate.

Current Status

Intermittent mandatory ventilation presently is the most widely used ventilatory technique in critical care in the United States.[54] Most patients with respiratory failure can be managed with IMV. Patients unable to be treated successfully probably will fail other techniques as well. However, no available scientific data proves that IMV produces a more favorable outcome in patients with respiratory failure.

Mandatory Minute Ventilation

Description

Mandatory minute ventilation is a ventilatory support technique designed to operate in a fashion similar to the function of an on-demand cardiac pacemaker. The original MMV circuit described by Hewlett et al.[8] could be added to several existent ventilators. It consisted of two reservoirs, one for spontaneous breathing and one for the ventilator, into which an adjustable total flow of fresh gas was delivered from a common source. If the patient's spontaneous minute ventilation was less than the fresh gas inflow, the spontaneous breathing reservoir filled to capacity, following which further flow was directed to the ventilator reservoir. When the ventilator reservoir filled to a certain volume, a mandatory positive-pressure breath directed its contents into the patient's lungs.

With MMV, an apneic patient receives the predetermined minute volume from the ventilator in a fashion indistinguishable from conventional CMV. If the patient breathes spontaneously, the ventilator still provides the difference between spontaneous ventilation and the preset mandatory minute ventilation. If the patient's minute ventilation matches the preselected level, the ventilator does not cycle, and the patient breaths without mechanical support.

The prefix "extended" was later added to MMV to denote a modification that allowed the patient to increase his minute ventilation above the selected value. However, Hewlett's original design included a safety valve that permitted the patient to breathe room air should his ventilatory requirement exceed the minute ventilation selected. Newer modifications of the MMV principle involve maintenance of the patient's respiratory rate below a set maximum value instead of assuring a minimum minute ventilation.[34] The mechanical breath during MMV can be delivered using any positive-pressure method. Originally ventilatory assistance was similar to IMV. Later, breath-to-breath assistance with PSV was introduced.

Documentation

Hewlett et al.[8] described the technical aspects of MMV in 1977. Two years later, Higgs and Bevan[55] published a case report regarding successful use of MMV in the postoperative management of a patient with myasthenia gravis. In these reports, MMV was proposed as a useful weaning technique to provide a smooth transition from CMV to spontaneous breathing after anesthesia and surgery. Subsequently, it was advocated as a general ventilatory support mode and an alternative to IMV, on the basis that it provides a higher back-up level of ventilation should the patient's spontaneous respiratory activity become inadequate.[56] No controlled studies to assess MMV effectiveness are available.

Advantages

Mandatory minute ventilation should provide a smooth recovery of spontaneous respiration in a patient recovering from anesthesia and surgery. Its use in other clinical situations requiring ventilatory assistance may be associated with problems related to its mechanism of operation.

Hazards

Weaning is unlikely to be accomplished by MMV without frequent adjustments in the level of minute ventilation. Since VD/VT should decrease as spontaneous breathing is augmented,[17] a reduction in mechanical support should decrease the total ventilatory requirement. Were the minute ventilation limit to remain unchanged, progress toward totally spontaneous breathing would stop at some intermediate level of assistance. Studies have not yet compared MMV with other weaning procedures.

The concept of MMV presents significant problems in the management of patients with respiratory failure caused by the adult respiratory distress syndrome (ARDS). Adequate ventilatory support in these patients is the amount that corrects respiratory acidosis and transfers a sufficient amount of respiratory work to the ventilator. Mandatory minute ventilation is designed to provide the portion of required minute ventilation the patient is unable to accomplish spontaneously. If the MMV is less than the spontaneous minute ventilation, the ventilator will not cycle until respiratory muscle fatigue ensues and spontaneous breathing is decreased. If the MMV exceeds that of the patient, CMV results. Therefore, MMV may not be useful in decreasing respiratory work, unless it is adjusted to control respiration entirely. In this respect, MMV differs from IMV, which may be adjusted to assume any portion of the patient's work of breathing.

Preliminary data indicate that control of the maximum respiratory rate instead of the minimum minute ventilation may be a more effective means of applying MMV in patients with increased respiratory work or variable CO_2 production.

Current Status

Insufficient scientific data are available to establish the value of MMV. Theoretically, the technique provides a viable alternative for the weaning of patients who have a neuromuscular induced inability to breathe adequately. It appears not to offer any advantages to patients with increased work of breathing and ventilatory insufficiency imposed by ARDS.

Inverse Ratio Ventilation

Description

Inverse ratio ventilation (IRV) denotes mechanical ventilation using an inspiratory-to-expiratory time ratio greater than 1. A variety of techniques are available by which the inspiratory time can be extended, each of which may result in different clinical effects. These include application of an end-inspiratory pause, retardation of inspiratory peak flow, or limitation of inspiratory pressure.

Most ventilators do not allow the patient to obtain additional fresh gas from the circuit when the ventilator is in its inspiratory phase. Hence, the long inspiratory phase of IRV usually makes this technique incompatible with spontaneous breathing, and respiratory depressants or muscle relaxants frequently must be administered to assure patient acceptance. In general, IRV is used to administer CMV, and weaning is accomplished using another technique. Pressure-limited IRV, when it is achieved with APRV, is almost identical to CMV. The relationship between IRV and APRV, therefore, is similar to that of conventional CMV and IMV.

Documentation

Inverse ratio ventilation initially was adopted for neonatal use during the late 1960s and 1970s.[57,58] Despite encouraging results in pediatric patients, IRV was not widely accepted in adult respiratory therapy, perhaps because of reports that compared its effects with those of PEEP.[59–61] The results of these experimental and clinical investigations indicated that the benefits produced by IRV were largely, if not completely, due to an elevation in mean airway pressure ($\overline{P_{AW}}$) and transpulmonary pressure. Because muscle paralysis frequently was required for IRV, IMV with CPAP appeared to represent a more promising approach. However, reports claiming improved oxygenation, lower peak inspiratory pressure (PIP), and enhanced efficacy of ventilation with reduction in V_D/V_T have appeared regularly.[62,63]

Improvement in gas exchange during IRV is attributed to more effective alveolar recruitment and better distribution of ventilation during the extended inspiratory phase. Tharratt et al.[63] reported the largest available clinical series comparing IRV and conventional positive-pressure ventilation in 31 patients with ARDS. In this study, a changeover from volume-limited conventional ventilation to pressure-limited IRV was followed by an average reduction in PIP of 20 cm H_20, PEEP of 12 cm H_20, and minute ventilation of 7 L/min. PaO_2 improved by 11 mmHg and $PaCO_2$ remained unchanged. Mean airway pressure increased by 5 cm H_2O. It is very difficult, however, to deduce from this study the true effect of the alteration in I:E ratio, since, simultaneously, the inspiratory flow pattern was changed and ventilation was transferred to a different part of the patients' lung-thorax pressure-volume curve. When expiratory time is shortened, air trapping may alter markedly the relationship between P_{AW} and V_L, with a resultant confounding effect on the findings. This fact was illustrated vividly by the 24 percent incidence of pneumothorax during IRV.

Advantages

The potential advantages of IRV are the result of alveolar recruitment, improved distribution of ventilation, and a decreased V_D/V_T. Alveolar recruitment should improve $\dot{V}/\dot{Q}$ matching, effect a reduction in venous admixture, and correct hypoxemia. Improved ventilatory efficiency often allows reduction of the peak P_{AW}. However, $\overline{P_{AW}}$ usually is increased or remains unchanged. Therefore, circulatory function frequently is identical to that during ventilation with a normal I:E ratio.

Hazards

Incompatibility with spontaneous breathing is a major limitation of IRV. The necessity of muscle paralysis or deep sedation and controlled ventilation often constitutes a significant obstacle. A restriction of expiratory time predisposes to air trapping in alveoli with long time constants for emptying. Regions so affected often become overdistended and are likely to rupture causing minor or major barotrauma.

Current Status

Available data indicate that in some patients with severe acute respiratory failure, IRV improves pulmonary gas exchange. This beneficial effect is inconsistent, and the exact role played by changing the I:E ratio, as opposed to alterations in $\overline{P_{AW}}$ or the incorporation of a decelerating inspiratory flow, is difficult to ascertain. Recent reports regarding the favorable effects of APRV support the concept of pressure-limited IRV.[64,65] In fact, APRV incorporates the favorable characteristics of IRV, spontaneous breathing, and partial ventilatory support into one technique with potentially widespread applicability.

Assisted Ventilation

Description

Assisted ventilation provides positive-pressure support in response to the patient's inspiratory effort. Triggering usually is initiated by a small drop in PAW at the start of a spontaneous inspiration (Fig. 6-5A). The ventilator breath may be delivered using any cycling method, inspiratory limit, and expiratory airway pressure. Because ventilation with AV requires a spontaneous breathing effort, total ventilatory support cannot be provided. Ventilatory assistance cannot be adjusted. Weaning is accomplished by disconnecting the patient from the ventilator.

Documentation

Originally, AV was believed to provide nearly full ventilatory support. However Marini et al.[66,67] demonstrated that patients receiving AV usually continue their spontaneous effort throughout the mechanical tidal volume delivery, thereby contributing significantly to the total ventilatory work. Marini's studies revealed that under favorable conditions the energy expended by the patient was 33 to 50 percent of that required for passive lung-thorax inflation. Under less favorable conditions, the patient's energy expenditure exceeded that of passive lung inflation. Therefore, AV must be regarded as a method of breath-to-breath partial ventilatory support, the amount of which is unknown.

Despite its limitations, AV was the first technique that permitted positive-pressure mechanical ventilatory support without a need to abolish the patient's spontaneous drive to breathe. The most important advantage of AV compared with CMV is easier adjustment of the ventilator to produce a more normal $PaCO_2$ and pH. However, when AV is adjusted to provide a large mechanical breath each time the patient triggers the ventilator, the $PaCO_2$ will be maintained close to the apneic threshold, and respiratory alkalosis usually cannot be avoided.[68] If, in contrast, the patient is allowed to regulate the spontaneous tidal volume independently, as is the case with IMV, the acid-base status will approach normal.[69]

When the assisting mechanical breath is flow-cycled and pressure-limited, AV is identical to PSV[70] (Fig. 6-7). No physiologic reason to use AV can be advanced if PSV is available. The advantage of PSV over AV is the ease with which the level of ventilatory support can be adjusted when necessary.

Advantages

There are no advantages to AV. Since AV provides a fixed amount of ventilatory assistance, we do not consider it a free-standing ventilatory technique in the full sense of the term. Breath-to-breath ventilatory support is better achieved by PSV (see Ch. 9).

Hazards

The disadvantage of AV is the unknown level of fixed ventilatory support. The patient performs one-third or more of the respiratory work to ventilate the lungs. In the absence of completely spontaneous respiratory cycles, pulmonary mechanics can be evaluated only by disconnection of the ventilator. Abrupt disconnection also is the only method of weaning possible. As previously discussed, sudden termination of ventilatory support may present a life-threatening cardiopulmonary stress to some patients with unstable circulatory function.

Safe application of AV requires meticulous attention to the triggering sensitivity to prevent undue respiratory effort on the one hand and autocycling of the ventilator on the other. The pulmonary and cardiovascular effects of AV do not differ from controlled positive pressure ventilation at similar tidal volumes and ventilator rates. Since AV requires patient effort, it provides no support if spontaneous respiration ceases.

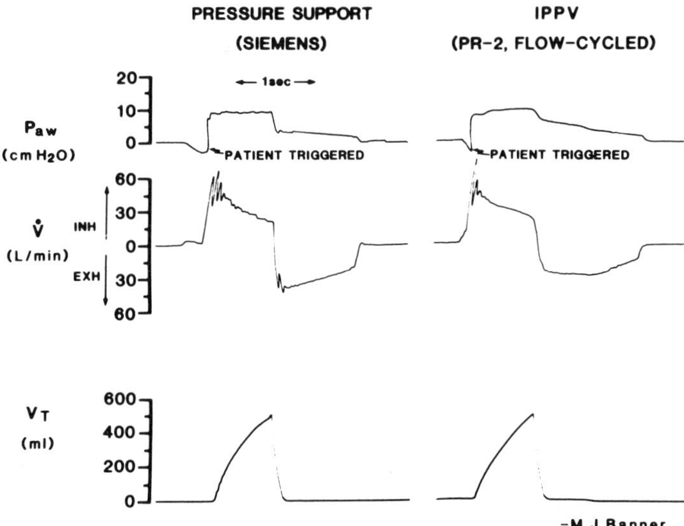

Fig. 6-7. Similarities between assisted ventilation with a patient-triggered, pressure-limited, flow-cycled ventilator (Puritan-Bennett PR-2) and a modern critical care ventilator designed to provide pressure support (Siemens 900 C). (Courtesy of M.J. Banner, Ph.D.)

Current Status

Assisted ventilation is still widely used as a primary mode of ventilatory support. Many patients can be managed safely with AV and weaned successfully with a T-piece. However, modern respiratory care should incorporate the option of adjustable partial ventilatory support, which is not available with AV. Intermittent mandatory ventilation, PSV, and perhaps APRV probably will supplant AV in the not-too-distant future.

Airway Pressure Release Ventilation

Description

Airway pressure release ventilation was introduced by Downs and Stock[10] in 1986. The unique feature of APRV is the augmentation of alveolar ventilation by a decrease in airway pressure and lung volume. Technically, the lung volume exchange is accomplished by intermittent release of CPAP. The APRV system includes a CPAP circuit in which baseline airway pressure is maintained above ambient with a threshold resistor valve and either a high gas flow or a pressurized volume reservoir (see Fig. 6-3A). A sufficiently sensitive demand valve also could be used to provide CPAP.

A release valve is situated in the expiratory limb of the CPAP circuit to allow rapid decrease in airway pressure. The release valve must have extremely low flow resistance to allow adequate empyting of the lungs during the period of pressure release. The release valve is controlled by a timing device that allows adjustment of the extent, duration, and frequency of pressure release.

A level of CPAP adjusted to optimize expiratory lung volume and pulmonary gas exchange is essential to the successful use of APRV. When the timer opens the release valve, airway pressure falls rapidly (Fig. 6-3B), gas flows from the lungs, and lung volume decreases below baseline, enhancing the excretion of CO_2. When the release valve closes, CPAP and lung volume are rapidly reestablished by the high, continuous gas flow (Fig. 6-3C). Augmentation of alveolar ventilation depends on the release volume and APRV rate. Release volume is determined by lung compliance, airway resistance, release time, and the gradient between CPAP and the release pressure level. The patient can breathe freely between or during the APRV breaths. If high enough release volume and rate are used, CMV results.

Weaning from APRV is accomplished by lowering the frequency of airway pressure release, until the patient is breathing with CPAP alone. From a synchronization standpoint, augmentation of ventilation during APRV is similar to conventional IMV.

Inverse ratio ventilation with a pressure limit closely mimics APRV. In fact, during CMV, the techniques are indistinguishable on the basis of PAW tracing. However, IRV seldom is combined with spontaneous breathing, and therefore is not used to provide partial support. If weaning is attempted during IRV, it is accomplished by decreasing the time of increased airway pressure, rather than increasing it, as is the case with APRV.

Documentation

Initial experimental and clinical investigations showed that alveolar ventilation and arterial oxygenation can be maintained effectively using APRV.[64,65] Experimental studies comparing APRV and conventional positive-pressure ventilation (PPV) found no significant differences in oxygenation or ventilation when similar airway pressure, tidal volume, and ventilator rate were administered to animals with normal lungs. However, in dogs with oleic acid-induced lung injury, APRV resulted in significantly lower $PaCO_2$ and higher PaO_2 compared with conventional support. These results suggest that the airway pressure pattern of APRV may favor a more uniform distribution in injured lungs.

A study comparing spontaneous breathing, APRV, and PPV with a similar level of CPAP in dogs with oleic acid-induced lung injury showed that ventilatory failure and arterial desaturation that existed during spontaneous breathing could be effectively corrected by either APRV or PPV.[25] In this study, PaO_2 was significantly better and venous admixture lower during PPV. The differences in oxygenation may have reflected a difference in mean transpulmonary pressure, which, by design was lower during APRV, or it may have resulted from reduction and redistribution of pulmonary blood flow during PPV. Systemic oxygen delivery, however, was superior during APRV, because circulatory function was better preserved.

Peak airway pressure during APRV is 30 to 75 percent of that during PPV. The extent of this reduction depends on lung mechanics and whether APRV and PPV have been adjusted to a similar $\overline{PAW}$ or to a similar level of CPAP. Not surprisingly, no differences in circulatory function have been observed between APRV and PPV in studies employing similar levels of $\overline{PAW}$.[64,65,71] This is true regardless of the presence or absence of acute lung injury or the intravascular volume status of the experimental animal or the patient. However, APRV originally was designed to be used as an adjunct to CPAP. When APRV and PPV are added to existing CPAP therapy, the hemodynamic advantages of the former become obvious. In dogs with induced lung injury, ventilation could be controlled using APRV, with no depression of stroke volume, cardiac output, and tissue oxygen delivery compared with spontaneous breathing with CPAP. When PPV was used in a similar fashion, stroke volume decreased by 42 percent, oxygen delivery diminished by 32 percent, and the oxygen utilization coefficient increased by 33 percent.

Advantages

The advantages of APRV compared with other forms of PPV are related to low peak and mean airway and intrathoracic pressures. Peak airway pressure during APRV never exceeds the CPAP level, and maximum lung volume corresponds to the FRC. Therefore, the incidence of barotrauma should be minimal.

Airway pressure levels up to 15 cm H_2O can be maintained safely using a tight-fitting mask in most patients who have intact protective airway reflexes. Since airway pressure during APRV never exceeds the CPAP level, it may be clinically feasible to commence APRV in a patient receiving mask-CPAP therapy without the need for tracheal intubation. Jousela et al.[72] have described a patient with myasthenia gravis, in whom postoperative weaning from mechanical ventilation and removal of the endotracheal tube was accomplished successfully by APRV delivered using a mask-CPAP circuit.

Changes in Ppl during APRV are similar to those that occur during spontaneous breathing with CPAP. Low mean Ppl may enable CMV to be delivered with little, if any, depression of cardiovascular function. Depression in circulatory performance during PPV is seen commonly and frequently cannot be avoided. Instead, it must be compensated for by lowering CPAP to a suboptimal level, by infusing large amounts of fluid to augment central blood volume, or by using inotropic agents to increase left ventricular contractility. All of these measures are potentially harmful and complicate therapy. Such compensatory support should be required less often during APRV.

Hazards

Currently available data do not allow conclusions to be made regarding potential adverse side effects of APRV. Low PAW and Ppl should minimize pulmonary and circulatory impairment from mechanical ventilation. Ventilatory assistance during APRV occurs in a nonsynchronized manner and the patient's spontaneous breaths are unassisted.

Current Status

Currently, APRV is an experimental technique with limited clinical use. No adult ventilator can reliably produce the rapid changes in airway pressure essential for successful ventilation using APRV. However, several neonatal ventilators incorporating IRV produce a similar but limited capability. Experimental and clinical investigations have shown that APRV can augment alveolar ventilation in dogs with or without lung injury and in postoperative patients with mild pulmonary insufficiency. Future studies in patients with varying degrees of respiratory insufficiency will establish or disprove the usefulness of APRV in clinical practice.

CONCLUSIONS

Evaluation of Ventilatory Techniques

The history of mechanical ventilation has seen the rise and fall of numerous techniques. A confusing array of methods has resulted in which slight modifications of old techniques claim, and are awarded, independent status without demonstrating significant applicability to clinical patient care. Superiority of a technique may lie in one or more of the following areas: therapeutic efficacy, safety, ease of operation, and cost. Evidence documenting the value of a new modality must be scientifically valid. Clearly the development of mechanical ventilation has not proceeded along these lines, and considerable future research is needed to delineate the role of existing approaches. Standard ventilatory techniques should be well documented, widely used, and applicable to all clinical situations requiring any level of mechanical ventilatory support. Four techniques meet most of these criteria: IMV, PSV, HFV, and APRV. Of these PSV and APRV lack sufficient documentation and general familiarity. High-frequency ventilation has generated volumes of scientific data but has not stood the test of time with respect to clinical use. Therefore, conventional PPV with IMV to provide ventilatory support is the most logical choice of a standard technique. IMV is widely used and accepted,[54] the equipment is readily available, and variables defining the level of ventilatory support are easily measured and communicated.

Once a standard ventilatory technique is chosen and accepted, controlled studies should be carried out to compare existing, alternative methods of ventilatory support. Comparisons should be made using comparable levels of support and equipment that are likely to maximize the efficacy of a given technique. There are no reliable data to permit conclusions regarding the superiority of one support over another. Were the results of such controlled studies ever to become available, mechanical ventilatory support would be greatly simplified.

REFERENCES

1. Barach Al, Martin J, Eckman M: Postive pressure respiration and its application to the treatment of acute pulmonary edema. Ann Intern Med 12:754, 1938
2. Frumin MJ, Bergman NA, Holaday DA: Alveolar-arterial O_2 differences during artificial respiration in man. J Appl Physiol 14:694, 1959
3. Ashbaugh DG, Petty TL, Bigelow DB, et al: Continuous positive pressure breathing (CPPB) in adult respiratory distress syndrome. J Thorac Cardiovasc Surg 57:31, 1969
4. Gregory GA, Kitterman JA, Phibbs RH, et al: Treatment of idiopathic respiratory distress syndrome with continuous postive airway pressure. N Engl J Med 284:1333, 1971
5. Kirby RR, Robison EF, Schulz J, et al: A new pediatric volume ventilator. Anesth Analg 50:533, 1971
6. Downs JB, Klein EF, Desautels DA, et al: Intermittent mandatory ventilation: a new approach to weaning patients from mechanical ventilators. Chest 64:331, 1973
7. Sjöstrand U: High frequency positive pressure ventilation (HFPPV): a review. Crit Care Med 8:345, 1980
8. Hewlett AM, Platt AS, Terry G: Mandatory minute volume: a new concept in weaning from mechanical ventilation. Anaesthesia 32:163, 1977
9. Norlander O: New concepts of ventilation. Acta Anesth Belg 33:221, 1982
10. Downs JB, Stock MC: Airway pressure release ventilation: a new concept in ventilatory support. Crit Care Med 15:459, 1987
11. Mushin WW, Rendell-Baker L, Thompson PW: Automatic Ventilation of the Lungs. Blackwell Scientific Publications, Oxford, 1959, p. 1980
12. Räsänen J: Conventional and high frequency controlled mechanical ventilation in patients with left ventricular dysfunction and pulmonary edema. Chest 91:225, 1987
13. Kilburn KH: Shock, seizures, and coma with alkalosis during mechanical ventilation. Ann Intern Med 65:977, 1966
14. Culpepper JA, Rinaldo JE, Rogers RM: Effect of mechanical ventilator mode on tendency towards respiratory alkalosis. Am Rev Respir Dis 132:1075, 1985
15. Hudson LD, Hurlow RS, Craig KC, et al: Does intermittent mandatory ventilation correct respiratory alkalosis in patients receiving assisted mechanical ventilation? Am Rev Respir Dis 132:1071, 1985
16. Froese AB, Bryan AC: Effects of anesthesia and paralysis on diaphragmatic mechanics in man. Anesthesiology 41:242, 1974
17. Douglas ME, Downs JB: Cardiopulmonary effects of intermittent mandatory ventilation. Int Anesthesiol Clin 18:97, 1980
18. Wolff G, Brunner JX, Gradel E: Gas exchange during mechanical ventilation and spontaneous breathing. Intermittent mandatory ventilation after open heart surgery. Chest 90:11, 1986
19. Pontoppidan H, Geffin B, Lowenstein E: Acute respiratory failure in the adult. N Engl J Med 287:743, 1972
20. Aubier M, Trippenbach T, Roussos C: Respiratory muscle fatigue during cardiogenic shock. J Appl Physiol 51:499, 1981
21. Cournand A, Motley HL, Werkö L, et al: Physiologic studies of the effects of intermittent positive pressure ventilation on cardiac output in man. Am J Physiol 152:162, 1948
22. Kirby RR, Downs JB, Civetta JM, et al: High level positive end-expiratory pressure (PEEP) in acute respiratory insufficiency. Chest 67:156, 1975
23. Räsänen J, Heikkilä J, Downs JB, et al: Continuous positive airway pressure by face mask in the treatment of cardiogenic pulmonary edema. Am J Cardiol 55:296, 1985
24. Räsänen J, Nikki P, Heikkilä J: Acute myocardial infarction complicated by respiratory failure: the effects of mechanical ventilation. Chest 85:21, 1984
25. Räsänen J, Downs JB, Stock MC: Cardiovascu-

lar effects of conventional positive pressure ventilation and airway pressure release ventilation. Chest 93:911, 1988
26. Peterson GW, Baier H: Incidence of pulmonary barotrauma in medical ICU. Crit Care Med 11:67, 1983
27. Mathru M, Rao TL, Venus B: Ventilator-induced barotrauma in controlled mechanical ventilation versus intermittent mandatory ventilation. Crit Care Med 11:359, 1983
28. Bartlett RH, Tomasian JM, Roloff DW, et al: Extracorporeal membrane oxygenation (ECMO) in neonatal respiratory failure: 100 cases. Ann Surg 204:236, 1986
29. Downs JB, Douglas ME: Intermittent mandatory ventilation: why the controversy? Crit Care Med 9:622, 1981
30. Petty TL: IMV vs. IMC. Chest 67:630, 1975
31. Weisman IM, Rinaldo JE, Rogers MH: Intermittent mandatory ventilation. Am Rev Respir 127:641, 1983
32. Hasten RW, Downs JB, Heenen TJ: A comparison of synchronized and nonsynchronized intermittent mandatory ventilation. Respir Care 25:554, 1980
33. Heenan TJ, Downs JB, Douglas ME, et al: Intermittent mandatory ventilation: is synchronization important? Chest 77:598, 1980
34. Boyer F, Jay S, Gaussorgues P, et al: A new approach to mandatory ventilation: Pressure support mandatory minute frequency (abstract). Intensive Care Med 14:262, 1988
35. Mecklenburgh JS, Latto IP, Al-Obaidi TAA, et al: Excessive work of breathing during intermittent mandatory ventilation. Br J Anaesth 58:1048, 1986
36. Pinsky MR, Summer WR, Wise RA, et al: Augmentation of cardiac function by elevation of intrathoracic pressure. J Appl Physiol 54:950, 1983
37. Curran FJ: Night ventilation by body respirators for patients in chronic respiratory failure due to late stage Duchenne. Arch Phys Med Rehabil 62:270, 1981
38. Braun SR, Sufit RL, Giovannoni R, et al: Intermittent negative pressure ventilation in the treatment of respiratory failure in progressive neuromuscular disease. Neurology (NY) 37:1874, 1987
39. Cropp A, DiMarco AF: Effects of intermittent negative pressure ventilation on respiratory muscle function in patients with severe chronic obstructive pulmonary disease. Am Rev Respir Dis 135:1056, 1987
40. Splaingard ML, Frates RC, Jefferson LS, et al: Home negative pressure ventilation: report of 20 years of experience in patients with neuromuscular disease. Arch Phys Med Rehabil 66:239, 1985
41. Simonds AK, Sawicka EH, Carroll N, et al: Use of negative pressure ventilation to facilitate the return of spontaneous ventilation. Anaesthesia 43:216, 1988
42. Chercik V, Vidyasagar D: Continuous negative chest wall pressure in hyaline membrane disease: one year experience. Pediatrics 49:753, 1972
43. Sanyal SK, Mitchell C, Hughes WT, et al: Continuous negative chest-wall pressure as therapy for severe respiratory distress in older children. Chest 68:43, 1975
44. Morris AH, Elliott CG: Adult respiratory distress syndrome: successful support with continuous negative extrathoracic pressure. Crit Care Med 13:989, 1985
45. Al-Saady N, Bennett ED: Decelerating inspiratory flow waveform improves lung mechanics and gas exchange in patients on intermittent positive pressure ventilation. Intensive Care Med 11:68, 1985
46. Kirby RR: Mechanical ventilation in acute ventilatory failure: Facts, fiction, and fallacies. Curr Probl Anesth Crit Care 1 (3):1, 1977
47. deLemos RA, McLaughlin GW, Diserens HW, et al: Assisted ventilation in the treatment of hyaline membrane disease: the use of CPAP with or without assisted ventilation utilizing a single ventilator system (abstract). Pediatr Res 6:406, 1972
48. Shapiro BA, Harrison RA, Walton JR: Intermittent demand ventilation (IDV): a new technique for support of ventilation in critically ill patients. Respir Care 21:521, 1976
49. Downs JB, Block AJ, Vennum KB: Intermittent mandatory ventilation in the treatment of patients with chronic obstructive pulmonary disease. Anesth Analg 53:437, 1974
50. Downs JB, Perkins HM, Modell JH: Intermittent mandatory ventilation. Arch Surg 109:519, 1974
51. Downs JB, Mitchell LA: Pulmonary effects of ventilatory pattern following cardiopulmonary bypass. Crit Care Med 4:295, 1976
52. Prakash O, Meij S: Oxygen consumption and blood gas exchange during controlled and inter-

mittent mandatory ventilation after cardiac surgery. Crit Care Med 13:556, 1985
53. Laaban JP, Lemaire F, Baron JF, et al: Influence of caloric intake on the respiratory mode during mandatory minute ventilation. Chest 87:67, 1985
54. Venus B, Smith R, Mathru M: National survey of methods and criteria used for weaning from mechanical ventilation. Crit Care Med 15:530, 1987
55. Higgs BD, Bevan JC: Use of mandatory minute volume ventilation in the perioperative management of a patient with myasthenia. Br J Anaesth 51:1181, 1979
56. Lamy M: Techniques of ventilatory therapy in the adult respiratory distress syndrome (ARDS). Acta Anesth Belg 33:243, 1982
57. Boros SJ, Matalon SV, Ewald R, et al: The effect of independent variations in inspiratory:expiratory ratio and end-expiratory pressure during mechanical ventilation in hyaline membrane disease: the significance of mean airway pressure. J Pediatr 91:794, 1977
58. Boros SJ: Variations in inspiratory:expiratory ratio and airway pressure waveform during mechanical ventilation: the significance of mean airway pressure. J Pediatr 94:114, 1979
59. Berman LS, Downs JB, VanEeden A, et al: Inspiration:expiration ratio: is mean airway pressure the difference? Crit Care Med 9:775, 1981
60. Gattinoni L, Marcolin R, Caspani ML, et al: Constant mean airway pressure with different patterns of positive pressure breathing during the adult respiratory distress syndrome. Clin Respir Physiol 27:273, 1983
61. Cole AG, Weller SF, Sykes MK: Inverse ratio ventilation compared with PEEP in adult respiratory failure. Intensive Care Med 10:227, 1984
62. Gurevitch MJ, VanDyke J, Young ES, et al: Improved oxygenation and lower peak airway pressure in severe adult respiratory distress syndrome. Treatment with inverse ratio ventilation. Chest 89:211, 1986
63. Tharratt RS, Allen RP, Albertson TE: Pressure controlled inverse ratio ventilation in severe adult respiratory distress syndrome. Chest 94:755, 1988
64. Stock MC, Downs JB, Frolicher DA: Airway pressure release ventilation. Crit Care Med 15:462, 1987
65. Garner W, Downs JB, Stock MC, et al: Airway pressure release ventilation (APRV). Chest 94:779, 1988
66. Marini JJ, Capps JS, Culver BH: The inspiratory work of breathing during assisted mechanical ventilation. Chest 87:612, 1985
67. Marini JJ, Rodriguez RM, Lamb V: Bedside estimation of the inspiratory work of breathing during mechanical ventilation. Chest 89:56, 1986
68. Downs JB, Douglas ME, Ruiz BC, et al: Comparison of assisted and controlled mechanical ventilation in anesthetized swine. Crit Care Med 7:5, 1979
69. Groeger JS, Levinson MR, Carlon GC: Assist control versus synchronized intermittent mandatory ventilation during acute respiratory failure. Crit Care Med 17:607, 1989
70. Banner MJ, Kirby RR: Similarities between pressure support ventilation and intermittent positive-pressure ventilation. Crit Care Med 13:997, 1985
71. Halpern P, Downs JB, Räsänen J: Hemodynamic effects of airway pressure release ventilation and positive pressure ventilation in hypovolemic dogs (abstract). Crit Care Med 16:452, 1988
72. Jousela IT, Nikki P, Tahvanainen J: Airway pressure release ventilation by mask. Crit Care Med 16:1250, 1988
73. Brunner EA: Current Problems in Anesthesia and Critical Care Medicine. Year Book Medical Publishers, Chicago, 1977
74. Eross B, Powner D, Grenvik A: Common ventilatory modes: terminology. In Kirby RR, Graybar GB (eds): Intermittent mandatory ventilation. Int Anesthesiol Clin 18(2):18, 1980
75. Graybar GB, Smith RA: Apparatus and techniques for mandatory ventilation. In Kirby RR, Graybar GB (eds): Intermittent mandatory ventilation. Int Anesthesiol Clin 18(2):73, 1980

7

Neonatal and Pediatric Ventilatory Support

Donald Null
Lawrence S. Berman
Reese Clark

NEONATAL VENTILATORY SUPPORT

Neonatal Respiratory Function

The physiology of respiration in the neonate has a direct bearing on the frequent requirement for assistance of ventilation in this group of patients. Respiratory failure continues to be the leading cause of morbidity and mortality in neonates.

Respiratory Control

Respiratory control mechanisms in the newborn are significantly different from those of the adult,[1] placing the newborn at a much higher risk of the development of respiratory failure. The preterm infant is at an even higher risk. Periodic breathing and short periods of apnea are very common in newborn infants, especially when they are preterm. These episodes predominate during sleep and may be associated with bradycardia and hypoxia.[2,3] It is not unusual for preterm infants to require frequent stimulation to resume spontaneous breathing. The severity of these episodes may be such as to warrant intervention with medications such as theophylline or caffeine, frequent external stimuli such as oscillating beds or bumper beds, nasal continuous positive airway pressure, or tracheal intubation with or without assisted ventilation. As many as 50 percent of preterm infants have apnea severe enough to require intervention.[2]

Premature infants have a demonstrated reduction in ventilatory response to carbon dioxide.[4,5] In addition, hypoxia appears to "flatten" the response to carbon dioxide, which is exactly opposite of the adult response.[6] A major difference between newborns and children or adults is their response to hypoxia.[7] More immature infants are less responsive to hypoxia. Term infants manifest a brief period of respiratory stimulation followed by apnea. The very-low-birthweight infant may respond solely with apnea. Therefore, a newborn, whether term or premature, who presents with apnea and/or periodic breathing, must be adequately evaluated for hypoxia. An arterial blood gas (ABG) measurement for immediate assessment, followed by pulse oximetry or transcutaneous oxygen monitoring for a longer period of assessment, are essential. Visual inspection of the newborn to ascertain the presence of hypoxia is not only useless, but also dangerous. Unlike the adult or child, the newborn with fetal hemoglobin generally does not appear cyanotic until the PaO_2 is less than 40 mmHg.

Mechanics of Breathing

A major disadvantage, particularly in premature infants, is the lack of chest wall rigidity, which results in a high chest wall compliance.[8] Premature infants are therefore at a mechanical disadvantage when they attempt to breathe. This problem is particularly accentuated when they have poor lung compliance due to hyaline membrane disease, congestive heart failure, or pneumonia. The latter entities necessitate generation of a high negative (subambient) intrathoracic pressure to move air into the lungs. In premature infants, inward collapse of the chest wall occurs, resulting in paradoxical motion of the chest wall and abdomen with associated intercostal and substernal retractions.

The airways of preterm infants are often functionally malacic. This lack of rigidity results in some areas of atelectasis and others of overinflation, leading to abnormal ventilation/perfusion ($\dot{V}/\dot{Q}$) relationships. The problem is severe enough in some infants to require positive-pressure ventilation. Airway resistance is high due to the extremely small airway diameters, and airway obstruction is a frequent complicating factor.[9] Finally, diaphragmatic muscle fatigue is felt to contribute to respiratory failure in both term and preterm infants. The exact etiology of this entity is unclear. It was originally believed to be due to a decreased number of type I muscle fibers.[10,11] Recent studies, however, have not confirmed this deficiency,[12] and its existence has been questioned.

Ventilatory Support

Selection of the proper management of the infant with respiratory failure is complicated by the various modalities of intervention available. It is made even more difficult because the definition of respiratory failure and the need for intervention are not precise. A single criterion of respiratory failure does not exist. One needs to look at multiple factors and the overall clinical course of the patient before making a decision to intervene.

The normal PaO_2 for a term infant should be 75 mmHg or higher and 65 mmHg or higher for a preterm infant during room air breathing.[13] The $PaCO_2$ should be less than 50 mmHg for the preterm and less than 40 mmHg at term.[14] A term infant might well require intervention if the previous $PaCO_2$ was 30 to 40 mmHg but has risen over the past 2 hours to 45 mmHg. Conversely, a term infant whose $PaCO_2$ is 45 mmHg but whose previous $PaCO_2$ was 48 to 50 mmHg can be observed safely for an additional period of time.

The chest radiograph provides important information in ascertaining the need for respiratory support. One should consider early intervention if poor inflation with a ground-glass appearance is present. Disease processes that are likely to worsen, for example hyaline membrane disease, require early intervention, whereas those that are not, such as transient tachypnea (wet lung disease), can be observed for a longer period of time. The overall goals of ventilatory support are to improve gas exchange, lung inflation, and $\dot{V}/\dot{Q}$ matching, and to decrease high inspired oxygen, work of breathing, and morbidity/mortality.

Continuous Positive Airway Pressure

Continuous positive airway pressure (CPAP) can be delivered to spontaneously breathing infants by nasal prongs, an endotracheal tube in the nasopharynx, or tracheal intubation. It is most useful in diffuse alveolar disease that is associated with deflation instability, low compliance, and loss of functional residual capacity (FRC). In order to use CPAP effectively, one must be cognizant of its benefits and risks (Table 7-1). First, CPAP does not recruit collapsed alveoli but rather assists in preventing collapse of alveoli that already have been recruited. The maintenance of recruited alveolar inflation leads

Table 7-1. Effects of CPAP

Potentially beneficial
Increased FRC
Reduced right-to-left intrapulmonary shunt
Improved PaO_2
Decreased work of breathing
Potentially detrimental
Increased $PaCO_2$ until FRC increases
If overdistention occurs:
Decreased compliance
Increased work of breathing
Increased pulmonary artery pressure
Increased right-to-left cardiac shunt (foramen ovale, PDA)
Increased barotrauma

FRC, functional residual capacity; PDA, patent ductus arteriosus.

to an overall increase in FRC. Second, the initial response to CPAP is to raise the $PaCO_2$ until the FRC is increased to normal. Third, CPAP may increase the work of breathing. Fourth, excessive CPAP results in alveolar overdistention, decreased compliance, increased work of breathing, pneumothorax, increased pulmonary artery pressure, and increased right-to-left shunt.[15]

For CPAP to be effective, it must be used early in the course of lung disease. Once diffuse atelectasis has developed with high $PaCO_2$ values, CPAP will only lead to further respiratory failure. Early use in lung diseases associated with low compliance enables the FRC to be restored as more alveoli are recruited by spontaneous or positive pressure breaths. It is most effective in babies weighing more than 1,200 g, since they generally have adequate respiratory effort to recruit collapsed alveoli.[16] However, CPAP is reportedly effective as well for very-low-birthweight infants (less than 1,250 g), if applied at birth, before alveolar collapse has occurred.[17]

The level chosen is that which prevents alveolar collapse without adversely affecting cardiac output or overdistending the lung. Generally, 4 to 8 cm H_2O for small premature infants and 6 to 12 cm H_2O for term infants suffices. The effect can be measured by improved blood-gas values, chest radiographs, and blood pressure. It can be used effectively following extubation to stabilize the upper airway until the edema secondary to endotracheal tube placement resolves. CPAP may also act to offset malacia.[18] This technique appears to be underused. Lack of success probably is related to late application and too little or too much pressure, rather than failure of CPAP, per se.

Conventional Mechanical Ventilation

Intermittent Mandatory Ventilation

Intermittent mandatory ventilation (IMV) is one of the most commonly employed methods of assisted ventilation used in the management of neonates with respiratory failure.[19] Time-cycled, pressure-limited, continuous-flow ventilators are almost always used (Fig. 7-1). They are relatively inexpensive and easy to adjust compared with their volume-regulated counterparts (see Figs. 15-69 to 15-74, Ch. 15). During IMV, several specific changes in ventilator parameters will improve gas exchange. When such changes are made, they should be directed toward accomplishment of specific therapeutic goals (Table 7-2). The risk of the change must be weighed against potential benefits. The most important variables are listed in Table 7-3.[20]

Positive Inspiratory Pressure. Positive-pressure breaths are used to recruit collapsed alveoli, decrease work of breathing, and improve ventilation. In the premature infant, and to a lesser degree in the term infant, the chest wall is very compliant. During spontaneous breathing, tidal volume is often inadequate. The newborn compensates by increasing respiratory frequency. If minute ventilation (tidal volume − dead space volume × rate) is maintained, hypercarbia does not develop. When fatigue occurs and the infant is no longer able to compensate, hypercarbia and respiratory acidosis develop. Intermittent positive-pressure breaths assist the infant's spontaneous ventilation, and also serve to recruit alveoli that have

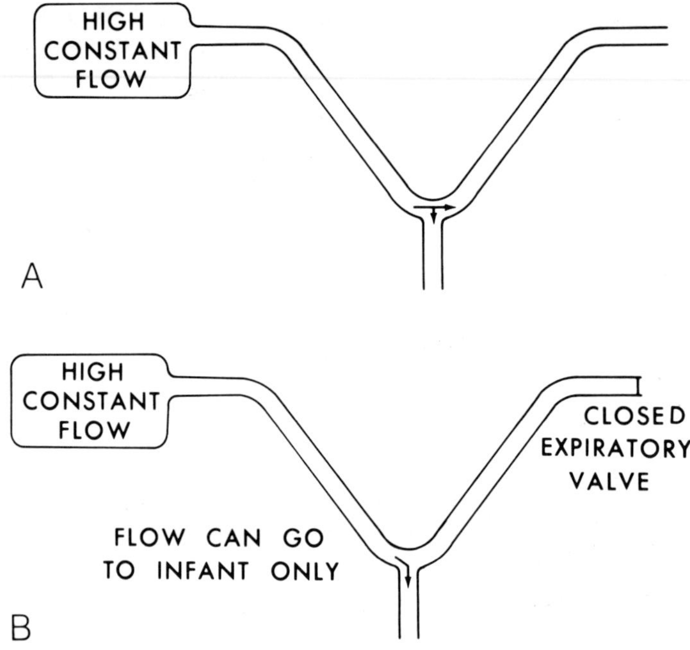

Fig. 7-1. Basic operation of a time-cycled, pressure-limited, continuous-flow infant ventilator. **(A)** A high flow of gas, generally 2 to 3 times the preselected minute ventilation, passes continuously through the circuit. The infant can breathe spontaneously using this flow. **(B)** A timing mechanism periodically closes the exhalation valve at a preselected frequency. When the valve is closed, the continuous gas flow is diverted into the infant's lungs, creating positive-pressure inflation. The combination of spontaneous and mechanical breaths is IMV. (See also Fig. 7-3.)

collapsed during expiration. When used with positive end-expiratory pressure (PEEP), these positive-pressure breaths increase the mean airway pressure applied to the lung and often result in improved lung inflation, decreased $\dot{V}/\dot{Q}$ mismatch, and improved oxygenation.[21] As collapsed alveoli are recruited, lung compliance improves, and efficiency of ventilation increases.

The negative effects of positive-pressure breaths are similar to and often worse than those of PEEP and CPAP. As no lung disease is entirely homogeneous, some airway and alveoli units are affected more than others. The less abnormal, hence more compliant, segments of the lung are at risk of overdistention and rupture. The association between the use of high positive inspiratory pressure and air leak syndromes is well known[22,23]; therefore, caution must be used in determining the optimal peak inspiratory pressure (PIP). As PIP is increased, mean airway pressure and mean lung volume increase. If the lung is overinflated, venous return to the heart is often decreased, pulmonary vascular resistance is increased, and cardiac output is impaired.

Table 7-2. Goals of Mechanical Ventilation in Neonatal Respiratory Failure

Alveolar recruitment
Increased CO_2 removal
Decreased work of breathing
Reduced exposure to high oxygen

Table 7-3. Variables of Importance in Ventilator Management

Peak inspiratory pressure (PIP)
Ventilator rate
Duration of positive pressure (I:E ratio)
Gas-flow rate
Postive end-expiratory pressure (PEEP)

Ventilator Rate. Adjustments in ventilator rate are directed at improving ventilation and decreasing work of breathing. The effect of increasing ventilator rate while holding tidal volume constant is to improve alveolar ventilation. The airway pressures and the ventilator inspiratory-to-expiratory (I:E) ratio are not changed.

Increases in ventilator rate also result in an increase of mean airway pressure and usually improve oxygenation. Compared with slow rate (20 to 40/minute) and long inspiratory time (at least 1 second) ventilation, rapid rate (50 to 60/minute) and short inspiratory time (0.5 second) ventilation reduces the incidence of pneumothorax.[24] However, the precise role of rapid rates in reducing the incidence of air leak is confounded by the shortened inspiratory time. A retrospective study[25] of factors associated with air leak suggested that the only component of positive-pressure ventilation which correlated with air leak was the inspiratory time. In that study, however, all infants were managed with relatively slow rates (~30 breaths/min) and long inspiratory time (0.9 to 1.5 seconds). The optimal ventilator rate is yet to be defined and certainly is disease-state and patient specific.

The principal adverse effects of rapid rate ventilation are gas trapping and the development of inadvertent (occult) PEEP[26] (Fig. 7-2). Lung emptying is dependent on respiratory compliance and impedance. The time constant (see Ch. 4) of the respiratory system during positive-pressure ventilation at rates of less than 100/min is defined as the respiratory compliance × airway resistance. Ninety-five percent lung emptying occurs after three time constants have elapsed. If the period of time allowed for expiration is less than four time constants, the gas delivered during inspiration will not be completely emptied before the next positive-pressure breath. When gas is trapped and expiratory volume increases, the lungs become overinflated, and lung compliance decreases. Eventually, the time constant of the lungs will decrease so that lung emptying occurs more rapidly and gas trapping decreases. However, the new equilibrium state is achieved only at the cost of an increased end-expiratory lung volume and the potential for baroinjury. In diseases with high airway resistance, air trapping is more of a problem than in those with reduced lung compliance. Gas trapping often can be reduced by increasing the expiratory time and reducing the I:E ratio.[27]

Another important but often unrecognized problem of high ventilator rates (more than 60 breaths/min) is loss of ventilator-delivered tidal volume despite maintenance of PIP. Boros et al.[28] showed that minute ventilation with some pressure-limited ventilators reaches a plateau

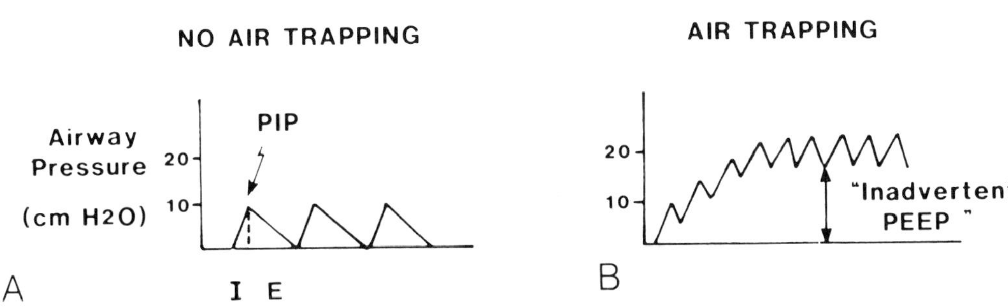

Fig. 7-2. Air trapping may result with insufficient expiratory time. **(A)** An I:E ratio of approximately 1:2.5 allows complete exhalation of gas before the subsequent ventilator cycle. **(B)** An increased rate and decreased I:E ratio to approximately 1:1 causes a retention of gas, overexpansion of the lungs, and an increase of inadvertent (occult) PEEP. This pressure occurs within the lungs and is not measured in the ventilator circuit. (From Banner,[157] with permission.)

or decreases at rates higher than 75/min and an I:E ratio of 1:2 as a result of decreased tidal volume delivery.

Inspiratory:Expiratory Ratios. The primary effects of an increased I:E ratio are increased airway pressure and improved oxygenation. So-called reverse I:E ratios to improve oxygenation have not been shown to reduce morbidity and mortality.[25] Increasing the inspiratory time of a pressure-limited, continuous flow ventilator will increase tidal volume delivery. Ventilation may improve if the expiratory time is adequate. However, this improvement is often insignificant.

The negative effects of long inspiratory times and high I:E ratios are caused by gas trapping similar to that which occurs with high ventilator rates. A high I:E ratio in patients with increased airway resistance predisposes to overinflation of the lungs and air leak.

Gas Flow. The primary effects of increased gas flow when a pressure-limited ventilator is used are to change the contour of the positive-pressure breath and to reduce the work of spontaneous breathing between sequential positive-pressure breaths. Increasing gas flow renders the contour less sinusoidal and more square[29] (see Ch. 15). This resulting increase in mean airway pressure may improve oxygenation. A sharp upstroke (square wave), however, also may increase turbulence, leading to decreased tidal volume delivery, worsened ventilation and oxygenation, and possible airway injury.

Between positive-pressure breaths, gas flow allows unencumbered spontaneous breathing. Such breathing negates some of the adverse circulatory effects of positive-pressure mechanical ventilation and is a major advantage of IMV (Fig. 7-3). However, if gas flow is inadequate, the infant must generate a larger negative intrathoracic pressure to achieve satisfactory tidal volume. An increased flow at a fixed end-expiratory pressure reduces the negative pressure required for spontaneous inspiration, and the work of breathing is decreased, as long as a threshold resistor PEEP/CPAP valve is used (see Ch. 15).

Controlled Positive-Pressure Ventilation

The use of controlled ventilation in the neonate is limited to paralyzed infants who, most often, have failed a trial of IMV. The most common indication for controlled ventilation is asynchronous breathing by the patient who thus "fights" the ventilator.[19] Perlman et al.[30] showed that paralysis with pancuronium and controlled positive-pressure ventilation was associated with a lower incidence of intraventricular hemorrhage (IVH) than occurred in preterm infants who breathed asynchronously with the ventilator and had fluctuating cerebral blood flow velocities.

Bancalari et al.[31] however, found that paralysis and controlled ventilation led to an increased incidence of IVH. Their assumption was that controlled ventilation led to a persistent elevation in venous pressure, increasing the risk of IVH, whereas IMV led to the facilitation of venous return and a decrease in venous pressure, thereby reducing the risk of IVH. In reality, both observations are probably correct, as Perlman was dealing with patients who were actively fighting the ventilator; this was not the case in Bancalari's study.

In term infants with asynchronous breathing, the risk of air leak is increased. Some investigators have suggested that paralysis results in improved gas exchange and reduces this risk.[32] However, controlled data demonstrating the effectiveness of this therapy is lacking. Recent studies have shown that paralysis reduces lung compliance and may even decrease the efficiency of gas exchange.[33] The most significant negative aspect of controlled ventilation is the loss of the patient's contribution to gas exchange. Invariably, the amount of ventilator support required is greater for controlled ventilation as compared with IMV.

Patient-Triggered (Assisted) Positive-Pressure Ventilation

Attempts at patient-triggered ventilation in neonates have been relatively unsuccessful. In large measure, the problem is due to the insensi-

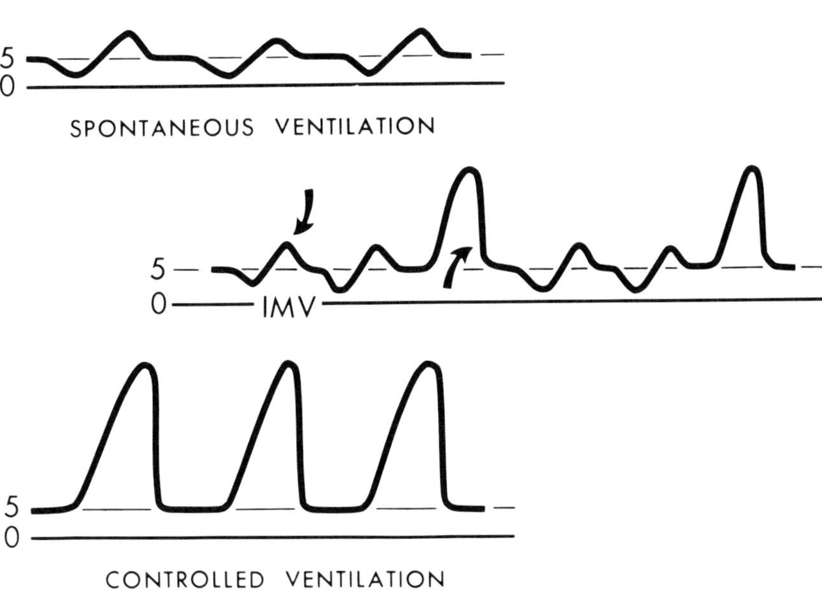

Fig. 7-3. IMV tends to offset the adverse circulatory effects of positive-pressure ventilation. Note that IMV has fewer high-pressure mechanical breaths than does controlled ventilation. In addition, the decrease in pressure associated with the spontaneous breaths augments venous return.

tivity of the trigger mechanism to detect the patient's inspiratory effort. If it is made too sensitive to offset this problem, body movements are often "confused" with breaths, and autocycling may occur. However, recent studies using esophageal pressure changes to cycle the ventilator suggest that this strategy improves oxygenationn and can be used in small prematures.[34] The exact role such technology will play in newborn ventilation is unclear.

Positive End-Expiratory Pressure

Most of the disease states causing acute respiratory failure in the neonate are associated with surfactant deficiency or dysfunction (e.g., hyaline membrane disease, meconium aspiration syndrome, and pneumonia). PEEP is used to prevent loss of FRC in conditions characterized by low lung compliance. In the absence of adequate surfactant amount or function, the neonate is unable to maintain alveoli open at the end of expiration. Progressive alveolar collapse develops, with increased $\dot{V}/\dot{Q}$ mismatch, decreased lung compliance, hypoxemia, and hypercarbia. When PEEP is employed with IMV, it serves to maintain open airway units recruited during the positive-pressure breaths, thereby reducing $\dot{V}/\dot{Q}$ mismatching and improving oxygenation.[35,36]

Problems associated with PEEP are related to the transmission of pressure to the pleural space, the right atrium, and the pulmonary arterioles. As PEEP is increased, FRC is increased, and more pressure is transmitted to the pleural space. The transmitted pressure can increase pulmonary vascular resistance and reduce venous return to the right atrium, causing diminished cardiac output and thereby compromised oxygen delivery.[15] If PEEP is too high, it may also be associated with overdistention of the alveoli and terminal airways, resulting in baroinjury of these structures. In addition, increasing

PEEP with a time-cycled, pressure-limited ventilator narrows the pressure amplitude delivered to the lung. If lung compliance remains constant, the delivered tidal volume will be reduced and ventilation will be decreased.

High-Frequency Ventilation

High-frequency ventilation (HFV) was introduced during the 1960s and 1970s by a number of investigators, including Sjöstrand,[37] Lunkenheimer et al.,[38] and Bohn et al.[39] By the early 1980s, a variety of types of high-frequency ventilators were being evaluated under experimental clinical protocols as alternatives to conventional ventilators for newborns with severe pulmonary problems. The theoretical aspects of HFV and how it works are well discussed in numerous other books and articles.[40–44] We focus on the different types of high-frequency ventilators and on the disease states in which they appear to be useful. At this writing, all high-frequency devices are still used under investigational protocols; however, we expect that by the early 1990s most, if not all, high-frequency devices will be licensed for general use in specific settings.

The definition of HFV is somewhat arbitrary but should be considered as ventilation occurring at frequencies at least twice the physiologic rate and with volumes that are near, equal to, or less than the anatomic dead space. Although many people consider HFV to be less tidal volume dependent than convention ventilation, such a perception is wrong. While HFV employs very small tidal volumes, it is more volume dependent than is conventional support, since ventilation is related approximately to the product of frequency and tidal volume squared. Additionally, increasing frequency limits the maximal tidal volume that can be delivered by most high-frequency ventilators.

Gas exchange during HFV is related to enhanced gas dispersion, increased turbulent flow, and augmented diffusion. For HFV to be effective, the airways need to be open, since pressure changes are significantly less than with conventional techniques. Thus, HFV is not an effective airway dilator. Three techniques of HFV commonly are described.

High-Frequency Positive-Pressure Ventilation

High-frequency positive-pressure ventilation (HFPPV) is achieved with conventional ventilators or specially designed, low compliance systems that deliver small volumes at rapid rates. These techniques are currently in use with most of the common newborn ventilators, at rates of 60 to 150 breaths/min. The major problem with such ventilators is that they are not specifically made to operate at these high rates. As a result, gas may become trapped within the lung, causing inadvertent PEEP, with resultant pulmonary hypertension, a fall in lung compliance, increased risk of air leak, and decreased cardiac output (Fig. 7-2).

Sjöstrand and co-workers developed specialized devices to avoid these problems and showed them to be useful in patients with hyaline membrane disease (HMD).[45]

High-Frequency Jet Ventilation and High-Frequency Flow Interruption

High-frequency jet ventilation (HFJV) and high-frequency flow interruption (HFFI) use ventilators that deliver gas from a pressurized source interrupted periodically by either pneumatic or electronic valves to produce a pulsatile flow. Volume is regulated by the duration of valve opening, the size of the valve orifices, and the gas source pressure. In jet ventilation, gas is delivered through a small catheter in a triple-lumen endotracheal tube directly into the trachea (Fig. 7-4). Flow interrupters deliver gas some distance from the airway and, in general, are connected to the endotracheal tube as are most standard ventilators.

The Bunnell jet ventilator has been used most

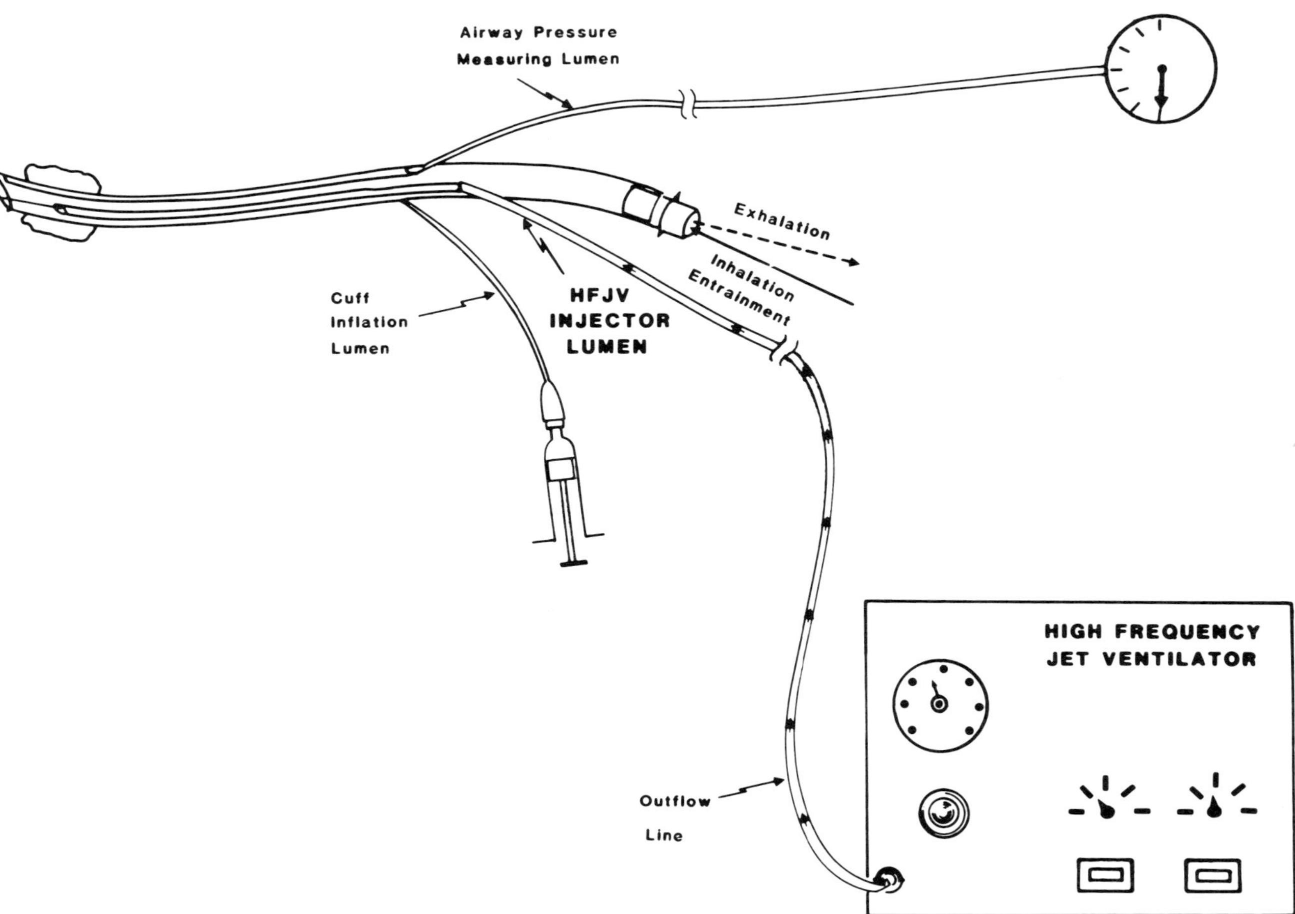

Fig. 7-4. Schematic depiction of a high-frequency jet ventilator. A high-pressure source gas passes intermittently through a rapidly opening/closing solenoid valve into an injector lumen. Additional gas (room air or a controlled FIO_2) is entrained (Bernoulli effect) to augment tidal volume. (From Banner & Smith,[158] with permission.)

frequently in neonatal ventilation. It appears to be most effective in pulmonary interstitial emphysema (PIE) and air leak syndromes.[46] Although its use has been limited in newborns with HMD, it appears to be as safe as conventional ventilators and is effective in maintaining adequate gas exchange at lower mean airway pressures.[47] To date, it has not proved useful in term infants with severe lung disease who fail conventional ventilation, and minimal success has been achieved in the management of diaphragmatic hernia.

The most important technical problem with HFJV is achieving adequate humidification. Even with adequate humidification, HFJV produces more acute tracheal inflammation and is associated with increased airway mucus.[48] Difficulty in ascertaining real airway pressure changes, critical positioning of the jet cannula within the airways, major airway or lung injury if obstruction to gas outflow occurs, and the fact that exhalation occurs passively (increasing the risk of air trapping and occult PEEP)[49] are other problems still needing resolution.

Flow interrupters, of which the Bird VDR and Infrasonics Infant Star are the two major examples, do not require any other special tubing or connectors. Their design results in less pressure dropoff and delivery of larger tidal volumes to the distal airways when compared to high frequency oscillatory ventilation. They are capable of both conventional and high-frequency modes, individually or in combination, and appear to be useful in the management of patients with air leak syndromes and possibly hyaline membrane disease.[50] Gas egress is generally passive, although some negative pressure is created in the airways that facilitates gas removal during exhalation. Because of its larger tidal volume capability, the Bird VDR appears to be a more effective device for larger neonates and young children. Because it is capable of higher pressure, it is more effective when airway plugging or blockage is present. The Infant Star does not generate a large enough tidal volume when used as a high frequency device to be effective in treating term or near-term infants with severe lung disease.

High-Frequency Oscillatory Ventilation

High-frequency oscillatory ventilation (HFOV) differs from all other types of high-frequency ventilation in that the net flow of gas from the ventilator to the patient is zero; that is, a volume of gas is delivered on the instroke and an equal volume of gas is removed on the outstroke. A continuous-bias gas flow is required to eliminate CO_2 and to provide oxygen, and a low-pass filter is necessary for gas egress (Fig. 7-5). The bias flow rate and the restriction of the bias flow egress with the low-pass filter determine the mean airway pressure in the system. Ventilatory amplitude is determined by the piston stroke or diaphragm movement. In general, patient oxygenation is determined by mean airway pressure and FIO_2, and ventilation is dependent on the stroke amplitude and frequency.

The Hummingbird (Senko Medical Instrument Mfg. Co., Ltd., Japan) and the high frequency oscillator manufactured by Sensor Medics Corporation have been used most extensively in newborn ventilation. The limitation of the oscillator is related to the volume that it is capable of delivering, the size of the patient, and the lung compliance. Oscillators in general are capable of rates that are significantly higher than other high-frequency ventilators.[41] In part, this capability results from the active exhalation phase, which minimizes gas trapping.[49]

A wider group of disease states have been treated with HFOV than with other forms of HFV. It has been evaluated extensively in the management of premature baboons with HMD and, if applied early, dramatically attenuates the disease course.[51] It has also been shown to be effective when used as a rescue technique in animals treated initially with conventional ventilation.[52]

During the past 4 years, we have offered HFOV as a rescue technique in the treatment of 242 infants with severe respiratory failure and in a controlled trial in patients with HMD. Most rescue patients (70 percent) have been referred from other level 3 nurseries for manage-

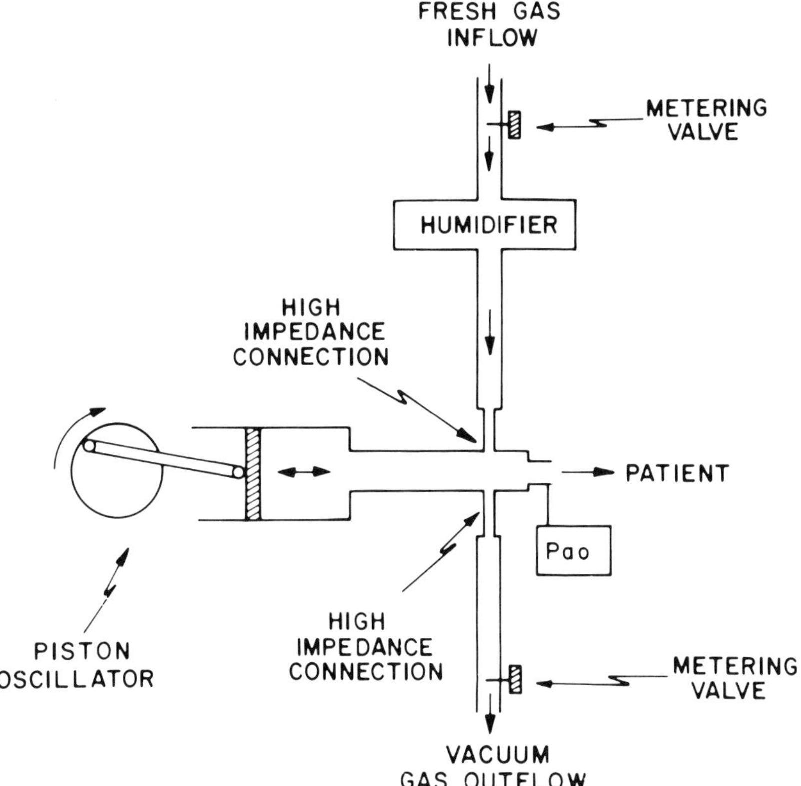

Fig. 7-5. High-frequency oscillator. In this example, a piston moves rapidly back and forth, alternately compressing and decompressing the gas column between it and the patient. The net result of such movement is zero gas delivery. However, an additional continuous gas inflow (bias flow) enters the circuit through a humidifier. When the piston moves forward (toward patient), this gas is delivered into the airway. Excess gas inflow is vented through the outflow metering valve (low-pass filter). Airway pressure and tidal volume are regulated by the balance between gas inflow and outflow. (From Banner,[157] with permission.)

ment of respiratory failure not responsive to maximal conventional modes of support. Survival in this population is 67 percent, with 51 percent of deaths occurring in infants weighing less than 1,000 g. In preterm infants, the most common diagnosis was persistent PIE. In term infants, diagnoses included meconium aspiration, pneumonia, and pulmonary hypoplasia caused by diaphragmatic hernia, oligohydramnios, and hydrops fetalis. This technique appears to be effective because it permits gradual inflation of the hypoplastic lung without associated lung injury. It also permits better oxygenation and ventilation than can be achieved with conventional management. Disease states that respond most dramatically to HFOV include HMD, pneumonia, air leak syndrome, shock lung, and pulmonary hypoplasia. The following report is illustrative of such a case:

> A 34-week gestational male infant was referred to us for extracorporeal membrane oxygenation (ECMO) therapy. He had been treated for more than 24 hours with 100 percent oxygen and high ventilator pressures at the referring hospital, but his condition had deteriorated. Upon arrival, PIP and PEEP were 55 cm H_2O and 6 cm H_2O, respectively. The ventilatory rate was 80 to 100/min and mean airway pressure was 20 cm H_2O. Arterial PO_2 was 40 to 50 mmHg (FIO_2 = 1.0), and $PaCO_2$ was 50 to

60 mmHg. A chest radiograph demonstrated diffuse alveolar infiltrates and poor inflation, even at these high pressures (Fig. 7-6A). The patient was treated with HFOV with a mean airway pressure of 22 cm H_2O. The first ABG measurement revealed a PaO_2 of 250 mmHg and a $PaCO_2$ of 38 mmHg. Within hours, the chest radiograph was improved markedly (Fig. 7-6B). Rapid weaning from HFOV was followed by tracheal extubation after 5 days of therapy.

We have found that approximately 50 percent of patients meeting ECMO criteria at our hospital can be rescued with HFOV without significant additional morbidity or mortality.[53,54] As HFOV is a much less invasive technique and lacks the long-term sequelae of right carotid artery ligation, we believe it should be offered to all patients before ECMO is initiated unless they are in cardiac failure.

The major problem with HFOV is related to the maintenance of cardiac output. Patients in a low output state do not tolerate this therapeutic approach.[55] Those whose disease is associated predominantly with airway problems also do not fare well, presumably because distal airway pressure changes are small during HFOV.

Although our experience with HFOV has been largely positive, a recent National Institutes of Health (NIH)-sponsored multi-institutional study presented less optimistic findings[56]; 327 infants treated with HFOV were compared with 346 infants treated with conventional mechanical ventilation. Mortality and the incidence of bronchopulmonary dysplasia (BPD) were the same in both groups. As compared with conventional ventilation, however, HFOV was associated with a higher incidence of pneumoperitoneum of pulmonary origin, grades 3 and 4 intracranial hemorrhage, and periventricular leukomalacia. In addition, more infants failed to respond to HFOV and had to be switched to conventional support than vice versa. The HIFI Study Group[56] concluded that HFOV, as used in their trial, offered no advantages over conventional support.

There are clear differences between our experience with HFOV and that reported by the NIH collaborative control trial. Many factors play a role in producing these differences. Not only is it difficult to compare different types of HFV, but it is difficult to compare similar types of HFOV that employ different strategies. Our ventilator has a variable I:E ratio, whereas the oscillator used in the NIH study has a fixed I:E ratio of 1:1. We generally use a 1:2 ratio. The 15-Hz and 1:1 I:E ratio in the NIH study potentially increases the risk of air trapping, air leak, and intravascular hemorrhage.

Patient selection also plays an important role in determining outcome. Most patients in the NIH study weighed less than 1,250 g. This group of patients has high morbidity and mortality, regardless of ventilator strategy; in our experience, they have a much less dramatic response to HFOV compared with children weighing more than 1,250 g. Finally, we have found that many patients with HMD require mean pressures of 15 to 20 cm H_2O. In the NIH trial, this characteristic could result in the patient failing HFOV, raising the question of whether crossover was balanced for the high-frequency and conventional treatment groups. If patients were crossed over to conventional support early, the study would be biased against HFOV.

While these concerns lead us to question the conclusions of this study, it nevertheless stands as the only controlled trial comparing HFOV and conventional support in the management of HMD.

Conclusions

When used properly, HFV appears to offer several potential advantages compared to conventional positive-pressure ventilation. These include decreased barotrauma, improved ventilation and oxygenation in specific disease states, and the maintenance of oxygenation and ventilation while decreasing air leaks. However, all types of HFV still require intensive investigation. While we believe these techniques are effective in the management of many respiratory conditions, the optimal strategies for the various

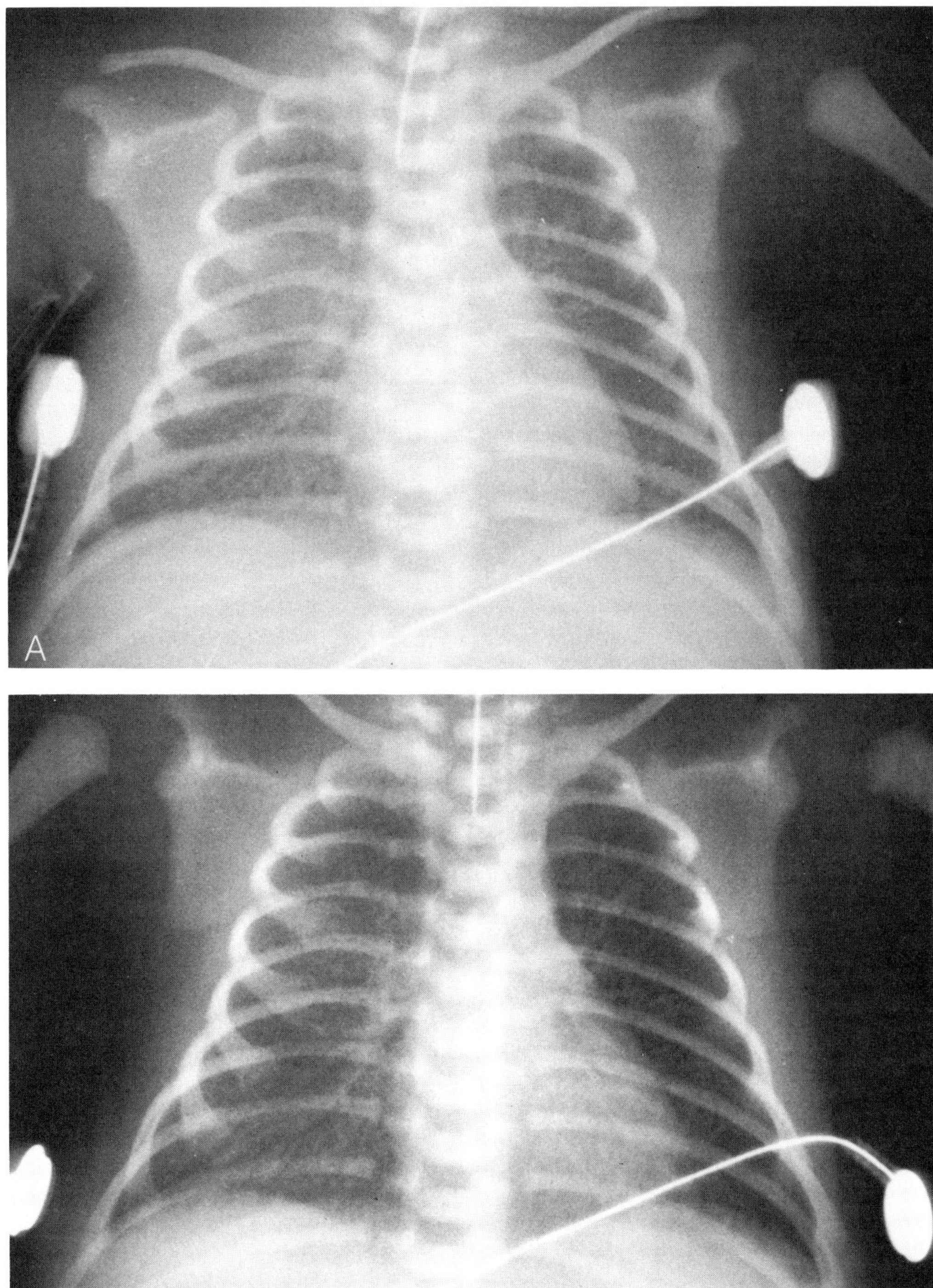

Fig. 7-6. (A) Chest radiograph of a 34-week gestional male infant treated for 24 hours with 100 percent oxygen and high-peak inspiratory pressure. Diffuse alveolar infiltrates are present. **(B)** The same patient after several hours of HFOV, the infiltrates have largely cleared. PaO_2 was markedly improved and successful weaning followed.

disease states and various devices still need to be established.

Ventilatory Strategies

Homogeneous Diffuse Pulmonary Disease

Several types of respiratory failure in the newborn are associated with the radiographic finding of diffuse pulmonary infiltrates. HMD, group B streptococcal pneumonia, pulmonary hemorrhage, and adult respiratory distress syndrome (ARDS) typically present with such involvement. The pathophysiologic component shared by these diseases is diffuse alveolar collapse, decreased lung compliance, and $\dot{V}/\dot{Q}$ mismatch.

The goal of assisted ventilation is to improve lung inflation, lung compliance, and $\dot{V}/\dot{Q}$ matching. Most commonly, PEEP/CPAP are used to accomplish this goal. PEEP maintains opening of recruited alveoli during expiration. Numerous studies have demonstrated that arterial oxygenation improves with PEEP.[57–60] However, if too much PEEP is added, cardiac output and oxygen delivery may fall.[15]

The definition of optimal PEEP remains an elusive goal. It requires the simultaneous estimation of cardiac output, transmitted pleural pressure, and arterial oxygen content. Using current technology, only the last of these three measurements can be made in an accurate and reproducible manner in the neonate. PEEP must be employed judiciously in very-low-birthweight infants and in term infants in septic shock due to their marginal cardiac reserve. Careful clinical assessment of changes in systemic perfusion, arterial blood pressure, heart rate, urine flow, central venous pressure, and arterial pH is helpful in estimating the effects of increasing PEEP on cardiac output.

Indications for the initiation of positive-pressure ventilation (PPV) should be disease- and patient-specific. Factors that indicate impending respiratory failure are physical signs of increased respiratory distress (tachypnea, nasal flaring, intercostal, subcostal, and sternal notch retractions, grunting, and intermittent apnea), a rising $PaCO_2$ associated with acidosis; and progressive hypoxemia despite oxygen and PEEP.

The PIP chosen when instituting ventilator support should produce good breath sounds and visual chest wall movement, and the ventilator rate should be sufficient to decrease the physical signs of respiratory distress and maintain a near normal $PaCO_2$. The I:E ratio must permit complete exhalation of the delivered breath and is assessed by observation of the chest wall and auscultation of breath sounds. If the chest is still deflating or if expiratory sounds are still heard when the next positive-pressure breath is delivered, the exhalation time is too short and gas trapping is likely to occur.

Although the approach to diffuse lung disease is patient-specific and therefore cannot be approached in a cookbook fashion, some global concepts can be applied.

First, it is easier to maintain an open alveolus than to recruit it. The pressure required to inflate a collapsed alveolus is often very near the pressure that will rupture the adjacent open, more compliant alveolus. Early intervention prior to the development of severe respiratory failure can decrease the pressure required to achieve adequate gas exchange and decrease the amount of ventilator-associated barotrauma.[35,61–63]

Second, oxygen toxicity is very likely an important cause of lung injury in neonates requiring assisted ventilation.[64,65] Neonates with diffuse lung injury will have some degree of intrapulmonary shunting of blood by poorly ventilated alveoli. Increasing the inspired oxygen will have no effect on delivery of oxygen to this blood. If pulmonary hypertension is absent, reducing the inspired oxygen decreases unnecessary (and ineffective) exposure to high FiO_2 values.

Third, while the ventilator rate, PIP, and inspiratory time all affect mean airway pressure and thereby improve oxygenation, PEEP is the most effective means of improving oxygenation.[21] The "safe" level to be used is dependent on lung compliance. In the very small premature infant with very mild HMD, levels of 2 to 4 cm H_2O may be adequate. In the term neonate with severe ARDS, levels of 8 to 12 cm H_2O may be required.

Finally, since lung disease is dynamic, ventilator strategies should be as well. Assessment and reassessment of the patient, the arterial blood gas measurements, and the vital signs are critical to optimal ventilator support. High PIP and longer inspiratory times may be necessary to recruit alveoli, but once this goal has been obtained and compliance improves, these strategies are likely to produce lung injury and therefore need to be changed.

Nonhomogeneous Pulmonary Diseases

Meconium Aspiration

Infants with meconium aspiration present a tremendous challenge from a ventilatory management standpoint. Approximately 9 percent of all newborns pass meconium prior to delivery.[66] Fortunately, meconium aspiration pneumonia only occurs in a small number of these patients. Passage of meconium may be associated with stress (hypoxia) in utero. If this problem has been longstanding, these patients are likely to have severe persistent pulmonary hypertension of the newborn (PPHN). The initial management of patients born with meconium-stained fluid includes proper airway suctioning by the obstetrician before the initiation of spontaneous breathing. Controversy surrounds the issue of whether tracheal suction should be performed on babies who are pink and who are crying vigorously. These patients are likely to suffer more morbidity from direct tracheal suctioning than if none is performed. However, babies who are depressed at birth, and therefore more likely to have aspirated meconium, should have their tracheas suctioned.

Because meconium-stained babies are at risk of PPHN, prevention of further hypoxia is critical. They should receive oxygen in the delivery room and be assessed for adequate oxygenation in the nursery. The decision to provide assisted ventilation may be a difficult one. Those infants not requiring intubation and assisted ventilation in the delivery room but demonstrating some degree of respiratory distress must be evaluated from a blood gas, oxygen lability, radiographic, and respiratory standpoint. The requirement for more than 50 percent oxygen, progressive increase in $PaCO_2$, labored respiration, and evidence of PPHN suggests the need for assisted ventilation.

Once ventilatory support is initiated, the infant must be followed carefully. Meconium aspiration is characterized by focal areas of atelectasis and air trapping that result in significant $\dot{V}/\dot{Q}$ mismatch. The goal of assisted ventilation is to decrease the mismatch without causing air leaks. In general, these patients benefit from slower rates, low PEEP, and reduced I:E ratios to permit lung emptying. Patients with meconium aspiration change from hour to hour. If air trapping is the major problem, the aforementioned pattern works best. However, if atelectasis predominates, longer inspiratory times and higher PEEP are necessary. By 24 hours, patients commonly develop a diffuse low lung volume state that may be due to a loss of surfactant.[67] When this problem is manifested, longer inspiratory times and higher PEEP become necessary.

Hyperventilation may be important for managing PPHN but poses the increased risk of barotrauma. During the early stages, when meconium in the airway produces both atelectasis and hyperinflation (ball-valve effect), HFV is rarely effective. In the later stages, when a more diffuse process associated with decreased compliance and loss of surfactant function supervenes, it may be very effective.

Excellent delivery room management and aggressive postdelivery intervention enable most meconium aspiration patients to be managed with low morbidity and minimal mortality. However, a subset remains who aspirate meconium well before delivery and have severe PPHN. This group of patients represent a maximal management challenge to the neonatologist.

Our experience suggests that HFV and ECMO should significantly decrease the mortality in this group of patients.[54]

Bronchopulmonary Dysplasia

Ventilatory management of the patient with BPD is difficult and often frustrating. These patients do not get well quickly. They act very much like adults with chronic obstructive pulmonary disease (COPD), except that lung function improves in most patients with time.

The picture of BPD has changed significantly over the past 10 years. During the 1970s, most patients with BPD had cystic-type lesions alternating with areas of atelectasis and overinflation. Reactive airway disease was common. Today, a large number of patients have what can best be described as hazy BPD. Their disease is more homogeneous and associated with low lung volumes. Patients with nonhomogeneous BPD require frequent and careful ventilatory management. In general, they do best with large tidal volumes, low PEEP (2 to 3 cm H_2O), and long expiratory times, to minimize air trapping. Those with severe air trapping often do best with no PEEP. Conversely, occasional patients with severe tracheobronchial malacia actually do better with PEEP of 4 to 8 cm H_2O, which seems to promote stabilization of the airways and reduce premature airway closure and air trapping. The predominant lung pathology (air trapping versus atelectasis) may vary from day to day. Therefore, some days longer inspiratory times and high PEEP are most effective, while on other days shorter inspiratory times and low PEEP are indicated.

Patients with very low birthweight who survive with hazy BPD and low lung volumes are often better from a blood gas standpoint than would appear to be the case radiographically. Ventilatory management involves increased PEEP (4 to 6 cm H_2O), and longer inspiratory times. They frequently tolerate ventilator weaning by the substitution of nasopharyngeal CPAP.

Of importance in the management of BPD patients is the maintenance of adequate oxygenation. Persistent hypoxia leads to cor pulmonale, a chief cause of mortality in these patients.[68] The pulmonary hypertension seen in BPD patients is responsive to an increase in arterial oxygen saturation.[69] We attempt to keep their PaO_2 values between 60 and 70 mmHg. If the patient develops cor pulmonale, the PaO_2 should be increased. Control of $PaCO_2$ can be equally important. We have noted several patients whose pulmonary artery pressure decreased when $PaCO_2$ was reduced from 60 to 70 mmHg to 40 to 50 mmHg, even though oxygenation remained the same.[70] An additional value of assisted ventilation in the BPD patient is to decrease the work of breathing, which decreases caloric expenditure and permits increased growth. Growth is extremely important to the overall survivability of the BPD patient.

Infection is a major concern in BPD patients and is commonly heralded by the need for increased ventilatory support. The most sensitive marker appears to be hypoxemia.[70] Any patient with a sudden increase in oxygen requirement and no specific cause should be considered infected. Bacterial and viral pneumonias are common causes of mortality in BPD patients.

Bronchodilators and diuretics are beneficial therapeutic adjuncts to assisted ventilation in BPD patients.[70] They are not without risk, however, and it is important to document their efficacy before continuing their use. Monitoring with pulse oximetry, transcutaneous PO_2 and PCO_2, and end-tidal PCO_2 may help decrease morbidity and mortality in these patients. Such noninvasive modalities are important, since an arterial puncture can produce agitation, leading to a blood gas result that does not adequately reflect the patient's steady state.

Nondiffuse Pneumonia

Most pneumonias in the newborn are diffuse, as the neonate tends not to localize infections well. The incidence of pneumonia is less than 1 percent in term infants but may be more than 10 percent in prematures.[71] Prematures are at increased risk because of their immature immune system and also the likelihood for nosocomial infections in the intensive care unit (ICU). Several organisms, however, can produce more localized pneumonia in neonates, including *Staphylococcus aureus*, *Klebsiella pneumoniae*, and *Escherichia coli*. Pneumococcal pneumonia, while frequently presenting with a diffuse HMD-like picture, may present with lobar disease.

Management in this group of patients must be directed at obtaining adequate ventilation and oxygenation with minimal barotrauma. Patients with focal pneumonia are at increased risk of barotrauma because of the nonhomogeneous nature of their lung disease. With lobar pneumonia, a significant intrapulmonary shunt leads to a relatively fixed PaO_2 that does not respond to increased FiO_2. High PIP and PEEP directed at the abnormal lobe(s) may be required. This approach, however, results in increased airway injury and risk to the portion of the lungs that are normal. Therefore, the goal should be to decrease FiO_2 to a level at which the PaO_2 is acceptable (approximately 50 mmHg). Ventilatory pressures and PEEP must be adjusted to avoid overexpansion of the normal lung parenchyma.

Pulmonary Hypoplasia

Patients with pulmonary hypoplasia can be divided into two categories: (1) those with diffuse hypoplasia, and (2) those with focal (usually unilateral) hypoplasia. Diffuse hypoplasia is most commonly the result of decreased amniotic fluid, either production (renal problems) or loss (prolonged rupture of the membranes). It is also seen in hydrops associated with pleural effusions and compression from abdominal masses or ascites. These patients generally have decreased total lung volume, and lung units may be decreased in number and size or be maldeveloped.[72] Abnormal $\dot{V}/\dot{Q}$ matching occurs along with a predisposition to lung injury with mechanical ventilation.

Extreme care must be taken when using assisted ventilation. Higher $PaCO_2$ and lower PaO_2 values should be accepted than for patients with more normal lungs. Newborn lungs differ from adult lungs in that the distal airways in certain circumstances are more compliant than the terminal air sacs or alveoli. During positive-pressure ventilation, marked airway distension and significant risk of injury can result.[73] The lowest possible pressures should be employed.

Positive end-expiratory pressure should be used for these patients but must be limited to avoid the previously discussed adverse effects. If PEEP is increased too much in the presence of a low PIP, the tidal volume delivered may not be enough to provide adequate ventilation. The precise pattern of ventilation must be individualized for each patient. Slow rate IMV with maximum spontaneous effort is best for some patients, while in others, rapid rate IMV with short inspiratory times and low peak pressures, may be optimal.

Patients with focal hypoplasia (diaphragmatic hernias, cystic adenomatoid malformation, other intrathoracic masses) are also difficult management problems. They generally have unilateral involvement, although the contralateral lung may also be hypoplastic. Persistent pulmonary hypertension is often present.[74] Ventilatory strategies are similar to those used for diffuse hypoplasia, using the least positive pressure to achieve acceptable PaO_2 and $PaCO_2$.

Treatment of PPHN involves manually or mechanically induced hyperventilation, which poses a significant risk of lung injury. Arterial PO_2 in a 50 to 60-mmHg range may worsen the PPHN. Therefore, the ventilatory management necessary to keep these patients alive can produce significant barotrauma, which ultimately will result in their death. Morbidity and mortality in patients with diffuse or focal pulmonary hypoplasia is predictably high.[75]

Newer modes of ventilatory assistance appear beneficial. We have used HFOV successfully in both forms of pulmonary hypoplasia.[53] Extracorporeal membrane oxygenation treatment, alone or in combination with HFOV, also enhances survival, particularly when PPHN is a complicating factor.[53] Patients with severe pulmonary hypoplasia who can be stabilized should be referred to centers capable of offering these therapies, since their prognosis is not as hopeless as previously thought.

Pulmonary Air Leak Syndromes

While pulmonary air leaks can occur in spontaneously breathing infants with minimal lung disease, they appear much more commonly in infants with severe lung disease requiring mechanical ventilatory support. Pulmonary air leak syndromes are a serious and often life-threatening complication of mechanical ventilation. The most important aspect of treatment is early diagnosis and, when possible, evacuation of the trapped air.

Common to the management of all pulmonary air leaks is the goal of reduced additional barotrauma. Once a hole in an airway has developed, the amount of gas that leaks through it will be dependent on its size and the pressure differential across it. Both are maximal at peak inflation. A reducton of the PIP should diminish the amount of air that escapes.[76] However, a reduction of PIP may decrease minute ventilation and can be associated with a rise in $PaCO_2$. This effect can be minimized by increasing the ventilator rate. Every effort should be made to prevent the development of further air leaks. In neonates with severe barotrauma, higher levels of arterial carbon dioxide and lower levels of arterial oxygen content should be accepted so as to reduce the amount of continued air leak.

Pneumothorax

If recognized early and treated quickly, the most easily managed air leak is a pneumothorax. Sudden decrease in chest wall movement, marked cyanosis and pallor, asymmetric breath sounds, and progressive hypotension suggest the diagnosis. Transillumination of the chest wall and/or a chest radiograph can be helpful in determining the site of the air leak. Immediate evacuation of trapped gas should be accomplished by a chest tube placed in any infant receiving positive-pressure support.

Pneumopericardium

A pneumopericardium is also easy to evacuate; however, its diagnosis can be more problematic. Most often, it is associated with sudden profound hypotension, evidenced by peripheral vasoconstriction, cyanosis, and pallor. Examination reveals distant heart sounds, crepitations during systole, absent pulses, and a decrease in the QRS size on the electrocardiographic (ECG) monitor. Breath sounds are usually equal over both lung fields and chest wall movement is not diminished during positive-pressure breaths. Again, immediate evacuation is the most important therapy.

Pneumomediastinum

A pneumomediastinum is most often diagnosed on the basis of radiographic findings. The presentation can be very similar to that of a pneumopericardium, except that the development of hypotension is usually less acute (and often is not present). Unlike air trapped in the pericardial sac or pleural space, air in the mediastinum is very difficult to evacuate. The mediastinum is separated into a number of small spaces by fascial septae; thus, gas is trapped in multiple separate pockets. It is nearly impossible to drain a pneumomediastinum effectively by placing a mediastinal tube.

Pulmonary Interstitial Emphysema

Pulmonary interstitial emphysema is associated with a high morbidity and mortality.[77] The diagnosis is based on the radiographic finding of hyperlucent bubbles radiating outward from the lung hilum.[78] Morphologic examination of the lungs of infants who die with PIE reveals gas trapped throughout the interstitium with dissection into the perivascular, peribronchial, and bronchiolar spaces.[73,78] This trapped gas often dissects further, progressing to pneumothorax, pneumomediastinum, or pneumopericardium. Even without extrapulmonary spread, PIE may compress adjacent structures, causing an increase in $\dot{V}/\dot{Q}$ mismatch, decreased lung compliance, increased airway resistance, and increased pulmonary vascular resistance. These changes often necessitate the use of higher ventilator settings to achieve adequate ventilation, which in turn perpetuates the PIE.

Various therapeutic approaches have been suggested, including selective bronchial intubation,[79] dependent positioning of the least affected lung,[80] surgical removal of the areas of major involvement,[81] visceral pleurotomy, rapid rate conventional ventilation (up to 150 breaths/min),[82] and HFV.[50,83] While all these interventions have been associated in selected patients with improvement in gas exchange and the radiographic appearance of PIE, their effectiveness in reducing long-term morbidity is unclear.

We have used HFOV to treat 68 patients with PIE and respiratory failure. Respiratory failure was defined as a $PaCO_2$ greater than 55 mmHg, with a pH less than 7.25, a PIP of 30 cm H_2O or higher, a PaO_2 of less than 55 mmHg (FIO_2 = 1.0), and a mean airway pressure greater than 12 cm H_2O. Seventy-five percent of these patients were referred from other level 3 centers. Four patients died shortly after arrival. Of the 64 remaining patients, 94 percent demonstrated improved ventilation and 60 percent demonstrated improved oxygenation. Overall survival was 70 percent. Approximately one-half the deaths were not directly related to pulmonary disease. Predictors of responsiveness to HFOV appear to be the degree of lung disease at admission and birth weight. Patients with bilateral tension PIE and/or a birthweight less than 1,000 g are least likely to respond to HFOV and have a high mortality rate.

Extracorporeal Membrane Oxygenation

Extracorporeal membrane oxygenation is a technique of long-term heart and lung bypass first employed in neonates by Dr. Robert Bartlett in 1975 for the management of intractable respiratory failure not responsive to conventional therapies.[84] Early success with ECMO was variable, in part because of poor patient selection. Wide acceptance was delayed for several reasons: (1) many infants selected for ECMO therapy were immature, and large numbers of them died because of bleeding (particularly intracranial) associated with the heparinization required, (2) ECMO is a complicated therapy that requires specialized personnel with extensive training, and (3) people were skeptical of the potential short-term and long-term morbidity.

Recent reports, however, indicate very impressive survival rates and acceptable morbidity, both of which are especially significant when judged in relationship to the severity of lung disease at the onset of therapy.[85,86] The very long-term morbidity of ECMO, however, remains to be seen. As more and more ECMO centers are opened and the criteria for initiating ECMO are relaxed, potential long-term sequelae must be carefully evaluated.

Two approaches are used to provide ECMO: venovenous (VV) or venoarterial (VA) perfusion. Venovenous perfusion is performed via the internal jugular vein with a single, double-lumen catheter or via the internal jugular and femoral or umbilical veins with two catheters. The advantage of VV perfusion is that the common carotid artery does not have to be ligated, thereby avoiding concomitant short-term and long-term morbidity. The disadvantages are that the patient requires heparinization, cardiac output cannot be fully supported, and oxygen delivery is significantly less than with VA perfusion. The VA approach generally uses the right internal jugular vein and right common carotid artery. It can fully support cardiac output and deliver high levels of oxygen to the systemic circulation. Its major disadvantages are that it also requires heparinization and carotid artery ligation.

Patient selection for ECMO remains an important issue (Table 7-4). In general, patients should have reached 34 weeks gestation or greater, since the high likelihood of intracranial hemorrhage in premature infants is increased by heparinization while receiving therapy. Birthweight should be at least 2 kg, to allow appropriate catheter size and the initiation of bypass. This indication is relative; patients who are small for gestational age should be considered for bypass even if they are less than 2

Table 7-4. Criteria for ECMO in Infants with Respiratory Failure

≥ 34 weeks gestation
≥ 2-kg birthweight[a]
≤ 7 days postgestation age[a]
Severe respiratory failure despite maximal support[a]
Cardiac decompensation
Absence of terminal or irreversible nonpulmonary disease

[a] Relative indication.

Table 7-5. PPHN Patients Treated with ECMO

Intrauterine growth retardation (IUGR)
Acquired immunodeficiency syndrome (AIDS)
Birth asphyxiation
Meconium aspiration
Sepsis (without DIC and capillary leak)
Infants of diabetic mothers
Hyperviscosity
Infants of mothers with chronic vascular disease

kg. Postgestational age should be 7 days or less.

Most patients who have been treated with 100 percent oxygen and high-pressure ventilator settings since birth and who are more than 7 days of age have sustained severe, irreversible pulmonary injury and, therefore, are not candidates for ECMO.[53] This requirement also is relative, since an infant who was doing reasonably well for 3 or 4 days may subsequently have higher levels of support only at 8 or 9 days. The infant must have severe respiratory failure in spite of aggressive conventional ventilatory and pharmacologic treatment. In the presence of cardiac decompensation, this criterion may be altered; that is, cardiac failure in the presence of less severe respiratory disease may still indicate the need for ECMO.

Contraindications to ECMO therapy include a gestational age of 34 weeks or less; evidence of severe lung injury with maximal ventilator support and 100 percent oxygen for more than 7 days; sepsis with disseminated intravascular coagulation (DIC) and capillary leak; renal failure; and a severe underlying nonpulmonary disease such as interventricular hemorrhage or bleeding into other closed spaces, chromosomal abnormality, some forms of congenital heart disease, renal agenesis, or any other nontreatable, terminal condition.[86]

Applications

Persistent Pulmonary Hypertension of the Newborn

Persistent pulmonary hypertension of the newborn, also called persistent fetal circulation, was first described in 1965.[88] It continues to be a major source of morbidity and mortality. Various therapies, both ventilatory and pharmacologic, have been used with generally good success. However, certain patients, despite maximal support, continue to die. This group appears to benefit from ECMO therapy.

The populaton at risk is summarized in Table 7-5. Patients with the most severe PPHN have longstanding intrauterine asphyxia resulting from uteroplacental dysfunction, maternal disease, or persistent cord compression. They have increased medial muscle in the small pulmonary vessels, and their pulmonary vascular bed appears to be overresponsive to factors that normally produce increased pulmonary vascular tone (acidosis, hypercarbia, and hypoxia).[89,90] Most patients with this syndrome can be managed with drugs, oxygen therapy, and mechanical ventilation to induce hypocarbia and alkalosis. Those patients who are unresponsive to this therapy usually die from persistent hypoxia and right heart failure, unless ECMO is used.

The major benefits of ECMO include (1) hyperoxia; (2) maintenance of alkalosis and hypocarbia; (3) reduced need for mechanical ventilation (decrease barotrauma); (4) decreased pulmonary blood flow; and (5) because of (1) through (4) may assist in stimulating regression of medial muscle. Survival with ECMO is better than 80 percent in the absence of complicating factors.

Meconium Aspiration

Patients with severe meconium aspiration and associated pulmonary failure may not respond to conventional mechanical ventilation. They suffer from severe $\dot{V}/\dot{Q}$ mismatch and persistent hypoxia. Air leaks of all types—pneumothorax, pneumomediastinum, pneumopericardium—are common and result in further hypoxia and acidosis. A significant number of these patients have PPHN, as one cause for meconium passage and aspiration is intrauterine asphxia. Placing the lungs at rest with ECMO decreases air leaks, permits healing, allows removal of particulate debris by pulmonary macrophages, and lessens the impact of PPHN. Following weaning from ECMO, these patients generally do well from a pulmonary standpoint.[86]

Hyaline Membrane Disease

Although predominantly a disease of prematurity, a number of patients are born at 34 to 37 weeks gestation and develop HMD. Often, because of their larger size, they are not managed early and aggressively, and develop significant atelectasis. Subsequently, after mechanical ventilation is begun, severe air leaks and refractory respiratory failure supervene. In such cases, ECMO can be used successfully. It permits adequate ventilation and oxygenation without the necessity to administer a high FiO_2. Healing usually occurs and, with adequate surfactant production, lung compliance improves and patients usually can be weaned effectively from ECMO and ventilator support.[86]

Sepsis and Pneumonia

Patients who have sepsis associated with DIC and capillary leak do not do well with ECMO, since the latter seems to result in additional capillary leak. However, a subset of patients with pneumonia and PPHN, particularly of group B streptococcal origin, respond very effectively to ECMO and do not appear to suffer major adverse effects. Patients with viral pneumonias and severe, intractable pulmonary disease may also be managed with ECMO until the disease resolves and the lung is cleared.[53] Some patients who are septic have profound cardiac dysfunction leading to death. They may be managed with ECMO for 2 to 3 days, until the factors responsible for cardiac depression are resolved.

Congenital Diaphragmatic Hernia

The survival of patients with congenital diaphragmatic hernia has changed very little, even with excellent ventilatory support.[74] Varying degrees of pulmonary hypoplasia result in severe PPHN and pulmonary failure. Patients whose condition deteriorates following surgical repair may respond well to ECMO.

The exact reasons that patients deteriorate following repair are not well defined but appear to be multifactorial. The hypoplastic lung has a contracted pulmonary vascular bed and a fixed increase in pulmonary vascular resistance. Additional increases in pulmonary vascular resistance result from at least two reasons. First, the small lung ''sees'' an increased blood flow following repair and responds to distention of the pulmonary artery by distal constriction of the pulmonary vascular bed.[91] Blood is shunted to the more normal lung, which also responds with vasoconstriction (similar to the pulmonary vascular response in the presence of a large VSD or PDA with increased left-to-right circulation). Second, when the small lung is mechanically ventilated, parenchymal injury may be followed by the release of various mediators that increase pulmonary vasoconstriction of both the normal and abnormal sides.

This group benefits from ECMO for several reasons. The lungs do not have to be overventilated (potential injury risk) in order to decrease pulmonary vascular resistance. A more gradual inflation of the hypoplastic lung can be employed. Gradual weaning from ECMO permits graded increases in pulmonary blood flow. The pulmonary vascular bed may accommodate better to this blood flow without a reflex vasospasm. We have seen one patient with a diaphragmatic hernia who was weaned rapidly from ECMO and developed severe pulmonary hypertension. This patient was treated again with high bypass settings for 24 hours, with a resulting decrease in pulmonary vascular resistance. Weaning was then accomplished over 72 hours, following which decannulation proceeded uneventfully.

Heart Disease

Patients with cardiomyopathy or myocarditis may benefit from ECMO because the heart is rested and allowed to recover during the perfusion period. Some forms of congenital heart disease, such as severe coarctation of the aorta, may benefit from ECMO prior to operation if the heart has suffered significant hypoxic injury before repair of the lesion. Postoperative ECMO support may prove to be of additional benefit to patients who undergo operative repairs. The heart can recover from the surgical procedure and be gradually reintroduced to its pumping requirements.

Complications

ECMO is a labor- and personnel-intensive procedure that is not suited for all nurseries. Bleeding is a likely problem that can occur at the incision sites where previous surgery was performed or where the cannulas are placed. It is also seen in the intrathoracic, gastrointestinal, genitourinary, and intracranial sites.[86,92] These common problems require early removal from ECMO.

Cannulation problems, including air or clot emboli and bleeding, occur, and arterial intimal injury may predispose to dissecting aortic aneurysm. Intracranial hemorrhage, brain edema, seizures, hemiparesis, and brain death all may be direct complications of ECMO. Circuit problems, including failure of the membrane lung or heat exchanger, tubing rupture, and air or clot embolization, can also occur during an ECMO run. Sepsis may result from the multiple sites for contamination. Pericardial tamponade, if it occurs, generally is related to catheter placement problems.[86]

In summary, ECMO is an invasive technique that should be reserved only for patients who fail all other modes of therapy, including, in our experience, HFOV. It is not indicated as early therapy to prevent potential lung injury. The long-term sequelae of unilateral carotid ligation are unknown. Future changes in technique may be expected to render ECMO more patient- and user-friendly. These probably will include circuits that no longer require heparinization and the use of alternative arterial sites so that common carotid ligation is not a necessity. ECMO should be reserved for patients who have a high probability of death unless it is employed.

Surfactant Replacement

Surfactant plays a central role in the transition of the lungs from fetus to newborn.[93] It promotes the development of uniform lung inflation by decreasing surface tension and increasing alveolar deflation stability. Lung compliance, work of breathing, and fluid resorption from the alveolus into the lung interstitium are optimized by the presence of surfactant.

The association between surfactant deficiency and HMD in premature humans and animals is well known. The goal of surfactant replacement is to restore surfactant sufficiency, thereby improving lung function and reducing the morbidity and mortality associated with this disease. Several controlled clinical trials of surfactant replacement therapy have demonstrated its effectiveness in improving gas exchange in infants with established lung disease.[94–97] Perhaps more importantly, the most recent multicenter collaborative effort showed that surfactant given to infants with severe neonatal respiratory distress syndrome was effective in reducing neonatal mortality, the incidence of pulmonary air leak, and the percentage of survivors in whom BPD developed.[98] Prophylactic administration of surfactant prior to the first breath in neonates at high risk of developing HMD produces similar if not better results. Unfortunately, there are no absolute predictors of who will develop HMD; thus, the prophylactic use of surfactant may be unnecessary in a significant number of patients identified as at risk.

While it is clear that surfactant will play an important role in the management of premature infants with HMD, several important questions remain to be answered. Basic issues concerning the dose, immunologic effects, best method of administration, benefits of repeated dosing, and the most efficacious type of surfactant (natural surfactant obtained from amniotic fluid, organic solvent extracts of heterologous surfactant, or artificial surfactants) remain ill defined and the subject of current research efforts.[99]

The potential therapeutic interaction between HFV to establish uniform lung inflation and subsequent administration of surfactant to help maintain this inflation at lower lung volumes remains to be explored. These are exciting areas in the arena of neonatal pulmonary research.

PEDIATRIC VENTILATORY SUPPORT

General Concerns

Pediatric respiratory care has received much less attention than that of neonates and adults. Techniques of mechanical ventilatory support have been modified from those employed in the latter two groups, often with less than satisfactory results. In recent years, however, increasing emphasis has been placed on disease conditions with a predilection for the pediatric population. Therapeutic modalities have been introduced that have had a major impact on selected problems, a few of which are discussed in this section.

Airway Maintenance

The first step in the respiratory support of the pediatric patient is the establishment and maintenance of the airway. Airway obstruction is relatively common and has many causes. These may be divided into congenital anomalies, infections, and trauma (Table 7-6). The airway should be secured expeditiously, usually by tracheal intubation. If it cannot be visualized, and the patient is at risk of hypoxia, steps should be taken to maintain oxygenation.

Table 7-6. Causes of Pediatric Airway Obstruction

Congenital
Choanal atresia
Sleep apnea, sudden infant death syndrome (SIDS)
Macroglossia (Beckwith-Wiederman syndrome, trisomy 21)
Facial malformations (Pierre-Robin syndrome)
Marquio dwarfism
Cystic fibrosis
Vascular rings
Infections/Allergies
Choanal stenosis
Enlarged tonsils and adenoids
Supraglottitis
Croup (laryngotracheobronchitis)
Bronchiolitis
Pneumonia
Asthmatic bronchitis/asthma
Trauma
Facial fractures
Foreign body
Tracheal stenosis
Postintubation croup
Tracheobronchomalacia

An emergency oxygen source may be provided by taking a 12-gauge intravenous cannula and placing it into the patient's trachea[100,101] (Fig. 7-7). The adaptor from a 3.0-mm ID endotracheal tube may then be placed on the catheter hub. Oxygen can be insufflated or positive-pressure ventilation delivered with a self-inflating bag. This technique will prevent hypoxemia even though $PaCO_2$ will increase and pH drop. In dogs, satisfactory oxygenation is maintained during spontaneous breathing or manual inflation[101] (Figs. 7-8 and 7-9). The position of the catheter tip relative to the carina is important, with better oxygenation and carbon dioxide elimination achieved as the carina is approached. Higher gas flow also improves ventilation.[102] Gas exchange appears to result both from turbulent flow and passive diffusion. Cardiac oscillations may help the latter.[101]

Humidification and oxygenation are essential following tracheal intubation or tracheotomy. Additional equipment attached to the circuit increases the possibility of a leak developing or of an accidental extubation. Water-borne bacteria, especially *Pseudomonas aeruginosa,* often

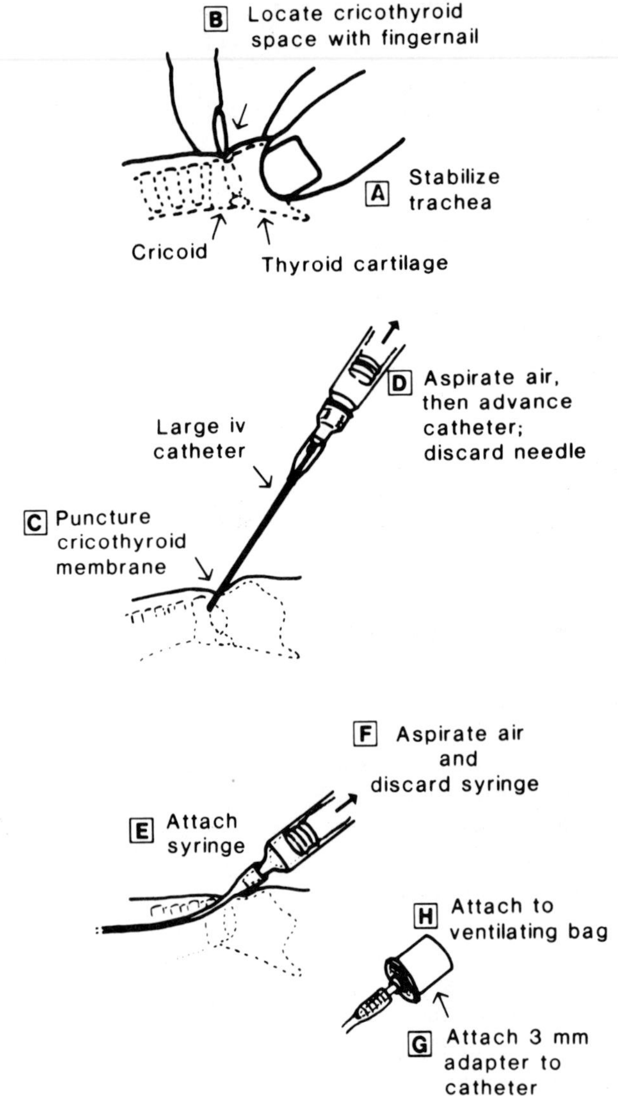

Fig. 7-7. Establishment of an emergency airway for oxygen delivery. (From Coté et al.,[101] with permission)

predispose to nosocomial infection. Frequent suctioning is necessary to prevent secretions from blocking the endotracheal tube. Patients may require sedation so they can tolerate the endotracheal tube. Care should be taken to avoid excessive sedation and possible cardiovascular depression.

Tracheotomy

When patients require prolonged tracheal intubation, the need for tracheotomy must be considered. Numerous factors must be considered before making this decision, including the need for a more stable airway, so that the patient

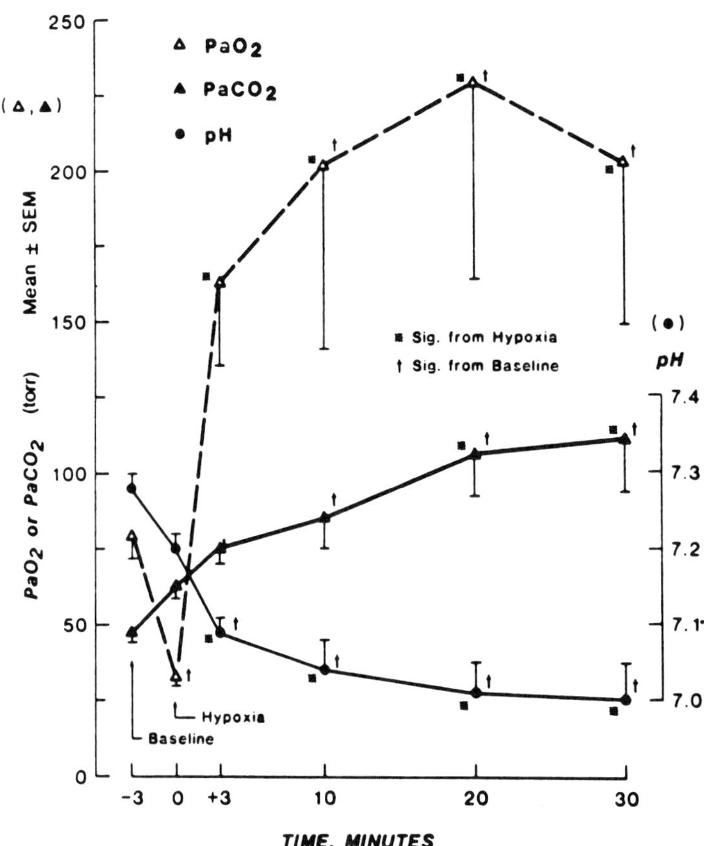

Fig. 7-8. Blood gas and pH values in six spontaneously breathing dogs with oxygen insufflation through a 12-gauge cannula. Oxygenation is satisfactory but severe respiratory acidemia is present. (From Coté et al.,[101] with permission.)

may be cared for on the floor or at home; the necessity for prolonged ventilatory support; excessive secretions; and the possibility of eventual extubation.[103]

Complications from tracheotomies range from 10 to 30 percent,[104,105] with the highest incidence in children under 1 year of age. The procedure is also associated with a mortality rate of 1.6 to 3 percent. Problems include subcutaneous emphysema, pneumothorax, pneumomediastinum, dislodging of the tube from the trachea, bleeding, and thyroid injury.[105–108] When performed under less controlled circumstances (e.g., without an endotracheal tube), the incidence of complications increases.[107] Care of the patient with a tracheotomy is similar to that of a patient with an endotracheal tube. A chest radiograph should be taken to verify the tube's position and the possibility for subcutaneous air. Humidification and oxygenation must be individualized. Frequent suctioning is necessary. The tube ties should be padded to prevent local neck trauma.

The most immediately life-threatening complication is obstruction, which may be acute or often presents with a gradual increase of the

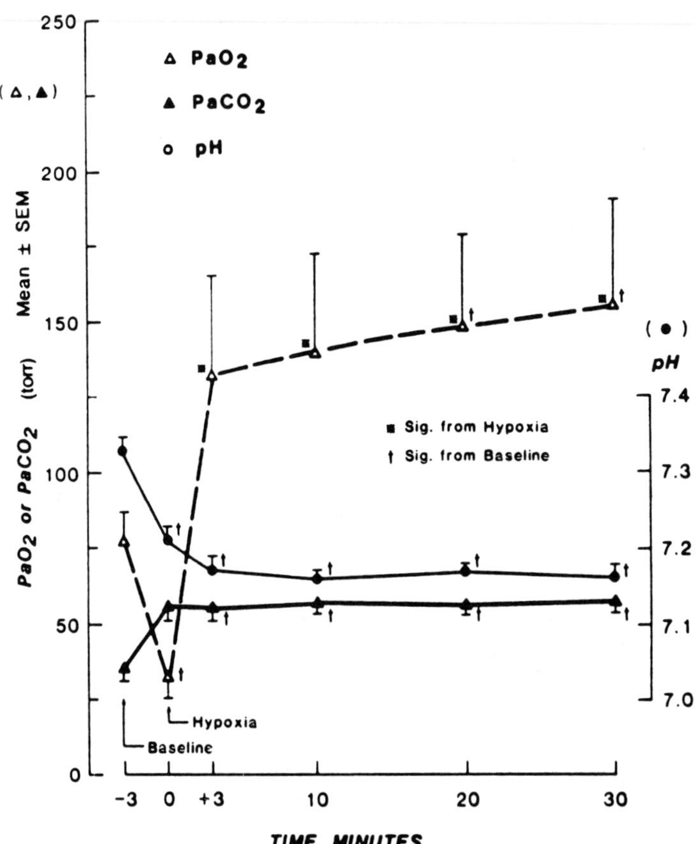

Fig. 7-9. Same measurements as in Figure 7-5 during manual inflation through a 12-gauge intratracheal cannula. The dogs were paralyzed to eliminate spontaneous breathing. Significant improvement in ventilation and acidemia are noted. (From Coté et al.,[101] with permission.)

respiratory rate or obvious cyanosis. Although this problem may be resolved with suctioning, a tube change may be necessary. At best, this is a dangerous procedure in a patient with a fresh tracheostomy stoma, and the insertion of a tracheotomy or endotracheal tube into the stoma may produce a false tract outside the trachea. If the patient cannot be ventilated through the tracheotomy tube, bag-mask ventilation, followed by orotracheal intubation, is indicated in view of the difficulty of replacement. In any event, occlusion of the stoma site leak is often necessary. Reoperation may be necessary for a definitive solution.

Respiratory Syncytial Virus Infections

Respiratory syncytial virus (RSV) is a common cause of life-threatening respiratory distress in young patients, although it also causes problems in other age groups. This medium-size RNA and lipid-containing virus[109,110] is destroyed at 55°C. A multiplicity of strains exist, several of which may be present during a disease outbreak.[111–114] Annual outbreaks occur, although the time and place vary from year to year.[115–117] Sixty to 90 percent of bronchiolitis and 10 to 30 percent of pediatric bronchitis[118]

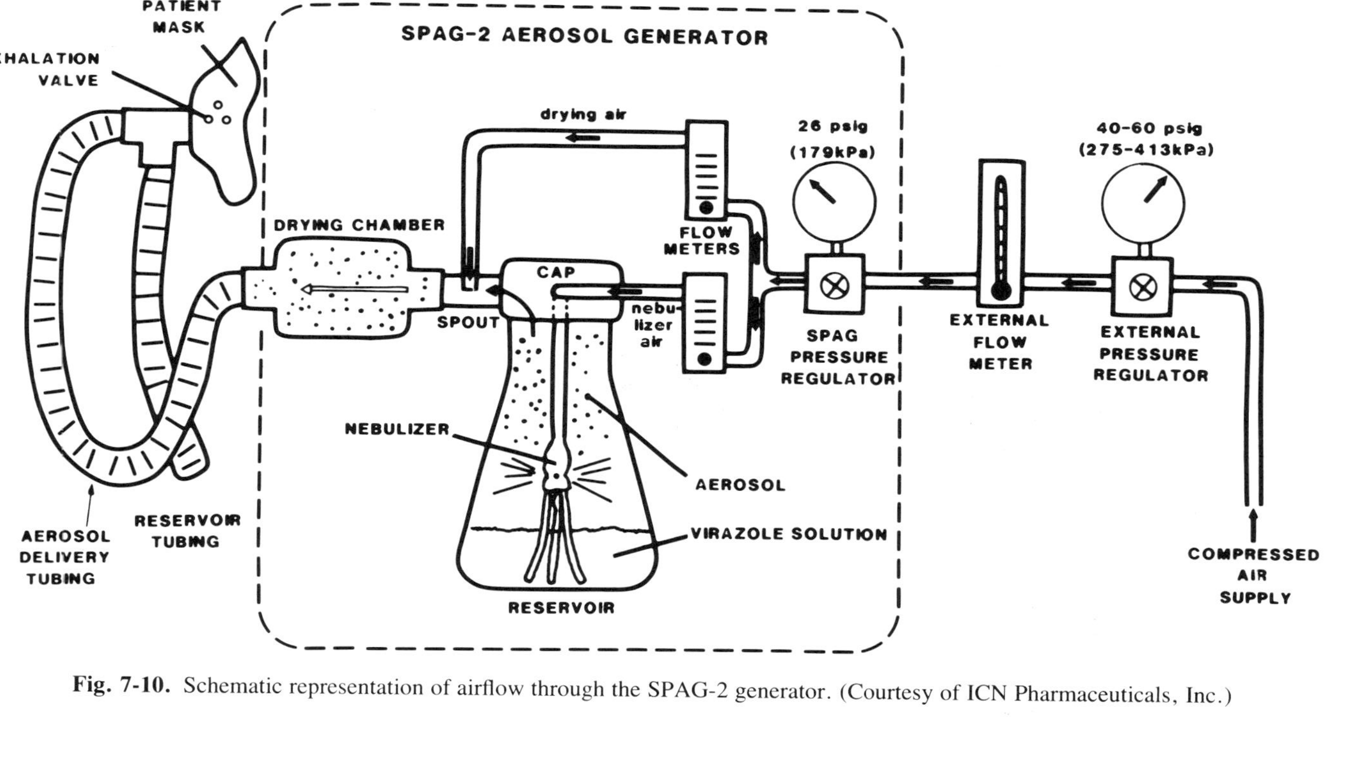

Fig. 7-10. Schematic representation of airflow through the SPAG-2 generator. (Courtesy of ICN Pharmaceuticals, Inc.)

are caused by RSV, but it does not play a significant role in croup. It is rare in patients without respiratory disease.[116] Infections are most common in children 2 to 5 months of age. They are unusual at ages under 4 months or over 2 years. Reinfections are common.[119] Transmission by droplets is rapid, often via an older child with a "cold."[120] Although RSV bronchiolitis is reasonably benign in normal infants, it may be deadly in patients with preexisting cardiac or pulmonary disease.[121,122]

Ribavirin, a synthetic nucleoside, counteracts replication of RSV in animals[123] and is approved for use in nonventilated hospitalized patients.[124] It is delivered through a face mask or hood, with oxygen concentrations varied as needed. The unit used to deliver ribavirin is called Small Particle Aerosol Generator Model 2 (SPAG-2, ICN Pharmaceuticals, Costa Mesa, CA), specifically designed for such application (Fig. 7-10). It is driven by pressurized gas regulated to 26 psig, which is directed to both the nebulizer and drying chambers. Particles in the fine aerosol are dried and reduced to a final size of approximately 1.3 μm. Flow through the nebulizer is controlled by the nebulizer orifice size, not by the flowmeter valve.

Patients requiring mechanical ventilation present special challenges[119,125] (Fig. 7-11). The SPAG-2 usually is not used in line with mechanical ventilators because of crystallization of ribavirin within the ventilator circuitry.[126] Aerosol tubing from the SPAG unit is inserted into the inspiratory limb of the ventilator circuit.[119] SPAG-2 nebulizer flows of 6 L/min, and drying flows of 3 to 4 L/min are adjusted so that the combined ventilator and SPAG outputs generate a PIP equal to that of the ventilator alone before

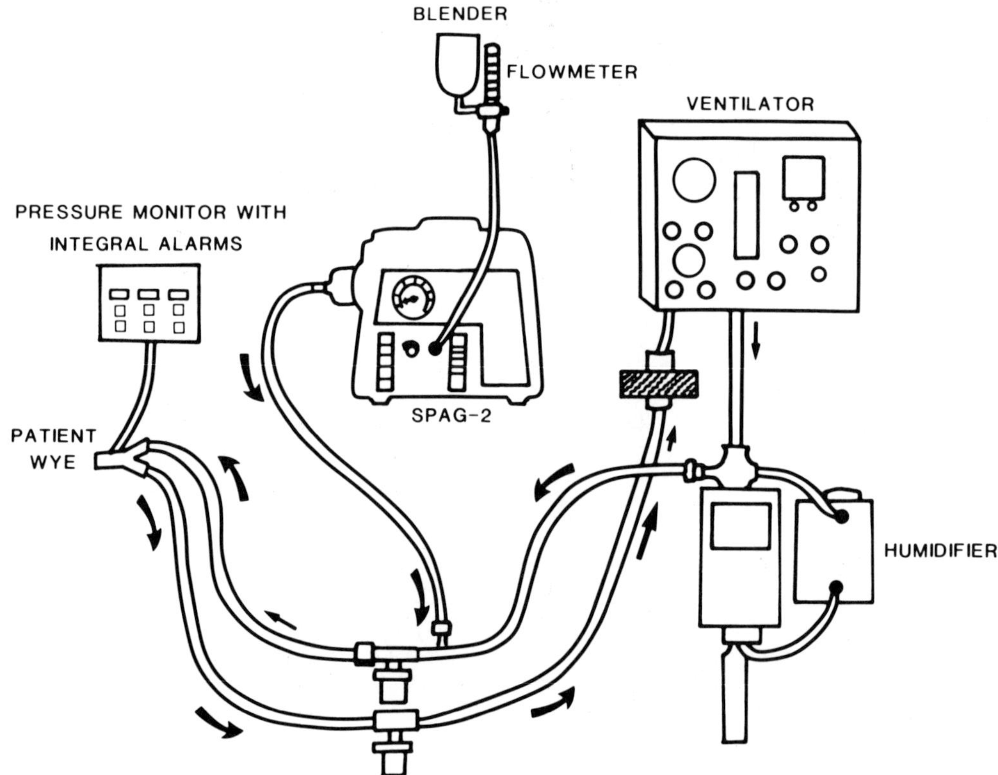

Fig. 7-11. Incorporation of the SPAG-2 generator into the ventilator circuit for treatment of a mechanically ventilated patient.

the SPAG unit was installed. A filter minimizes crystalline deposition of ribavirin on the exhalation valve, which is changed frequently. Although some crystallization occurs, the crystals have not been seen in the endotracheal tube.[125] The PEEP level must be checked frequently because of the continuous gas flow and the increasing resistance through the filter.

Airway Obstruction

Asthma

Acute asthma is a reversible airway disease in childhood. It is frequently triggered by allergens, although exercise, infections, and other factors may play a role.[127] During the acute episode, bronchospasm, airways edema, and secretions may combine to cause acute obstruction.

Initially, patients often manifest increased ventilation and hypocapnia within a few minutes of the beginning of the episode. As the patient tires, ventilation decreases, and hypercapnia and respiratory acidemia supervene. With further deterioration, a life-threatening combination of respiratory acidemia, hypoxemia, and metabolic (nonrespiratory) acidosis result (status asthmaticus).[128] The differential diagnosis of asthma includes other entities, such as foreign body aspiration, viral bronchiolitis, croup, and pneumonia. A known history of asthma and allergy help to confirm the diagnosis.

The physical examination generally reveals a patient in respiratory distress who in all probability is using the accessory muscles of respiration. Beware of the patient who previously presented with wheezing, but now does not, particularly if treatment has not been rendered. The strong possibility exists that absence of wheezing reflects exhaustion and absence of ventilation. Oxygen saturation should be evaluated, and appropriate steps taken to ensure adequate oxygenation. Frequently, these patients are hypovolemic, and restitution of intravascular volume is of paramount concern.[129]

The general approach to any patient in respiratory distress must be followed in this disease. Early treatment is important to reduce morbidity.[130] Supplemental oxygen must be given as needed. Oral feedings should be avoided initially since tracheal intubation is a potential intervention, and aspiration of gastric contents is a major problem. Stomach emptying is slowed, and patients may retain large amounts of gastric fluids.

Prevention of the initial episode for the most part is beyond the scope of this text. Allergic triggering agents should be avoided. Efforts to remove allergens from the patient's environment or to modify them to decrease their effect have met with limited success. Avoidance of upper airway infections and pneumonia should be attempted and emotional stress minimized whenever possible.

For the patient in respiratory distress, the goal is to reverse the airways obstruction. Epinephrine, 0.01 mg/kg intramuscularly (IM), is the most commonly used drug in the emergency room or office, but aerosolized β_2-adrenergic agents have been shown to be as effective in speed of onset, effect, and duration as epinephrine (Table 7-7).

Aerosolized agents are administered with a nebulizer and mouthpiece or mask over a few minutes, and may be repeated every 20 to 30 minutes. More specific β_2-adrenergic drugs produce fewer systemic adverse reactions, such as vomiting, tachycardia, or dysrhythmias, than does epinephrine.[131] Oxygen should be given with the inhalation agents.[129] If the patient does not improve after two doses, atropine or ipratroprium bromide may be used,[132] followed in particularly resistant cases by aminophylline, 6 mg/kg (equivalent to 5 mg/kg theophylline), intravenously (IV) over 20 minutes. Since a dose of 5 mg/kg theophylline should increase the preexisting level of theophylline by no more than 10 μg/ml, and the initial theophylline level usually is less than 5 μg/ml, the patient should be able to tolerate this increase. If there is a question, the loading dose may be decreased by 50 percent.

Additional therapy should include steroids.[129,133] Methylprednisolone, 2 to 3 mg/kg/

Table 7-7. Pharmacologic Agents for the Treatment of Asthma in Children

Drug	Parenteral	Aerosol
ADRENERGIC		
Epinephrine	Subcutaneous (1 : 1,000) 0.01 ml/kg/dose Maximum 0.5 ml q15–20 min Maximum 3 times	Not used
Sus-Phrine	Subcutaneous (1 : 200) 0.005 ml/kg/dose Maximum 0.15 ml q6h	Not used
Terbutaline	Subcutaneous (0.05%) 0.01 mg/kg/dose Maximum 0.25 mg, q20–30 min	1% solution 0.03 ml/kg Maximum 1 ml q4–6h
Albuterol (salbutamol)	Intravenous (0.1%) 0.2 μg/kg/dose Maximum 2 μg/kg/min or 10 μg/kg over 10 min	0.5% solution 0.01–0.03 mg/kg dilute with 1.5 ml saline q4–6h
Isoproterenol	Intravenous (0.02%) 0.05–0.1 μg/kg/min Increase by 0.05–0.1 μg/ml/min q15 min	0.5% solution 0.01–0.02 ml/kg Maximum 0.5 ml q6h
Isoetharine	Not used	1% solution 0.01 ml/kg Maximum 0.5 ml, q2–6h
Metaproterenol	Subcutaneous (0.1%) 0.01 ml/kg for 3 doses q20–30 min	5% solution 0.005–0.01 ml/kg Maximum 0.4 ml, q4–6h
Theophylline	Intravenous 25 mg/ml Loading 6–7.5 mg/kg over 20 min Modify by levels	Not used
ANTICHOLINERGIC		
Atropine	Not used	0.03–0.05 mg/kg
Ipratropium	Not used	20–40 μg metered dose q6h (> 6 year old)
CORTICOSTEROIDS		
Hydrocortisone	Loading: 5–7 mg/kg Maintenance: 5 mg/kg q6h	No
Methylprednisolone	Loading: 1 mg/kg Maintenance: 0.8 mg/kg q4–6h	No
Beclomethasone	Not used	50–100 μg q6h (inhaler)

(Modified from Chantarojanasiri,[159] with permission.)

day in four divided doses, is typical. This dose may be tapered after 48 hours if the patient improves. Antibiotics are used, if indicated, to treat infection. If the child deteriorates or fails to improve, admission to the ICU is indicated for closer monitoring of therapy.

Isoproterenol infusion has been used to treat respiratory failure in patients with status asthmaticus.[130,134,135] Continuous ECG monitoring is mandatory and an arterial cannula advisable. Isoproterenol is started at 0.1 μg/kg/min and increased every 15 to 30 minutes by 0.1 μg/mg/min. The progressive increase is stopped if the patient improves or if tachycardia above 200/min, cardiac abnormality, or hematemesis is evident.[134] Myocardial ischemia has been reported with higher doses of IV isoproterenol,[136] and caution should be exercised. The continuous aerosolization of β_2-agents appears to represent improvement in the handling of status asthmaticus and may obviate some of the side effects of continuous intravascular administration. Such therapy is not yet approved in the United States; thus, frequent administration (i.e., every 20 minutes) seems advisable.[137]

Indications for mechanical ventilation include severe hypercapnia (more than 60 mmHg), deterioration of mental status, decreased respiratory effort, or cardiac instability.[130] Initial ventilator settings include a tidal volume of 10 to 12 ml/kg and an I:E ratio of 1:2. After stabilization, subsequent changes in tidal volume, rate, or oxygenation are indicated by blood gas analysis. If PEEP/CPAP is used, a low level of 2 to 4 cm H_2O should be employed in order to prevent air trapping. Bronchodilator therapy should continue, and chest physiotherapy with frequent suctioning may be necessary if mucus and other secretions obstruct the airway. If the patient cannot be managed satisfactorily, muscle relaxants may be necessary to ensure oxygenation and ventilation. Sedation and pain relief are essential to the therapeutic regimen.

Heliox

Air is primarily a mixture of oxygen and nitrogen. As early as 1936, it was suggested that helium be mixed with oxygen rather than nitrogen to assist patients with upper airway obstruction.[138] Gas flow varies depending on the characteristics of tubes through which it flows. Significant reductions in the diameter of the tube often cause turbulence. As flow becomes turbulent, gas density rather than viscosity plays an important part in determining the volume flow. Thus, a "lighter" gas (lower density) will flow through a fixed orifice at a higher rate than one with a greater density.[139] Oxygen and helium have the same viscosity but lower density than oxygen and nitrogen (air). A helium-oxygen mixture (79 percent/21 percent), heliox, has a volume flow through a restricted orifice almost three times that of air. Conversely, only one-third the pressure differential is necessary for heliox to produce equal volume flow (Fig. 7-12).

Since heliox has a lower density than air, an increase in expiratory flow may be expected with the former.[140] However, in persons with severe and diffuse obstructive airway disease

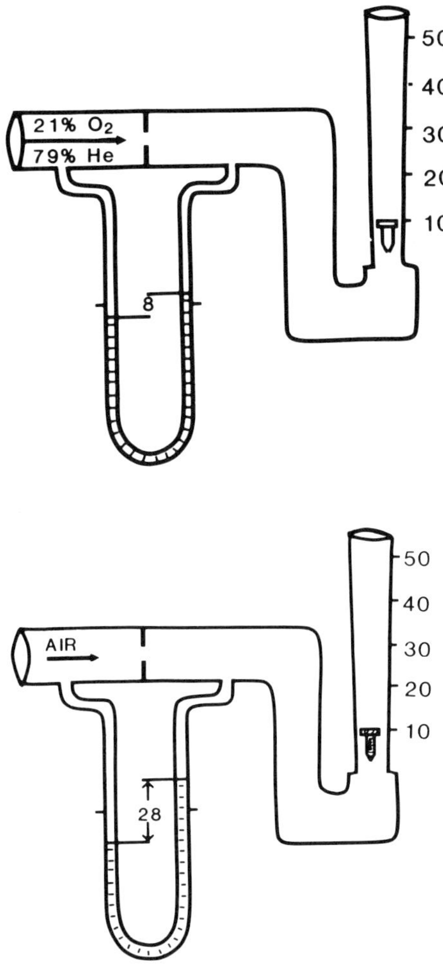

Fig. 7-12. Comparison of air and a 70 percent He-21 percent O_2 (heliox) flow through a 4-mm orifice. At a constant flow rate of 10 L/min, the pressure differential necessary to drive the heliox is approximately one-third that necessary for air (8 versus 28 cm H_2O, respectively). If the same pressure differential was employed for both gases, the heliox flow would be three times that of air.

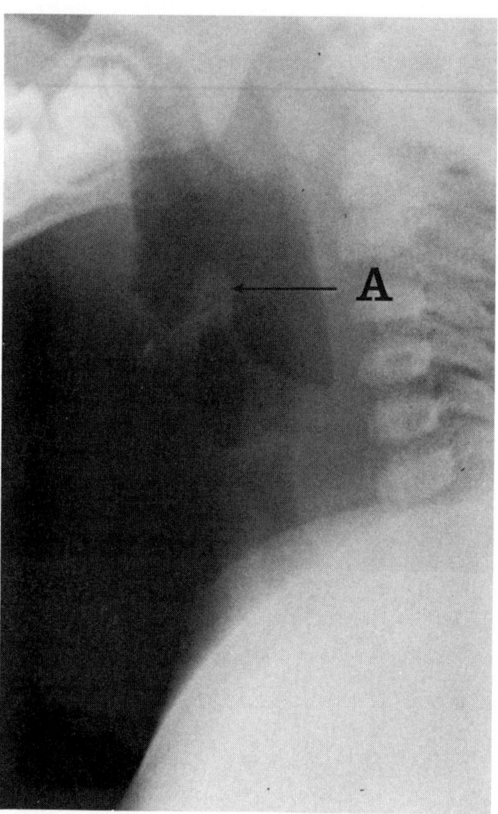

Fig. 7-13. Lateral radiograph of neck showing normal anatomy of airway and epiglottis with distinct margins (A).

and a very low gas flow that is laminar rather than turbulent, little or no difference may be noted. Heliox has been shown to increase the volume of ventilation without a change in compliance in experimental animals,[141] possibly due to dilation of the peripheral bronchial tree.

Croup and Supraglottitis

The differentiation of upper airway obstruction is critical. While many diseases predispose to obstruction (Table 7-6), common causes include croup and supraglottitis (epiglottitis). Hospitals should have a defined protocol to handle these patients.

Differentiation of patients into those with probable croup versus those with probable supraglottitis usually is possible (Table 7-8). Normal and abnormal radiographs to differentiate supraglottitis are shown in Figures 7-13 and 7-14. It is important to remember, however, that the cause of the obstruction is not radiologic and that it is not necessary to send the patient for radiographic studies to confirm the diagnosis. Indeed, patients may have life-threatening complications while awaiting studies when the diagnosis could have been made on the basis of the history and other physical clues.[142] Patients with croup may be evaluated according to the scoring system in Table 7-9. A patient who shows moderate croup scores (7 or greater) should be observed in a pediatric ICU, and treatment with racemic epinephrine may be beneficial.

Table 7-8. Differentiation Between Croup and Epiglottitis

Characteristic	Croup	Epiglottitis
Age	6 mo–3 yr	2–6 yr
Onset	Gradual	Rapid
Etiology	Viral	Bacterial
Cough	Hoarse	None
Posture	Any	Sitting
Fever	Absent/High	High
Appearance	Usually not ill	Anxious, acutely ill
Recurrence	Sometimes	Rarely
Season	Winter	None

The diagnosis of acute supraglottitis is of paramount importance. This life-threatening disease of acute onset usually occurs in patients 2 to 6 years of age.[143] The child acutely presents with respiratory distress, fever, dysphagia, and apprehension. A muffled voice, stridor, assumption of the sitting position with mouth open and chin thrust forward, and drooling are common.

The diagnosis may be confirmed radiographically, although such confirmation should be eliminated if the patient exhibits respiratory distress or cyanosis. The typical radiologic picture shows an enlarged epiglottitis and aryepiglottic folds with obliteration of the valleculae and pyriform sinuses (Figs. 7-13 and 7-14). Glottic and sublottic regions are normal.

Table 7-9. Clinical Evaluation of Croup

Symptom	0	1	2
Stridor	None	Inspiratory	Inspiratory/expiratory
Cough	None	Hoarse	Bark
Air entry	Normal	Decreased	Markedly decreased
Flaring/retractions	None	Flaring/suprasternal	Suprasternal, subcostal, intercostal
Color	Normal	Cyanosis (room air)	Cyanosis (40% oxygen)

If the diagnosis of supraglottitis is even suspected, the patient should be accompanied at all times by a physician knowledgeable in pediatric airway management and tracheal intubation. Equipment for emergency intubation, cricothyrotomy, and a tracheostomy must be available. A source of oxygen and a means of providing ventilation are also essential.

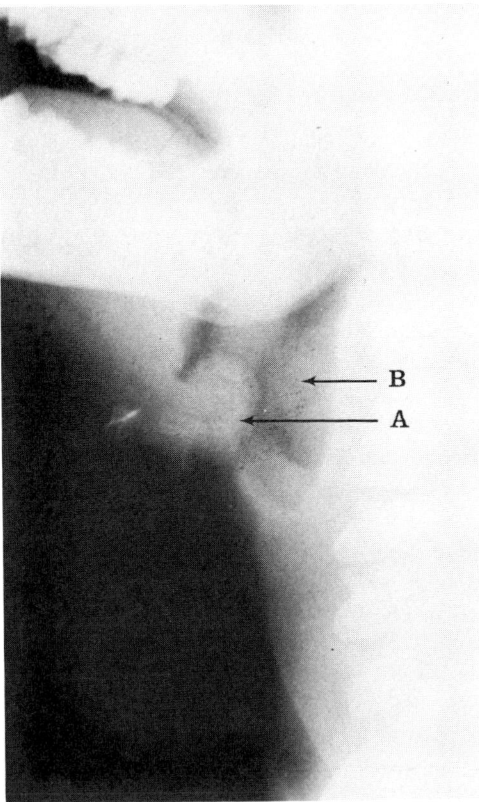

Fig. 7-14. Lateral radiograph of neck demonstrating swollen epiglottis (A) and partial obstruction of upper airway, probably caused by lymph node enlargement (B).

Examination and airway management for supraglottitis should be performed only in the operating room with general anesthesia. Examination of a nonanesthetized child anywhere else may precipitate total airway obstruction. Even waiting to start an IV infusion until the patient is in the operating room and safely anesthetized is preferable.

General anesthesia is induced most commonly by inhalation of oxygen and halothane through a mask with the child in a sitting position. Monitoring should include an oxygen saturation monitor. As anesthesia is induced, the patient usually can be placed in a supine position. Following induction, assisted ventilation usually is relatively easy. When the anesthetic depth is sufficient to permit laryngoscopy, the throat and epiglottis are evaluated. If the diagnosis of supraglottitis is confirmed, an orotracheal tube is inserted, followed by a nasotracheal tube, once IV access is obtained and any other necessary monitors are placed.

Because supraglottitis is frequently caused by *Hemophilus influenzae,*[144] type B, antibiotics should be started. Pharyngolaryngotracheal cultures are positive in 20 to 40 percent of patients, and blood cultures are positive in 50 to 90 percent. *H. influenzae* is often resistant to ampicillin; thus, broad-spectrum agents, including chloramphenicol, should be used until sensitivities are available. Racemic epinephrine and steroids are not of benefit in this disease.

With adequate treatment in the pediatric ICU, patients normally are extubated after 1 to 2 days. They should not have oral intake prior to extubation. Direct observation of the epiglottis should be performed using sedation and muscle relaxants,[145] if necessary, to facilitate inspection. Following extubation, the patient should be observed for 24 hours before transfer to the floor.

Racemic Epinephrine

Studies of croup and of postintubation croup have shown that a racemic mixture of epinephrine delivered by intermittent positive-pressure ventilation (IPPB) reduces edema and dilates the airway. Corkey et al.[146] evaluated children with acute infectious croup. After the diagnosis was made, the patients were given either racemic epinephrine or saline by IPPB followed by examination 15 minutes later. Significant improvement occurred after the epinephrine therapy.

A 2.25 percent solution of racemic epinephrine in a 1:8 dilution is commonly administered.[147] The minimum time between doses is 30 minutes, and they may be repeated as needed or until the response becomes minimal.[133] Although a rapid response usually occurs, relief may be temporary and repeated courses of therapy are common.[149] Routine administration of racemic epinephrine probably is not advisable, since paroxysmal supraventricular tachycardia has been reported.[150] Racemic epinephrine is of no demonstrated value in supraglottitis.

Home Ventilation

Improved medical care permits long-term survival of children with respiratory insufficiency who previously would have died. Some do not require continuous hospitalization but have sufficient residual pulmonary disease to require home support, varying from added oxygen to full mechanical ventilation.[151–156]

Planning the discharge of a patient to home care is not an easy job.[151] Such care is expensive (although not as much as hospitalization) and may require extensive changes to make the home environment suitable.[152] A team of physicians, respiratory therapists, and nurses must be available. Parents should be extensively trained to care for these patients and to develop such skills as tracheal suctioning, changing of tracheotomy tubes, and chest physiotherapy. Knowledge of CPR is essential.

The patient mix is variable and includes primary neurologic diseases, BPD, and congenital heart disease. Equipment needs are variable and many different ventilators have been used. At least two complete circuits should be prepared, and spare parts must be readily available. Other necessary equipment is outlined in Table 7-10.

Table 7-10. Equipment for Home Ventilator Care

Mechanical ventilator
2 circuits, including humidifier
Pressure and volume alarm
Oxygen source (when applicable)
Oxygen analyzer (when applicable)
Self-inflating resuscitator bag
Suction unit
Tracheostomy care items
Cannulas
Ties
Foam
Hemostat
Hydrogen peroxide
Cotton/Telfa pads
Saline vials
Stethoscope
Apnea/cardiac monitor
Intercom

(From Downes & Hersir,[136] with permission.)

Most patients with chronic neuromuscular problems eventually die while receiving home ventilation. Nevertheless, home care provides comfort to them and their families and gives them a sense of belonging. Causes of death in home ventilator patients include ventilator disconnection, accidental decannulation, airway obstruction, hemorrhage, sepsis, pneumonia, progression of the primary disease, recurrent malignancy, and congestive heart failure.[152] Home mechanical ventilation for as long as 20 years has been reported.[153]

REFERENCES

1. Rigatto H: Control of ventilation in the newborn. Annu Rev Physiol 46:661, 1984
2. Martin RJ, Miller MJ, Carlo WA: Pathogenesis of apnea in preterm infants. J Pediatr 109:733, 1986
3. Lee D, Caces R, Kwiatowski K, et al: A developmental study on types and frequency distribu-

tion of short apneas in term and preterm infants. Pediatr Res 22:334, 1987
4. Gerhardt T, Bancalari E: Apnea of prematurity. I. Lung function and regulation of breathing. Pediatrics 74:58, 1984
5. Gerhardt T, Bancalari E: Apnea of prematurity: II. Respiratory reflexes. Pediatrics 74:63, 1984
6. Rigatto H, de la Torre-Verduzco R, Cates DB: Effects of O_2 on the ventilatory response to CO_2 in preterm infants. J Appl Physiol 39:896, 1975
7. Jansen AH, Chernick V: Development of respiratory control. Physiol Rev 63:437, 1983
8. Motoyama EK, Brody JS, Colten HR, et al: Postnatal lung development in health and disease. Am Rev Respir Dis 137:742, 1988
9. Polgar G: Mechanical properties of lung and chest wall. p. 49. In Thibeault DW, Gregory GA (eds): Neonatal Pulmonary Care. 2nd Ed. Appleton-Century-Crofts, E. Norwalk, CT, 1986
10. Keens TG, Bryan AC, Levison H, et al: Developmental pattern of muscle fiber types in human ventilatory muscles. J Appl Physiol 44:909, 1978
11. Muller N, Volgyesi F, Bryan MH, et al: The consequences of diaphragmatic muscle fatigue in the newborn infant. J Pediatr 5:793, 1979
12. Maxwell L, McCarter RJM, Kuehl TJ, et al: Development of histochemical and functional properties of baboon respiratory muscles. J Appl Physiol 54:551, 1983
13. Koch G, Wendel H: Adjustment of arterial blood gases and acid base balance in the normal newborn infant during the first week of life. Biol Neonate 12:136, 1968
14. Orzalesi MM, Mendicini M, Bucci G, et al: Arterial oxygen studies in premature newborns with and without mild respiratory distress. Arch Dis Child 42:174, 1967
15. Witte MK, Galli SA, Charburn RL, et al: Optimal positive end-expiratory pressure therapy in infants and children with acute respiratory failure. Pediatr Res 24:217, 1988
16. Bancalari E, Eisler E: Neonatal respiratory support. p. 243. In Kirby RR, Smith RA, Desautels DA (eds): Mechanical Ventilation. Churchill Livingstone, New York, 1986
17. Avery ME, Tooley WH, Keller JB, et al: Is chronic lung disease in low birthweight infants preventable? A survey of eight centers. Pediatrics 79:26, 1987
18. Engelke SC, Roloff DW, Kuhns LR: Post-extubation nasal continuous positive airway pressure. A prospective controlled study. Am J Dis Child 136:359, 1982
19. Boros SJ: Principles of ventilator care. p. 367. In Thibeault DW, Gregory GA (eds): Neonatal Pulmonary Care. 2nd Ed. Appleton-Century-Crofts, E. Norwalk, CT, 1986
20. Carlo WA, Martin RJ: Principles of assisted ventilation. Pediatr Clin North Am 33:221, 1986
21. Stewart AR, Finer NN, Peters KL: Effects of alterations of inspiratory and expiratory pressures and inspiratory/expiratory ratios on mean airway pressure, blood gases, and intracranial pressure. Pediatrics 67:474, 1981
22. Greenough A, Dixon AK, Roberton NRC: Pulmonary interstitial emphysema. Arch Dis Child 58:612, 1983
23. Hart SM, McNail M, Gamsu HR, et al: Pulmonary interstitial emphysema in very low birthweight infants. Arch Dis Child 58:612, 1983
24. Heicher DA, Kasting DS, Harrod JR: Prospective clinical comparison of two methods for mechanical ventilation of neonates: rapid rate and short inspiratory time versus slow rate and long inspiratory time. J Pediatr 98:957, 1981
25. Primhak R A: Factors associated with pulmonary air leak in premature infants receiving mechanical ventilation. J Pediatr 102:764, 1983
26. Simbruner G: Inadvertent positive end-expiratory pressure in mechanically ventilated newborn infants: detection and effect on lung mechanics and gas exchange. J Pediatr 108:589, 1986
27. Bancalari E: Inadvertent positive end-expiratory pressure during mechanical ventilation. J Pediatr 108:567, 1986
28. Boros SJ, Bing DR, Mammel MC, et al: Using conventional infant ventilators at unconventional rates. Pediatrics 74:487, 1984
29. Boros SJ: Variations in inspiratory:expiratory ratios and airway pressure wave form during mechanical ventilation. The significance of mean airway pressure. J Pediatr 94:114, 1979
30. Perlman JM, Goodman S, Kreusser KL, et al: Reduction in intraventricular hemorrhage by elimination of fluctuating cerebral blood flow velocity in preterm infants with respiratory distress syndrome. N Engl J Med 312:1353, 1985
31. Bancalari E, Gerhardt T, Feller R, et al: Muscle

relaxation during IPPV in prematures with RDS. Pediatr Res 14:590, 1980
32. Stark AR, Bascom R, Frantz ID: Muscle relaxation in mechanically ventilated infants. J Pediatr 94:441, 1979
33. Bhutani VK, Abbasi S, Sivieri EM: Continuous skeletal muscle paralysis: effect on neonatal pulmonary mechanics. Pediatrics 81:419, 1988
34. Greenough A, Greenall F: Patient triggered ventilation in premature neonates. Arch Dis Child 63:78, 1988
35. Corbet A, Adams J: Current therapy in hyaline membrane disease. Clin Perinatol 5:299, 1978
36. Gregory GA: Continuous positive airway pressure. p. 349. In Thibeault DW, Gregory GA (eds): Neonatal Pulmonary Care. 2nd Ed. Appleton-Century-Crofts, E. Norwalk, CT, 1986
37. Sjöstrand U: Experimental and clinical evaluation of high frequency positive pressure ventilation. Acta Anaesthesiol Scand [Suppl] 64:1, 1977
38. Lunkenheimer P P, Rafflebeaul W, Keller A, et al: Application of transtracheal pressure oscillations. Br J Anaesth 44:627, 1972
39. Bohn DJ, Miyasaka K, Marchak BE, et al: Ventilation by high-frequency oscillation. J Appl Physiol 48:710, 1980
40. Smith RB: Ventilation at high respiratory frequencies. Anaesthesia 37:1011, 1982
41. Froese AB, Bryan AC: High frequency ventilation. Am Rev Respir Dis 135:1363, 1987
42. Chang HK: Mechanisms of gas transport during ventilation by high frequency oscillation. J Appl Physiol 56:553, 1984
43. Drazen JM, Kamm RD, Slutsky AS: High-frequency ventilation. Physiol Rev 64:505, 1984
44. Ackerman NG, Null DM, deLemos RA: High-frequency ventilation: history, theory and practice. p. 307. In Kirby RR, Smith RA, Desautels DA (eds): Mechanical Ventilation. Churchill Livingstone, New York, 1985
45. Heijman K, Sjöstrand U: Treatment of the respiratory distress syndrome. A preliminary report. Opuscula Medica 19:235, 1974
46. Boros SJ, Mammel MC, Coleman JM, et al: Neonatal high-frequency jet ventilation: four years' experience. Pediatrics 75:657, 1985
47. Carlo WA, Chatburn RL, Martin RJ: Randomized trial of high-frequency jet ventilation versus conventional ventilation in respiratory distress syndrome. J Pediatr 110:275, 1987
48. Ophoven JP, Mammel MC, Gordon MJ, et al: Tracheobronchial histopathology associated with high frequency jet ventilation. Crit Care Med 12:829, 1984
49. Bancalari A, Gerhardt T, Bancalari E, et al: Gas trapping with high frequency ventilation: jet versus oscillatory ventilation. J Pediatr 110:617, 1987
50. Gaylord MS, Quissell BJ, Lair ME: High-frequency ventilation in the treatment of infants weighing less than 1500 grams with pulmonary interstitial emphysema. A pilot study. Pediatrics 79:915, 1987
51. deLemos RA, Coalson JJ, Gerstmann DR, et al: Ventilatory management of infant baboons with hyaline membrane disease: the use of high frequency ventilation. Pediatr Res 21:594, 1981
52. deLemos RA, Coalson JJ, deLemos JA, et al: Rescue with high frequency oscillatory ventilation "normalizes" the lung inflation pattern in hyaline membrane disease. Am Rev Respir Dis (In press)
53. Carter JM, Gerstmann DR, Clark RH, et al: The roles of high frequency oscillatory ventilation and extracorporeal membrane oxygenation in the treatment of acute neonatal respiratory failure. (Submitted for publication)
54. Cornish JD, Gerstmann DR, Clark RH, et al: Extracorporeal membrane oxygenation and high frequency oscillatory ventilation: potential therapeutic relationships. Crit Care Med 15:831, 1987
55. deLemos RA, Gerstmann DR, Clark RH, et al: High frequency ventilation—The relationship between ventilator design and clinical strategy in the treatment of hyaline membrane disease and its complications. Pediatr Pul 3:370, 1987
56. HIFI Study Group: High-frequency oscillatory ventilation compared with conventional mechanical ventilation in the treatment of respiratory failure in preterm infants. N Engl J Med 320:88, 1989
57. Gregory GA, Brooks J, Wiebe H, et al: The time course changes in lung function after a change in CPAP. Clin Res 25:193, 1977
58. Gregory GA, Kitterman JA, Phibbs RH, et al: Treatment of the idiopathic respiratory distress syndrome with continuous positive airway pressure. N Engl J Med 284:1133, 1971
59. Pollack MM, Fields SI, Holbrook PR: Cardiopulmonary parameters during high PEEP in children. Crit Care Med 7:372, 1980
60. Fox WW, Berman LS, Downes JJ, et al: The

therapeutic application of end-expiratory pressure in meconium aspiration syndrome. Pediatrics 56:214, 1975
61. Gerard P, Fox WW, Outerbridge EW, et al: Early versus late introduction of continuous negative pressure in the management of the idiopathic respiratory distress syndrome. J Pediatr 87:591, 1975
62. Kromstop RM, Brown EG, Sweet AY: The early use of continuous positive airway pressure in the treatment of idiopathic respiratory distress syndrome. J Pediatr 87:263, 1967
63. Allen LP, Reynolds EOR, Rivers RPA, et al: Control trial of continuous positive airway pressure given by face mask for hyaline membrane disease. Arch Dis Child 52:373, 1977
64. deLemos RA, Coalson JJ, Gerstmann DR, et al: Oxygen toxicity in the premature baboon with hyaline membrane disease. Am Rev Respir Dis 136:677, 1987
65. O'Brodovich HM, Melting RB: Bronchopulmonary dysplasia. Am Rev Respir Dis 132:694, 1985
66. Gregory GA, Gooding CA, Phibbs RH, et al: Meconium aspiration in infants—a prospective study. J Pediatr 85:848, 1974
67. Clark DA, Nieman GF, Thompson JE, et al: Surfactant displacement by meconium-free fatty acids: an alternative explanation for atelectasis in meconium aspiration syndrome. J Pediatr 110:765, 1987
68. Anderson WR, Engle RR: Cardiopulmonary sequelae of reparative stages of bronchopulmonary dysplasia. Arch Pathol Lab Med 107:603, 1983
69. Abman SH, Wolfe RR, Accurbo FJ, et al: Pulmonary vascular response to oxygen in infants with severe bronchopulmonary dysplasia. Pediatrics 75:80, 1985
70. Null DM, Yoder B: Bronchopulmonary dysplasia. p. 91. In Kirby RR, Taylor RW (eds): Respiratory Failure. Year Book Medical Publishers, Chicago, 1986
71. Harbison RW, deLemos RA: Neonatal pneumonia. Compr Ther 11:33, 1985
72. Langston C, Thurlbeck WM: Conditions altering normal lung growth and development. p. 1. In Thibeault DW, Gregory GA (eds): Neonatal Pulmonary Care. 2nd Ed. Appleton-Century-Crofts, E. Norwalk, CT, 1986
73. Ackerman NB, Coalson JJ, Kuel TJ, et al: Pulmonary interstitial emphysema in the premature baboon with hyaline membrane disease. Crit Care Med 12:512, 1984
74. Bohn D, Tamura M, Perrin D, et al: Ventilator predictors of pulmonary hypoplasia in congenital diaphragmatic hernia, confirmed by morphologic assessment. J Pediatr 11:423, 1987
75. Swischuk LE, Richardson CJ, Nichols MM, et al: Primary pulmonary hypoplasia in the neonate. J Pediatr 95:573, 1979
76. Cole R, Miodownik S, Carlon G, et al: Pneumatic to electrical analog for high frequency jet ventilation in disrupted airways. Crit Care Med 12:711, 1984
77. Heneghan MA, Sosulski R, Alarcon MB: Early pulmonary interstitial emphysema in the newborn: a grave prognostic sign. Clin Pediatr 7:361, 1987
78. Swischuk LE: Bubbles in hyaline membrane disease: differentiation of types. Radiology 122:417, 1977
79. Brooks JB, Bustamante SA, Koops BL, et al: Selective bronchial intubation for the treatment of severe localized pulmonary interstitial emphysema in newborns. J Pediatr 91:643, 1977
80. Swingle AM, Eggert LD, Bucciarelli RL: New approaches to management of unilateral tension pulmonary emphysema in premature infants. Pediatrics 74:354, 1984
81. Levine DH, Trump DS, Waterkotte G: Unilateral pulmonary interstitial emphysema: a surgical approach to treatment. Pediatrics 68:510, 1981
82. Eyal FC, Arad ID, Godder K, et al: High frequency positive pressure ventilation in neonates. Crit Care Med 12:793, 1984
83. Pokora T, Bing DR, Mammal MC, et al: High frequency jet ventilation. Pediatrics 72:27, 1985
84. Bartlett RH, Gazzaniga AB, Fong SW, et al: Extracorporeal membrane oxygenator support for cardiopulmonary failure: experience in 28 cases. J Thor Cardiovasc Surg 73:375, 1977
85. Kirkpatrick BV, Krummel TM, Mueller D G, et al: Use of extracorporeal membrane oxygenation for respiratory failure in term infants. Pediatrics 72:872, 1983
86. Bartlett RH, Toomasian J, Roloff D, et al: Extracorporeal membrane oxygenation (ECMO) in neonatal respiratory failure. Ann Surg 204:236, 1986
87. Cornish JD: ECMO Clinical Specialist Training Manual. 2nd Ed. The San Diego Regional ECMO Program, 1987
88. Chu J, Clements JA, Cotton E, et al: The pulmo-

nary hypoperfusion syndrome. Pediatrics 35:733, 1965

89. Murphy JD, Rabinovitch M, Goldstein JD, et al: The structural basis of persistent pulmonary hypertension of the newborn. J Pediatr 99:62, 1981
90. Drummond WH: Persistent pulmonary hypertension of the neonate (persistent fetal circulation syndrome). Adv Pediatr 30:61, 1983
91. Geggel RL, Murphy JD, Langleben D, et al: Congenital diaphragmatic hernia: arterial structural changes and persistent pulmonary hypertension after surgical repair. J Pediatr 107:457, 1985
92. Schumacher RE, Barks JDE, Johnston MV, et al: Right-sided brain lesions in infants following extracorporeal membrane oxygenation. Pediatrics 82:155, 1988
93. Jobe A: The role of surfactant in neonatal adaptation. Sem Perinatol 12:113, 1988
94. Hallman M, Merritt TA, Iarvenpaa AL, et al: Exogenous human surfactant for treatment of severe respiratory distress syndrome: a randomized prospective clinical trial. J Pediatr 106:963, 1985
95. Enhorning G, Shennan A, Possmager F, et al: Prevention of neonatal respiratory distress syndrome by tracheal instillation of surfactant. A randomized clinical trial. Pediatrics 76:145, 1985
96. Kwong MS, Egan EA, Notter RH, et al: Double blind clinical trial of calf lung surfactant extract administered at birth to very premature infants for prevention of respiratory distress syndrome. Pediatrics 76:593, 1985
97. Gitlin JD, Soll RF, Parad RB, et al: Randomized controlled trial of exogenous surfactant for the treatment of hyaline membrane disease. Pediatrics 79:31, 1987
98. Collaborative European Multicenter Study Group: Surfactant replacement therapy for severe neonatal respiratory distress syndrome. An international randomized clinical trial. Pediatrics 82:683, 1988
99. Jobe A, Ikegami M: Surfactant for the treatment of respiratory distress syndrome. Am Rev Respir Dis 136:1256, 1987
100. Bjoraker DG, Kumar NB, Brown ACD: Evaluation of an emergency cricothyrotomy instrument. Crit Care Med 15:157, 1987
101. Coté CJ, Eavey RD, Todres ID, et al: Cricothyroid membrane puncture: oxygenation and ventilation in a dog model using an intravenous catheter. Crit Care Med 16:615, 1988
102. Slutsky AS, Watson J, Leith DE, et al: Tracheal insufflation of O_2 (TRIO) at low flow rates sustains life for several hours. Anesthesiology 63:278, 1985
103. Filston HC, Johnson DG, Crumrine RS: Infant tracheostomy: a new look with a solution to the difficult cannulation problem. Am J Dis Child 132:1172, 1978
104. Friedberg J, Morrison MD: Paediatric tracheostomy. Can J Otolaryngol 3:147, 1974
105. Guadet PT, Peerless A, Sasaki CT, et al: Pediatric tracheostomy and associated complications. Laryngoscope 88:1633, 1978
106. Carter P, Benjamen B: Ten-year review of pediatric tracheotomy. Ann Otol Rhinol Laryngol 92:398, 1983
107. Tepas JJ, Heroy JH, Shermeta DW, et al: Tracheostomy in neonates and small infants: problems and pitfalls. Surgery 89:635, 1981
108. Allen TH, Steven IM: Prolonged endotracheal intubation in infants and children. Br J Anaesth 37:566, 1965
109. Fenner F: The classification and nomenclature of viruses: summary of results of meetings of the international committee on taxonomy of viruses in Madrid, September 1975. Virology 71:371, 1976
110. Waterson AP, Hobson D: Relationship between respiratory syncytial virus and Newcastle disease—Parainfluenza group. Br Med J 2:1166, 1962
111. Forsyth BR: Identification of respiratory syncytial virus antigen by agar gel diffusion and immunoelectrophoresis. Proc Soc Exp Biol Med 133:568, 1970
112. Beem M: Repeated infections with respiratory syncytial virus. J Immunol 98:1115, 1967
113. Coates HV, Alling DW, Chanock RM: An antigenic analysis of respiratory syncytial virus isolates by a plague reduction neturalization test. Am J Epidemiol 83:299, 1966
114. Suto T, Yano M, Ikeda M, et al: Respiratory syncytial virus infection and its serologic epidemiology. Am J Epidemiol 82:211, 1965
115. Gardner PS: How etiologic, pathologic, and clinical diagnoses can be made in a correlated fashion. Pediatr Res 11:254, 1977
116. Kim HW, Arrobio JO, Brandt CD, et al: Epidemiology of respiratory syncytial virus infection

in Washington, DC. Am J Epidemiol 98:216, 1973
117. Mufson MA, Levine HD, Wasil RE, et al: Epidemiology of respiratory syncytial virus among infants and children in Chicago. Am J Epidemiol 98:88, 1973
118. Jackson GG, Muldoon RL: Viruses causing common respiratory infections in man. III. Respiratory syncytial viruses and coronaviruses. J Infect Dis 128:674, 1973
119. Coates HV, Channock RM: Clinical significance of respiratory syncytial virus. Postgrad Med 35:460, 1964
120. Berglund B: Respiratory syncytial viruses in families. Acta Paediatr Scand 56:395, 1967
121. Hall CB, Powell KR, MacDonald NE, et al: Respiratory syncytial viral infection in children with compromised immune function. N Engl J Med 315:77, 1986
122. Hall CB, McBride JT, Gala CL, et al: Ribavirin treatment of respiratory syncytial viral infection in infants with underlying cardiopulmonary disease. JAMA 254:3047, 1985
123. Hermans PE, Cockerill FR: Antiviral agents. Mayo Clin Proc 58:217, 1983
124. Isaacs D: Ribavirin. Pediatrics 79:289, 1987
125. Frankel LR, Wilson CW, Demers RR, et al: A technique for the administration of ribavirin to mechanically ventilated infants with severe respiratory syncytial virus infection. Crit Care Med 15:1051, 1987
126. Hicks RA, Olson LC, Jackson MA, et al: Precipitation of ribavirin causing obstruction of a ventilation tube. Pediatr Infect Dis 5:707, 1986
127. Fletcher CM, Pride NB: Definitions of emphysema, chronic bronchitis, asthma, and airflow obstruction: 25 years on from the Ciba symposium. Thorax 39:81, 1984
128. Wagner PD, Dantzker DR, Iacovoni VE, et al: Ventilation perfusion inequality in asymptomatic asthma. Am Rev Respir Dis 118:511, 1978
129. Robotham JL: Obstructive airway disease in infants and children. p. 69. In Kirby RR, Taylor RW (eds): Respiratory Failure. Year Book Medical Publishers, Chicago, 1986
130. Downs JJ, Heiber MS: Status asthmaticus in children. p. 107. In Gregory GA (ed): Respiratory Failure in the Child: Clinics in Critical Care Medicine. Churchill Livingstone, New York, 1981
131. Becker AB, Nilson NA, Simmons FER: Inhaled salbutamol (albuterol) vs. injected epinephrine in the treatment of acute asthma in children. J Pediatr 102:465, 1083
132. Mann NP, Huller EJ: Ipratropium bromide in children with asthma. Thorax 37:72, 1982
133. Leffert F: Asthma: a modern perspective. Pediatrics 62:1061, 1978
134. Downes JJ, Wood DW, Harwood I, et al: Intravenous isoproterenol infusion in children with severe hypercapnia due to status asthmaticus: effects on ventilation and clinical score. Crit Care Med 1:63, 1973
135. Wood DW, Downes JJ, Harwood I, et al: Intravenous isoproterenol in the management of respiratory failure in childhood status asthmaticus. J Allergy Clin Immunol 50:75, 1972
136. Downes JJ, Hersir MS: Status asthmaticus in children. p. 107. In Gregory GA (ed): Respiratory Failure in the Child. Churchill Livingstone, New York, 1981
137. Robertson CF, Smith F, Beck R, et al: Response to frequent low doses of nebulized salbutamol in acute asthma. J Pediatr 106:672, 1985
138. Barach AL; The therapeutic use of helium. JAMA 107:1273, 1936
139. MacIntosh R, Mushin WW, Epstein HG: Physics for the Anesthetist. Blackwell Scientific Publications, Oxford, 1963, p. 192
140. Mink SN, Wood DH: How does HeO_2 increase maximum expiratory flow in human lungs. J Clin Invest 66:720, 1980
141. Berend N, Christopher KL, Voelkel NF: Breathing HeO_2 shifts the lung pressure-volume curve of the dog. J Appl Physiol 54:576, 1983
142. Flashburgh MH, Ramesh I, Patel RI, et al: Pulmonary edema and cardiac arrest in a patient with acute epiglottitis. Anesth Rev 12:42, 1985
143. Daum RS, Bates JR, Smith AL: Epiglottitis (supraglottitis): infection of specific organ systems. p. 138. In Cherry JD, Feigen RD (eds): Textbook of Pediatric Infectious Diseases. WB Saunders, Philadelphia, 1981
144. Sinclair SE: *Hemophilus influenzae* type B in acute laryngitis with bacteremia. JAMA 117:170, 1941
145. Rothstein P, Lister G: Epiglottitis. Anesth Analg 62:785, 1983
146. Corkey CWB, Barker GA, Edmonds JF, et al: Radiographic tracheal diameter measurements in acute infectious croup. Crit Care Med 9:587, 1981

147. Krusela AL, Vesikari T: A randomized double-blind placebo-controlled trial of dexamethasone and racemic epinephrine in the treatment of croup. Acta Paediatr Scand 77:99, 1988
148. Westley CR, Cotton EK, Brooke JG: Nebulized racemic epinephrine by IPPB for the treatment of croup. Am J Dis Child 132:484, 1978
149. Jordan WS, Graves CL, Elwyn RA: New therapy for postintubation laryngeal edema and tracheitis in children. JAMA 212:585, 1970
150. Caldwell CC, Leukoff AH, Purohit DM: Paroxysmal supraventricular tachycardia in a neonate. Clin Pediatr 16:579, 1977
151. Ad Hoc Task Forces on Home Care of Chronically Ill Infants and Children: Guidelines for home care of infants, children, and adolescents with chronic disease. Pediatrics 74:434, 1984
152. Schreiner MS, Donar ME, Kettrick RG: Pediatric home mechanical ventilation. Pediatr Clin North Am 34:47, 1987
153. Frates RC, Splaingard ML, Smith EO, et al: Outcome of home mechanical ventilation in children. J Pediatr 106:850, 1985
154. Burr BH, Guyer B, Todres ID, et al: Home care for children on ventilators. N Engl J Med 309:1319, 1983
155. Goldberg AI, Faure EAM, Vaughn CJ, et al: Home care for life-supported persons: An approach to program development. J Pediatr 104:785, 1984
156. Alexander MA, Johnson EW, Petty J, et al: Mechanical ventilation of patients with late stage duchenne muscular dystrophy: Management in the home. Arch Phys Med Rehabil 60:289, 1979
157. Banner MJ: Technical aspects of high frequency ventilation. Curr Rev Respir Ther 7:89, 1985
158. Banner MJ, Smith RA: Mechanical ventilation. p. 1178. In Civetta JM, Taylor RW, Kirby RR (eds): Critical Care. JB Lippincott, Philadelphia, 1988
159. Chantarojanasiri: Lower airway disease: bronchiolitis and asthma. p. 216. In Rogers M (ed): Textbook of Pediatric Intensive Care. Williams & Wilkins, Baltimore, 1987

8

Special Ventilatory Techniques and Considerations

Michael J. Banner
David A. Desautels

Conventional ventilatory techniques and principles are usually appropriate for conditions that arise daily in the intensive care unit (ICU). Occasions do occur, however, when special ventilatory techniques are indicated. Under these conditions, conventional methods of ventilation may fail, necessitating specialized methods, such as independent lung ventilation (ILV) and high-frequency jet ventilation (HFJV). Indications for mechanical ventilation and life support may also arise in environments other than the ICU. Safety, reliability, practicality, and logistical considerations should be addressed when providing ventilatory support in atypical environments, such as during transport and in a hyperbaric chamber.

INDEPENDENT LUNG VENTILATION

On occasion, pulmonary parenchymal involvement may be confined to one lung or lobe; atelectasis, aspiration pneumonia, or contusion are common examples (Fig. 8-1). Attempts to use conventional techniques, such as continuous positive airway pressure (CPAP) or mechanical ventilation to restore lung volume and improve oxygenation, may fail. Instead, more specialized methods are needed.[1,2]

Simple alterations of body position can directly influence blood gas exchange. In the upright position, dependent alveoli are maximally compressed at end-exhalation compared with those in the nondependent portions of the lung. However, the dependent alveoli receive a greater proportion of total gas flow during inspiration. The majority of pulmonary blood flow is also partitioned to the dependent lung areas and thereby maximizes the optimal alveolar ventilation to perfusion ratio ($\dot{V}A/\dot{Q}$).

In cases of unilateral lung involvement, when the goal is to improve gas exchange, the patient should be moved into the lateral decubitus position. This maneuver can be simplified using a special bed.[3] With the uninvolved lung down, inspired gas and blood are preferentially distributed to that side during spontaneous breathing. Confirmation of optimal positioning can be elicited by turning the patient 180 degrees and placing the involved lung down. Blood gases should then deteriorate.

Unfortunately, positioning does not always substantially improve oxygenation, and lung volume may need to be increased. Application of CPAP and mechanical ventilation can actually cause further deterioration. Compliance of the diseased lung is decreased so that positive airway pressure preferentially influences the

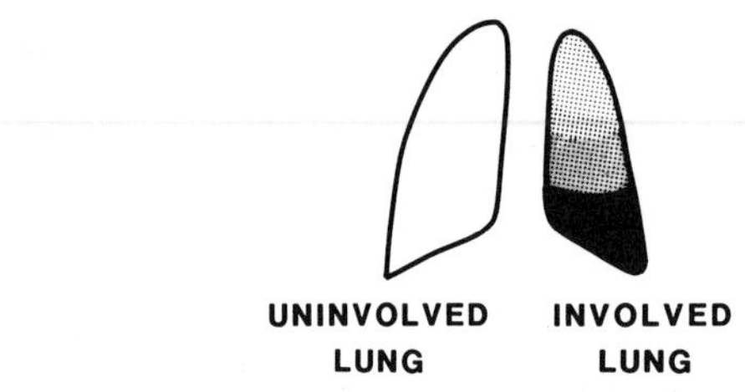

	UNINVOLVED LUNG	INVOLVED LUNG
COMPLIANCE	NORMAL	↓
FRC	NORMAL	↓
$\dot{V}_A/\dot{Q}$	NORMAL	↓

Fig. 8-1. Unilateral pathophysiology: atelectasis, pneumonia, aspiration, or contusion occurring in only one lung. Compliance, functional residual capacity (FRC), and alveolar ventilation/perfusion matching ($\dot{V}A/\dot{Q}$) are decreased only in the involved lung.

healthy lung and produces overdistention and an abnormally high $\dot{V}A/\dot{Q}$. Not only are these alveoli now overdistended, but the resulting increase in pressure shifts blood away from the normal lung to diseased areas with a decrease of $\dot{V}A/\dot{Q}$ (Fig. 8-2). Under such circumstances, if CPAP does not restore appropriate function, ILV is initiated to prevent the previously described problems of $\dot{V}A/\dot{Q}$ mismatch.

Normally, the right lung receives 60 percent of the tidal volume (VT), and attempts are made to maintain that ratio during ILV. Devices are currently available for ILV.[1,2,4,5] All provide complete control and isolation of VT and CPAP to each lung by synchronizers attached to separate ventilators or a single ventilator. These synchronizers may not be necessary, however, as long as inspiration to each lung is not more than 90 degrees out of phase.

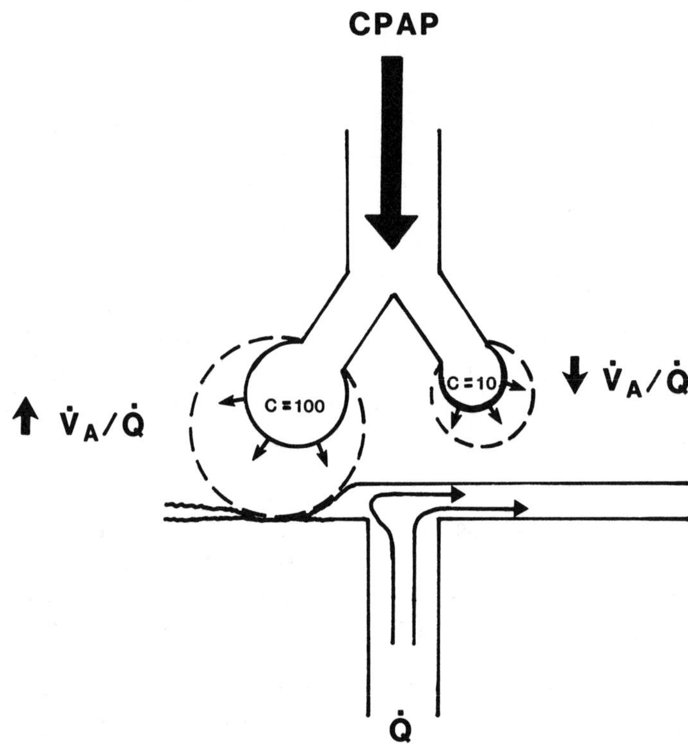

Fig. 8-2. Ventilation maldistribution with conventional application of CPAP to lungs with differential compliance (C). Grossly overdistended healthy lung with a C of 100 ml/cm H_2O compresses pulmonary capillaries and directs perfusion to the low compliant involved lung, predisposing to severe alveolar ventilation/perfusion ($\dot{V}A/\dot{Q}$) mismatching. Thus, conventionally applied CPAP is inappropriate for treating unilateral pathophysiology.

A double-lumen endotracheal tube permits isolation of each lung and permits independent lung therapy. CPAP and mechanical ventilation [e.g., intermittent mandatory ventilation (IMV)] can then be directed only when needed to provide the appropriate support necessary to restore function to each lung (Fig. 8-3). This tube should be treated with great care; the narrow lumen on each side is more difficult to suction, and there is a greater likelihood of obstruction by mucus plugs. Correct placement can be confirmed by clamping one lumen of the double-lumen endotracheal tube, both of which are attached to a conventional self-inflating bag. Breath sounds should stop in the lung on the clamped side but continue on the contralateral side. Not all cuffs on double-lumen tubes are of the preferred high-volume/low-pressure type; therefore, care must be taken to select a proper size and not to overinflate the cuff.

Independent lung ventilation is continued until the disease process is corrected enough that the difference in CPAP levels between the two lungs is 5 cm H_2O. At this point, the double-lumen endotracheal tube is removed and a standard single-lumen tube is inserted in order to apply CPAP and IMV in the conventional manner.

HIGH-FREQUENCY JET VENTILATION

The term *high-frequency ventilation* is a generic one encompassing three primary techniques: high-frequency positive-pressure ventilation (HFPPV), high-frequency jet ventilation (HFJV), and high-frequency oscillation (HFO). Most clinical experience in the United States is with HFJV, which has received considerable attention as an alternate mode of mechanical ventilation. Gas is accelerated through a 14-gauge injector cannula and lateral pressure decreases below the ambient level at the nozzle or outlet of the injector. The result is gas entrain-

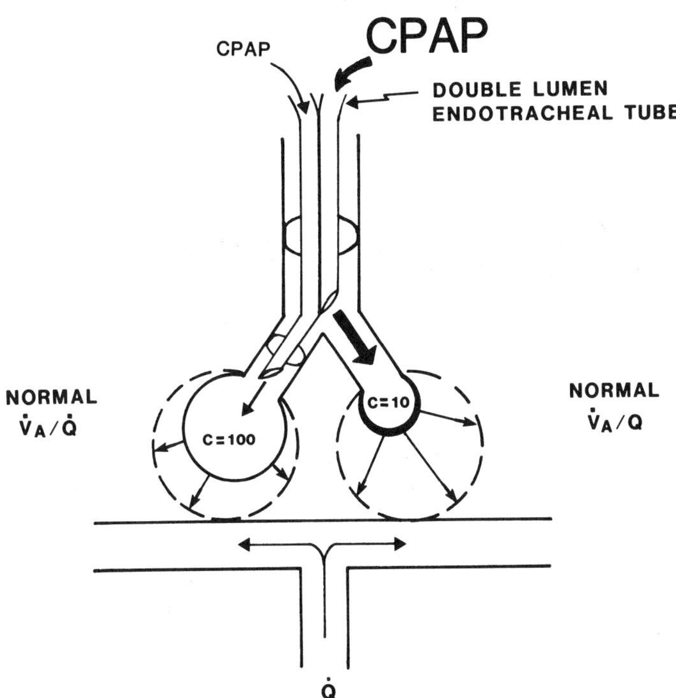

Fig. 8-3. Independent lung ventilation. Lungs are isolated with a double-lumen endotracheal tube, and a greater level of CPAP is applied only to the involved lung. Thus, overall normal alveolar ventilation/perfusion ($\dot{V}_A/\dot{Q}$) matching is maximized. FRC is restored to the involved lung (see text). C, compliance.

ment, which contributes significantly to the inspiratory flow rate and V_T[6,7] (Fig. 8-4).

Inspiratory flow and pressure waveforms with HFJV presumably are rectilinear and linear, respectively; however, as lung-thorax compliance (C_{LT}) decreases and/or airway resistance (R_{AW}) increases, peak flow rate delivery and V_T are decreased and airway pressure is increased[8] (Fig. 8-5). Tidal volume also decreases as the level of PEEP/CPAP is increased,[9] and jet entrainment is inhibited by increased airway/alveolar backpressure.[10,11]

Most HFJV systems are electrically and pneumatically powered with a conventional 50-psig gas power source. An adjustable pressure regulator, built into the ventilator, is used to adjust

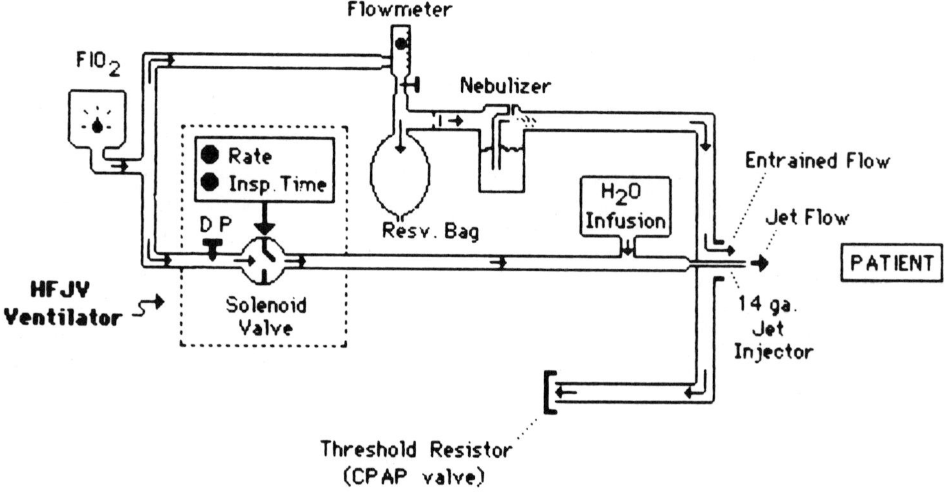

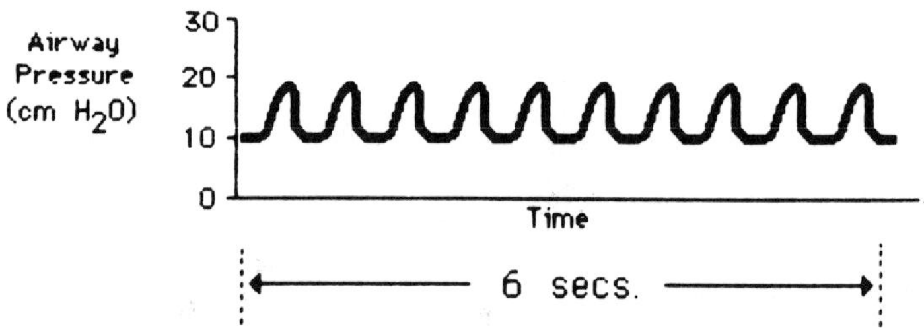

Fig 8-4. High-frequency jet ventilation (HFJV) system. Gas under pressure (50 psig) at a known F_IO_2 is directed to the HFJV ventilator and a flowmeter. Drive pressure, adjustable from 5 to 50 psig, is directed into the ventilator's solenoid valve. The opened/closed rate (ventilator rate) and the duration the solenoid valve is open (inspiratory time) are electronically controlled. V_T is directly proportional to the drive pressure and inspiratory time settings. A continuous flow rate from the flowmeter (15 to 20 L/min) is sent through the circuit. During inhalation, gas is accelerated through a 14-gauge injector that creates subatmospheric pressure at its outlet and causes additional gas to be entrained. V_T equals injector volume plus entrained volume. Airway pressure is measured in the endotracheal tube about 15 cm distal to the injector outlet (not shown). Humidification is provided by infusing water (20 to 30 ml/h) directly into the jet stream and entraining nebulized water. A threshold resistor valve is used to control the level of CPAP. An HFJV rate of 100 breaths/min with a CPAP of 10 cm H_2O is shown above.

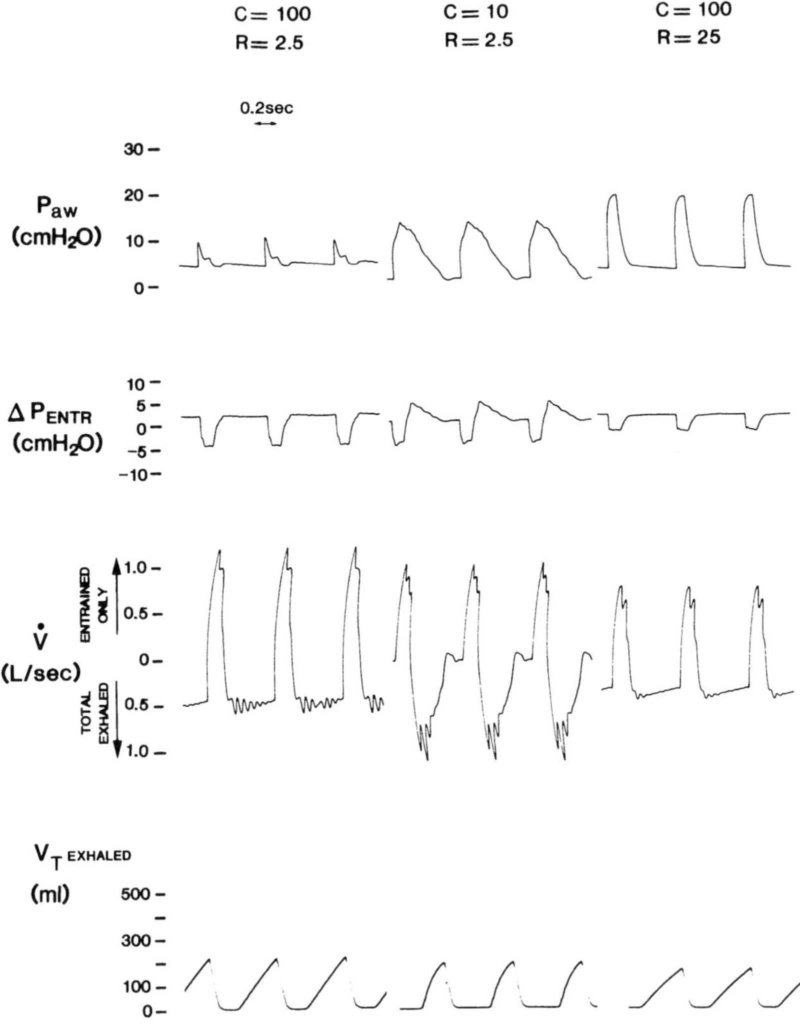

Fig. 8-5. Airway pressure (PAW), the change in jet entrainment pressure (Δ Pentr), entrained and total exhaled flow rate (V̇), and exhaled volume (VT) during HFJV under various conditions of compliance (C) (ml/cm H_2O) and resistance (R) (cm H_2O/L/sec). The HFJV rate was 100 breaths/min, at a 20 percent inspiratory time, and a jet drive pressure of 25 psig. When C was decreased, PIP increased, the Δ Pentr and entrained V̇ decreased and as a result, VT decreased from 220 ml to 190 ml, representing a 3-L decrease in minute ventilation. When R was increased, PIP increased further, in turn, resulting in a lower Δ Pentr, entrained V̇ and thus VT, (i.e., 160 ml), representing a 6-L decrease in minute ventilation.

the driving pressure from 5 to 50 psig. A solenoid valve-actuated system is used to control frequency and inspiratory time; this type of cycling mechanism is reliable and easy to operate. The simple design provides independent control of ventilator rate and inspiratory time (Fig. 8-4).

Three controls are common to HFJV: drive pressure, rate, and percentage of inspiratory time (%TI). The drive pressure directly affects VT and peak inflation pressure (PIP) (i.e., increased drive pressure increases VT and PIP). The %TI control regulates the duration of inspiration. At a rate of 100 breaths/min, the entire

Table 8-1. Characteristics of High-Frequency Jet Ventilation

Frequency	100–150 breaths/min
Injector type	1. 14-gauge steel cannula (internal diameter = 1.7 mm; length = 10 2. Lumen embedded in side wall of endotracheal tube
Cycling mechanism	Time
% Inspiratory time	20–30% respiratory cycle
Drive pressure	5–50 psig (directly affects peak inflation pressure, tidal volume, and minute ventilation)
Tidal volume	Injector flow plus entrained flow (100–300 ml)
Inspiratory flow pattern	Square
Exhalation	Passive

(From Civetta et al.,[39] with permission.)

ventilatory cycle is 0.6 second; if a 20 percent TI is selected, inspiratory time is 0.12 second and expiratory time is 0.48 second. Thus, the inhalation-to-exhalation time ratio (I:E) is approximately 1:4 or 0.25. Such values commonly are employed in adult and pediatric patients. The overall characteristics of HFJV are summarized in Table 8-1.

A special endotracheal tube with a jet injector lumen embedded in its side wall has been used for HFJV in lieu of the "traditional" 14-gauge jet injector. At the same ventilator settings, the latter demonstrates significantly greater PIP, peak-entrained flow, and exhaled VT than is found in the injector lumen endotracheal tube.[12]

Another technique employs a sliding Venturi device (Percussionaire Corp., Sandpoint, ID).[13] A pulsatile jet flow is delivered into a Venturi tube that provides gas entrainment. Comparisons of the sliding Venturi device, the 14-gauge injector, and the injector lumen endotracheal tube methods at identical ventilator settings in subjects with acute respiratory failure revealed that VT was greatest with the sliding Venturi, less with the 14-gauge injector, and least with the injector lumen endotracheal tube. Arterial PCO_2 ($PaCO_2$) showed the converse relationship; that is, $PaCO_2$ was lowest with the sliding Venturi and greatest with the injector lumen endotracheal tube.[14] The sliding Venturi has also been used to provide HFJV with inhalational anesthesia during extracorporeal shock-wave lithotripsy (ESWL).[15]

Indications

Indications for HFJV are summarized in Table 8-2. Two deserve special mention.

Table 8-2. Indications for and Complications of High-Frequency Jet Ventilation

Established indications
- Bronchopleural fistula
- Bronchoscopy
- Laryngoscopy

Possible indications
- Excessive PIP—may predispose to pulmonary barotrauma, decreased cardiac output, and increased intracranial pressure; lower airway pressures with HFJV might minimize these problems.
- Hyaline membrane disease—Low PIP with HFJV may decrease the incidence of bronchopulmonary dysplasia.
- Emergency percutaneous transtracheal jet ventilation—for upper airway obstruction, crushed larynx, and similar conditions.

Complications
- Inadequate humidification
- Damage to tracheal mucosa—shear forces from the high-velocity jet pulses may damage these tissues.

(From Civetta et al.,[39] with permission.)

Airway Disruption

Critically sick patients in respiratory failure are at risk of the development of forms of airway disruption, such as bronchopleural fistula (BPF). A BPF is an abnormal passage or communication between the pulmonary parenchyma and the intrapleural space. Patients in whom this complication occurs as a result of positive-pressure ventilation (PPV) present a significant therapeutic challenge, which has been met with variable success.[16–18] Pneumonectomy, lobectomy, barotrauma, and intrapleural infections are predisposing factors for a BPF. Loss of a substantial amount of inspired V_T results, so that the effectiveness of mechanical ventilation is reduced. V_T with conventional mechanical ventilation (CMV) takes the path of least resistance during mechanical inhalation, which is observed as air bubbling through the underwater trap in the suction apparatus. When air is leaking and a major portion of the ventilator V_T exits via the chest tube, there is a decrease in the effective V_T available to inflate uninvolved portions of the lungs. The detrimental effects of the air leak predispose the patient to progressive atelectasis, decreased $\dot{V}_A/\dot{Q}$, and gas exchange.

With CMV, high PIP is generated when large tidal volumes are delivered to patients with decreased lung compliance and BPF. Airway pressures greater than the critical opening pressure of the BPF (airway pressure level associated with the onset of flow leakage through the fistula site) promote opening of the fistula and egress of flow through the BPF (Fig. 8-6), resulting in a loss of V_T. In addition to high PIP, inspiratory time is a factor in affecting fistula leak flow. The portion of the mechanical inspiratory phase spent at pressures higher than the critical opening pressure of the BPF directly affects the amount of tidal volume loss through the fistula. Thus, both the pressure gradient across the fistula site and the time during which the area of the BPF is open and enlarged adversely affect ventilation and promote even greater enlargement of the BPF, exacerbating the problem.

Ventilation of patients with airway disruption, such as a BPF, is a major indication for HFJV. The ability of HFJV to maintain adequate gas exchange and minimize fistula leak flow in the presence of large BPF and other sources of airway disruption has been well documented.[8,19–21] Lower PIP and smaller tidal volumes, relative to CMV, are characteristic of HFJV. Airway inflation pressures less than the critical opening pressure of the BPF precludes opening of the fistula and loss of inspired V_T (Fig. 8-6A). However, gas flow leakage through the fistula during HFJV persists when the PIP is greater than the critical opening pressure of the BPF (Fig. 8-6B). Only when PIP with HFJV is less than the critical opening pressure of the BPF will egress of flow through the fistula be prevented. Minimizing/preventing fistula leak flow may hasten granulation and healing and, thus, spontaneous closure of the fistula.

Lower Airway Pressures

The theoretical advantages of HFJV over CMV are less barotrauma due to lower PIP (Fig. 8-6) and less interference with the cardiovascular system by mechanical cycling.[21] Tilden et al.[22] used HFJV successfully to ventilate a pediatric patient in postoperative respiratory failure who could not be adequately ventilated on CMV and required high PIP. PIP on CMV was up to 80 cm H_2O, pneumomediastinum was diagnosed, and arterial blood gas (ABG) analysis revealed PaO_2 and $PaCO_2$ of 82 and 59 mmHg, respectively. After switching to HFJV, PIP decreased to 23 cm H_2O (71 percent decrease), the pneumomediastinum resolved over time, and the PaO_2 and $PaCO_2$ improved to 186 and 44 mmHg, respectively, on the same fractional concentration of inspired oxygen (F_IO_2) as during CMV.

Reasons cited for instituting HFJV include a PIP greater than 70 cm H_2O with barotrauma.[21] Tilden's patient met these criteria and lower airway pressures, resolution of the pneumomediastinum, and substantial improvements in oxygenation and carbon dioxide elimination resulted when HFJV was instituted.

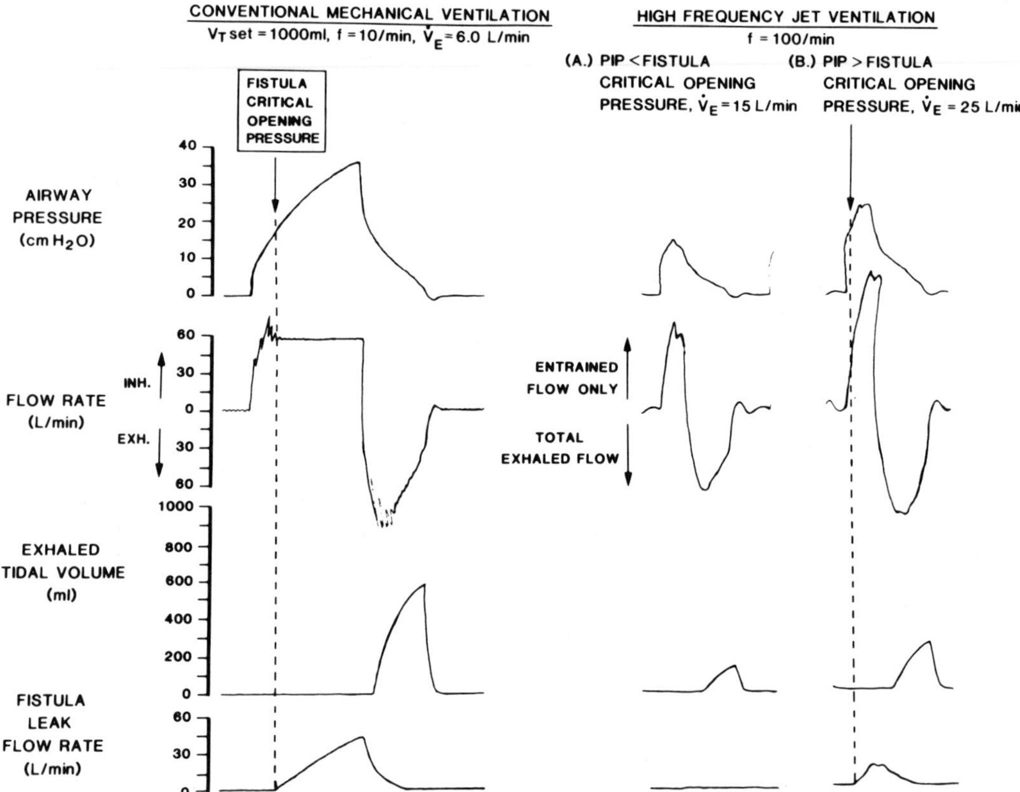

Fig. 8-6. Comparison of conventional mechanical ventilation (CMV) and HFJV under conditions of a bronchopleural cutaneous fistula (BPF). The critical opening pressure of the BPF (airway pressure level associated with the onset of flow leakage through the BPF) was approximately 20 cm H_2O. During CMV at a frequency (f) of 10 breaths/min, the PIP exceeded the critical opening pressure, resulting in a substantial leak. Set/delivered VT was 1,000 ml, while exhaled VT was 600 ml (400 ml leak through the BPF). Note that the exhaled minute ventilation ($\dot{V}E$) was 6 L/min rather than the expected 10 L/min. **(A)** During HFJV, at a frequency of 100 breaths/min and an exhaled VT of 150 ml, PIP was less than the critical opening pressure of the BPF; as a result, no leak through the BPF occurred and $\dot{V}E$ increased to 15 L/min. **(B)** Even though HFJV was used at the same frequency, PIP was greater than the critical opening pressure of the BPF, resulting in a leak through the fistula. HFJV is effective in ventilating the patient and preventing egress of flow through the fistula only when PIP is less than the critical opening pressure of the BPF.

Complications

Complications of HFJV are listed in Table 8-2. Inadequate humidification is one of the more common problems reported.[6] Anhydrous gas, delivered at high flow rates, causes secretions to inspissate, particularly in the endotracheal tube; in some instances, total occlusion has occurred, requiring immediate extubation and reintubation.[6] Deleterious effects on the respiratory mucosa and the airways result from breathing dry gas. To minimize this problem, water is infused into the jet stream and nebulized directly into the airway (Fig. 8-4). Humidity is easily controlled by regulating the drip rate of the water infusion pump; however, care must be taken to avoid fluid overload. An infusion rate of approximately 20 to 30 ml/h appears satisfactory for most patients.[7]

Another potential complication arises with

the injector lumen endotracheal tube. If the tip of the endotracheal tube and the orifice of the injector lumen is at or near the carina, and the orifice of the injector lumen is "aimed" toward a mainstem bronchus, the bulk of the inhaled flow is directed to one lung, predisposing to maldistribution of ventilation. This problem can be minimized by positioning the endotracheal tube an appropriate distance (approximately 5 to 10 cm) from the carina.[23]

VENTILATORY SUPPORT DURING TRANSPORT

Selection of mechanical ventilatory devices, oxygen power systems, and other respiratory life-support equipment to transport patients suffering acute respiratory failure demands careful attention. Requirements for inter- and intrahospital transport arise daily.

In most instances, self-inflating bags suffice for transferring the intubated, postoperative patient from the operating room to the recovery room or ICU. A patient with acute respiratory failure may need to be moved from the ICU to other areas for diagnostic procedures, such as fluoroscopy, angiography, or computed tomography (CT) scans. During intrahospital transport, supplemental oxygen, CPAP, CMV, or IMV may be necessary. Interhospital transportation of the critically ill often involves aircraft ambulances. For transporting a mechanically ventilated patient, a transport ventilator, adequate oxygen supply, and emergency airway equipment are required.[24] Therefore, maintaining life-support during intra- and interhospital transport is a critical aspect of mechanical ventilatory therapy.

Choice of Ventilator

Mechanical ventilation during transport is often administered with a manual self-inflating bag (e.g., Ambu), a flow-inflating (Mapleson) system, or an oxygen-powered breathing device (Elder demand valve or similar device). However, because the VT, respiratory rate, minute ventilation, PIP, and FIO_2 delivered by these manually operated devices may vary from breath to breath, a portable time-cycled ventilator is a better alternative (Table 8-3 and Fig. 8-7). Mechanical ventilators typically used in the ICU are large and cumbersome and therefore impractical for the transportation of ventilator-dependent patients. Certain characteristics are desirable for a transport ventilator (Table 8-4). It must be light enough for one person to carry easily, compact enough to be stored in a locker or on a bed, and suitable both for adults and for children.[25,26] In addition, the ventilator controls must be easily identified and used. The IMV bird (Bird Products Corp., Palm Springs, CA), a time-cycled ventilator that incorporates a demand-flow valve CPAP system, satisfies the

Table 8-3. Characteristics of a Time-Cycled Ventilator

Mechanical inhalation is terminated after a preselected inspiratory time (TI) elapses.

Tidal volume (VT) = TI (sec) × inspiratory flow rate (ml/sec)

$$\text{Peak inflation pressure (PIP)} = \frac{\text{TI} \times \text{inspiratory flow rate}}{\text{lung-thorax compliance}}$$

$$\text{For example, PIP} = \frac{2 \text{ sec} \times 500 \text{ ml/sec}}{20 \text{ ml/cm } H_2O} = 50 \text{ cm } H_2O$$

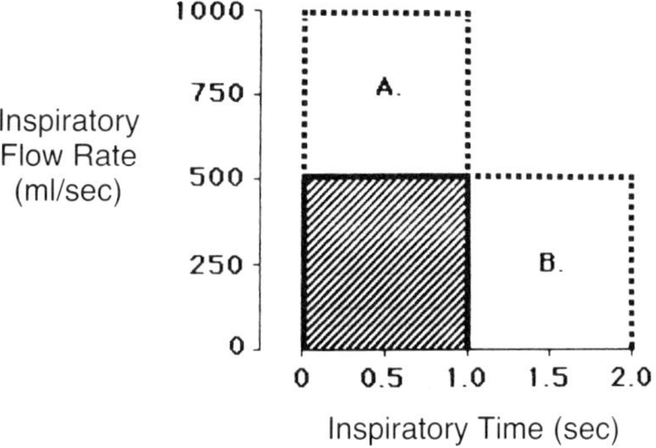

Fig. 8-7. With a time cycled ventilator, mechanical inhalation is terminated after a preselected inspiratory time elapses. Tidal volume is the product of inspiratory flow rate and inspiratory time, and is represented as the area under the curve. The shaded curve represents a VT of 500 ml. Tidal volume may be increased to 1,000 ml either by increasing flow rate **(A)** or by increasing inspiratory time **(B)**.

Table 8-4. Characteristics of a Transport Ventilator

CPAP ≤ 30 cm H_2O (an upper limit has not been established)
Demand flow rate capabilities ≤ 120 L/min during spontaneous ventilation
Time-cycled (see Table 8-3 and Fig. 8-8)
Range of IMV of 2–45 breaths/min
PIP ≤ 150 cm H_2O
Peak mechanical inspiratory flow rate ≤ 120 L/min
A range of FIO_2 of 0.21–1.0
Humidification capabilities
Pneumatically powered
Lightweight (approximately 10–20 lb)
Gas consumption should be minimal

CPAP, continuous positive airway pressure; IMV, intermittent mandatory ventilation; PIP, peak inflation pressure.

criteria listed in Table 8-4 for transferring adult and pediatric patients within the hospital and for interhospital flights. We have transported more than 100 patients with this ventilator (Fig. 8-8). The Bear Cub infant ventilator (Bear Medical, Riverside, CA) is recommended for the transportation of newborn patients with acute respiratory failure. This ventilator satisfies the criteria listed in Table 8-4, with the exceptions that it requires both pneumatic and electronic power sources and that lower levels of CPAP (up to 30 cm H_2O), peak inspiratory flow rates (up to 30 L/min), VT (up to 200 ml), and higher ventilator rates (up to 60/min) are capable of being provided.

A variety of portable ventilators have been designed specifically for transporting ventilator-dependent patients. These ventilators range in cost, size, complexity of operation, and modalities of ventilation that can be provided (Table 8-5). The Hamilton adult/pediatric transport ventilator (Max) typifies this group of miniature ventilators (Fig. 8-9). The ventilator is small (2.5 in. × 7.5 in. × 5.5 in.), lightweight (4 lb), and is pneumatically (e.g., E size O_2 cylinder) and battery-powered. It is time-cycled and can provide IMV, CMV, expiratory positive airway pressure (EPAP), and continuous positive-pressure ventilation (CPPV) at an FIO_2 of 1.0. (Variable FIO_2 may be provided if a pneumatic power system as shown in Fig. 8-8 is used.)

Simplicity of operation is essential for the safe and efficient use of a transport ventilator.[26]

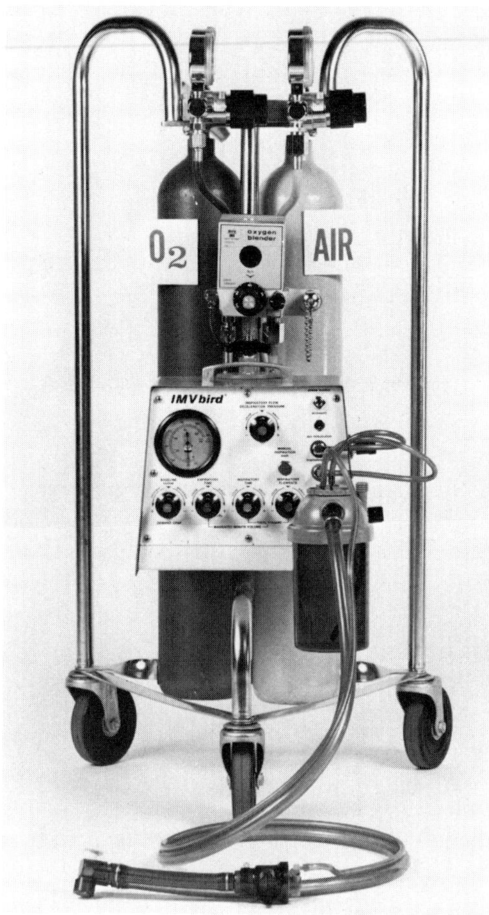

Fig. 8-8. IMV bird is a time-cycled, pneumatically powered ventilator. Two E-sized cylinders (one oxygen and one air), yoked together and connected to an oxygen/air blender, provide pneumatic power; FIO_2 is regulated by an air/oxygen blender.

The aforementioned ventilator, for example, has two control knobs: one for the ventilator rate (range 6 to 30 breaths/min) and the other for the delivered tidal volume (range 100 to 1,500 ml). The operator merely sets the breathing rate and then adjusts the tidal volume control knob to ensure adequate chest rise and fall during ventilator cycling. The ventilator has an adjustable overpressure governor that limits the PIP from about 20 to 150 cm H_2O. A demand-flow valve is incorporated into the ventilator to provide gas-flow rate for spontaneous breathing.

Table 8-5. Representative Listing of Adult/Pediatric (Not Infant) Transport Ventilators

	Hamilton	IMV Bird	Bird Transport	Ohmeda Logic	Healthdyne 105	Penlon 350	Bio-Med IC-2A	Newport 1100	PneuPac
Size (in.)	3 × 11.5 × 6	9 × 10 × 9	2.5 × 2.8 × 3.5	8.5 × 7.25 × 4.8	11.8 × 10 × 6.7	6.5 × 6.6 × 3	3.4 × 6.3 × 10.2	9.5 × 7 × 6	7 × 3.4 × 2.5
Weight (lb)	5	10	3.1	10.6	21	8.8	9	12	3
Modalities of ventilation	IMV, CMV, CPPV, spontaneous PEEP	CMV,IMV CPAP,CPPV	CMV	CMV,CPPV	IMV,CMV, CPPV,CPAP	CMV,CPPV	IMV,CMV, CPPV,CPAP	IMV,CMV, CPPV,CPAP	CMV,CPPV
Tidal volume range (ml)	100–1,500	50–2,000	10–2,700	100–2,000	10–4,000	10–2,300	160–2,800	110–2,570	35–1,000
Peak mechanical inspiratory flow rate (L/min)	90	110	200	70	70	60	75	90	40
Demand-flow capability	Demand-flow valve	Demand-flow valve	None	None	Continuous flow rate	None	Available flow for spontaneous breathing[c]	Continuous flow rate	None
Peak spontaneous inspiratory flow rate on demand (L/min)	120	120	—	—	60	—	75	15	—
Inspiratory time (sec)	1.0	0.5–3.0	0.1–4.0	0.25–2.0	0.1–5.0	0.2–2.0	0.4–2.0	0.1–3.0	0.3–1.4
Peak inflation pressure (cm H_2O)	>150	120	135	90	85	80	100	150	80
Airway pressure manometer (cm H_2O)	0–150	0–120	0–120 (optional)	0–100	0–100	0–100	0–100	0–80	None
FiO_2	1.0[a]	1.0[a]	1.0[a]	0.5 or 1.0[a]	1.0[a]	1.0[a]	1.0[a]	1.0[a]	1.0[a]
Cycling mechanism	Time	Time	Time	Time	Time	Time	Time	Time or pressure	Time
CPAP/PEEP range (cm H_2O)	5–20[b]	1–35	None	1–20	1–25	1–20	1–20	1–25	1–20
Alarms	Yes	None	None	Yes	Yes	None	None	Yes	None

[a] FiO_2 is 1.0 when powered by an O_2 cylinder, variable FiO_2 may be provided using an air/O_2 blender with air and O_2 sources.

[b] End-expiratory pressure is provided using a threshold resistor valve (Vital Signs, Totawa, NJ).

[c] During spontaneous inhalation, the ventilator switches on, but the exhalation valve remains depressurized to allow venting of gas to the atmosphere. Depending on the inspiratory flow rate, and time settings, gas flow rate for a specific duration of time is available for spontaneous breathing. The system does not function as a demand-flow valve system.

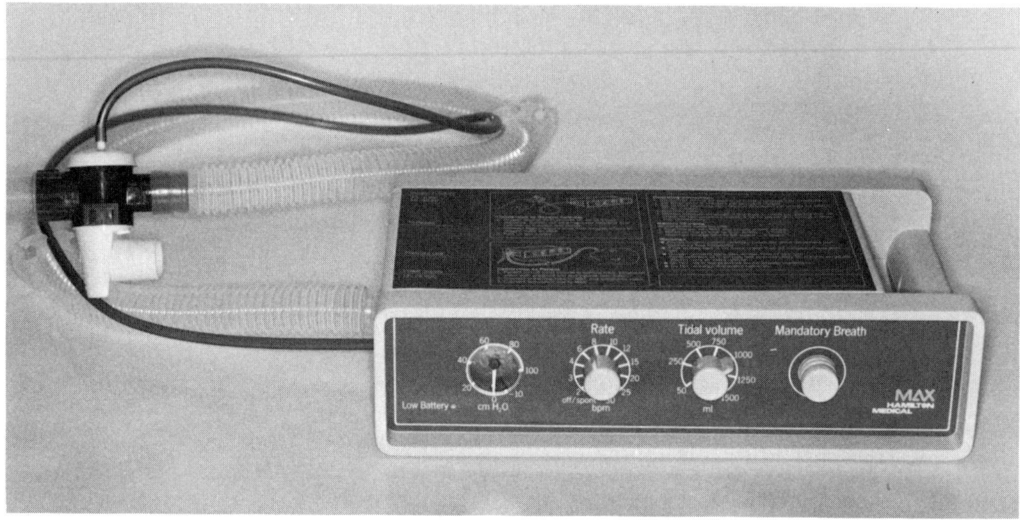

Fig. 8-9. An example of a portable, easy to operate, transport ventilator for adult and pediatric (not newborn) patients (Max, Hamilton Medical, Reno, NV). One control sets the ventilator rate, and the other, the VT. A demand-flow valve automatically provides gas flow for spontaneous breathing.

Peak flow rates up to 120 L/min may be provided on demand.

Transport- and ICU-type ventilators should be capable of generating high PIP and constant inspiratory flow waveforms with minimal flow rate deterioration when ventilating patients with decreased CLT and/or increased RAW (Fig. 8-10). Hypercapnia and hypoxemia will result when using a transport ventilator that is unable to generate sufficient airway pressure and flow rate. Therefore, we recommend that clinicians choose a transport ventilator that can ventilate adult and pediatric patients under conditions of high, as well as low, CLT and RAW.

Oxygen Supply

A self-contained oxygen supply for transport ventilators can be provided in one of three ways: gaseous, liquid, and solid (chemically produced) states. Since the duration of intrahospital transport rarely exceeds 15 minutes, an E-sized oxygen cylinder with a capacity of approximately 660 L is sufficient. For example, if the patient is connected to a demand CPAP-IMV ventilator and gas consumption is 30 L/min, oxygen power can be provided for more than 20 minutes. If additional gas consumption is anticipated, two E-sized cylinders can be yoked together (Fig. 8-8).

By contrast, a gas supply for interhospital transport (and sometimes intrahospital as well) requires an H-sized oxygen cylinder with a capacity of approximately 6,660 L. Depending on transport time, two to three such large cylinders may sometimes be necessary. The only disadvantages of the H-sized cylinder are its height (5 ft) and weight (approximately 150 lb).

A more efficient way to provide pneumatic power for interhospital transport is to use a liquid oxygen reservoir from which 860 ft^3 of gaseous oxygen can be converted from 1 ft^3 of liquid oxygen. One unit (Mark II Liquid Oxygen Reservoir, Union Carbide Corp. Cryogenic Equipment, Danbury, CT) provides 13,800 L gaseous oxygen, which is equivalent to two large H-sized cylinders. The unit is approximately 3 ft high, weighs only 70 lb when full, and occupies 0.25 m^2 of floor space (Fig. 8-11). It provides enough oxygen to power a ventilator for approximately 7 hours at a minute ventilation

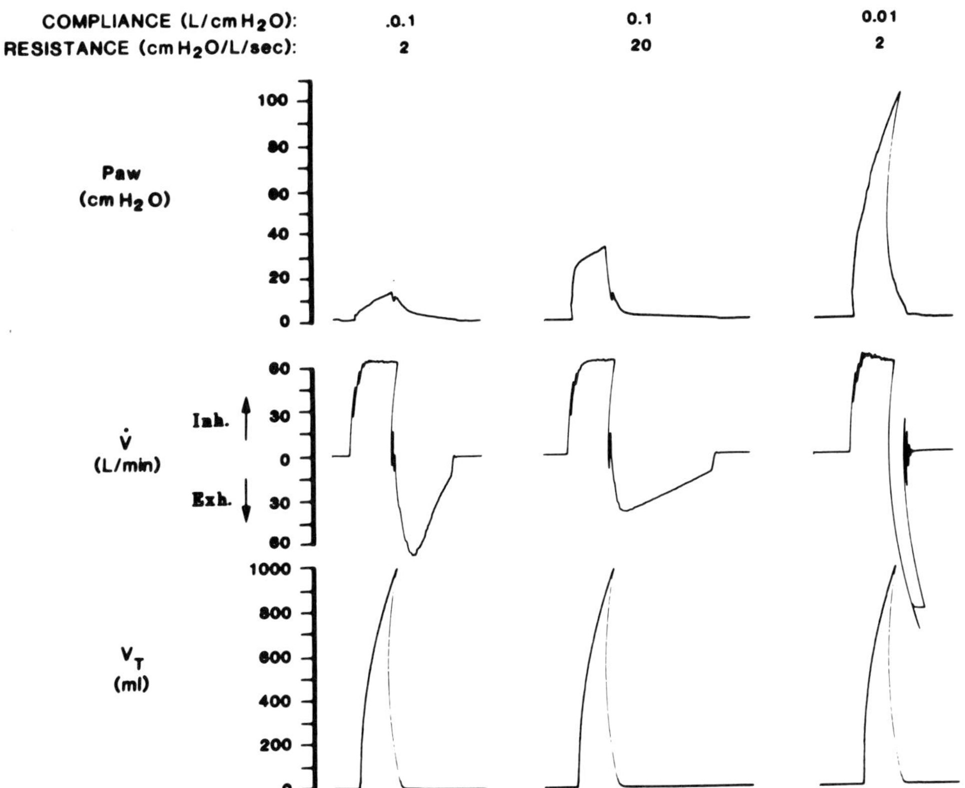

Fig. 8-10. Airway pressure (PAW), flow ($\dot{V}$), and VT recordings using a portable transport ventilator (Max, Hamilton Medical, Reno, NV) under conditions of varying compliance and airways resistance. Transport ventilators should be capable of generating high PIP and fairly constant inspiratory flow waveforms and tidal volumes when ventilating patients with low CLT and increased RAW.

of 30 L/min. The unit has a standard oxygen connector that supplies 50 psig for ventilator operation. In the ambulance, a 20-ft length of high-pressure oxygen tubing from the reservoir to the ventilator allows the patient to be moved into and out of the vehicle without being disconnected from the ventilator.

Another method of providing oxygen for emergency use during transport is by means of a chemical oxygen generator.[27,28] This self-contained portable system provides oxygen without high-pressure oxygen storage (AVOIX, Scott Aviation, Lancaster, NY) (Fig. 8-12). Oxygen is produced chemically by the thermal decomposition of solid sodium chlorate ($NaClO_3$), which yields oxygen (O_2) and sodium chloride (NaCl) under controlled reaction temperatures:

$$2\ NaClO_3 \rightarrow 3\ O_2 \uparrow +\ 2\ NaCl$$

The heat required to trigger the chemical reaction is initiated when an igniting (firing) pin is pulled, after which oxygen flow rates up to 8 to 10 L/min (STP) of 99.5 percent oxygen are produced for approximately 20 minutes.

The chemical oxygen generator is equipped with an oxygen outlet to an oxygen mask or self-inflating ventilation bag device (e.g., Ambu bag, Airshield). A solid-state chemical oxygen generator is a means of providing an efficient and reliable source of oxygen that is easily handled and has the advantage of long term storage life. Oxygen in this configuration is not subject to slow leakage as would be the case in a pressurized cylinder, but is instead bound in the stable

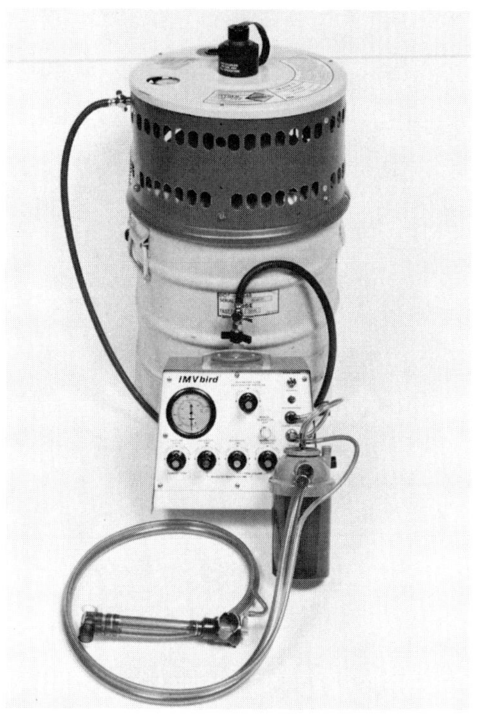

Fig. 8-11. This IMV bird is powered by a liquid oxygen reservoir unit that has a capacity of 13,800 L of gaseous oxygen.

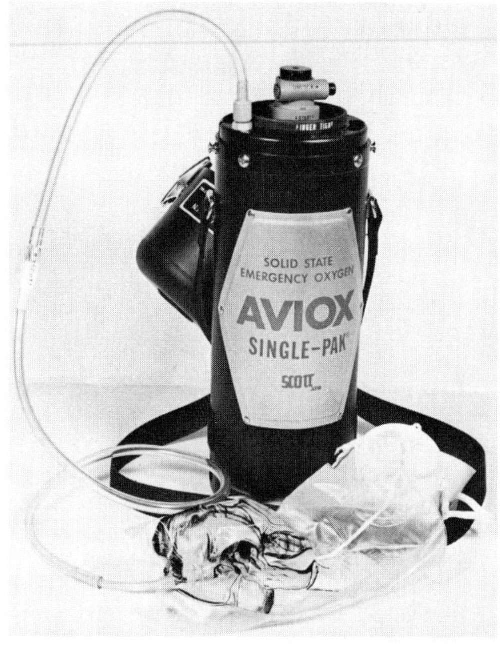

Fig. 8-12. Solid-state chemical oxygen generator (Scott Aviation, Lancaster, NY). Oxygen is produced chemically by the thermal decomposition of solid sodium chlorate.

chemical compound, $NaClO_3$. Gilstad[29] reported using a solid chemical oxygen generator to power a portable mechanical ventilator for battlefield casualties. Currently, $NaClO_3$ oxygen generators are used as an emergency oxygen source on jet aircraft and by the U.S. Navy on nuclear submarines.[28] Because of the size (14.8 in. × 9.8 in. × 4.75 in.) and weight (8.55 lb), $NaClO_3$ oxygen generators appear ideally suited as a backup system to provide emergency oxygen for use during transport.

Ancillary Equipment

During transport, an alternate means of ventilation with a hand-operated squeezable bag that provides CPAP is necessary. A 100 percent oxygen, flow-inflating Mapleson D system is preferable to the conventional self-inflating Ambu-type bag[30] (Fig. 8-13). The FIO_2 can be set as high as 1.0, the patient can breathe spontaneously with up to 30 cm H_2O of CPAP, and positive inspiratory pressure can be regulated manually by squeezing the bag. We have used this particular flow-inflating manual ventilation system successfully for transporting adults and children with acute respiratory failure. The major disadvantage is the gas consumption (i.e., a continuous high rate of flow, up to 20 to 25 L/min, must be provided); however, the liquid oxygen system minimizes this disadvantage.

In addition to portable mechanical ventilators, other respiratory support equipment is required. A kit containing airway management paraphernalia is essential (Table 8-6). Two examples of possible life-saving interventions with equipment from such a kit include replacing an endotracheal tube with a ruptured cuff to maintain ventilation or inserting a McSwain dart or Heimlich valve to treat a pneumothorax. This equipment should be given the same care as the transport ventilator.

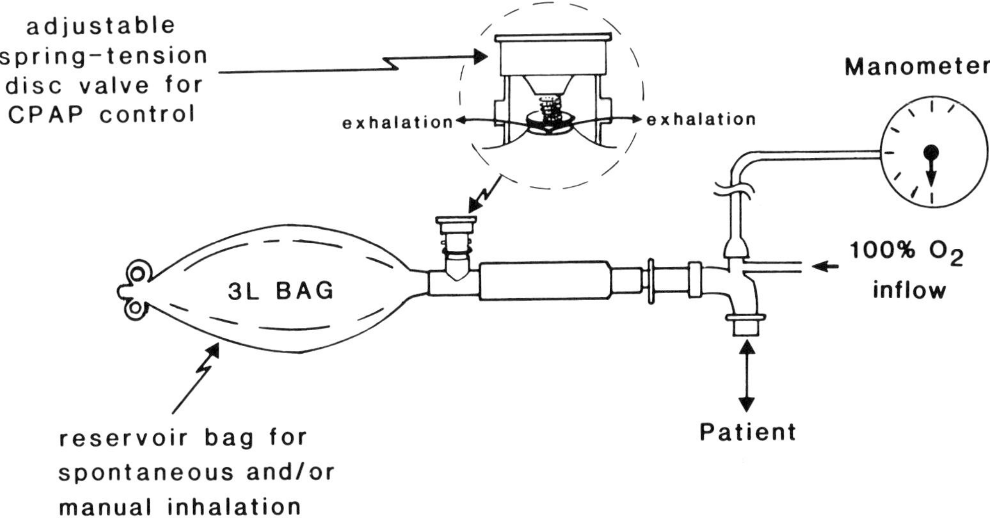

Fig. 8-13. Mapleson D, 100 percent oxygen flow-inflating manual ventilation device. Patients can breathe spontaneously with up to about 30 cm H_2O of CPAP. IMV is regulated by squeezing the bag. A manometer records the levels of CPAP and IMV peak inflation pressure.

A functional readily available system for suctioning is equally vital. Portable or installed suction equipment must have a vacuum adequate to develop −300 mmHg.[31] It should be fitted with large-bore nonkinking tubing with a rigid suction tip. Sterile catheters of various sizes should also be available for suctioning through an endotracheal or tracheotomy tube. A nonbreakable collection bottle and a supply of water for rinsing the tubes must be provided. The suction force should be easily adjustable, especially for use with children.

Table 8-6. Airway Management Kit for Ventilation During Emergency Transport

Laryngoscope with curved and straight blades in various sizes with spare batteries and bulbs
Endotracheal tubes of various sizes
Adaptors for attaching endotracheal tubes to ventilators and gas sources
Forceps
Magill forceps
Oral and nasal airways
Esophageal obturator airway with gastric suction capability
McSwain dart or Heimlich valve
Syringes (10- and 50-ml sizes)
Cetacaine
Surgical lubricant (water soluble)
Adhesive tape (1- and 2-in. sizes)
Suction catheters (various sizes)

Monitoring

The severity of the patient's illness and the duration of the transport determine the type of physiologic monitoring equipment that will be required during intra- and interhospital transport. Continuous observation by qualified personnel is an essential safety element during medical transport and is important for detecting signs of clinical deterioration (pallor, cyanosis, diaphoresis) or changing mental status. Visualization, palpation, and auscultation of the chest to ascertain the adequacy of ventilation should be performed whenever repositioning of the intubated patient is necessary.

Other basic monitoring routines include electrocardiography (ECG) and measurements of arterial blood pressure. During transport or during special procedures, the ECG monitors the presence of dysrhythmias or ischemia. Immediate availability of a defibrillator and pharmacologic support is also essential.

Arterial blood pressure can be monitored either invasively or noninvasively. Invasive arterial monitoring is popular in the ICU because it provides the ability to monitor blood pressure continuously and provides access to ABG analysis. If invasive monitoring has already been instituted, it can be continued during transport. Although availability of specimens for ABG analysis is usually not an issue during transportation, the arterial blood pressure of any hemodynamically unstable patient should nevertheless be monitored continuously.

Adequate information can also be obtained by combining an automated noninvasive blood pressure device with an oximeter. Electronic noninvasive blood pressure devices sense pressure oscillation as a cuff is deflated and display the systolic, diastolic, and mean arterial blood pressures and the pulse rate. These devices can be programmed to repeat measurements from every minute to every 30 minutes. We have found these devices to be reliable and accurate.

The continuous measurement of arterial oxygen saturation can be monitored by reliable lightweight oximeters that are currently available. Refinement of these devices and the use of microprocessors have resulted in equipment that has little tendency to drift and is easily calibrated. Both ear oximeters and pulse oximeters are effective. However, under conditions of hypotension and in the presence of vasoactive drug infusions, spurious information may be displayed. Nevertheless, we have found these devices to be useful, especially in children. All children being transported in our institution are monitored with an oximeter or, in infants, with transcutaneous PO_2 and PCO_2 electrodes.

Other patients may require central venous and pulmonary capillary wedge pressure and cardiac output measurements. Again, the severity of the illness and the duration of the transport define the necessity for more invasive methods. Such monitoring is usually not necessary unless these methods have already been initiated for a critically ill patient about to undergo transport.

Electromagnetic interference may present a problem. No medical device that interferes with aircraft navigation or communications equipment should be used, and medical equipment should be tested to ensure that this problem does not arise.

Altitude-Related Problems

Altitude-related pressure changes pose specific problems and are always a threat to patients transported in aircraft, whether cabins are pressurized or not. The effects on a patient flying at 35,000 to 40,500 ft in a pressurized cabin are the same as those at 8,000 ft in an unpressurized cabin. At sea level on an average day, the cabin pressure in an aircraft will be 760 mmHg (14.7 psig). At 8,000 ft, the barometric pressure decreases approximately 25 percent to 564.6 mmHg (11.9 psig). Any gas in a closed space within the body expands by more than a fourth of its initial volume (Boyle's law). Personnel must be aware of these hazards, as they relate to volume changes in the thorax, lung, gut, central nervous system (CNS), and other body spaces. For example, a nonfunctioning thoracostomy tube can be fatal. Gastric distention should be relieved before transport, and the pressure in endotracheal tube cuffs and pneumatic splints should be monitored and adjusted according to changes in altitude.

A decrease in atmospheric pressure reduces the partial pressure of inspired oxygen ($P_{I}O_2$), although the proportion of oxygen in the air remains the same (21 percent) at all altitudes. The $P_{I}O_2$ at any altitude is calculated by multiplying the barometric pressure at that altitude by the constant volume percentage of oxygen (i.e., 0.21). At sea level, the $P_{I}O_2$ is 760 mmHg $\times$ 0.21 = 160 mmHg, while the partial pressure of alveolar oxygen ($P_{A}O_2$) is 105 mmHg, and that of arterial oxygen (PaO_2) is 95 mmHg (Fig. 8-14). At 8,000 ft, $P_{I}O_2$ is 116 mmHg, $P_{A}O_2$ is 70 mmHg, and PaO_2 is 60 mmHg in a healthy person with normal cardiac and pulmonary function. However, a patient with mild hypoxemia who has impaired oxygenation can sustain a life-threatening decrease in PaO_2, which predisposes to myocardial ischemia and arrhythmia. Supplemental oxygen should therefore be provided for such patients, for example, those with chronic obstructive pulmonary disease (COPD), a history of myocardial infarction or anemia

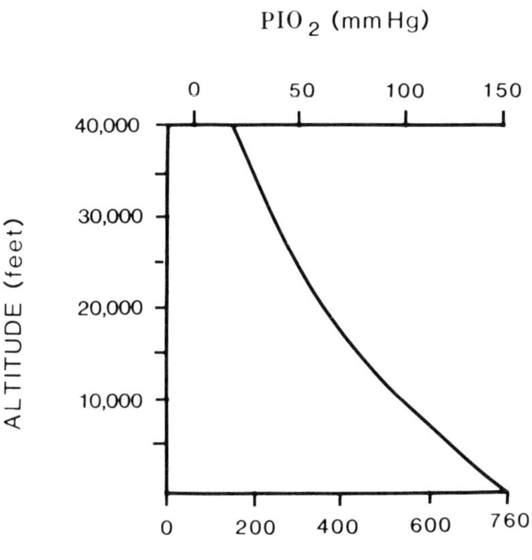

Fig. 8-14. Relationship between the partial pressure of inhaled oxygen (P_{IO_2}), altitude, and the total ambient pressure is indicated by the isopleth. As altitude increases, the total ambient barometric pressure decreases, thus P_{IO_2} decreases since $P_{IO_2} = 0.21 \times$ total ambient pressure. (Modified from West,[41] with permission.)

(Hb of less than 7 g/dl) who are transported in either unpressurized or pressurized cabin aircraft.

MECHANICAL VENTILATION IN A HYPERBARIC OXYGEN ENVIRONMENT

Hyperbaric medicine is the use of special gas mixtures, including oxygen in a high-pressure environment to produce alterations in the normal physiologic responses of the body. Examples of hyperbaric oxygen (HBO) applications are (1) to increase dissolved oxygen in the blood in cases of hemoglobin poisoning, such as poisoning by carbon monoxide, cyanide, or methemoglobin (e.g., insecticide exposure); (2) to provide a greater pressure differential for inert gas removal from tissues, such as in diving accidents (e.g., nitrogen); (3) to increase the partial pressure of oxygen to facilitate wound healing, such as osteoradionecrosis; and (4) to combat bactericidal effects, such as occurs in gas gangrene, mucormycosis, and other diseases (Table 8-7).

Basic Principles

Hyperbaric chambers are generally cylindrically shaped containers in which a patient is placed and the pressure increased. Hyperbaric chambers are of two general types: multiplace chambers with room for two or more patients, with attendants inside the chamber, and monoplace or single-person chambers. In multiplace chambers, the patient can be administered an F_{IO_2} of 1.0 or other gas mixtures by oronasal mask or endotracheal tube. In monoplace chambers, the patient breathes the treatment gas (usually an F_{IO_2} of 1.0) from the chamber environment.[32] Pressure inside a hyperbaric chamber is increased by adding additional air or oxygen to the chamber. Chamber pressure may be expressed in units of atmospheres absolute (ATA) or millimeters of mercury (mmHg). For every 33 feet seawater (fsw) depth simulated in a hyperbaric chamber, pressure increases by 1 ATA, or 760 mmHg. For example, prior to compression, at sea level, the simulated depth is 0 fsw, and the chamber pressure is 1 ATA, or 760 mmHg. At 33 fsw, chamber pressure is 2 ATA or 1,520 mmHg, respectively.

Like underwater divers, the patient, equipment, and medical personnel inside a hyperbaric chamber are subject to the same basic physical principles and gas laws. Clinicians must be aware of these gas laws and be vigilant in order to avert catastrophes associated with changes in physiology and pressures.

Boyle's law is the most common gas law associated with hyperbaric medicine. When the temperature is held constant, volume (V) will vary inversely with the pressure (P) (V =

Table 8-7. Clinical Applications of Hyperbaric Oxygenation

Established indications
Air or gas embolism (acute)
Carbon monoxide poisoning and acute smoke inhalation
Crush injury, compartment syndrome, and other acute traumatic ischemia
Cyanide poisoning (acute)
Decompression sickness
Enhancement of healing in selected problem wounds
Exceptional blood loss (anemia)
Gas gangrene (clostridial)
Necrotizing soft tissue infections
Crepitant anaerobic cellulitis
Progressive bacterial gangrene
Necrotizing fascitis
Nonclostridial myonecrosis
Miscellaneous necrotizing infections in the compromised host
Osteomyelitis (refractory)
Radiation necrosis
Selected refractory anaerobic infections
Skin grafts or flaps (compromised)
Special considerations
Burns (thermal)
Potential indications
Anaerobic and mixed brain abscesses
Carbon tetrachloride poisoning (acute)
Cerebrovascular accident (acute)
Head injury (cerebral edema)
Fracture healing and bone grafting
Hydrogen sulfide poisoning
Pyoderma gangrenosum
Sickle cell anemia crises
Spider bite (brown recluse)

(Adapted from Hyperbaric Oxygen Therapy,[40] with permission.)

1/P), an important fact to remember both on compression and decompression. For example, if a patient holds his breath while the chamber is compressed, the surrounding pressure will compress his lungs. Compression to depths in excess of 132 fsw or 5 ATA result in compression of the lungs below that of residual volume, producing what is referred to as a "squeeze." As a result, fluid attempts to fill the lung to occupy the remaining "space." If the patient holds his breath during decompression, the surrounding pressure decreases, and the lungs expand to their limits, beyond which they tear, and gas leaks into the vascular system, and intrapleural or mediastinal spaces. Dissection of air into the vascular system precipitates to gas embolism, which can be fatal. Ironically, the best treatment for arterial gas embolism is immediate compression in a hyperbaric chamber.

Side Effects and Potential Problems

Side effects and other potential problems of HBO therapy exist as a result of alterations in physiology that occur during hyperbaric exposure. If the consequences of a patient's disorder outweigh the risks of any possible side effects, then HBO therapy should proceed. Side effects and potential problems of HBO therapy include the following:

1. *Upper respiratory infection (URI) or sinusitis:* These disorders are associated with the risk of ear drum rupture or sinus tear from pressure changes. Should HBO therapy be indicated, myringotomies may be required.
2. *Pneumothorax:* Pneumothoraces occurring at depth should be treated prior to decompression. Trapped air between the lung and chest wall expands during decompression, resulting in further compression on the lung and mediastinum.
3. *Chronic obstructive pulmonary disease (COPD)*: Rupture of blebs or bullae during decompression have occurred in patients with COPD. Thus, greater caution should be exercised during decompression by carefully monitoring these patients.
4. *Confinement anxiety:* Patients who are claustrophobic, for example, present problems to the medical staff, especially when using monoplace hyperbaric chambers. Patients with severe forms of confinement anxiety may become so anxious that HBO therapy should be discontinued or withheld altogether.
5. *Seizure disorders:* Patients with a history of seizure disorders may be predisposed to experiencing a seizure when breathing high concentrations of oxygen under pressure.
6. *Ocular effects in premature infants:* HBO is not recommended in premature infants because of the risk of retrolental fibroplasia.

Potential fire hazards occur when oxygen, fuel, and ignition sources are present; therefore, reducing any one of these components reduces the risk of fire. In multiplace hyperbaric chambers, air is used for compression, and oxygen concentration is maintained no greater than 23 percent.[33] To maintain the oxygen concentration inside the chamber as low as possible, a mechanical ventilator or respiratory therapy device (e.g., O_2 mask) should be equipped with a scavenger, which can retrieve exhaled gas with O_2 concentrations greater than 21 percent, and direct these gases out of the hyperbaric chamber. If a scavenger system is not used, the chamber should be vented at specific intervals, depending on the gas mixtures used. Monoplace chambers use oxygen for compression, thereby making fire safety a critical concern.

Blood Gas Measurements

Arterial blood gas measurements are tedious and difficult in a hyperbaric chamber. If a blood specimen is drawn while the chamber is compressed (at depth), the increased gas tensions in the blood will decrease as the sample is removed from the chamber for analysis, due to equilibration with the lower ambient pressure. Thus, the validity of blood gas measurements is questionable unless a blood gas machine is available inside the hyperbaric chamber. However, since the electronic components of the blood gas machine can create a spark, potentially causing a fire, the machine should be encased in an airtight seal and purged with nitrogen; this, however, makes it impractical to operate.

Other methods used for obtaining information on blood oxygen and carbon dioxide are (1) transcutaneous oxygen[34] and carbon dioxide, which are helpful for trending information; (2) single-cell oxygen probes, which have been evaluated with reported difficulties[35]; and (3) pulse oximetry and capnography, which are useful for measuring oxygen saturation and end-tidal CO_2, respectively. These monitors are not built to be used inside the hyperbaric chamber. Monitoring is done from the outside, with connections to the patient through a penetration port in the chamber.

Choice of Ventilators

Indications for mechanical ventilation in the hyperbaric environment are the same as in the ICU. However, since the environment is obviously different, so is the operation of a mechanical ventilator; therefore, unique factors affecting the patient and the ventilator should be considered.

Patient Factors

Confined air spaces, such as an endotracheal tube cuff, change volume as the hyperbaric chamber is compressed and decompressed (Boyle's law). During compression, pressure increases and the volume in the endotracheal tube cuff decreases, resulting in a leak of pressure and volume from the lungs when the ventilator attempts to deliver a tidal volume. Conversely, if such a leak is compensated for at depth, then the cuff volume will expand during decompression, and the endotracheal tube cuff will distend and burst. In monoplace hyperbaric chambers, it is difficult to alter the endotracheal tube cuff volume as the chamber pressure is varied. In these situations, inflation of an endotracheal tube cuff with air could be fraught with serious problems due to leaking (hypercapnia, hypoxemia, aspiration, and cardiac arrest). Since liquids are incompressible, this problem is averted by infusing normal saline solution, rather than air, into the cuff.

Suctioning, auscultation of the lungs, and monitoring of ventilatory parameters are also problematic when monoplace chambers are used, since access to the patient is precluded.

Ventilator Characteristics

Spontaneous and mechanical positive-pressure ventilation should be possible with ventilators used in hyperbaric chambers. As in the

ICU, patients suffering acute lung injury may require CPAP and IMV or CMV. Levels of CPAP up to about 30 cm H_2O may be required (an upper limit has not been established) and PIP up to about 100 cm H_2O may be necessary to ventilate the patient mechanically. Tidal volume range should be adjustable from about 100 to 1,500 ml in order to ventilate pediatric and adult patients. The F_{IO_2} should also be adjustable from 0.21 to 1.0. Volume-cycled or pressure-cycled ventilators should be employed rather than time-cycled ventilators. Volume-cycled type ventilators deliver more consistent tidal volumes from breath to breath, and are thus preferable. Full humidification of inhaled gases during spontaneous and mechanical ventilation are essential, especially for patients where humidity therapy is indicated (e.g., large amounts of inspissated secretions, pulmonary burns). Other desirable characteristics of a mechanical ventilator for use in a hyperbaric chamber are listed in Table 8-8.

Access to the ventilator is also restricted in a monoplace hyperbaric chamber. Once the patient and ventilator have been sealed inside the chamber and pressurized, the ventilator life-support system is inaccessible to the operator. For example, it is difficult to change the ventilator setting, adjust or reconnect the airway connections, or suction the patient. A ventilator used within a monoplace chamber must either be adjusted prior to compression to settings required during hyperbaric conditions, or should have its controls accessible from outside the chamber.

Exhaled gases from the ventilator should be directed outside the chamber. This is easily done by directing exhaled gas to a scavenger, and then to the outside through an exit port in the chamber. Since the pressure in a hyperbaric chamber is greater than the outside pressure, a bias valve exit port is required to maintain the appropriate pressure differential and to vent exhaled gas outside the chamber. Should the patient be inadvertently connected directly to the outside, a profound pressure differential occurs and results in evacuation of the patient's lungs. The bias valve is therefore essential in maintaining a safe pressure differential.

Table 8-8. Desirable Characteristics of a Mechanical Ventilator in a Hyperbaric Environment

Cycling mechanism: Pressure- or volume-cycled ventilators may be used in a hyperbaric chamber.

Modalities of ventilation:
Mechanical positive-pressure ventilation: IMV and assisted and controlled mechanical ventilation are options that should be available.
Spontaneous positive-pressure ventilation: A demand-flow valve CPAP system should be capable of delivering CPAP up to about 30 cm H_2O.

Airway pressure, flow rate, and tidal volume characteristics: PIP up to about 150 cm H_2O, peak inspiratory flow rate up to about 120 L/min, and tidal volume range from 100–1,500 ml should be available.

F_{IO_2} capability: An F_{IO_2} of 0.21 or 1.0 is used for most hyperbaric treatment schedules; however, the ability to deliver nitrox or heliox should be available.

Humidification: Humidification of inhaled gases may not be necessary for short periods of ventilation, but may be required for protracted periods.

Power source: A pneumatically-powered ventilator is preferred over an electrically powered one, since the latter may predispose to a fire.

Ventilator monitors: Real time displays of airway pressures (PIP, CPAP), F_{IO_2}, tidal volume, and ventilator rate should be provided. In addition, high PIP and low-pressure disconnect alarms are essential.

Consistency: As pressure in the hyperbaric chamber increases and decreases, ventilators should operate in a consistent fashion with no alterations in tidal and minute volume, breathing frequency, CPAP, F_{IO_2}, and inspiratory time.

Gas compression: Factors affecting gas compression volume in the breathing circuit should be minimized as much as possible.

Ease of operation: The ventilator should be simple to operate by a wide range of personnel.

Gas consumption: Gas consumption should be minimal.

Physical dimensions: The ventilator should be small in size and as light as possible due to the confined area of the hyperbaric chamber.

Sterilization/disinfection: Disassembly and reassembly of the breathing circuit should be easily performed to facilitate sterilization and disinfection procedures.

Transportability: The ventilator should be capable for use during the transport of patients from the hyperbaric chamber to other areas of the hospital (e.g., ICU, operating room).

Cost: The ventilator should be relatively inexpensive and affordable.

The major differences in operating a ventilator in a hyperbaric chamber as opposed to normal conditions are (1) the alterations in pressure in the chamber and the driving pressure powering the ventilator; (2) gas densities; (3) the different gases used; and (4) the confined area of the chamber. These factors often preclude the respiratory therapist from having precise control of the ventilator.

A mechanical ventilator must be adjusted in accordance with the changes in pressure that occur in a hyperbaric chamber, which are increased and decreased during therapy. The ventilator should operate in a consistent fashion with no alterations in tidal and minute volume, breathing frequency, CPAP, FIO_2, and other factors. Most often, a pressure differential regulator is used to provide a 50-psig ventilator driving pressure source, regardless of the pressure in the chamber. There is some question whether the appropriate ventilator driving pressure differential should be maintained at this or a higher driving pressure. If the latter is the case, a significantly greater pressure should be supplied to the ventilator. Second, there is an increase in gas density as pressure increases in the system. This increased density inhibits gas movement through the normal pneumatic cartridges, altering their function.

In our evaluations, only specific types of gas-powered ventilators, such as the Penlon and a prototype Emerson model, operated without altering their set parameters when the chamber pressures were varied. Pneumatically-powered, time-cycled ventilators are subject to alterations in VT, inspiratory time, expiratory time, breathing rate, and inspiratory flow rate as chamber pressure is varied. Ross and Manson reported that VT delivery decreased significantly in pneumatic, time-cycled ventilators when pressure

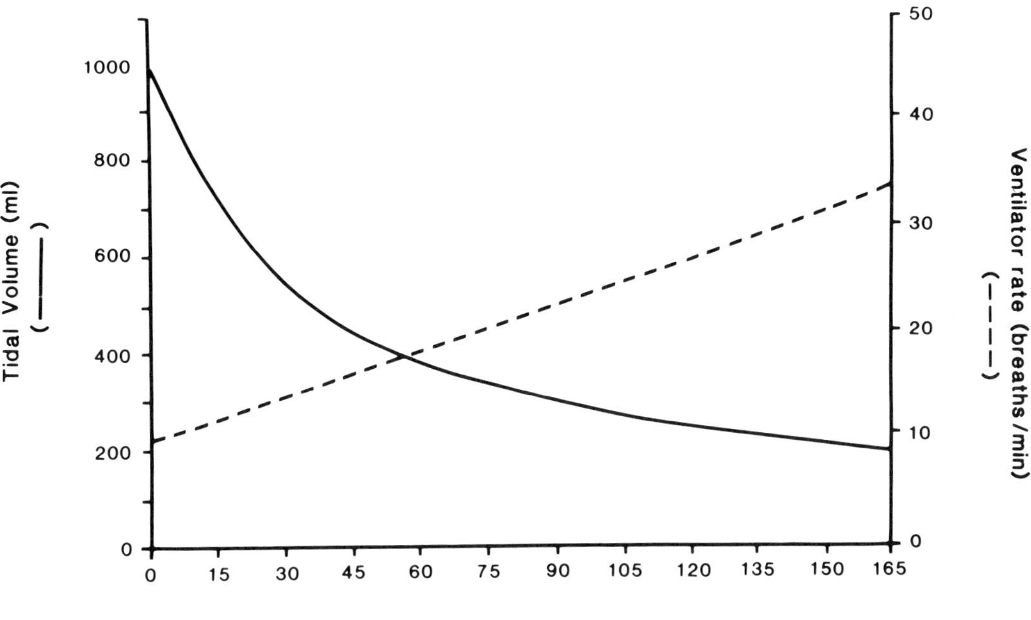

Fig. 8-15. Relationships of ventilator tidal volume and breathing rate for pneumatically powered, time-cycled mechanical ventilators in a hyperbaric chamber. Tidal volume delivery decreases exponentially, while ventilator rate increases linearly as pressure is increased in a hyperbaric chamber (the greater the simulated depth in feet seawater, the greater the pressure in the chamber). In contrast, tidal volume delivery and rate are relatively constant with volume- and pressure-cycled ventilators (not shown) as pressure in the chamber is increased.

was increased in the hyperbaric chamber. In addition, ventilatory frequency increased with depth[36]; subsequent studies have reaffirmed these findings[37,38] (Fig. 8-15). All ventilators should have a drive pressure at least 50 psig greater than that of the chamber pressure. This would mean that a patient at a depth of 165 fsw (6 atm total pressure) should have a ventilator driving pressure of 123.5 psig (5 × 14.7 psi = 73.5 psig + 50 psig), although at such high driving pressures, the ventilator's internal pneumatic circuitry can rupture. For this reason and the factors cited above, caution should be exercised when operating a mechanical ventilator in a hyperbaric environment.

Alterations in gas density, beyond the normal increase from pressure, result when special or exotic gases are used (e.g., nitrox, heliox, oxygen and air, neon), and can affect ventilator operation. For example, a gas mixture of 79 percent helium and 21 percent oxygen has a density about one-third that of air; thus, greater inspiratory flow rates from a ventilator result at the same driving pressure as compared with using air. If the ventilator's inspiratory time is unchanged, this will result in an increase in tidal volume (VT = inspiratory flow rate × inspiratory time) and PIP (PIP = VT ÷ CLT). As the hyperbaric chamber is compressed, gas density increases, and flow rate from the ventilator diminishes. Pneumatic time-cycled ventilators alter VT delivery, as well as inspiratory and expiratory times, due to changes in gas density that occur during compression. Also,

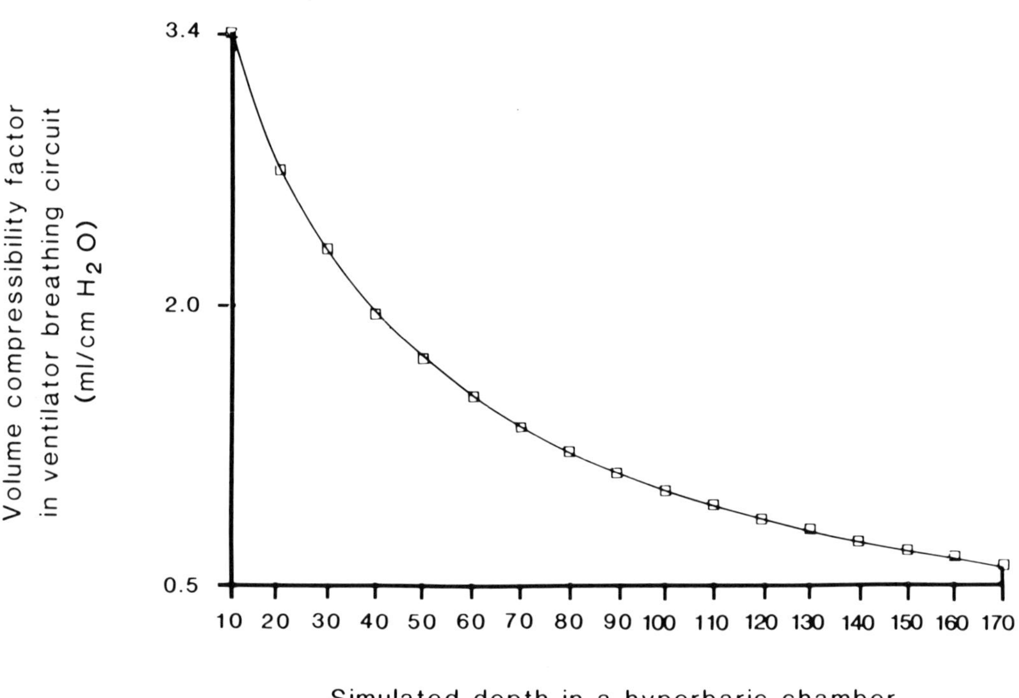

Fig. 8-16. Relationship between the volume compressibility factor (ml/cm H_2O) in a ventilator breathing circuit and simulated feet seawater (fsw) depth in a hyperbaric chamber. As depth increases, chamber pressure increases and the volume compressibility factor decreases in an exponential manner. Larger decreases in the volume compressibility factor occur at depths up to about 66 fsw or 3 ATA pressure relative to greater depths.

the ventilator rate changes significantly since inspiratory and expiratory times are affected by changes in gas density.[37]

Another factor to consider is the change in compression volume in the ventilator breathing circuit as a result of compression and decompression in a hyperbaric chamber (Fig. 8-16). Variations in the volume compressibility factor in a ventilator breathing circuit are due to the variations between the pressure in the hyperbaric chamber and the PIP. As pressure in the chamber increases, the volume compressibility factor of the breathing circuit decreases.

REFERENCES

1. Carlon CG, Ray C, Klein R: Criteria for selective positive end-expiratory pressure and independent synchronized ventilation of each lung. Chest 74:501, 1978
2. Gallagher TJ, Banner MJ, Smith RA: A simplified method of independent lung ventilation. Crit Care Med 8:396, 1980
3. Schimmel L, Civetta JM, Kirby RR: A new mechanical method to influence pulmonary perfusion in critically ill patients. Crit Care Med 5:277, 1977
4. Ray C, Carlon CG, Miodownik S: A method of synchronizing two MA-1 ventilators for independent lung ventilation. Crit Care Med 6:71, 1978
5. Sayer DM, Jung RC, Koons R: A unilateral lung ventilator. Respir Ther 3:41, 1973
6. Froese AB: High frequency ventilation. A critical assessment. p.V(A):1. In Shoemaker WC (ed): Critical Care: State of the Art. Vol 5. Society of Critical Care Medicine, Fullerton, CA, 1984.
7. Banner MJ: Technical aspects of high frequency ventilation. Curr Rev Respir Ther 7:91, 1985
8. Carlon GC, Miodownik S, Ray C: High frequency jet ventilation. p. 77. In Carlon GC, Howland WS (eds): High Frequency Ventilation in Intensive Care and During Surgery. Marcel Dekker, New York, 1985
9. Banner MJ, Gallagher RC, Desautels DA, et al: A manifold to measure exhaled tidal volume during high frequency jet ventilation. Crit Care Med 14:730, 1985
10. Schlacter MD, Perry ME: Effect of continuous positive airway pressure on lung mechanics during high frequency jet ventilation. Crit Care Med 12:755, 1984
11. Hamilton LH, Londino JM, Linehan JH: Pediatric endotracheal tube designed for high frequency ventilation. Crit Care Med 12:988, 1984
12. Banner MJ, Boysen PG: Comparison of two flow injector devices to deliver high frequency jet ventilation. Crit Care Med 14:374, 1986
13. Mikhail MS, Banner MJ: Hemodynamic effects of positive end-expiratory pressure during high frequency ventilation. Crit Care Med 13:733, 1985
14. Gallagher RC, Banner MJ, Modell JM: Comparison of delivery systems for high frequency jet ventilation. Crit Care Med 13:313, 1985
15. Weber W, Alpen E, Gravenstein N, et al: Inhalational anesthesia during high frequency jet ventilation for extracorporeal shock wave therapy of gallbladder stones. Anesth Analg 66:187, 1987
16. Downs JB, Chapman RL: Treatment of bronchopleural fistula during continuous positive pressure ventilation. Chest 69:363, 1976
17. Gallagher TJ, Smith RA, Kirby RR, et al: Intermittent inspiratory chest tube occlusion to limit bronchopleural cutaneous airleaks. Crit Care Med 4:328, 1976
18. Phillips YY, Lonigan RM, Joyner LR: A simple technique for managing a bronchopleural fistula while maintaining positive pressure ventilation. Crit Care Med 7:351, 1979
19. Carlon GC, Ray C, Klain M, et al: High frequency positive pressure ventilation in the management of a patient with a bronchopleural fistula. Anesthesiology 52:160, 1980
20. Ray C, Miodownik S, Carlon G, et al: Pneumatic-to-electric analog for high frequency jet ventilation of disrupted airways. Crit Care Med 12:711, 1984
21. Carlon GC, Ray C, Griffin J: Tidal volume and airway pressure on high frequency jet ventilation. Crit Care Med 11:83, 1983
22. Tilden SJ, Berman LS, Banner MJ, et al: Prolonged use of HFJV for a pediatric patient. Crit Care Med 13:508, 1985
23. Kessler H: High frequency jet ventilation. p. 175. In Carlon GC, Howland WS (eds): High Frequency Ventilation in Intensive Care and During Surgery. Marcel Dekker, New York, 1985
24. Harless KW, Morris AH, Cengiz M, et al: Civilian ground and air transport of adults with acute respiratory failure. JAMA 240:361, 1978

25. Murphy EJ, Desautels DA, Modell JH: A compact headboard and ventilator transport system. Crit Care Med 6:387, 1978
26. Downs JB, Marston AW: A new transport ventilator: an evaluation. Crit Care Med 5:112, 1977
27. Unfer SM, Bozynski ME: Solid state oxygen for use in emergency evacuation of neonates. Crit Care Med 12:475, 1984
28. Harwood V: Chemical Oxygen Generators for Business and Utility Aircraft. Society of Automotive Engineers, 1971, p. 1494
29. Gilstad DW: Casualty resuscitation on the chemical battlefield. p. 27. In Newball HH (ed): Proceedings of the Symposium on Respiratory Care of Chemical Casualties. U.S. Army Medical Research and Development Command, McLean, VA, 1983
30. Berninger GT, Forrette MJ: Adult manual resuscitators. Curr Rev Respir Ther 1:115, 1979
31. Committee on Allied Health: Emergency Care and Transportation of the Sick and Injured. 2nd Ed. American Academy of Orthopaedic Surgeons, Chicago, 1977, p. 358
32. Davis JC: Hyperbaric medicine: critical care aspects. In Shoemaker WC (ed): Critical Care: State of the Art. Vol 5. Society of Critical Care Medicine, Fullerton, CA, 1984
33. Davis JC, Hunt TK: Hyperbaric Oxygen Therapy. Undersea Medical Society, Bethesda, MD, 1977
34. Sheffield PJ, Workman WT: Noninvasive tissue oxygen measurements in patients administered normobaric and hyperbaric oxygen by mask. HBO Rev 6:47, 1985
35. Sheffield PJ: Tissue oxygen measurements with respect to soft-tissue wound healing with normobaric and hyperbaric oxygen. HBO Rev 6:18, 1985
36. Ross JAS, Manson HJ: Behavior of three resuscitators under hyperbaric conditions. Aviat Space Environ Med 48:26, 1977
37. Gallagher TJ, Smith RA, Bell GC: Evaluation of the IMV bird and modified mk 2 bird in a hyperbaric environment. Respir Care 22:501, 1977
38. Gallagher TJ, Smith RA, Bell GC: Evaluation of mechanical ventilators in a hyperbaric environment. Aviat Space Environ Med 49:375, 1978
39. Civetta JM, Taylor RW, Kirby RR (eds): Critical Care. JB Lippincott, Philadelphia, 1988
40. Hyperbaric Oxygen Therapy: Committee Report. Undersea Medical Society, Bethesda, MD, 1986
41. West JB: Respiratory Physiology. Williams & Wilkins, Baltimore, 1976

9

Weaning Mechanical Ventilatory Support

Neil R. MacIntyre
M. Christine Stock

The need for mechanical ventilation is usually the result of an imbalance between the patient's ventilatory demand (or load) and the patient's inherent ventilatory capabilities[1] (Fig. 9-1). Thus, the safe withdrawal of such support can take place only when the patient reestablishes a tolerable balance between load and capability. Since the "reestablishment" rate can vary widely, so also can the rate of withdrawal. The requirement for ventilator support ceases quickly after the resolution of transient neurological dysfunction (e.g., anesthesia, drug overdose) or reversible load increases (e.g., asthma). Conversely, more gradual withdrawal may be needed during recovery from more permanent neurologic dysfunction (e.g., central nervous system infarcts or trauma), from chronic load increases (e.g., chronic obstructive lung disease), or from disease complicated by malnutrition and other debilitating conditions. The concept of weaning should probably be reserved for this latter group.

Table 9-1 cites the relative proportions of patients whose mechanical ventilatory support can be withdrawn in either less than or more than 24 hours.[2] These data demonstrate that the majority of ventilated patients experience only brief periods of load/capability imbalance and thus tolerate rapid removal of mechanical ventilatory support. In this setting, weaning is not an issue. By contrast, approximately one-third of patients requiring mechanical ventilatory support experienced periods of load/capability imbalance exceeding 24 hours. For these patients, a longer withdrawal process frequently is required. This chapter focuses primarily on the needs of such patients and on the various techniques and approaches available.

GOALS OF MECHANICAL VENTILATION DURING WEANING

During the acute phase of respiratory failure, the primary goals of ventilatory support are adequate gas exchange and ventilatory muscle rest. However, once reversal of the process that precipitated failure begins, weaning from ventilatory support becomes an additional primary goal. To this end, two secondary goals become important: optimization of ventilatory muscle function and provision of smooth, comfortable interactions between the patient's breathing efforts and the mechanical ventilatory pattern; referred to as patient-ventilator synchrony.

Optimization of Ventilatory Muscle Function

Weaning returns the breathing loads to the patient's ventilatory muscles. For ultimate success, however, the loads must be reduced to

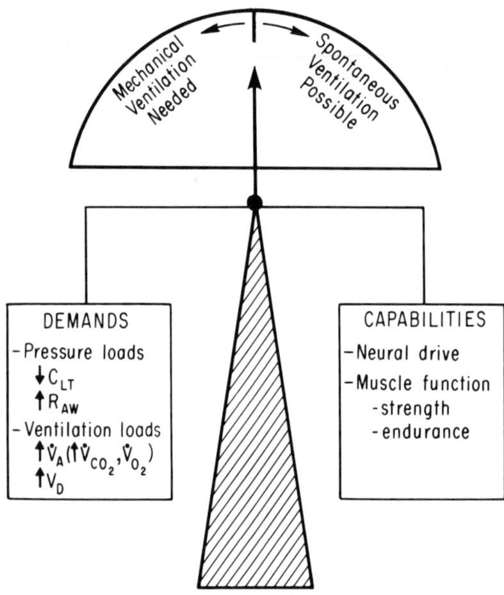

Fig. 9-1. Schematic representation of the balance between ventilatory demands and ventilatory capabilities involved in determining the need for mechanical ventilatory support.

tolerable levels, and the muscles must have adequate strength and endurance (Fig. 9-1). Even though increased loads may have precipitated ventilatory failure, impaired muscle function can become the rate-limiting step during ventilator withdrawal. Impaired muscle function may result from residual muscle fatigue, from malnutrition, and from direct effects of the primary disease. In addition, disuse atrophy may develop in ventilatory muscles that have been paralyzed or unused for prolonged periods.[3]

Mechanical ventilation should maximize muscle function by providing an appropriate load quantity with favorable load characteristics. Load quantity is the amount of inspiratory pressure generation, or mechanical work (and thus energy expenditure), that is required on the ventilatory muscles (Fig. 9-2). Small load quantities should be supplied early during recovery to forestall atrophy.[4] Recent data further suggest that near-normal workloads (2 to 5 J/min) will be tolerated well during recovery from ventilatory failure.[5] Belman[6] argues that additional short periods of near-fatiguing workloads may be a useful conditioning stimulus. As the primary therapeutic modalities improve ventilatory mechanics, weaning consists of returning increasing proportions of the ventilatory load to the patient's muscles.

A given ventilatory load quantity can be characterized by its pressure and volume change components (Fig. 9-2). The relationship between pressure/volume changes impacts on both energy efficiency and conditioning. Normal ventilatory muscles operate under pressure and volume change characteristics that appear optimal for muscle energy efficiency (i.e., work/muscle oxygen demand).[7]

Shifts to high-pressure low-volume characteristics (Fig. 9-2), as often occur in low-compliance high-resistance lungs, reduce this

Table 9-1. Duration of Mechanical Ventilatory Support Requirements

	Number of Patients[a] (% of Total)	Duration Mean Days of Ventilatory Support
Ventilatory Support <24h	583 (64)	<1
Postanesthesia		
Drug		
Asthma		
Ventilatory Support >24h	327 (36)	11.8
Prolonged postoperatively	113 (12.4)	3.8
Acute lung injury	20 (2.2)	13.3
Chronic lung disease	54 (5.9)	23.2
Multisystem failure	60 (6.5)	18.5
Trauma	28 (3.1)	10.8
Other	52 (5.7)	9.3

[a] N = 910.

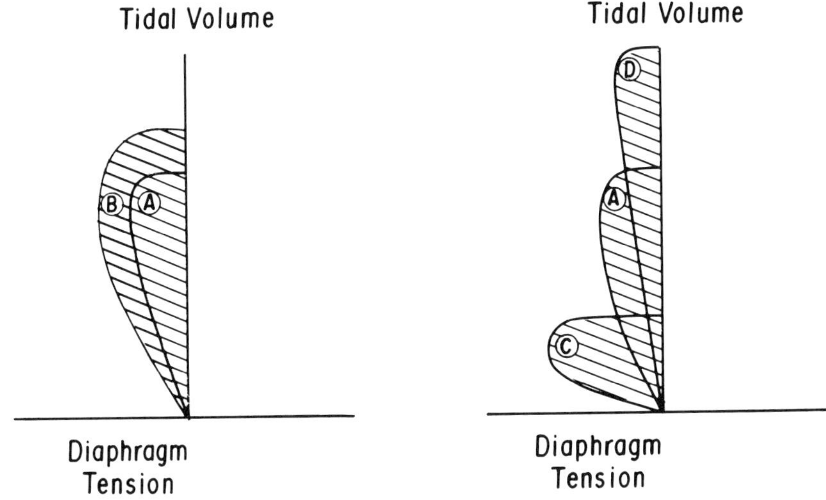

Fig. 9-2. Quantity and characteristics of ventilatory muscle loads. In both panels, load is represented by a ventilatory muscle tension (pressure)/tidal volume curve. The area within each curve represents work. The left panel depicts changes in work quantity. Curve A is a normal resting breath and curve B represents normal hyperventilation with increases in both volume and muscle tension (i.e., the pressure-volume relationship remains balanced). The right panel depicts changes in work characteristics. Again, curve A is a normal resting breath. Curve C, however, represents a breath against high impedance loads (e.g., ARDS, COPD). Note the increase in pressure requirements relative to volume change under these circumstances. Although the quantity of load/breath in curve C is similar to the normal curve A, many more breaths/min are needed for adequate ventilation and thus work/minute is increased markedly when curve C represents the actual tidal breath. Curve D represents a breath against very low impedances (e.g., through a tracheostomy) and a much lower pressure-volume change relationship.

efficiency. From a muscle-conditioning perspective, loads with high-pressure low-volume characteristics emphasize sarcomere development but deemphasize mitochondrial development,[8] a situation that may be undesirable for an endurance-oriented muscle such as the diaphragm. Because of these efficiency and conditioning effects, the desirable load characteristic during muscle recovery probably is a relatively normal balance between pressure and volume changes.[9,10]

Patient-Ventilator Synchrony

A mechanical ventilatory pattern that is not coordinated with a patient's ventilatory drive increases oxygen consumption and carbon dioxide production, necessitating a higher minute ventilation.[11] Furthermore, this dysynchrony may lead to the clinician's use of excessive sedation, a common cause of prolonged weaning.[1] Therefore, a ventilatory pattern that is synchronized with the patient's mechanoreceptors and inspiratory flow demands is desirable. This goal applies not only to appropriately selected mechanical ventilation parameters but also to minimizing the high-pressure loads imposed by ventilator circuits, endotracheal tubes, and demand valves.

MEASURING POTENTIAL FOR WEANING

No ideal combination of measurements and observations allows us to decide reliably that a patient is ready to assume spontaneous alveolar ventilation. Nevertheless, important objective and subjective parameters are useful in determining the need for continued mechanical ventilatory support. Measurements of mechanical pulmonary function, neuromuscular function, and the respiratory pattern, together with the patient's subjective impressions are all important as reflections of the ability to breathe. So also is the measurement of gas exchange as it affects discontinuation of mechanical ventilation will be covered.

Mechanical Pulmonary Function

With the advent of microprocessor-controlled ventilators, we can determine static compliance, resistance, breath-by-breath tidal volumes, and a host of other variables. Many of these are of definite academic interest. However, no data suggest that a knowledge of these variables enhances the prediction of weaning success, although they may quantitate the progression or regression of disease.

The airway pressure pattern may give information regarding increased airways resistance and/or decreased pulmonary compliance as the etiology of high peak airway pressure. A typical airway pressure pattern from a single conventional positive-pressure breath is depicted in Figure 9-3. When the expiratory valve remains closed 0.25 second beyond the initial delivery of the mechanical breath, gas distributes more evenly throughout the lungs[12] and a plateau pressure (Pplat) results. The difference between the peak inflation pressure (PIP) and plateau airway pressure is a reflection of RAW, whereas the difference between Pplat and positive end-expiratory pressure (PEEP) is related to the static lung compliance:

$$C_{LT} = \frac{V_T}{\text{Pplat} - \text{PEEP}} \qquad (1)$$

where C_{LT} is lung-thorax compliance and V_T is exhaled mechanical tidal volume. This calculation has significance only if the patient makes no ventilatory effort during the pressure measurements. As patients recover from acute restrictive pulmonary disease, C_{LT} increases. Normal C_{LT} in spontaneously breathing, upright adults is 100 ml/cm H_2O. The C_{LT} threshold, which produces ventilatory failure or precludes weaning from mechanical ventilation is unknown.

Airway resistance is calculated by dividing change in pressure by flow. The pressure gradient of interest is from the distal airways (ideally, intra-alveolar pressure) to either the large airways or the proximal tracheal tube. If airway pressure is measured distal to the tracheal tube, the calculation reflects only the patient's intrinsic resistance and excludes that of the tube. When pressure is measured proximal to the tracheal tube (in the ventilator circuit), the calculated resistance includes that introduced by the tube. Alveolar pressure can be approximated from the Pplat (Fig. 9–3). Subtraction of Pplat from PIP represents the pressure change to overcome RAW and is necessary in its calculation. Airway resistance is difficult to quantitate without microprocessor capability to measure inspiratory gas flow. However, it can be approximated by using a constant inspiratory flow waveform and determining the average primary flow rate from a pneumotachograph or other flow-sensing device:

$$R_{AW} = \frac{\text{PIP} - \text{Pplat}}{\dot{V}_I} \qquad (2)$$

where $\dot{V}_I$ is inspiratory flow rate. Calculating changes in airway resistance can document quantitatively the progression of disease and healing. As was mentioned previously, however, whether this information is a useful predictor of successful weaning from mechanical ventilation is unclear.

Measurements of peak and plateau pressures associated with a ventilator-delivered V_T may be used for calculation of inspiratory work (W_I) performed on the lung and thorax, power ($\dot{W}_I$/min), and tension time index (TTI), all of which are indices of total muscle load when the patient breathes spontaneously. Requirements are a constant inspiratory flow waveform and no spontaneous inspiratory effort.[13] Under such conditions, pressure-time plots agree closely with pressure-volume plots, which usually are employed to calculate $\dot{W}_I$. A rather complex mathematical analysis based on the geometric

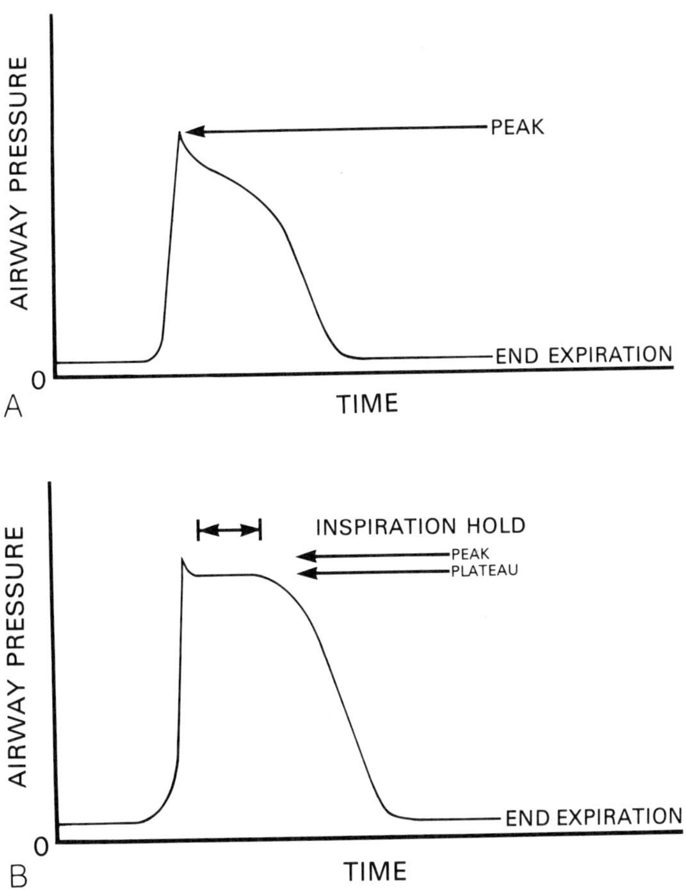

Fig. 9-3. (A) Airway pressure pattern of a typical positive-pressure breath over time. **(B)** Airway pressure pattern when 0.25 second inspiratory hold is applied to a typical positive-pressure breath. Plateau airway pressure becomes distinct during inspiratory hold. Thus, peak, plateau, and end-expiratory airway pressures can be distinguished.

configuration of the pressure-volume (and hence, pressure-time) profiles leads to the following equations:

$$W_I = (PIP - \tfrac{1}{2}\,Pplat) \times V_T \qquad (3)$$

$$\dot{W}_I = W_I \times f/min \qquad (4)$$

$$TTI = (PIP - \tfrac{1}{2}Pplat) \times T_I/Ttot \qquad (5)$$

where $T_I/Ttot$ is inspiratory time as a fraction of total ventilatory cycle time. These total load indices can also be expressed in terms of C_{LT}, R_{AW}, and $\dot{V}_I$:

$$W_I = (\dot{V}_I \times R_{AW} - \tfrac{1}{2}V_T/C_{LT}) \times V_T \qquad (6)$$

$$TTI = (\dot{V}_I \times R_{AW} - \tfrac{1}{2}V_T/C_{LT}) \times T_I/Ttot \qquad (7)$$

They may give predictive information for weaning, especially if indexed to muscle strength.[14,15] Unfortunately, large doses of sedatives or muscle-relaxants are frequently needed to ablate spontaneous ventilation to make these measurements properly. Such drugs usually are not justified solely for the purpose of measuring mechanical function, especially in the patient for whom weaning is imminent.

As an alternative to complex measurements of mechanical function, the spontaneous respiratory rate is an exquisitely sensitive reflection of changes in pulmonary mechanics.[16] Respiratory rate changes within less than 1 second after a lung compliance change.[17] With augmented pressure loads from decreased CLT or increased RAW, larger drops in intrapleural pressure (Ppl) are required to produce the same spontaneous tidal volume. The patient responds by taking shallower breaths to minimize the work expended per breath. To maintain adequate alveolar ventilation, respiratory rate must increase.

Neuromuscular Function

Muscle strength and muscle endurance influence the successful discontinuation of mechanical ventilation. Muscle strength allows the patient to inspire, an important consideration for breathing and coughing, while endurance ensures that the patient will continue to breathe indefinitely.

Strength can be assessed by the measurement of maximum voluntary ventilation (MVV), vital capacity, and peak negative pressure (PNP). The first two are effort-dependent; thus, it is possible to obtain a falsely low, but not falsely high, value. Patients who require mechanical ventilation for less than 7 days can be judged ready for discontinuation of mechanical ventilation from measurements of respiratory muscle strength only. Using resting minute ventilation, PNP, and MMV, Sahn and Lakschminarayan[18] prospectively found that 76 of 100 such patients were successfully weaned and extubated if they met the criteria in Table 9-2.

On the other hand, the prediction of weaning success for patients who require protracted ventilatory support is more complex. They frequently have multiple-system disease and nutritional deficiencies. Vital capacity alone does not predict success in weaning. Morganroth and co-workers[20,21] retrospectively examined the combination of PNP vital capacity to tidal volume ratio, respiratory rate, and minute ventilation to predict weaning success. They found that this combination of variables did not predict successful weaning and did not change between the time the patients could not and could be weaned from ventilatory support. Thus, conventional measurements of muscle strength poorly reflected the patient's ability to assume spontaneous ventilation in this more severely disabled population.

Table 9-2. Indices of Respiratory Muscle Strength that Predict Successful Weaning for Patients Ventilated Less than 7 Days

Variable	Value
Negative inspiratory pressure	More negative than 30 cm H_2O
Minute ventilation	< 10 L
Maximum voluntary ventilation	> twice minute ventilation

Combining measurements of total load and of muscle function might better reflect the need for ventilatory support than either measurement alone. Dividing TTI by the maximum diaphragmatic pressure (PDI_{max}) predicted fatigue in normal adults breathing against high resistances.[22–24] PDI_{max} is measured best by placing transducers on either side of the diaphragm. Clinically, it can be approximated from properly performed PNP pressure measurement.[1] When the TTI/PDI_{max} exceeds 0.15 in normal adults, muscle fatigue develops. Milic-Emili[14] and Kline et al.[15] successfully predicted the onset of respiratory muscle fatigue by calculating TTI/PDI_{max} in a small number of mechanically ventilated patients. Whether the development of respiratory muscle fatigue necessarily precludes weaning from ventilatory support has not been determined.

Experimental approaches to the assessment of neuromuscular function include diaphragmatic electromyographic (EMG) patterns, which are technically difficult to perform. A shift in the high- to low-power spectrum ratio is associated with muscle overload and inpending fatigue.[25] Simpler approaches worthy of future investigation include scalene and sternocleidomastoid muscle observations[5] and the measurement of airway pressure 100 msec after the initiation of a spontaneous breath taken from a closed circuit.[26]

Gas Exchange

Carbon Dioxide Elimination

A primary purpose of mechanical ventilation is to eliminate CO_2. Thus, to be weaned from ventilator support, the patient must be able to breathe so that the pHa is within normal limits and the $PaCO_2$ is acceptable. Respiratory acidemia is one indication of weaning failure. Only two variables determine $PaCO_2$: alveolar ventilation and CO_2 production. Factors that increase dead-space ventilation or CO_2 production necessitate a larger minute ventilation to keep $PaCO_2$ normal, thus imposing an increased ventilation load (Fig. 9-1, Table 9-3). These abnormalities should be treated aggressively before making any attempts at weaning.

Arterial Oxygenation

Mechanical ventilation rarely is instituted solely to reverse hypoxemia. Rather, supplemental oxygen and PEEP/continuous positive airway pressure (CPAP) are indicated to support arterial oxygenation. However, if the mechanically ventilated patient requires an $FIO_2 > 0.50$ to keep $PaO_2 > 65$ mmHg (or $SaO_2 > 0.90$), the underlying disease process probably is not reversed sufficiently to permit discontinuation of ventilator support. For patients with acute restrictive pulmonary defects (acute lung injury), PEEP/CPAP may decrease the requirement for supplemental oxygen and improve pulmonary mechanics sufficiently to obviate mechanical ventilation.[27] The application of PEEP/CPAP does not reverse the disease process, but the underlying defect in pulmonary function, a decreased functional residual capacity (FRC), can be corrected by such therapy. As a general guideline, ventilated patients who need a high FIO_2 despite appropriate PEEP/CPAP therapy usually are not ready to assume totally spontaneous ventilation.

Table 9-3. Circumstances that Require Larger Minute Ventilation

Increased dead space
Pulmonary gas trapping (COPD or asthma)
Low cardiac output
Excessive (more than is needed) positive end-expiratory pressure
Pulmonary emboli
Increased CO_2 production
Fever
Shivering
Agitation/exercise
Diet with high carbohydrate-to-lipid nonprotein calorie ratio
Hypermetabolism-thyroid storm, malignant hyperthermia)

Ventilatory Pattern

Once mechanical ventilation is discontinued, the pattern of breathing that the patient adopts should be tolerable indefinitely. Respiratory rate, tidal volume, and regularity determine this pattern. Most critically ill patients cannot tolerate respiratory rates in excess of 30 to 35 breaths/min. This degree of tachypnea often reflects underlying pathology. The clinical situation and the medical history will usually allow discrimination between the various causes of an abnormally rapid respiratory rate.

Tachypnea must be distinguished from alveolar hyperventilation (an abnormally low $PaCO_2$ accompanied by respiratory alkalemia). Although tachypnea and hyperventilation may coincide, their differential diagnosis is important. Problems that result in tachypnea with normocarbia are summarized in Table 9-4. Tachypnea is one of the earliest signs that weaning has been unsuccessful. Tobin and co-workers[28] found that patients who failed a weaning trial exhibit a rapid, shallow ventilatory pattern immediately after cessation of mechanical ventila-

Table 9-4. Differential Diagnosis of Tachypnea with Normocarbia

Acute restrictive pulmonary defect/decreased FRC
Pulmonary edema (cardiogenic, noncardiogenic, or ARDS)
Mechanically decreased FRC
Pleural fluid
Pneumothorax
Ascites
Obesity
Supine position (worse head down)
Central nervous system
Abdominal splinting
Pain
Muscular weakness
Generalized (e.g., muscle relaxant drugs, myasthenia)
Quadriplegia
Ventilatory muscle fatigue
Acutely increased physiologic dead-space ventilation
See Table 9-3

ARDS, adult respiratory distress syndrome.

tion. Thus, the respiratory rate may be the most consistent predictor of weaning success.[29]

Narcotic administration is the most common cause of bradypnea. Narcotics typically induce a ventilatory pattern with a slow rate and a large tidal volume. Spontaneous rates below 10 breaths/min usually result from narcotic ventilatory depression and are a possible reflection of iatrogenic ventilatory failure. Mental status correlates poorly with the degree of ventilatory depression. Thus, narcotic administration to suppress "agitation" easily can result in a sedate patient with depressed ventilatory drive. Further, narcotics can render the patient wakeful enough to follow commands, yet apneic unless instructed to breathe.

In summary, very low or very high spontaneous respiratory rates often reflect processes that will preclude discontinuation of mechanical ventilation. Other specific patterns of ventilation may impart information regarding respiratory muscle status. For example, respiratory alternans, alternate abdominal and thoracic accessory muscle use heralds early respiratory muscle fatigue.[29] Patients who develop respiratory muscle fatigue probably will fail attempts at weaning from mechanical ventilation. For all of the stated reasons, ventilatory rate and pattern should receive vigilant attention before, during, and after weaning.

Subjective Sensation of Ventilation

William Osler might be relieved to hear that critical care specialists also have learned that listening to the patient is of value. Patients who indicate that breathing is uncomfortable or that they feel short of breath probably will fail trials of weaning. The converse, however, is not always true; patients who are not ready for weaning or who fail weaning trials may be very comfortable. Clinicians should ensure that the patient's dyspnea is caused by the disease and not by the equipment through which the patient is breathing (see Chs. 14 and 15).

Tracheal Extubation

Although discontinuation of mechanical ventilation and tracheal extubation are frequently discussed simultaneously, the patient may not be ready for extubation, even though he can breathe without ventilator support. Mechanical ventilation is the most common reason for tracheal intubation in critically ill patients. However, four other indications must be considered prior to tracheal extubation (Table 9-5). When none of these five indications is present, extubation is appropriate.

Positive-pressure ventilation can be delivered with a mask, but this technique is impractical in the ICU other than for emergency measures. Most critically ill patients who require ventilatory support also need tracheal tubes. Once weaning is achieved, the tube should remain in place until all other indications are ruled out—a process that usually takes less than five minutes. The majority of patients who do not have airway obstruction prior to intubation will not develop obstruction when they are extubated. However, a small but significant number acquire sufficient vocal cord edema to cause problems. Patients with abscesses or tumors of the face or neck should be evaluated carefully prior to extubation. Similar considerations apply to those with facial trauma.

If the patient cannot prevent foreign material from passing through the vocal cords, a cuffed tracheal tube should be used to protect the airway. The three primary, primitive airway protective reflexes are gag, swallow, and cough. Of the three, cough reflex is the most important, but also requires the most strength. Airway protection can be present in the absence of gag or swallow reflexes. Extubating a patient who is unable to protect the airway increases the

Table 9-5. Indications for Tracheal Intubation in the Critically Ill

Mechanical ventilation
Pulmonary toilet
Airway protection
Airway obstruction
CPAP (when mask CPAP is inappropriate)

risk for pulmonary aspiration of gastric contents.

A tracheal tube also allows suctioning of secretions from the large airways. Pulmonary toilet for the patient who is unable or unwilling to cough can be performed safely through a tracheal tube. Patients may be able to breathe, but unable to cough effectively. High-level quadriplegics frequently retain artificial airways for pulmonary toilet, even though they do not need mechanical ventilation. Occasionally, patients who can breathe and who retain airway protective reflexes lack the "desire" to cough spontaneously or on command, because of an altered level of consciousness. The variables which reflect ventilatory muscle strength, vital capacity, and PNP are excellent predictors of the patient's ability (not desire) to cough.[30] Although nasotracheal suctioning can be performed, a high incidence of dysrhythmias and complications may result which are preventable with proper suctioning through an artificial airway.[31–33]

Finally, CPAP without ventilatory support may be needed in a patient for whom mask CPAP is inadvisable. Up to 12 to 15 cm H_2O CPAP can be delivered effectively with a mask.[24] However, mask CPAP should be restricted to patients who are able to remove the close-fitting mask if they must vomit.

In summary, to be ready for extubation, patients should be successfully weaned from mechanical ventilation, not require in excess of 5 to 10 cm H_2O CPAP and 0.50 FIO_2, not be at high risk of developing airway obstruction, have intact airway protective reflexes, and be able and willing to cough.

WEANING TECHNIQUES

No randomized, prospective investigation demonstrates the superiority of one weaning technique over another. Emotion, rather than intellect, frequently dominates debate concerning the choice of a weaning mode. Weaning should be considered only when the patient's underlying cause of ventilatory failure has resolved, when the nutritional status is favorable, and when a metabolically and hemodynamically stable state is achieved. This section describes how the two most common techniques for weaning, T-piece, and intermittent mandatory ventilation (IMV),[35] are employed together with their advantages and drawbacks. A newer approach to weaning, pressure support ventilation (PSV), is also considered.

T-Piece

Weaning using the T-piece method alternates full ventilatory support and no ventilatory support until the patient can sustain spontaneous ventilation indefinitely. The patient undergoes short "T-piece periods," initially lasting 5 to 10 minutes, at intervals throughout the day. The T-piece periods are separated by at least 1 to 2 hours of continued mechanical ventilation to allow the patient to rest.[2] Furthermore, patients usually receive full nocturnal ventilatory support until weaning is nearly complete. The T-piece periods are lengthened and/or increased in frequency until the patient assumes his own work of breathing entirely. During T-piece periods, gas exchange and early signs of ventilatory muscle fatigue should be monitored closely. When such fatigue occurs, mechanical ventilation should be resumed. Weaning is successful when the patient requires no ventilatory support for 24 hours.

Using this weaning technique, Morganroth and co-workers[21] studied 11 patients who were mechanically ventilated for more than 30 days. Nine were weaned successfully over periods ranging from 11 to 43 days. The time spent during T-piece periods each day was predictive of the fraction of the entire weaning process that was completed. Patients who breathed through a T-piece for a total of 10 h/day, on the average, had progressed 60 percent of the way to complete weaning. If 12 days were required to reach this point, an additional 8 days to completely discontinue ventilatory support probably would be necessary.

Rather than having patients breathe at ambient pressure during T-tube weaning, high-flow

CPAP systems can be used. This technique allows the patient with abnormally stiff lungs to maintain a higher FRC and thereby decrease the elastic work of breathing. A demand-valve CPAP system should not be used for this purpose, since it may introduce sufficient work to make the technique fail.

The T-piece weaning method requires relatively simple equipment. Only a T-piece, connecting tubing, and an oxygen source are needed. However, the patient who is transferred suddenly from full to no ventilatory support must be observed closely and continuously for early signs of failure. To achieve success with this technique, the observer must interrupt each T-piece period after the patient has breathed for as long as possible without experiencing excessive muscle fatigue. Thus, although the equipment is simple, the process is labor intensive.

Intermittent Mandatory Ventilation

Intermittent mandatory ventilation allows unrestricted spontaneous ventilation punctuated by positive pressure breaths at predetermined intervals.[36] It is one of the few methods of positive-pressure ventilation that allows partial support in graded increments (or decrements) to suit individual patient requirements. Unlike the T-piece method, where the weaning process is abrupt, the onset of weaning during ventilatory support with IMV is gradual.

Successful application of IMV necessitates the use of appropriate equipment. Currently marketed demand valves frequently offer high resistance and create a lag between the patient's initial inspiratory effort and the delivery of gas. As a result the inspiratory work of breathing is increased. Spontaneous inspiratory work is lessened if gas is delivered by high continuous flow, usually 40 to 60 L/min, with a low-compliance reservoir bag in the inspiratory limb.[37,38]

Weaning with IMV requires more sophisticated equipment than does the T-piece technique. However, IMV affords the opportunity to withdraw ventilatory support gradually, so that only the required level of support is provided at any given time. When the patient is ready for weaning, the rate of mechanical breaths is decreased commensurate with the recovery of spontaneous breathing. The patient's clinical course should dictate the rate at which mechanical support is withdrawn. Arranging rigid schedules by which to decrease the ventilatory frequency defeats the purpose of the technique and is likely to prolong the process. As with the T-piece method, vigilance for early signs of failure allows intervention before the patient becomes overtly distressed, fatigued, or hemodynamically compromised.

Although neither IMV nor T-tube weaning is definitely superior, indirect evidence suggests that in selected populations, IMV possesses certain advantages. Räsänen and co-workers[39] compared full and partial ventilatory support with IMV and CPAP to controlled mechanical ventilation and PEEP in patients with left ventricular failure. These investigators found that abrupt discontinuation of ventilatory support at the onset of a T-piece trial affected cardiac function detrimentally. However, when ventilatory support was withdrawn gradually using IMV, cardiac function did not change.

When a switch from full ventilatory support to a T-piece occurs, mean airway pressure drops significantly, causing an increase in intrathoracic blood volume. Conversely, mean airway pressure falls gradually with IMV, thus avoiding rapid redistribution of blood volume. Thus, for patients with compromised left ventricular function in whom abrupt centralization of blood volume is potentially deleterious, IMV appears to be the preferred weaning technique.

Pressure Support Ventilation

Pressure support ventilation is a relatively new technique of mechanical ventilatory support that can be used for weaning process. It provides an adjustable, preselected level of inspiratory pressure assist with every spontaneous breath effort. Depending upon the level of pressure assistance, ventilatory muscle loads with each breath are either partially or totally eliminated.[40] Weaning is accomplished by decreasing the inspiratory pressure assist from high to progressively lower levels as ventilatory failure resolves.[10]

A protocol for weaning with PSV is outlined in Table 9-6. This approach begins at an inspiratory pressure that virtually completely unloads the ventilatory muscles. This level is termed PSV_{max} and is defined as the inspiratory pressure that results in a VT of 10 to 12 ml/kg.[40] Gradual and progressive reduction of this pressure allows an increasingly greater proportion of the work/breath to be assumed by the ventilatory muscles. The rate of decrease in the inspiratory pressure assist is determined from conventional parameters, especially the patient's respiratory rate, which is an excellent guide to the intrinsic "load sensors." Mechanical ventilatory support is weaned when the level of inspiratory pressure is just that required to overcome the resistance load imposed by the endotracheal tube (generally 5 to 10 cm H_2O).

Pressure support ventilation weaning differs from IMV or T-piece techniques in several important aspects. First, the quantity of work is returned to the patient gradually with every breath. This is in contrast to the intermittent return of total load/breath that occurs with approaches that alternate full machine support with spontaneous unsupported breathing. This more regular workload probably contributes to the improved comfort reported with PSV.[40] Second, ventilatory work is characterized by a more normal pressure-volume relationship during PSV weaning than during IMV weaning (Fig. 9-4 and Table 9-7). This difference may explain the increased muscle efficiency and promote endurance conditioning.[7,8,40] Finally, because the inspiratory pressure assist is designed to persist as long as the patient demands flow, better patient-ventilator synchrony may result, thereby improving comfort and reducing sedation needs.

This approach has not been compared with conventional weaning techniques in any systematic study. Moreover, such a study is not likely to occur given the clear historical success rate of conventional approaches and because hundreds of patients would need to be randomized to properly address the question. Thus the application of a PSV weaning approach must be justified primarily on other rationale, including improved comfort and more physiologic loads on the ventilatory muscles. Further studies on ventilatory reflexes and muscle function during the weaning process are needed to more fully address these issues.

Table 9-6. Pressure Support Weaning Protocol

1. *Patient selection:* Slowly resolving pulmonary process, reliable respiratory drive.
2. *Initial settings:* Start at PSV_{max} (VT = 10–12 ml/kg; work to inflate the lungs is provided by the ventilator)
   a. Reduce pressure support level as tolerated, that is, gradually increase patient work while simultaneously decreasing ventilator work (respiratory rate reflects tolerance)
   b. Extubate at 5 cm H_2O pressure support
3. *Considerations:*
   a. PSV_{max} pressure $>$ 50 cm H_2O is rarely needed (higher pressures indicate an unstable patient).
   b. Backup controlled ventilation should be used as "safety net."

PSV_{max} is highest level of inspiratory pressure assist required to deliver a tidal volume of 10–12 ml/kg and to eliminate the patient's contribution of work to each breath.

SUMMARY

Readiness for the discontinuation of mechanical ventilatory support is probably more important than the method of weaning employed. Unfortunately, the prediction of weaning success is difficult, even when combining information that reflects respiratory muscle strength, mechanical pulmonary function, neuromuscular function, gas exchange, and ventilatory pattern. The respiratory rate may be the best easily available guide to success.

The two most commonly employed weaning techniques, T-piece trials and IMV, do not appear to differ in their rate of success, although they have variable physiologic effects. Appropriate equipment is essential for the success of any technique. A newer approach employing PSV may return breathing work to the patient

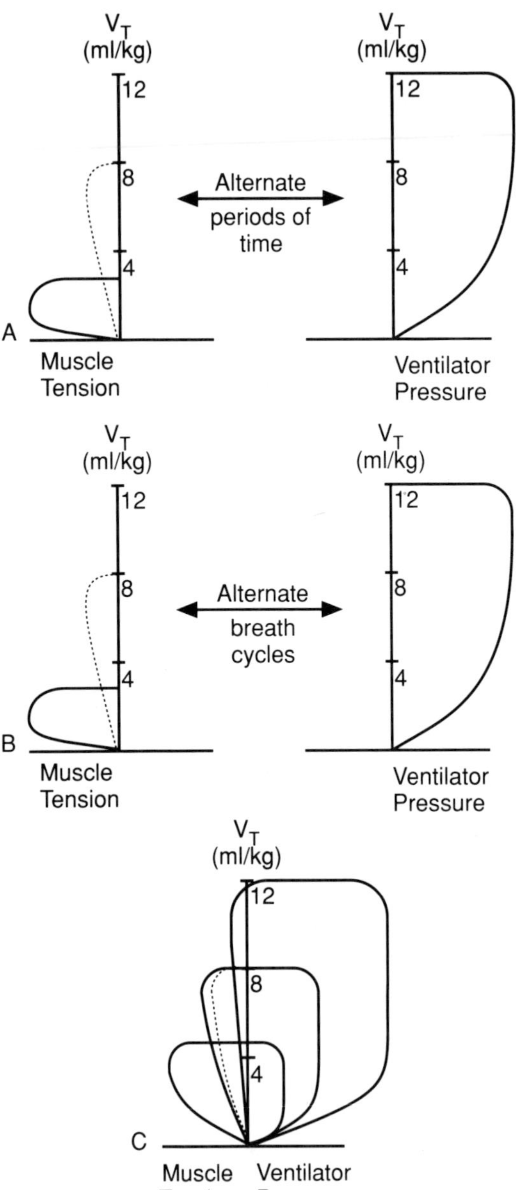

Fig. 9-4. Schematic diagrams representing quantity and characteristics of the patient's and the ventilator's contributions to work of breathing during various modes of mechanical ventilatory support. Work/tidal breath is the area inscribed by the pressure-volume relationship during that breath. Spontaneous breaths are depicted with leftward directed muscle tension or intramuscular pressure; ventilator breaths are depicted with rightward directed airway pressure. The dashed line represents a normal pressure-volume relationship. **(A)** Control/T-tube ventilation. This approach enables patients to work only during T-tube trials. Patient work quantity is controlled by the duration of the T-tube trial while work characteristics are fixed as a higher than normal pressure/volume configuration reflecting abnormal impedances imposed by disease. **(B)** Intermittent mandatory ventilation with a demand valve system. This approach allows patients to work between mandatory ventilator breaths. Patient work quantity is thus controlled by the number of mandatory breaths given; work characteristics are again fixed in a higher than normal pressure/volume configuration. **(C)** Pressure support ventilation. Patient work quantity is controlled by the level of pressure applied with every breath. Unlike other volume-cycled ventilator modes, work characteristics are changed with PSV to a more normal configuration.

Table 9-7. Comparison of T-Piece, IMV, and PSV Weaning Techniques

	T-Piece	IMV	PSV
Work quantity	All or none	Adjust by number of mandatory breaths	Adjust by level of applied pressure
Work characteristics	Fixed as high P/V by ET tube and disease	Fixed as high P/V by ET tube and disease	P/V reduced by applied pressure
Synchrony	Regular periods of constant load; variable is determined by patient	Irregular loads; V_T of mandatory breaths set by clinician	Regular loads; patient interacts with applied pressure to determine V_T
Minute ventilation	Variable	Mandatory breath rate to guarantee minimum minute ventilation	Variable

P/V, pressure-volume relationship; ET, endotracheal.

on a breath-by-breath basis with a more normal load configuration. Randomized controlled studies comparing weaning modes do not exist.

ACKNOWLEDGMENTS

We thank Ms. E. Lawrence and Ms. B. Powell for expert secretarial assistance.

REFERENCES

1. Marini JJ: The physiologic determinants of ventilator dependence. Respir Care 31:271, 1986
2. Gillespie DJ, Marsh HMM, Divertie MB, et al: Clinical outcome of respiratory failure in patients requiring prolonged (>24 hours) mechanical ventilation. Chest 90:364, 1986
3. Glenn WWL, Hogan JF, Loke JSO: Ventilatory support by pacing of the conditioned diaphragm in quadriplegia. N Engl J Med 310:1150, 1984
4. Marini JJ: Exertion during ventilator support: how much and how important? Respir Care 31:385, 1986
5. Brochard L, Harf A, Lorino H, et al: Pressure support prevents diaphragmatic failure during weaning from mechanical ventilation (MV). Am Res Respir Dis 139:513, 1989
6. Belman MJ: Respiratory failure treated by ventilatory muscle training (VMT). Eur J Respir Dis 62:391, 1981
7. Mommaerts WFHM: Energetics of muscular contraction. Physiol Rev 49:427, 1969
8. Leith DE, Bradley M: Ventilatory muscle strength and endurance training. J Appl Physiol 41:508, 1976
9. MacIntyre NR, Leatherman NE: Mechanical loads on the ventilatory muscles: a theoretical analysis. Am Rev Respir Dis (In press, 1989)
10. MacIntyre NR: Weaning from mechanical ventilatory support: volume-assisting intermittent breaths versus pressure-assisting every breath. Respir Care 33:121, 1988
11. Marini JJ, Smith TC, Lamb VJ: External work output and force generation during synchronized intermittent mechanical ventilation: effect of machine assistance on breathing effort. Am Rev Respir Dis 138:1169, 1988
12. Fuleihan SF, Wilson RS, Pontoppidan H: Effect of mechanical ventilation with end-inspiratory pause on blood-gas exchange. Anesth Analg 55:122, 1976
13. Marini JJ, Rodriguez RM, Lamb V: Bedside estimation of the inspiratory work of breathing during mechanical ventilation. Chest 89:56, 1986
14. Milic-Emili J: Is weaning an art or a science? Am Rev Respir Dis 134:1107, 1986
15. Kline JL, Zimnicki GL, Antonenko DR, et al: The use of calculated relative inspiratory effort as a predictor of outcome in mechanical ventilation weaning trials. Respir Care 32:870, 1987
16. Weled BJ, Winfrey D, Downs JB: Measuring exhaled volume with continuous positive airway pressure and intermittent mandatory ventilation: techniques and rationale. Chest 76:166, 1979
17. Rose DM, Downs JB, Heenan TJ: Temporal responses of functional residual capacity and oxygen tension to changes in positive end-expiratory pressure. Crit Care Med 9:79, 1981
18. Sahn SA, Lakschminarayan MB: Bedside criteria for the discontinuation of mechanical ventilation. Chest 63:1002, 1973
19. Gilbert R, Auchincloss JH, Peppi D: The first few hours off a respirator. Chest 65:152, 1974
20. Morganroth ML, Grum CM: Weaning from mechanical ventilation. J Intens Care Med 3:109, 1988
21. Morganroth ML, Morganroth JL, Nett LM, et al: Criteria for weaning from prolonged mechanical ventilation. Arch Intern Med 144:1012, 1984
22. Collett PW, Perry C, Engel LA: Pressure time product, flow, and oxygen cost of resistive breathing in humans. J Appl Physiol 58:1263, 1985
23. Roussos C, Fixley M, Gross D, et al: Fatigue of inspiratory muscles and the synergic behavior. J Appl Physiol 46:897, 1979
24. McGregor M, Becklake MR: The relationship of oxygen cost of breathing to respiratory mechanical work and respiratory force. J Clin Invest 40:971, 1961
25. Cohen CA, Zagelbaum G, Gross D, et al: Clinical manifestations of inspiratory muscle fatigue. Am J Med 73:2308, 1982
26. Montgomery AB, Holle RHO, Neagley SR, et al: Prediction of successful ventilator weaning using airway occlusion pressure and hypercapnic challenge. Chest 91:496, 1987
27. Räsänen J, Heikkila H, Downs JB, et al: Continuous positive airway pressure by face mask in acute cardiogenic pulmonary edema. Am J Cardiol 55:296, 1985
28. Tobin MJ, Perez W, Guenther SM, et al: The pattern of breathing during successful and unsuccessful trials of weaning from mechanical ventilation. Am Rev Respir Dis 134:1111, 1986

29. Macklem PT: Respiratory muscles: the vital pump. Chest 78:753, 1980
30. Shapiro BA, Harrison RA, Kacmarek RM, et al: Clinical Application of Respiratory Care. Year Book Medical Publishers, Chicago, 1985, p. 544
31. Anesthesia Study Committee of the NY State Society of Anesthesiologists: Clinical Anesthesia Conference: endotracheal suction and death. NY State J Med 68:565, 1968
32. Demers RR: Complications of endotracheal suctioning procedure. Respir Care 27:453, 1982
33. Shim C, Fine N, Fernandez R, et al: Cardiac arrhythmias resulting from tracheal suctioning. Ann Intern Med 71:1149, 1969
34. Stock MC, Downs JB: Administration of continuous positive airway pressure by mask. Acute Care 10:184, 1984
35. Venus B, Smith RA, Mathru M: National survey of methods and criteria used for weaning from mechanical ventilation. Crit Care Med 15:530, 1987
36. Downs JB, Klein EF, Desautels D, et al: Intermittent mandatory ventilation: a new approach to weaning patients from mechanical ventilation. Chest 64:331, 1973
37. Gibney RTN, Wilson RS, Pontoppidan H: Comparison of work of breathing on high flow and demand valve continuous positive airway pressure breathing systems. Chest 82:692, 1982
38. Henry WC, West GA, Wilson RS: A comparison of the oxygen cost of breathing between a continuous-flow CPAP system and demand-flow CPAP system. Respir Care 28:1273, 1983
39. Räsänen J, Nikki P, Heikkila J: Acute myocardial infarction complicated by respiratory failure: the effects of mechanical ventilation. Chest 85:21, 1984
40. MacIntyre NR: Respiratory function during pressure support ventilation. Chest 89:677, 1986

10

Ventilation During Anesthesia

Nikolaus Gravenstein
Samsun Lampotang

Mechanical ventilation during anesthesia gained its primary impetus as a result of the difficulties in maintaining adequate gas exchange during thoracic surgical procedures and the introduction of muscle relaxants.[1]

During anesthesia, ventilatory requirements often are considerably different from those in the intensive care unit (ICU). The intensivist is confronted with a patient who is in respiratory distress and needs ventilator support, or is already receiving such support which must be maintained or weaned. In contrast, the patient presenting for surgery under anesthesia typically has no preoperative requirement for ventilator therapy. A change in the anesthetized patient's ventilation is iatrogenic, normally expected to be transient, and is acutely reversible.

Ventilatory support during anesthesia is necessitated (1) by the administration of drugs which depress normal ventilatory drive (e.g., anesthetics, narcotics) and alter physiologic responses (e.g., muscle relaxants), (2) by unusual positions (e.g., prone), (3) by the surgical incision (e.g., thoracotomy), or (4) by the placement of rctractors, packs and so forth, which inhibit or prevent the muscular response to any ventilatory drive that may still be present. Potent inhalation and intravenous anesthetics all suppress spontaneous ventilation. The facilitation of tracheal intubation by muscle relaxants, the enhanced operating conditions which they provide, and the availability of specific drugs to reverse them, make their use (and the depression of ventilation) virtually standard in anesthesia care.

Consider a typical anesthetic for a cholecystectomy. An otherwise healthy patient comes to the operating room (OR) breathing spontaneously. Following preoxygenation by mask, a barbiturate and a rapid-acting muscle relaxant are administered. While awaiting onset of sufficient muscular relaxation to allow easy visualization of the airway, the anesthesiologist delivers the tidal volume (V_T) manually. This procedure is followed by tracheal intubation, whereupon V_T is again delivered manually and bilateral breath sounds verified to confirm proper tube placement. Subsequently, the ventilation mode is converted from manual to mechanical, and inhalation anesthetics are added to the respired gas. Prior to the surgical incision, supplemental muscle relaxant is administered to facilitate surgical exposure and is continued until closure of the wound is begun. At this point, delivery of the inhalation anesthetic is gradually diminished in preparation for awakening the patient. Any residual muscle relaxant activity is reversed, and rapid weaning from complete ventilatory support to manually-assisted ventilation, and spontaneous breathing proceeds as tolerated. When all goes well, the patient is awake at this stage, breathing spontaneously, and ready for extubation. The entire process often takes less than 1 hour, is managed by a single individual in full time attendance, and is repeated (in different patients) many times each day.

Anesthesia ventilator systems are, therefore, designed to provide acute, short duration support in concert with an anesthesia machine and breathing circuit. This chain of events, which facilitates repeated transitions from spontaneous to manual to mechanical to manually-assisted spontaneous and finally to spontaneous ventilation again is unusual in the ICU. Furthermore, unlike the ICU ventilator, virtually all anesthesia ventilators are designed to work in parallel (integrated) with an anesthesia machine.

MISSION PROFILES

The American Society of Anesthesiologists (ASA) basic monitoring standards dictate that the patient under anesthesia is cared for continuously on a one-on-one basis by the anesthesia provider.[2] The ICU nurse or physician, in contrast, usually cares for two or more patients simultaneously. The difference in requisite and available human monitoring of ventilator and ventilator equipment in these two environments offers an intuitive explanation for the greater sophistication of the automated alarms and internal monitoring available in ICU ventilators compared to those used during anesthesia.

The different mission profiles of ICU and anesthesia ventilators are evident in their respective design and function (Table 10-1). The underlying pathology (ICU), or typical lack thereof (OR), dictate the ''bells and whistles'' considered necessary and desirable in each setting. The typically longer duration of ventilatory support and more gradual weaning of the ICU patient suggest the need for more flexibility in an ICU ventilator than is normally necessary in the OR.

Historically, anesthesia ventilators have been relatively ''bare-bones'' devices, functioning primarily to replace the anesthesiologist's hand on the breathing bag (Fig. 10-1). Note the limited and simple control panels in Figure 10-1B. The shorter duration of intraoperative ventilation makes the use of humidification devices less common and thus not normally a part of an anesthesia ventilator. When necessary, they are added into the anesthesia breathing circuit. The premium placed on space is also evident; anesthesia ventilators are typically hardly larger than a bread box (Fig. 10-2).

Continuous positive airway pressure (CPAP) requires a breathing circuit to provide continuous gas flow in the range of the peak inspiratory flow rate.[3] However, such high flow rates are not feasible in the OR because the respired gas mixture also contains expensive anesthetics, much of which would be wasted and would lead to OR contamination.[4] Accordingly, the ventilator and breathing circuit are routinely ''scavenged'' to limit such contamination.[5] The current trend in anesthesia practice employs ever lower fresh-gas flow rates to minimize heat and humidity losses, as well as anesthetic consumption and pollution. Since the bulk of ventilation during anesthesia is controlled, spontaneous breathing with high flow CPAP is of little benefit when compared to positive end-expiratory pressure (PEEP), in conjunction with mechanical ventilation.

Table 10-1. Ventilator Mission/Application Profile

	Anesthesia	ICU
Patient respiratory status	Normal	Abnormal
Duration of support	Acute (<8 hr)	Chronic (>8 hr)
Humidification	No	Yes
Physical size	Small, integrated	Flexible, stand alone
Human monitor	Continuous	Intermittent
Alarms	Low pressure/apnea	Low pressure/apnea/high pressure
CPAP capability	No	Yes
Scavenger	Yes	No
PEEP	Add on	Yes

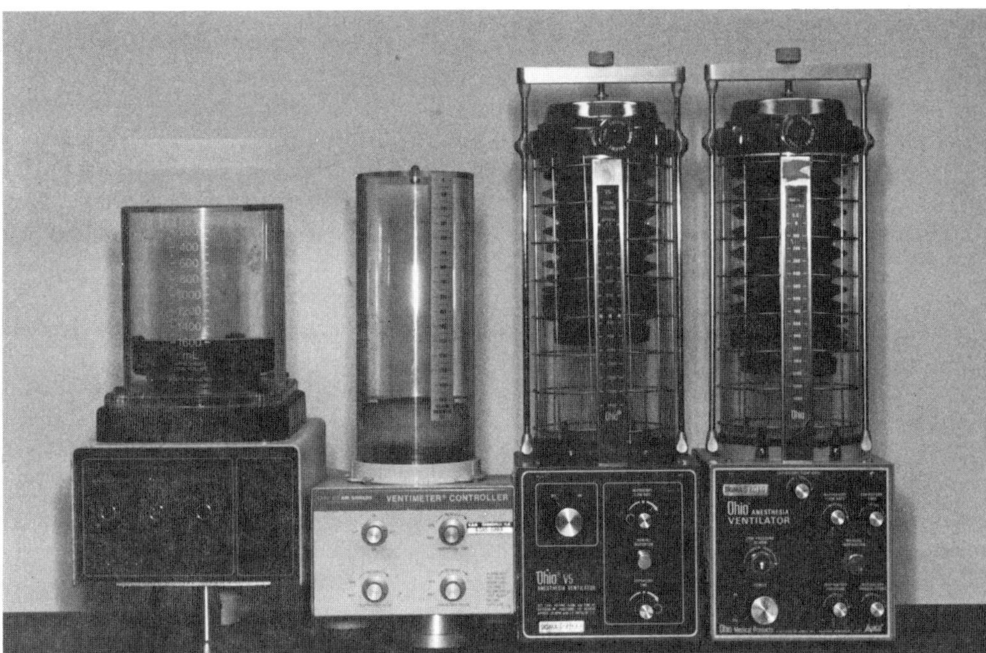

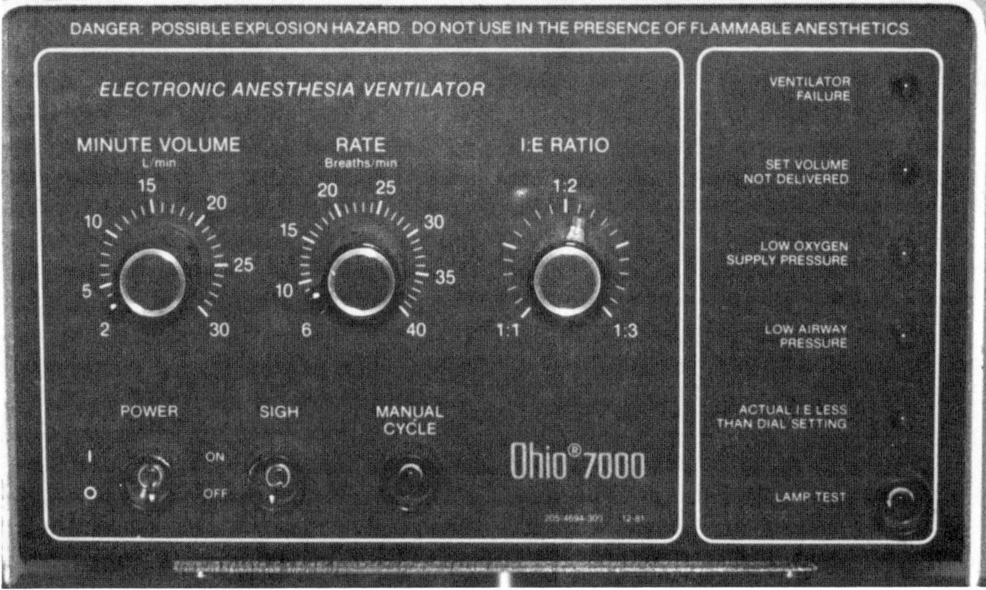

Fig. 10-1. **(A)** Typical anesthesia ventilators in current use. The two on the left are ascending bellows types and the two on the right are descending bellows types. **(B)** Close-up view of one anesthesia ventilator control panel. Note that there are only six controls.

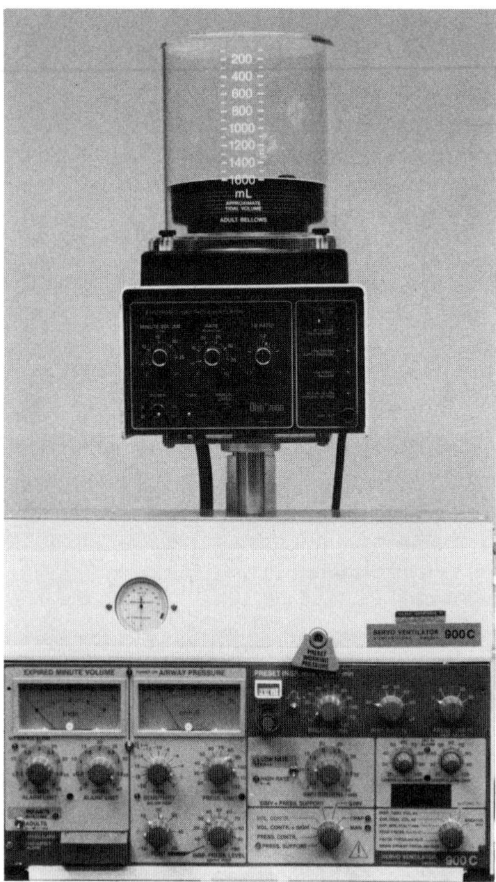

Fig. 10-2. ICU ventilator with an anesthesia ventilator placed on top of it. Note the difference in size and complexity.

EQUIPMENT COMPARISONS: ANESTHESIA VERSUS ICU VENTILATORS

According to Schreiber's criteria,[6] most anesthesia ventilators are classified as (1) controllers (start of inspiration and expiration are controlled by the ventilator setting, regardless of patient effort); (2) pneumatically-powered (power to cycle the ventilator is derived from a compressed gas rather than a mechanical source); (3) time-cycled (initiation of mechanical inspiration and expiration is based solely on elapsed time); (4) volume-limited (inspired V_T is a function of bellows excursion, rather than a preset delivery pressure); and (5) indirect power transmitters (gas powering the ventilator moves a bellows, which in turn delivers the V_T to the patient (Table 10-2).

Although many ICU ventilators allow assisted ventilation (i.e., the ventilator completes a breath initiated by the patient), this feature is lacking in most anesthesia ventilators (Table 10-2). In the ICU, ventilators can be electronically- or pneumatically-powered. No anesthesia ventilators are electronically-powered. On the other hand, pneumatic, electronic, or combination control circuitry are common features of both ICU and OR ventilators. Both types of ventilators typically use time-cycling, whereas permutations of inspiratory flow rate (constant versus variable) and circuit pressure (e.g., inspiratory hold) are common additional features of ICU, but not anesthesia, ventilators. ICU ventilators are usually volume-limited, with an adjustable high-pressure limit. In contrast, almost all anesthesia ventilators incorporate only a fixed low-pressure limit. Anesthesia ventilators do not provide adjustable PEEP. When PEEP is used, it is as an add-on component to the anesthesia breathing circuit rather than integrated into the ventilator. Most modern ICU ventilators do not incorporate a bellows; therefore, V_T is controlled by adjustment of the inspiratory flow rate and inspiratory time, or by piston excursion. With anesthesia ventilators, V_T is determined by a combination of the ventilator bellows excursion plus the fresh gas flow of the anesthesia machine.

Virtually all anesthesia ventilators, as mentioned, incorporate an indirect power transmission (i.e., a housing around the ventilator bellows is pressurized to empty the contents into the circuit), whereas piston and continuous flow-type ICU ventilators transmit the V_T directly to the patient.

ANESTHESIA BREATHING CIRCUITS

Breathing circuits link the ventilator to the patient. The two most common anesthesia

Table 10-2. Ventilator Classification[a]

	Anesthesia	ICU
Mode	Controlled	Assisted/controlled
Power source	Pneumatic	Pneumatic, electronic
Cycling control	Time	Time, patient inspiratory effort
Flow pattern	Constant	Adjustable
Safety limit	Volume, time	Volume, time, pressure
Power transmission	Indirect (bellows)	Direct (piston/fresh gas)

[a] A comparison of attributes common to the majority of anesthesia and ICU ventilators in use.
(Based on Schreiber's Classification Scheme,[6] with permission.)

breathing circuits are the circle system and the Bain circuit. Circle systems are employed most frequently. In both systems, the fresh gas source which provides oxygen and inhalational anesthetic agents to the breathing circuit is the anesthesia machine (Fig. 10-3).

Circle System

Unlike an ICU ventilator breathing circuit, the circle breathing system used during anesthesia contains a carbon dioxide absorber (Fig. 10-3). This system uses valves to provide intermittent, unidirectional gas flow. Fresh gas is continuously added to the system at the absorber, usually at total flow rates considerably less than the minute ventilation. This arrangement is possible because carbon dioxide in the exhaled gas is filtered through the CO_2 absorber and removed, allowing the "scrubbed" exhaled gases to be rerouted to the patient. Thus, rebreathing of gases (except carbon dioxide) occurs.

Unidirectional gas flow is accomplished via one-way valves located in the inspiratory and expiratory limbs of the breathing circuit at the absorber canister. CO_2 removal by the absorbant is so efficient that, in principle, the total fresh gas flow required is as little as that necessary to supply oxygen for metabolic needs—on the order of 4 ml O_2/kg/min with a leak-free circuit. In practice, however, many potential leakage sites must be compensated for by additional fresh gas flow to the breathing circuit (Fig. 10-4). Quite commonly, monitoring of respiratory gases during anesthesia (e.g., capnometry) is desirable; if done with a sidestream sampling device, another "leak" is imposed, and an additional flow requirement equal to the gas sampling rate of the monitor, usually 100 to 200 ml/min, must be provided unless the sampled gas is rerouted back into the circle system.

Ventilation may be spontaneous, manual, or mechanical. It is helpful to consider both circuit pressure and venting of excess gas from the circuit to further delineate the difference between the modes of ventilation (Table 10-3).

For spontaneous breathing, a reservoir bag is positioned on the CO_2 absorber side of the expiratory valve (Fig. 10-3). Inspiratory "negative" pressure opens the inspiratory valve and seals the expiratory valve. CO_2-free gas is drawn from the inspiratory limb of the circle, the absorber, and the fresh gas inlet in the absorber. An inspiratory gas flow rate in excess of the fresh-gas flow rate is provided from the breathing bag reservoir positioned between the expiratory valve and the absorber. This arrangement requires that the breathing bag/ventilator hose selector switch is set for breathing bag use. The bag contains exhaled gases which pass through the absorber where CO_2 is removed during spontaneous inspiration. During exhalation, positive circuit pressure closes the inspiratory valve and opens the expiratory valve. Exhaled gases then refill the reservoir bag. Any excess volume (i.e., added fresh gas flow in excess of the gas consumed) is vented from the circle system through an adjustable pressure-limiting (APL) valve located at the reservoir bag on the absorber side of the expiratory valve.

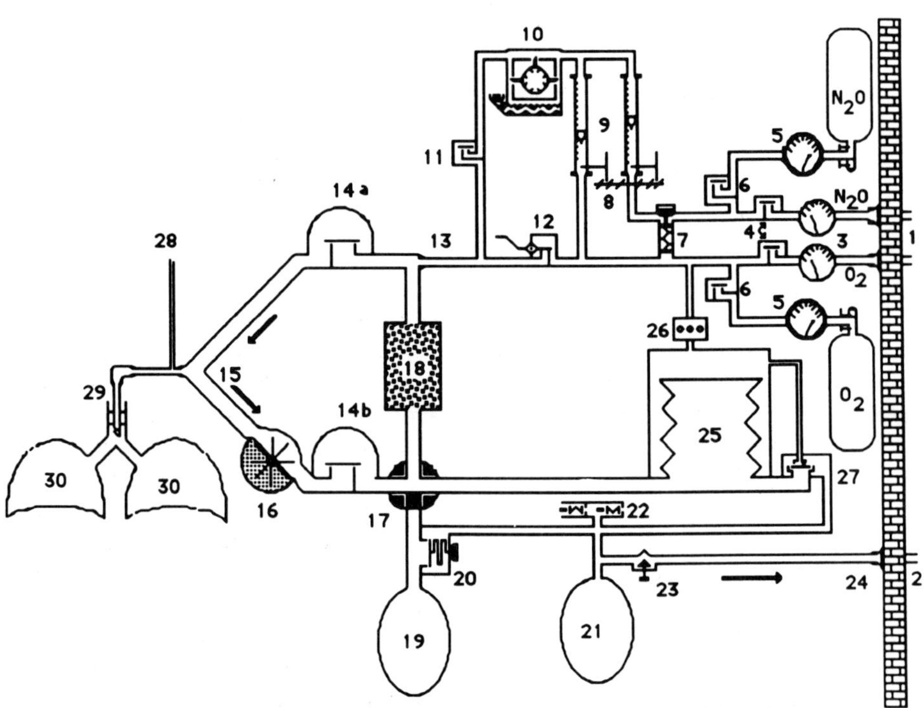

Fig. 10-3. Schematic of gas supply and anesthesia machine with a circle system. Anesthesia machine (1–13), breathing circuit (14–20), scavenging system (21–24), anesthesia ventilator (25–27), and patient interface (28–30).

Gas Supply and Anesthesia Machine

1, central gas supply; 2, central vacuum; 3, pressure gauges for piped oxygen and nitrous oxide; 4, one-way valve preventing loss of gas when piped gas is disconnected; 5, pressure gauges for oxygen and nitrous oxide cylinders; 6, valves preventing flow from cylinders while piped gas is connected and pressurized; 7, oxygen pressure failure protection (stops nitrous oxide flow when oxygen pressure falls); 8, oxygen proportioning device (prevents delivery of less than preset proportion of oxygen in gas mixture); 9, flowmeter tubes and floats; 10, anesthetic vaporizer; 11, device minimizing pressure transmission from breathing circuit to vaporizer; 12, oxygen flush valve; 13, common gas (fresh gas) outlet.

Breathing Circuit

14a, inspiratory valve; 14b, expiratory valve; 15, patient hoses and Y-piece; 16, spirometer; 17, breathing bag/ventilator hose selector-switch set for ventilator use; 18, CO_2 absorber; 19, breathing bag; 20, adjustable pressure limiting (APL) or "pop-off" valve.

Scavenging System

21, scavenging reservoir bag; 22, valve to compensate for excess positive or negative pressure; 23, suction control; 24, connection to central vacuum; 25, ventilator bellows (ascending type); 26, ventilator housing and power supply (here oxygen) and controls; 27, ventilator spill valve.

Patient Interface

28, gas sampling site for monitoring inhaled and exhaled gas composition; 29, endotracheal tube; 30, lungs. (Modified from Gravenstein,[31] with permission.)

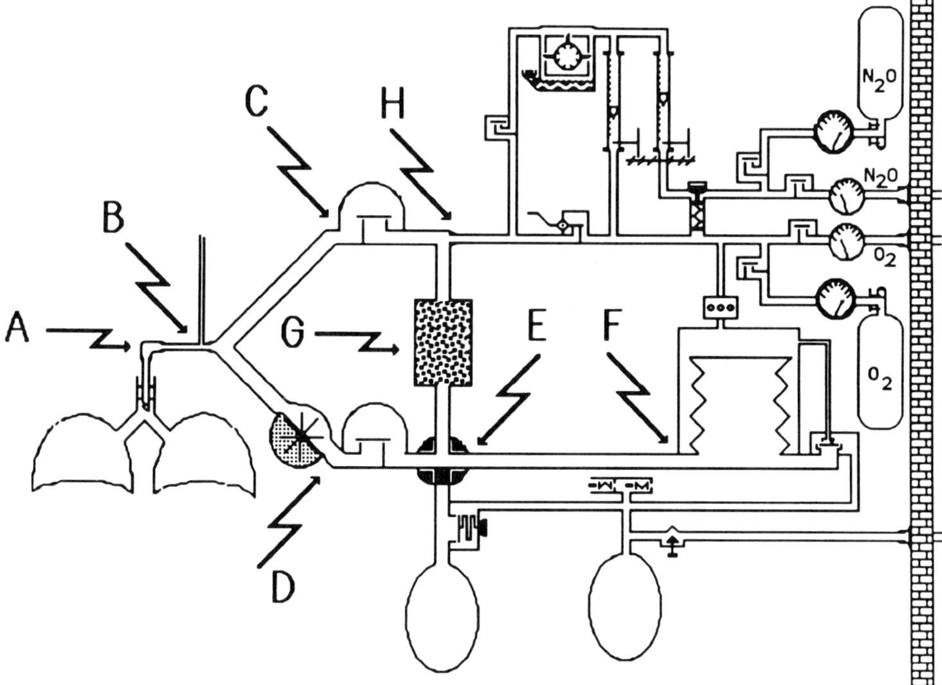

Fig. 10-4. Schematic of Figure 10-3 showing common leak and disconnect sites. A, elbow connecting endotracheal tube and breathing circuit Y-piece; B, gas sampling line attachment; C, inspiratory hose attachment to circle system; D, expiratory hose attachment to circle system; E, ventilator hose attachment to circle system; F, ventilator hose attachment to ventilator; G, CO_2-absorber gaskets; H, common gas outlet connection to circle system. (Modified from Gravenstein,[31] with permission.)

Normally, the APL valve is set to offer minimal resistance to exhalation during spontaneous ventilation (i.e., it is fully open). Fresh gas flow, which is added to the circuit during the expiratory pause, flows through the absorber and out the APL valve.

Manual ventilation is distinguished from spontaneous breathing because it occurs when compression of the reservoir bag adds positive pressure to the absorber canister from which it is transmitted to the circuit during inspiration. This pressure opens the inspiratory valve while sealing the expiratory valve. The gas flow path is otherwise identical to spontaneous ventilation, except that excess gas in the circuit is vented out of the APL valve during inspiration. Manual ventilation is pressure limited by the APL valve. When it is adjusted to a partially closed setting, sufficient inspiratory pressure is generated to deliver the desired V_T, while excess gas (and pressure) are vented from the breathing circuit.

Mechanical ventilation is achieved by replac-

Table 10-3. Circuit Gas Pressure and Venting from Anesthesia Circuits

	Inspiratory phase		Expiratory phase	
	Pressure	Venting	Venting	Vent site
Spontaneous	0	0	+	APL valve
Manual	+	+	0	APL valve
Mechanical	+	0	+	Ventilator spill valve

ing the reservoir bag (literally or in effect via the selector switch) with a coupling hose and ventilator (Fig. 10-3). During mechanical inspiration, gas flow from the ventilator bellows into the absorber canister raises circuit pressure, seals the expiratory valve, and opens the inspiratory valve. Both the APL and ventilator spill-valves are completely closed; hence, no venting of gas occurs, in contrast to manual inspiration. Passive exhalation takes place when the inspiratory valve seals and the expiratory valve opens as breathing circuit pressure increases above that of the absorber canister. Once the ventilator bellows is refilled, excess gas from the continuous fresh-gas flow vents only out of the ventilator bellows spill-valve (the APL valve is completely closed). This valve opens only during exhalation and is a built-in safety mechanism that prevents a circuit pressure increase. Because 2 to 4 cm H_2O pressure is required to activate the ventilator spill-valve, this amount of "PEEP" is always present during mechanical ventilation with bellows anesthesia devices. This threshold pressure ensures that the bellows is completely refilled before the excess gas is vented.

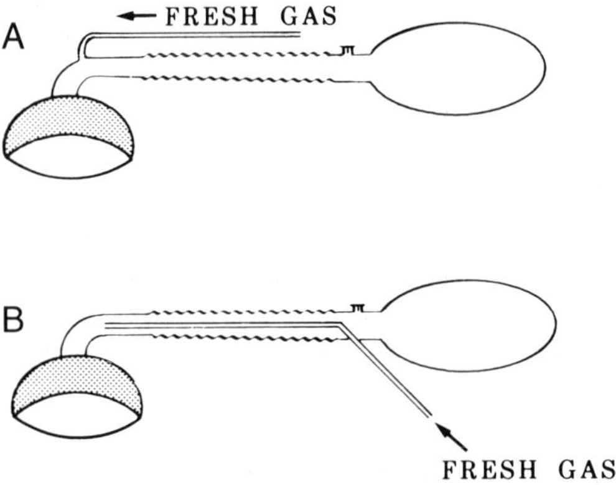

Fig. 10-5. **(A)** Mapleson D. **(B)** Coaxial version thereof (Bain). During mechanical ventilation, the adjustable pressure-limiting valve located at the reservoir bag is closed and the reservoir bag is replaced by the ventilator hose.

Bain Circuit

The Bain circuit is a coaxial version of the Mapleson D circuit (Fig. 10-5). It is classified as a partial rebreathing circuit. Unlike the circle system, it does not include a CO_2 absorber or unidirectional valves. Fresh gas flow through the inner tubing is provided by the anesthesia machine and is continuous and unidirectional. CO_2 is eliminated by the flushing effect of the fresh gas flow on the gases in the outer tube (Fig. 10-6).

During spontaneous breathing, the inspired breath consists of a mixture of the fresh gas flow from the anesthesia machine plus the gas in the proximal portion of the outer tubing of the Bain circuit. The VT contribution from the outer tubing is related to the time and amount by which the inspiratory flow rate exceeds the fresh-gas flow rate provided through the inner tube. Exhalation reverses gas flow in the outer tubing which fills with exhaled VT containing CO_2 and the fresh gas flow. The reservoir bag is refilled, followed by venting of excess gas through the fully open APL valve. During the expiratory pause, fresh gas flow from the inner tube to the outer tube continues (Fig. 10-6B). This gas flow clears the gas containing CO_2 from the patient-end of the Bain circuit.

Manual ventilation is distinguished from spontaneous breathing by the venting of excess gas that occurs during inspiration when the inspiratory pressure exceeds the setting of the APL valve. Thus, part of the reservoir bag volume is returned to the patient (after passing through the outer tubing) and the rest is vented out the APL valve. Fresh gas flow during manual inspiration also contributes to inspired VT. Exhalation proceeds as during spontaneous breathing, the expiratory pause again serving to allow the fresh gas to purge some of the exhaled gas containing CO_2 from the outer tube of the circuit.

Mechanical ventilation is characterized by gas flow patterns similar to those of spontaneous breathing, except that inspiration is a positive-pressure event. Exhalation differs in that excess gas is vented through the ventilator spill valve,

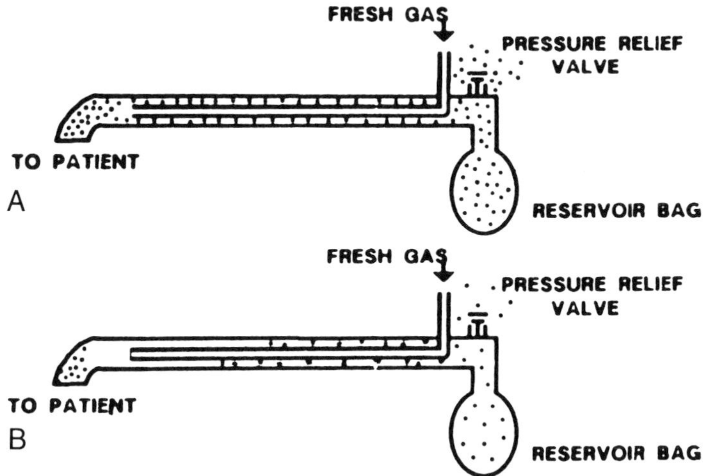

Fig. 10-6. Bain system showing dilution and flushing of exhaled CO_2 during mid-expiration **(A)** and during the expiratory pause **(B)**. The amount of CO_2 (stippling) remaining in the circuit at the beginning of the next breath is inversely related to the fresh-gas flow rate. (Modified from Gravenstein et al.[32] with permission.)

instead of the APL valve, once the bellows is refilled.

Inspired gas normally contains some CO_2 during ventilation with a Bain circuit. This characteristic is in direct contrast to the circle system (CO_2 absorber) and ICU ventilator (nonrebreathing) where it is distinctly abnormal to find CO_2 in the inspired gas. The Bain circuit is designed to provide a predictable $PaCO_2$[7] when a VT of 12 to 15 ml/kg, respiratory rate of 12 to 15 breaths/min, and fresh gas flow of 70 ml/kg/min are provided. In a normal adult patient, this combination results in a $PaCO_2$ in the mid-thirties (Fig. 10-7).

Considerable flexibility is provided in terms of the respiratory rate and VT settings to achieve a particular $PaCO_2$ because of the rebreathing of CO_2 with this circuit. Figure 10-8 demonstrates the relationship between minute volume and PCO_2. The recommended ventilation settings place a patient on the flat portion of this curve, allowing considerable latitude in minute ventilation while keeping PCO_2 in a narrow range. This feature has important implications for the patient who requires either hyperventilation, or who has higher than normal CO_2 production. Unlike other circuits, once ventilation places the patient on the flat portion of the depicted curve (Fig. 10-8), increasing minute ventilation will not decrease PCO_2. The only way to decrease $PaCO_2$ at this point is to increase fresh gas flow (i.e., move to a higher curve in Fig. 10-8). Thus, the $PaCO_2$ is independent of minute ventilation and dependent on fresh gas flow once the flat portion of a curve in Figure 10-8 is reached, in contrast to both circle and ICU ventilator breathing circuits in which $PaCO_2$ is dependent on minute ventilation and independent of fresh gas flow.

The independence of PCO_2 at higher minute ventilations with the Bain circuit arises because of progressively greater amounts of inspired CO_2 present. As minute ventilation increases, the amount of CO_2 cleared during each respiratory cycle decreases if the fresh-gas flow rate is held constant. Stated another way, at higher minute ventilation with a Bain circuit, both effective (gas without CO_2) and ineffective (gas with CO_2) ventilation occurs. Although total minute ventilation may be increased, effective (alveolar) ventilation remains relatively unchanged, as do P_ACO_2 and $PaCO_2$ (Fig. 10-8). CO_2 monitoring is consequently the best way to insure adequate ventilation with this circuit.

To achieve a lower $PaCO_2$ (i.e., to move to a higher curve in Fig. 10-8) a higher fresh-gas

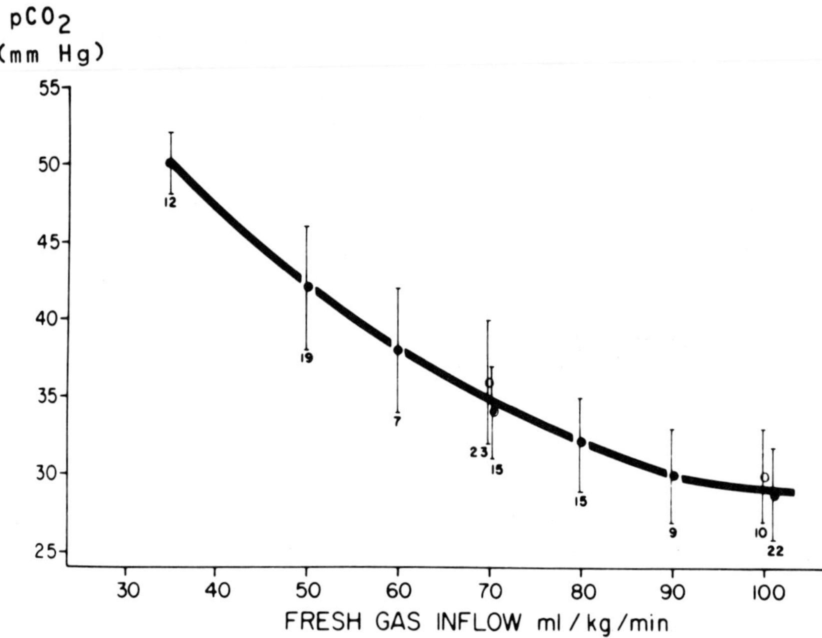

Fig. 10-7. Fresh gas inflow in relation to arterial PCO_2. The figures indicate the number of patients at a given inflow of fresh gas. The bar (I) indicates standard deviation. At inflow rates of 70 and 100 ml/kg body weight, male (○) and female (●), have been separated. Ventilation was mechanical with a VT at least 10 ml/kg and a respiratory rate of 12 to 16/min. (From Bain and Spoerel,[7] with permission.)

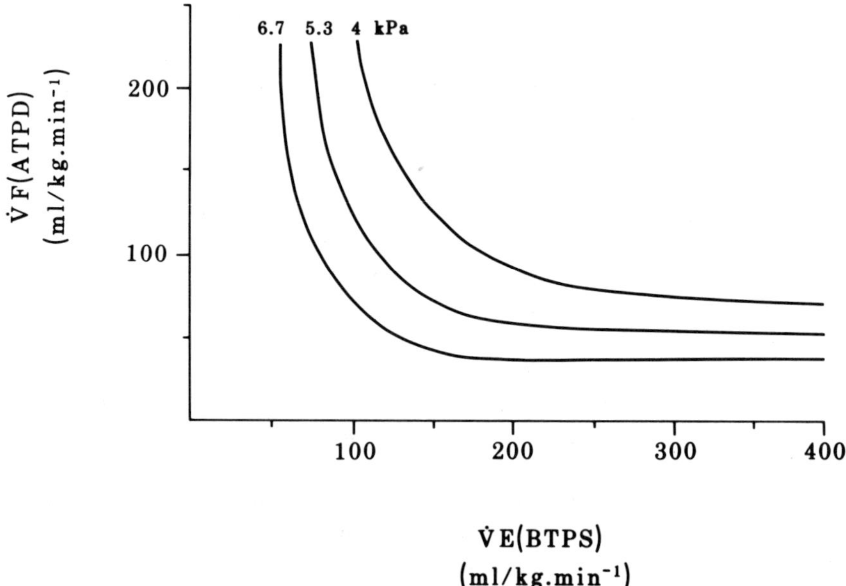

Fig. 10-8. Nomogram predicting $PaCO_2$ at any combination of fresh gas flow (V̇F) and exhaled minute ventilation (V̇E) when the Bain circuit is used with controlled ventilation in humans. The three curves are PCO_2 isopleths at 4, 5.3, and 6.7 kPa (30, 40, 50 mmHg, respectively). (From Seeley et al.,[8] with permission.)

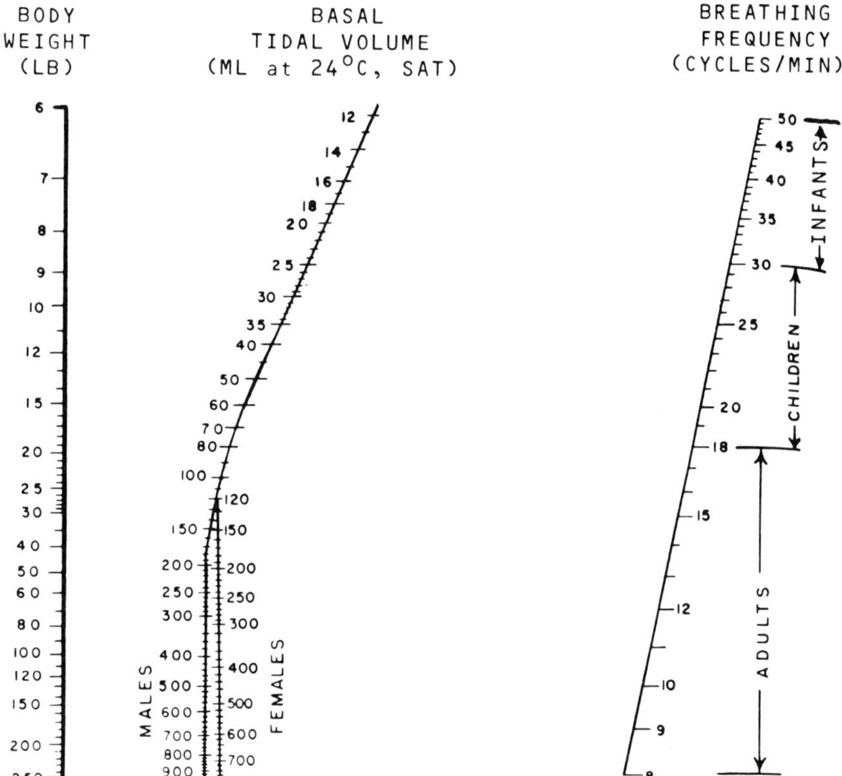

Fig. 10-9. Nomogram from which the standard (basal) ventilation can be obtained from the breathing frequency, body weight, and gender. Corrections to be applied as required: daily activity, add 10%; fever, add 5% for each degree F above 99°F (rectal); altitude, add 5% for each 2,000 ft above sea level; metabolic acidosis during anesthesia, add 20%; tracheotomy and endotracheal intubation, subtract a volume equal to 0.5 of the body weight; added dead space with anesthesia apparatus, add volume of apparatus and mask dead space. (From Radford,[33] with permission.)

flow rate must be used. Conversely, to obtain a higher $PaCO_2$, either a lower fresh-gas flow rate or a lower minute ventilation is used. If the latter approach is chosen, it must be sufficiently low so that $PaCO_2$ becomes minute ventilation dependent (i.e., on the steep portion of the curves in Fig. 10-8). An alternative is to use excess fresh gas flow (e.g., 100 ml/kg/min or greater) to keep the patient on the minute ventilation-dependent portion of the curve. Ventilation can then be adjusted as with the circle system or an ICU ventilator, using the Radford nomogram (Fig. 10-9). The excess fresh gas flow method commonly is employed when an ICU patient is ventilated with a Mapleson D circuit and fresh-gas flow rates of 10 L/min or higher.

SCAVENGING

A properly functioning ICU ventilator provides a VT consisting of oxygen and nitrogen whenever the FIO_2 is less than 1.0. Exhaled gas consists of oxygen, nitrogen, and carbon dioxide. Anesthesia ventilators must be able to deliver not only oxygen with or without nitrogen, but also anesthetic gases and/or vapors; therefore, they are interfaced with an anesthesia machine. With some breathing circuits, the inspired VT can also include CO_2 (see above). Anesthesia ventilator breathing circuits may use very low fresh-gas flow rates (up to 1 L/min in a circle system) or low flow rates (usually less than 10 L/min in a Bain circuit). In compari-

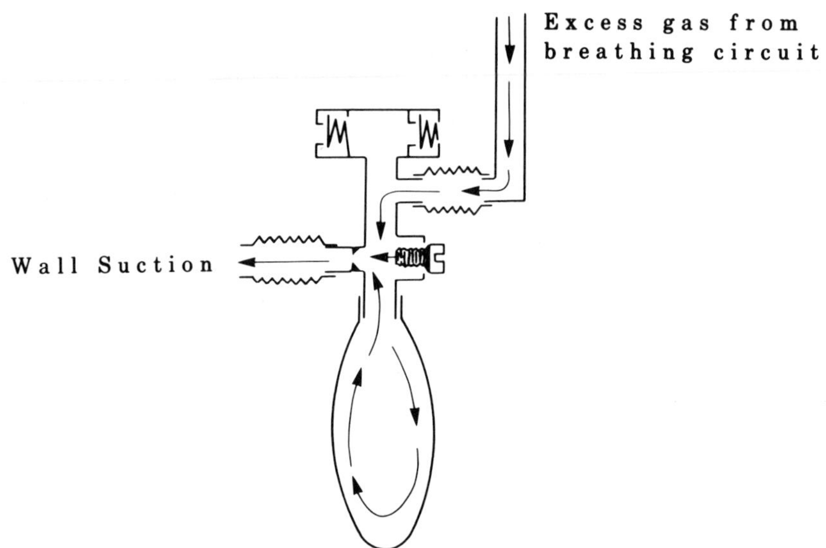

Fig. 10-10. Anesthesia scavenger system. Note the incorporation of a positive pressure (overpressure) governor (right) and a negative pressure valve (left) to prevent either positive or negative pressure being transmitted from the scavenger system to the ventilator or breathing circuit. (Modified from Schreiber,[34] with permission.)

son, ICU ventilators frequently use high continuous-gas flow rates (i.e., more than 20 L/min) and all use fresh-gas flow rates at least equal to the patient's minute ventilation. High flow systems, as noted previously, are undesirable in the OR because of the high cost of inhalational anesthetic agents and concerns about OR pollution. They are unnecessary because the motivation for high continuous fresh-gas flow systems in the ICU is to minimize the spontaneous work of breathing with CPAP, a mode used infrequently in the OR.

Intensive care unit ventilators can spill the excess high fresh-gas flow as well as the exhaled VT to ambient air with a negligible effect on the ICU environment. In the OR, the situation is quite different. Here, the spilled gases also contain anesthetic agents, 70 percent or more of which may be nitrous oxide. To limit pollution, these gases are collected into a scavenger reservoir and evacuated from the room.[11]

The scavenging system is attached to the APL and ventilator spill-valves (Fig. 10-3). Because gas delivery to the scavenger is intermittent (Table 10-3), most systems contain a reservoir bag to accommodate periods of higher flow. Scavengers must function without risk to the patient and cannot allow scavenger-related negative or positive pressure to reach the breathing circuit.[12,13] To accomplish this goal, positive and negative pressure-relief valves are incorporated into the system (Fig. 10-10). Scavenger tubing and component connections use 19 mm fittings, making it difficult to attach them incorrectly to a breathing circuit that employs 15 and 22 mm internal diameter fittings.

CONTROL OF F_{IO_2}

The method by which the F_{IO_2} is regulated in ICU and OR ventilators differs significantly. The former rely primarily on proportional flow control valves or blenders that usually are adjusted by a single control with the approximate F_{IO_2} inscribed on the dial. Anesthesia circuit F_{IO_2} adjustment occurs independently of the ventilator. In most anesthesia systems, the respired gas mixture is adjusted by flowmeter tandems arranged in series. This configuration

Table 10-4. Summary of Monitors and Alarms

Device	Machines with device (%)	Working (%)
Oxygen monitor	75.1	85.8
Ventilator rate monitor[a]	19.5	83.3
Ventilator low-pressure alaram[a]	87.0	97.2
Ventilator high-pressure alarm[a]	25.2	93.5
Oxygen: nitrous oxide-flow ratio alarm	18.9	100
Oxygen pressure fail-safe	100	100

[a] Machines with ventilators.
(From Kumar et al.,[14] with permission.)

allows greater precision of very low (less than 1 L/min) through high flow rates. Oxygen flow is manipulated in relation to another gas (e.g., air or nitrous oxide). This arrangement creates potential problems, the most notable of which is the possibility of setting, and thereby also delivering, a hypoxic gas mixture when the second gas is not air. Hypoxic gas settings are considerably less likely with newer anesthesia machines that have a mechanical linkage between the oxygen and nitrous oxide flow controls. This linkage, when functioning properly, physically prevents an F_{IO_2} of less than 0.25 from being set. However, these linkages are not incorporated into the flow controls of other gases, such as helium, which are available on some anesthesia machines.

Anesthetic administration is routinely associated with many more manipulations of the F_{IO_2} in a short period of time than is usual in the ICU. For example: preoxygenation, F_{IO_2} equals 1.0; maintenance, F_{IO_2} equals 0.4, balance equals N_2O; early emergence, F_{IO_2} equals 0.3, balance equals N_2O; and emergence, F_{IO_2} equals 1.0. Such frequent changes highlight the need for and utility of continuous oxygen monitoring. To guard against undetected hypoxic mixtures, the ASA basic monitoring standards dictate continuous F_{IO_2} monitoring using an analyzer with an audible alarm at all times.[2] Despite such recommended basic monitoring standards, many anesthesia practitioners still do not adhere to them (Table 10-4).[14]

When air-oxygen mixtures are used, as is common during intra-abdominal procedures, the setting of a desired F_{IO_2} based on air- and oxygen-flowmeter readings is not intuitive. A method for predicting the ratio of air:oxygen-flowmeter settings is presented in Figure 10-11. The approximate ratio is determined by calculating the differences between the desired F_{IO_2} and the oxygen concentration in air (0.21) (denominator), and oxygen (1.0) and desired F_{IO_2} (numerator). An easy rule-of-thumb is that the F_{IO_2} is 0.6 whenever the oxygen- and air-flow rates are equal.

PRACTICAL CONSIDERATIONS

Anesthesia ventilators can be likened to a bag in a box.[15] The bag is the bellows and the box the bellows housing. The drive mechanism, or power for ventilation, is derived from compressed gas (usually oxygen) that pressurizes the bellows housing (Table 10-5). The

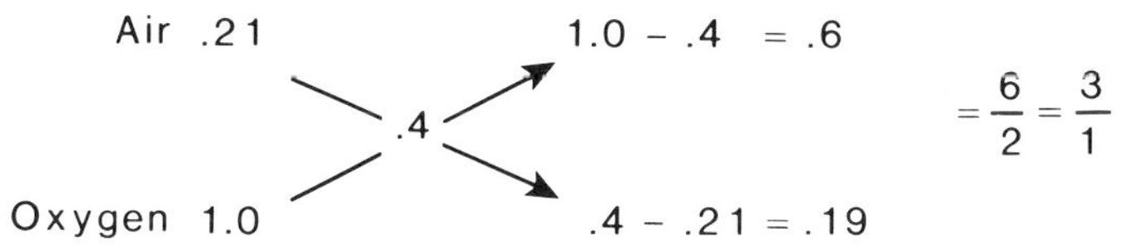

Air .21 → .4 → 1.0 − .4 = .6

Oxygen 1.0 → .4 → .4 − .21 = .19

$$= \frac{6}{2} = \frac{3}{1}$$

Fig. 10-11. Method for determining the ratio of air- to oxygen-flowmeter settings to obtain a desired F_{IO_2}—in this example, desired F_{IO_2} = 0.4.

Table 10-5. Selected Anesthesia Ventilator Specifications

	Ohio 7000 Electronic Anesthesia Ventilator[a]	Ohio[b]	Ohio V5 Ventilator[c]	Dräger AV-E[d]	Air shields Ventimeter[e]
Mode	Controlled	Controlled/assisted	Controlled/assisted	Controlled	Controlled
Cycling	Electronic	Fluidic	Fluidic	Electronic	Fluidic
Driving	Pneumatic	Pneumatic	Pneumatic	Pneumatic	Pneumatic
Low-pressure Alarm (cm H_2O)	6	8	8	Adjustable: 5–30	Not specified
Inspiratory flow rate (L/min)	4–60	30–90	30–90	10–30	1.5–60
PIP (cm H_2O)	75	65	60	Not specified	60
V_T	0–1500	0–1400	0–1400	50–150	0–1500
Bellows	Ascending	Descending	Descending	Ascending	Ascending
Driving Gas	O_2 (Venturi)	O_2/Air (Venturi)	O_2/Air (Venturi)	O_2/Air	O_2

[a] Ohio 7000 Electronic Anesthesia Ventilator, Operation Maintenance. Ohmeda, The BOC Group, Inc., Madison, WI, 1985.

[b] Ohio Anesthesia Ventilator. Operation and Maintenance Manual. Ohio Medical Products, The BOC Group, Inc., Madison, WI.

[c] Ohio V5 Anesthesia Ventilator. Operation and Maintenance Manual. Ohio Medical Products, The BOC Group, Inc., Madison, WI, 1986.

[d] Narkomed 3. Technical Service Manual. North American Dräger, Telford, PA, 1988.

[e] Air Shields Ventimeter Ventilator. User Service Instructions. Narco Air Shields, Hatboro, PA 1974.

bellows is thereby compressed partially or completely from its preselected volume, emptying its contents into the breathing circuit. Gas to fill the bellows and breathing circuit comes from the anesthesia machine by way of the fresh-gas supply hose (which enters the breathing circuit at the CO_2 absorber; Fig. 10-3). To prevent gas accumulation, and hence, pressure buildup in the circuit, excess gas is vented from either the APL valve (during spontaneous and manual ventilation) or the ventilator spill-valve (during mechanical ventilation). The APL valve must be securely closed to prevent VT loss during mechanical ventilation. In some newer models, the APL valve is automatically "taken out" of the system during mechanical ventilation. This mechanism prevents VT loss if the APL valve is not completely sealed.

The ventilator spill-valve is closed by the same gas that pressurizes the bellows housing during mechanical inspiration, creating a closed system (Fig. 10-3). A closed ventilation system may predispose to barotrauma whenever additional gas is provided after activation of the oxygen flush valve during inspiration or from obstruction of the ventilator hose or scavenger system. The latter situations create a closed system by isolating the breathing circuit, with its continuous fresh gas inflow, from the ventilator spill-valve (obstructed ventilator hose) or by inactivating the ventilator spill-valve (obstructed scavenger). The oxygen flush valve (not on ICU ventilators) provides an unmetered high flow rate of gas (35 to 75 L/min) to the fresh-gas inflow hose. This valve, present on all anesthesia machines, is commonly used to quickly refill the circuit after it has been opened (e.g., after disconnection and reconnection to the endotracheal tube). To avoid barotrauma, it should not be activated during mechanical inspiration, and its use should always be accompanied by monitoring of circuit pressure.

CIRCUIT PRESSURE MONITORING

Monitoring of breathing circuit pressure is an integral part of mechanical ventilation for two reasons: (1) to monitor ventilator function (e.g., attainment of adequate positive pressure in the breathing circuit); and (2) to identify changes in the circuit or patient as reflected by increased peak inflation pressure (PIP) (e.g., kinked or obstructed endotracheal tube, decreased thoracic or lung compliance) or, conversely, decreased PIP (e.g., leak, disconnection, or inadequate VT).

The ideal site for pressure monitoring is at the airway. This location is routinely used in the ICU. The airway-pressure monitoring tube is routed back to the ICU ventilator where it is transduced and displayed, either by an aneroid manometer, or analogue or digital meter. Microprocessor-controlled ICU ventilators incorporate adjustable high- and low-pressure audible alarms. Older ICU ventilators are often upgraded by a supplemental add-on pressure-monitoring unit.

Anesthesia ventilators differ in several respects. They should routinely monitor breathing circuit pressure and emit an audible alarm when the low pressure threshold is not met.[2] Pressure is usually measured at a site remote from the airway, most often in the expiratory limb of the breathing circuit. This location is as satisfactory as sensing at the airway, since flow through anesthesia systems is intermittent, unrestricted, and of relatively low velocity. The anesthesia circuit design, however, makes it inappropriate and incorrect to locate the ventilator pressure-sensing site in either the ventilator or ventilator hose. Older anesthesia ventilators with their low-pressure sensing transducer in these locations should be upgraded. This is an important consideration because a common error in switching from spontaneous or manual ventilation to mechanical ventilation is to forget to change the bag/ventilator selector switch from bag to ventilator (Fig. 10-3); activation of the ventilator results in the transmission of intermittent positive-pressure to both the ventilator and ventilator hose. A pressure-sensing site in either of these locations will sense positive pressure and fail to alarm, even though the patient is not ventilated.

Since 1986, the ASA basic monitoring stan-

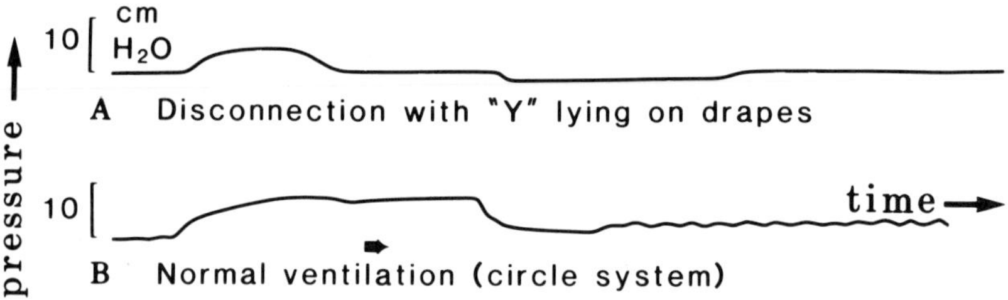

Fig. 10-12. Circuit pressure tracing with a disconnection **(A)**, as compared with normal ventilation **(B)**. This highlights the limitations of a nonadjustable low-pressure disconnect alarm. In this example, if the alarm threshold were 5 cm H_2O or less, no alarm would have occurred, despite a disconnection. (Modified from McEwen et al.,[35] with permission.)

dards have dictated that anesthesia ventilators be equipped with low-pressure (disconnect) alarms.[2] It has been argued that the term *disconnect alarm* should be abandoned because the alarm is not functional during spontaneous or manual ventilation (the ventilator is not engaged).[16] Furthermore, sufficient airway pressure to prevent the alarm from sounding can still occur with ventilator cycling if the disconnected portion of the circuit is partially obstructed by an object (e.g., a surgical drape, operating table). When a smaller endotracheal tube is dislodged from the airway, the flow resistance of the tube creates sufficient pressure changes when the ventilator cycles to prevent the low-pressure alarm from sounding (Fig. 10-12).

Most anesthesia ventilator low-pressure alarms have a fixed limit (Table 10-5) and few systems display the monitored pressure, which severely limits diagnostic possibilities. However, the CO_2 absorber-mounted manometer provides a site for pressure monitoring in the breathing circuit. This analogue manometer measures and displays pressure in the absorber canister, providing a good indication of circuit pressure during the respiratory cycle. It is limited when a PEEP device is used because the canister and expiratory valve are isolated by the inspiratory and PEEP valves. Thus, end-expiratory pressure in the absorber, but not the circuit, is displayed. This shortcoming has been resolved with newer absorber manometers in which the opening of the pressure-sensing tubing is on the breathing circuit (i.e., patient side, not absorber side) of the inspiratory absorber valve.

ANESTHESIA MACHINE AND VENTILATOR INTERACTION

ICU ventilators function autonomously, whereas anesthesia-ventilator function is integrated with the anesthesia machine. The anesthesia machine provides continuous fresh gas to ventilate and anesthetize the patient through the breathing circuit. From a ventilation perspective, it can be viewed as a constant flow generator in parallel with the ventilator. This arrangement generates a component of the delivered VT, independent of the ventilator bellows excursion, a noteworthy fact since most clinicians interpret the bellows excursion as the VT and adjust it according to the inscribed scale on the external housing. In point of fact, the VT delivered to the breathing circuit with an anesthesia ventilator and machine system is determined by several factors:

$$V_{T_{del}} = V_{T_{set}} + FGF \times T_I \qquad (1)$$

where $V_{T_{del}}$ (ml) is the tidal volume delivered to the breathing circuit; $V_{T_{set}}$ (ml) is the ventilator bellows excursion; FGF (ml/sec) is the fresh gas flow; and T_I (sec) is the inspiratory time. This formula should be considered with the range of commonly used fresh gas flow rates: 10 L/min (167 ml/sec) on induction and emer-

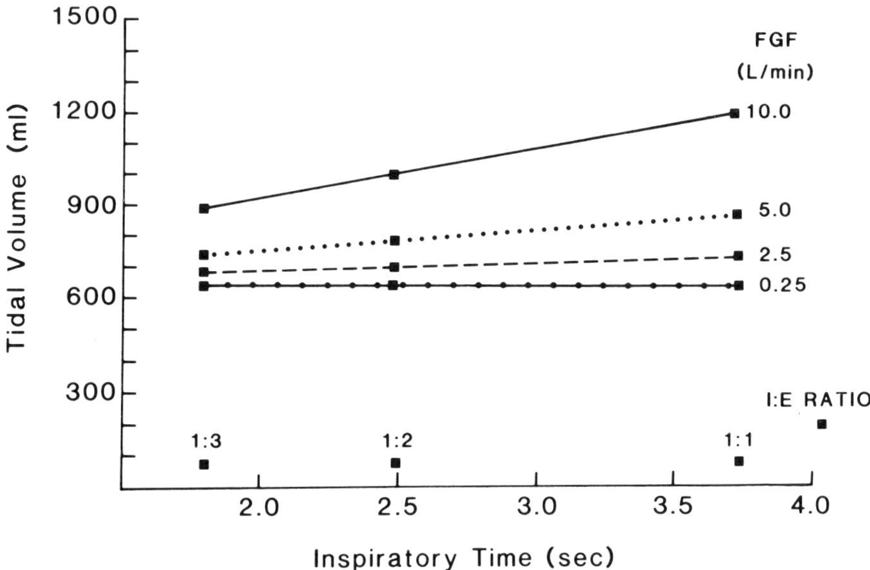

Fig. 10-13. The effect of the inspiratory-to-expiratory time ratio (I:E) and fresh-gas flow (FGF) on the delivered VT as determined with a test lung. The ventilator was set for a VT of 600 ml by observing the bellows excursion at 8 breaths/min. I:E was 1:3, 1:2, and 1:1 at the corresponding inspiratory times. Data are means ± SD. (From Gravenstein et al.,[17] with permission.)

gence and often only 1 to 2 L/min (17 to 34 ml/sec) or less during the maintenance phase of anesthesia.

Figure 10-13 shows the impact of the fresh-gas flow contribution on delivered VT as a function of TI and fresh-gas flow. In the adult patient, VT changes of several hundred ml may be of no great consequence. The pediatric patient, on the other hand, can be adversely affected by failure to appreciate the magnitude of these effects.

Consider a 5-kg infant with the bellows set to deliver a 50 ml VT. Fresh gas flow is 10 L/min (167 ml/sec) during induction. For a frequency of 20 breaths/min, with an inspiration: expiration (I:E) ratio of 1:2, the TI is 1 second. Therefore, according to Eq. (1):

$$\begin{aligned} V_{T_{del}} &= 50 \text{ ml} + (167 \text{ ml/sec} \times 1 \text{ sec}) \\ &= 50 \text{ ml} + 167 \text{ ml} \\ &= 217 \text{ ml} \end{aligned}$$

More than four times the indicated VT (bellows excursion) is delivered to the breathing circuit because of the magnitude and duration of fresh-gas flow. The TI is increased at decreased frequencies and at higher I:E ratios. To prevent unintentional hyperventilation, real-time measurements of VT are helpful. Barotrauma related to excessive VT should also be considered and is largely preventable by verifying that the PIP is acceptable after any changes in fresh gas flow, I:E ratio, or ventilator frequency.

It is distinctly unusual to have high circuit/airway pressure alarms incorporated in anesthesia circuits; as noted, even the low-pressure alarms are usually not adjustable. The anesthesia clinician must rely on direct observation of the absorber manometer, the "feel" of the bag, subtle changes in breath sounds, and/or the sounds of ventilator cycling to detect major increases or all but total loss of circuit pressure, or both.

Tidal Volume Assessment During Anesthesia

It is apparent that VT assessment during anesthesia is desirable. A variety of techniques

Table 10-6. Tidal Volume Assessment During Anesthesia

Auscultation	Subjective
Inspection	Subjective
Peak inspiratory pressure	Objective (not quantitative)
Palpation	Subjective
Airway spirometry	Objective, ideal
Circuit spirometry	Objective (overestimation bias)
Capnometry	Objective for adequacy but not volume

are employed (Table 10-6). Clinical methods are limited, and bellows excursion alone can be misleading. As a result, clinical assessment is often supplemented by spirometers. Most commonly, spirometry is performed in the breathing circuit rather than at the airway, thereby limiting the additional dead space, bulk, and weight of a spirometer connected to the airway. Spirometry done in either the inspiratory or expiratory limbs will accurately measure the VT delivered to the circuit, but systematically overestimates the VT delivered to the patient during mechanical ventilation. This inaccuracy is due to the compression of gases within the circuit and distension of the circuit by positive pressure ventilation.[18,19] Coté and co-workers have measured this compression volume, which reflects wasted ventilation, (that going into the circuit, but not the patient) in a number of anesthesia circuits (Fig. 10-14).[19] Overall, the Mapleson D (Bain) type of circuit had the lowest compression volume at all pressures. The addition of a humidifier to any circle system increased the compression volume.[19]

Any spirometric measurement in the inspiratory or expiratory limbs is incorrect by the magnitude of the compression volume for the PIP observed and reflects only the circuit VT. This leads to a modification of the formula previously presented:

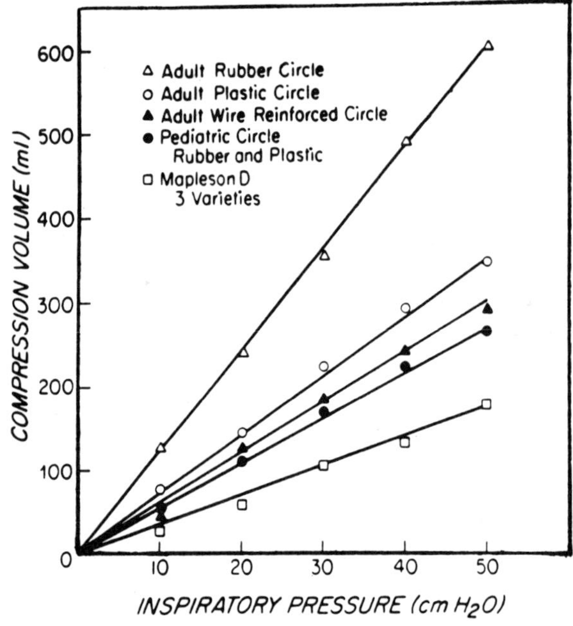

Fig. 10-14. Compression volume (ml) versus peak inspiratory pressure (cm H_2O) as determined with a 1,000-ml calibrated respiratory syringe. The Mapleson D circuits as a group had the lowest compression volume and the lowest ventilation losses. The pediatric rubber and plastic circle systems had the next lowest compression volume and were nearly identical to the adult wire-reinforced circuit. The adult plastic circuit had the second-largest compression volume losses, while the adult rubber circuit was the least efficient and had the largest compression volume. (From Coté et al.,[19] with permission.)

$$VT_{delp} = VT_{set} + (FGF \times TI) - V_{ccv} \quad (2)$$

where VT_{delp} (ml) is the tidal volume delivered to the patient, and V_{ccv} (ml) is the circuit compression volume at PIP.

Determination of VT with a Bain circuit may be even more inaccurate if performed at a site remote from the airway. In addition to the V_{ccv}, if the inspired VT is measured, it does not include the fresh gas-flow contribution (underestimation); if the expired VT is measured, it includes the fresh gas flow (overestimation) during the expiratory pause.

Capnometers are also used indirectly to assess VT. They report respiratory rate as well as CO_2 values in the respired gas, allowing inferences as to the adequacy of ventilation.

ANESTHESIA VENTILATORS

Anesthesia ventilators with bellows are classified as ascending or descending, based on the movement of the bellows during the expiratory phase (see Fig. 10–1). With both types, inspiration is effected by pressurizing the bellows housing, compressing the bellows and delivering the VT. During expiration, the bellows is refilled by the return of exhaled gas from the breathing circuit. However, a descending type may also refill in the presence of a leak or disconnection, since the weight of the bellows will entrain air.

The potential of continued ventilator function in spite of refilling of the bellows with entrained room air makes descending bellows ventilators less desirable than the ascending type. A spirometer, placed in either limb of the circle system or in a Bain circuit when a descending-type bellows ventilator is used, will not show a decreased VT associated with a leak anywhere between the spirometer and the patient. In contrast, an ascending bellows ventilator will not refill passively; therefore, if a leak in excess of the fresh-gas flow rate occurs, it is immediately evident by inspection of either the spirometer or the bellows, or both. The spirometer will indicate a decreased VT, and the bellows will no longer rise to the top of the bellows housing at the end of the expiratory phase.

The gas used to compress the bellows is oxygen in most ventilators or an air-oxygen mixture. Because the driving gas is at higher pressure than the anesthesia circuit, it can leak through a hole in the bellows, resulting in hyperventilation, pulmonary barotrauma, and a change in FIO_2.[20–22] The change in FIO_2 may be either increased or decreased, depending on the ventilator driving gas composition in relation to the fresh gas flow.

Anesthesia Ventilator Oxygen Consumption

Any pressurized gas can be used to power anesthesia ventilators. Most manufacturers use compressed oxygen as a power source (Table 10-5). This gas is inexpensive, free of dust and particles, and is readily available in the OR. In addition, if there is a leak in the bellows, a nonoxygen drive gas may flow through it and dilute the circuit gas, creating a potentially hypoxic mixture.

Although a pipeline supply of bulk oxygen is readily available in all operating rooms, it will fail on occasion or anesthesia and ventilation will be required at a site remote from the pipeline source. For these reasons, each anesthesia machine is equipped with at least one E cylinder as an accessory O_2 source, that contains 660 L O_2 at 2,200 psig. With manual or spontaneous ventilation, this supply will last for a predictable time based on the oxygen flow set on the anesthesia machine (Fig. 10-3). The time to oxygen-cylinder depletion is markedly decreased during mechanical ventilation because the oxygen consumption of most anesthesia ventilators is in excess of the minute ventilation (Table 10-7).[23] The Dräger Narkomed uses a Venturi-drive-gas system, and thus the driving gas is a mixture of air and oxygen, resulting in lower oxygen consumption. In the event of a pipeline-oxygen-source failure, oxygen conservation is best accomplished by switching from mechanical ventilation to manual or spontaneous ventilation.

Table 10-7. Ventilator Oxygen Consumption (L/min)[a]

Minute Volume (L)	I:E	Air shield	Ohio anesthesia	Ohio V5	Ohio 7000	Dräger Narkomed 3
5	1:1	8.7	[b]	15.2	5.6	3.9
5	1:3	8.1	19.8	11.0	6.0	3.2
10	1:1	12.6	26.2	14.8	10.2	5.0
10	1.3	12.4	18.7	10.9	10.3	4.1

[a] Includes 2 L/min fresh-gas flow rate.
[b] Unable to set.
I:E, inspiratory to expiratory ratio.
(Modified from Raessler et al.,[23] with permission.)

Functional Limitations of Anesthesia Ventilators

During the typical surgical procedure, ventilation provided by an anesthesia ventilator is perfectly adequate. However, some patients in acute respiratory failure require ventilatory support that exceeds the capabilities of most anesthesia ventilators.[24] Before the anesthesia ventilator is abandoned in such circumstances, it should be reasonably clear that the outcome

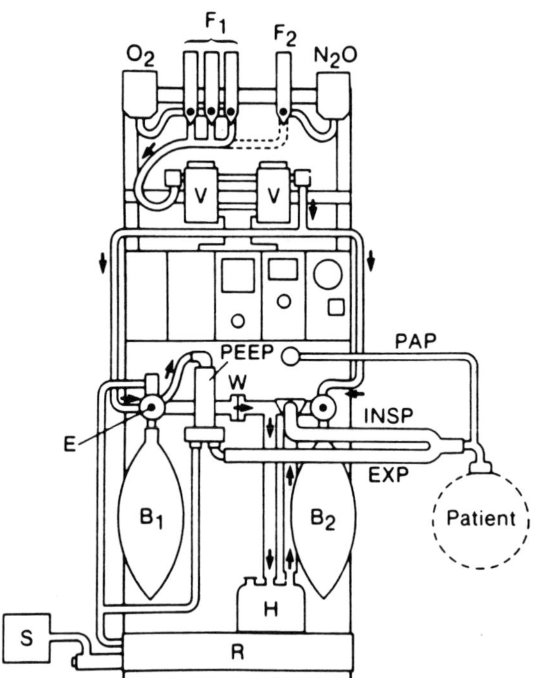

Fig. 10-15. Emerson 3MV modified for anesthesia use. Arrows indicate the direction of gas flow. The location of the PEEP column and the inspiratory limb connection have been reversed to ease interpretation. B_1, ventilator reservoir bag (5 L); B_2, spontaneous breathing reservoir bag (5 L); E, entrainment valve; EXP, expiratory tubing; F_1, oxygen-air flowmeters; F_2, nitrous oxide flowmeter; H, humidifier; INSP, inspiratory tubing; N_2O, nitrous oxide/oxygen blender; O_2, oxygen-air blender; PAP, proximal airway pressure line; PEEP, PEEP column; R, exhaust gas reservoir; S, suction connection for scavenging; V, vaporizer; W, one-way valve. (From Brown et al.,[26] with permission.)

will be improved by such a change. Schapera, et al. suggested that patients with acute respiratory failure who are mechanically ventilated with an ICU ventilator (Siemens) maintained better intraoperative pulmonary gas exchange than those ventilated with a conventional anesthesia ventilator (Ohio).[25] The Siemens 900C ventilator used in that study is, in fact, a combination ICU ventilator/anesthesia machine (perhaps best viewed as an ICU ventilator with anesthetic delivery capabilities).

Modification of an existing critical care ventilator to provide anesthetic capabilities has been proposed by others as a less expensive method (less than $10,000 versus more than $20,000) of achieving the same goal (Fig. 10-15).[26] These authors, however, noted that ventilation with this modified device occurred only 18 times in a 2-year period. This approach, therefore, still represents a considerable expense. Perhaps the most economical and least physiologically disruptive solution is simply to bring the ICU ventilator to the OR for those patients in respiratory failure. Although many anesthesiologists may be unfamiliar with the ICU ventilator, per se, a member of the respiratory care or ICU team can be present to assist with management. During these cases, anesthesia may be provided by an intravenous technique.

One way to assess the limitations in ventilator function is to observe the mean inspiratory flow or maximum minute ventilation under conditions of altered compliance and resistance. Marks, et al.[27] evaluated a number of anesthesia ventilators and observed that all generated a decreasing flow with increasing airway (back) pressure. The ICU/Anesthesia Siemens 900D ventilator in this study had the best performance overall (Fig. 10-16).

Decreased anesthesia ventilator performance with increased airway pressure is due in large part to decreased output of the flow generator, especially in those ventilators using a Venturi mechanism, wherein Venturi entrainment is decreased as the pressure differential (drive pressure − airway pressure) decreases. Another

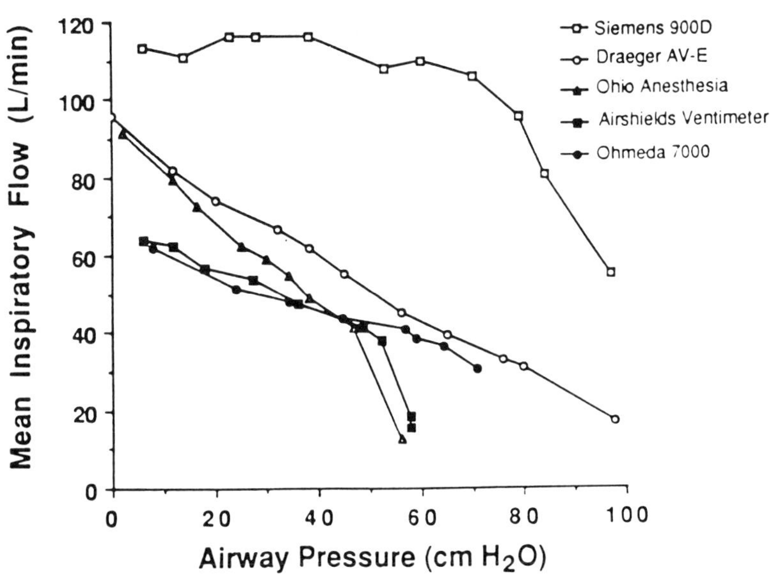

Fig. 10-16. Effect of increasing airway pressure on mean inspiratory flow for each ventilator/anesthesia machine. The Siemens 900D delivered pressure-independent flow at airway pressures less than 80 cm H_2O. All other anesthesia ventilators showed decreasing flow with increasing airway pressure. (From Marks et al.,[27] with permission.)

possible source of decreased function is the greater distensibility of some anesthesia versus ICU breathing circuits. In such cases, decreased lung compliance is associated with a greater volume loss to the patient.

HIGH FREQUENCY JET VENTILATION

High frequency jet ventilation (HFJV), which has gained a small following in the ICU environment, has also been suggested as a useful form of support during anesthesia for surgery of the brain, lung, or kidney. The reason most often cited is minimizing motion at the respective sites. During anesthesia, HFJV is no different than when applied in the ICU.

Anesthesia can be provided by either an intravenous technique, in which case the anesthesia machine and its breathing circuit become superfluous, or with an inhalational agent as during conventional mechanical ventilation. HFJV has considerable impact on anesthetic delivery when inhalational techniques are used. With conventional ventilation, the anesthetic concentrations set by the flowmeters and vaporizers are delivered to the circle system, and then to the patient with each V_T. By contrast, HFJV provides a V_T consisting of two components, the jet volume, containing no anesthetic, and the entrained volume, which contains anesthetic if its origin is the circle system.[28] Anesthetic concentrations in the HFJV circle system never equilibrate with those delivered to the circle system from the anesthesia machine because the jet volume contains only oxygen or an air-oxygen mixture. This portion usually comprises 55 to 60 percent of the total V_T.[29] With each exhalation, this gas dilutes the anesthetic in the circle system.

An in vitro evaluation of the relationship between drive pressure, anesthesia machine fresh-gas flow rate, and anesthetic concentration set on the anesthesia machine vaporizer is summarized in Figure 10-17. The results indicate that a 14 gauge injector inserted at the proximal endotracheal tube, in combination with a 5 L/min fresh gas flow, produces a delivered anesthetic concentration approximately one-fourth of that set on the vaporizer.[30]

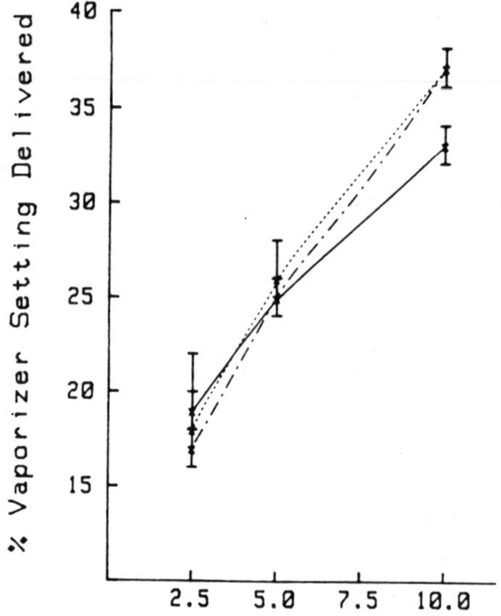

Fig. 10-17. Effect of fresh-gas flow rate and drive pressure of 20 psig (solid line), 30 psig (dotted line), and 40 psig (dashed line) on the concentration of anesthetic delivered to the lung as a percentage of that set on the anesthesia machine vaporizer during HFJV with entrainment of anesthesia agents from a circle system. (From Gravenstein et al.,[30] with permission.)

SUMMARY

An anesthesia ventilator, its breathing circuit, and its interaction with the anesthesia machine are quite different from the ICU ventilator and its breathing circuit. The two systems have evolved to satisfy different needs. Any time a patient's ventilation needs are more reminiscent of those typically seen in the ICU, consider upgrading the ventilatory support available in the OR by exchanging the anesthesia ventilator for its ICU counterpart.

REFERENCES

1. Mörch ET: History of mechanical ventilation. p. 1. In Kirby RR, Banner MJ, Downs JB (eds): Mechanical Ventilation. Churchill Livingstone, New York, 1985
2. ASA Standards for Basic Intraoperative Monitoring. p. 590. In 1989 Directory of Members. American Society of Anesthesiologists, Park Ridge, IL, 1988
3. Douglas M, Downs JB: Special correspondence. Anesth Analg 57:347, 1978
4. Matjasko J: Economic impact of low-flow anesthesia. Anesthesiology 67:863, 1987
5. Virtur RW, Escobar A, Modell JH: Nitrous oxide levels in operating room air with various gas flows. Can Anaesth Soc J 26:313, 1979
6. Schreiber PJ: Anesthesia Equipment Performance, Classification, and Safety. Springer-Verlag, New York, 1972
7. Bain JA, Spoerel WE: Prediction of arterial carbon dioxide tension during controlled ventilation with a modified Mapleson D system. Can Anaesth Soc J 22:34, 1975
8. Seeley HF, Barnes PK, Conway CM: Controlled ventilation with the Mapleson D systems. A theoretical and experimental study. Br J Anaesth 49:107, 1977
9. Katz JA, Marks JD: Inspiratory work with and without continuous positive airway pressure in patients with acute respiratory failure. Anesthesiology 63:598, 1985
10. Usubiaga L, Aldrete JA, Fiserova-Bergerova V: Influence of gas flows and operating room ventilation on the daily exposure of anesthetists to halothane. Anesth Analg 51:968, 1972
11. National Institute for Occupational Safety and Health, DHEW (NIOSH): Criteria for a recommended standard. Occupational exposure to waste anesthetic gases and vapors. Publication No. 77–140, 1977
12. Mor ZF, Stein ED, Orkin LR: A possible hazard in the use of a scavenging system. Anesthesiology 47:302, 1977
13. American National Standard for Anesthesia Gas Pollution Control. American National Standards Institute, New York, 1982
14. Kumar V, Hintze MS, Jacob AM: Anesthesia gas delivery systems and ancillary monitors—a survey of Iowa Hospitals. Anesth Analg 67:S121, 1988
15. Andrews JJ: Understanding your anesthesia machine and ventilator. p. 59. In International Anesthesia Research Society Review Course Lectures. 1989
16. Epstein RA: Anesthesia Patient Safety Foundation Newsletter. p. 39. December 1988
17. Gravenstein N, Banner MJ, McLaughlin G: Tidal volume changes due to the interaction of anesthesia machine and anesthesia ventilator. J Clin Monit 3:187, 1987
18. Newbower RS: The physics of ideal gases. J Clin Anesth 1:232, 1989
19. Coté CJ, Petkau AJ, Ryan RF, et al: Wasted ventilation measured in vitro with eight anesthetic circuits with and without inline humidification. Anesthesiology 59:442, 1983
20. Feeley TW, Bancroft ML: Problems with mechanical ventilators. Int Anesth Clin 20:83, 1982
21. Rendell-Baker L, Meyer JA: Accidental disconnection and pulmonary barotrauma. Anesthesiology 58:286, 1983
22. Waterman PM, Pautler S, Smith RB: Accidental ventilator-induced hyperventilation. Anesthesiology 48:141, 1978
23. Raessler KL, Kretzman WE, Gravenstein N: Oxygen consumption by anesthesia ventilators. Anesthesiology 69:A271, 1988
24. Gallagher TJ, Civetta JM: The multiple trauma patient: assessment and anesthesia. p. 89. In Gallagher TJ (ed): Advances in Anesthesia. Vol. 1. Year Book Medical Publishers, Chicago, 1984
25. Schapera A, Marks JD, Minagi H, et al: Perioperative pulmonary function in acute respiratory failure: effect of ventilator type and gas mixture. Anesthesiology 71:396, 1989
26. Brown DL, Schulz J, Kirby RR: Modification of a critical care ventilator for anesthesia use. Crit Care Med 15:1055, 1987
27. Marks JD, Schapera A, Kraemer RW, et al: Pressure and flow limitations of anesthesia ventilators. Anesthesiology 71:403, 1989
28. Baraka A, Mansour M, Abou Jaoude C, et al: Entrainment of oxygen and halothane during jet ventilation in patients undergoing excision of tracheal endobronchial tumors. Anesth Analg 65:191, 1986
29. Bellefleur M, Berman LS: Factors affecting gas entrainment with high-frequency jet ventilation. Anesth Analg 65:S15, 1986
30. Gravenstein N, Weber W, Banner MJ: Entrainment of anesthetic agents from the circle system

during high frequency jet ventilation and anesthesia. Anesthesiology 65:A148, 1986

31. Gravenstein JS: Gas Monitoring and Pulse Oximetry. Butterworths, Boston, (in press)
32. Gravenstein JS, Paulus DA, Hayes TJ: Capnography in Clinical Practice. p. 38. Butterworths, Boston, 1988

artificial respiration. J Appl Physiol 7:456, 1955

34. Schreiber P: Anesthesia Systems, North American Dräger. p. 49. Merchants Press, Boston, 1985
35. McEwan JA, Small CF, Saunders BA, et al: Hazards associated with the use of disconnect monitors. Anesthesiology 53:S391, 1980

11

Monitoring Respiratory and Hemodynamic Function in the Patient with Respiratory Failure

Roger C. Bone
Nikolaus Gravenstein
Robert R. Kirby

Care of a critically ill patient requires that data be gathered, stored, and analyzed in a logical fashion. Monitoring is repeated or continuous observation to detect change in a patient's condition. It is a fatiguing, repetitive task that machines do well and people do poorly. Invasive monitoring requires meticulous manual skills for placement of sensors, costly equipment, and sterile procedures. Patient discomfort and potential complications of invasive procedures should limit them to the few in whom benefits are likely.[1] The spectrum from noninvasive to highly invasive monitoring is shown in Table 11–1.

Respiratory emergencies are commonplace in the care of critical care patients. Zwillich et al.[2] found 400 complications in a prospective analysis of 354 consecutive mechanically ventilated patients with a variety of causes of respiratory failure. Monitoring may increase our ability to detect complications of mechanical ventilation[3] and should complement the clinician's clinical acumen through data acquisition by objective measurements. If used as an adjunct to clinical care rather than as a substitute, such monitoring should improve patient care. Certain techniques might also help define the resolution or progression of lung disease and the results of therapeutic maneuvers during the course of respiratory failure. Measurement of hemodynamic parameters is essential for proper management of critically ill patients; access to certain measurements of respiratory function in acute respiratory failure may also improve decision-making capabilities.

Arterial blood gas (ABG) partial pressures are available routinely in most hospitals. However, exclusive reliance on blood gas measurements as an index of respiratory function is unwise because they are obtained intermittently, and a variable time lapses before the results are available. In addition, ABG values offer an incomplete definition of pathological physiology. For example, most respiratory complications in the patient with respiratory failure cause the arterial oxygen partial pressure (PaO_2) to decrease. Thus changes in PaO_2 alone do not usually help to make a diagnosis. However,

Table 11–1. Monitoring Procedures

Noninvasive procedures
Physical examination
Electrical sensing with surface electrodes, (e.g., ECG and EEG)
Gas sampling using skin surface probes
Radiological examination
Pulse oximetry, capnography
Invasive procedures
Intravenous injection and blood sampling from capillaries and peripheral veins
Cutaneous needle electrodes for ECG and EEG
Rectal probe
Bladder catheter
Tissue oxygen probe
Intra-arterial and venous gas tension and pH analysis
Highly invasive
Arterial central venous and pulmonary artery catheters
Intracardiac probes
Intracranial probes

the PaO_2 is essential in ascertaining the severity of disease and guiding treatment once the diagnosis is made.

The overall importance of clinical and metabolic measurements is obvious. Daily weight, intake and output, and blood chemistries are important measurements that are usually available. Intermittent determinations are usually satisfactory because changes occur at a gradual rate. Rapidly changing respiratory measurements (e.g., gas flow rate and pressure) might, if frequently monitored, provide clues dictating immediate therapeutic intervention. Information obtained from measurements at a patient's airway cannot substitute for blood gas measurements or chest roentgenograms, but it can have special advantages. The measurements are noninvasive, and with appropriate equipment the information can be provided continuously and without significant time delay.

DIAGNOSTIC STUDIES

The simplest and most valuable patient monitoring is intelligent observation by experienced personnel. In the evaluation of pulmonary competence over short or long time intervals, physical and radiological examination continue to be of prime importance. As more sophisticated diagnostic studies become available, there is a tendency for clinical specialists to neglect these fundamental techniques. The time has not yet arrived when it is safe to do so, and it probably never will. Newer techniques should supplement, not supplant, the basic methods.

Symbols for measurements that are appropriate for the patient with respiratory failure and that directly or indirectly provide information about respiratory function in most intensive care unit (ICU) settings are listed in Table 11–2. Not all these measurements are necessary in every patient treated for respiratory failure. Selection of tests should be based on the likelihood of their providing information valuable for clinical decision-making. Selected variables, their units, formulas, and normal values are presented in Tables 11–3 and 11–4.

Physical Examination

Heart Rate and Blood Pressure

Tachycardia is an abnormality often suggesting blood volume or flow deficits. The increase

Table 11–2. Symbols

$\bar{}$ Dash above any symbol indicates a mean value
$\dot{}$ Dot above any symbol indicates a time derivative
Primary symbols

- V = gas volume
- $\dot{V}$ = gas volume/unit time
- P = gas pressure
- F = fractional concentration in dry gas phase
- (f) = respiratory frequency (breaths/unit time)
- $\dot{Q}$ = volume of blood/unit time
- C = concentration of gas in blood phase
- S = percent saturation of hemoglobin with O_2 or CO_2

Examples

- V_A = volume of alveolar gas; V_T = tidal volume
- $\dot{V}_E$ = minute volume; $\dot{V}O_2$ = O_2 consumption
- P_AO_2 = alveolar O_2 pressure; $P\bar{c}O_2$ = mean capillary O_2 pressure
- F_IO_2 = fractional concentration of inspired O_2
- $\dot{Q}s$ = shunt blood flow; $\dot{Q}t$ = cardiac output
- $R = \dot{V}CO_2/\dot{V}O_2$
- CaO_2 = ml O_2/ml arterial blood
- $S\bar{v}O_2$ = saturation of Hb with O_2 in mixed venous blood

Table 11–3. Bedside Measurements

Physical examination
Body weight
Urine output, plasma and urine osmolality, specific gravity, osmolar and free water clearance
Radiological examination
Electrocardiogram (ECG)
Hematocrit and hemoglobin
Arterial blood gases
Intra-arterial monitoring
Tidal volume (V_T) expired minute volume ($\dot{V}_E$), and peak inspiratory pressure (PIP)
Physiologic dead space (V_D) or the ratio of dead-space to tidal volume (V_D/V_T)
Bedside measurements of lung mechanics
Hemodynamic monitoring
Physiologic shunt oxygen delivery
Inspired and expired gas measurements

in heart rate is usually proportional to the degree of cardiac impairment and/or hypovolemia; however, an increased heart rate is not specific and may result from such factors as anxiety, stress, and fever. Bradycardia in the face of low cardiac output is an ominous sign suggesting inadequate coronary blood flow.

The blood pressure is usually measured with a sphygmomanometer or an arterial catheter. The sphygmomanometer is not applicable for situations in which continuous monitoring is required. However, frequent measurement is available with mechanical devices that inflate the cuff and record the blood pressure automatically at preselected intervals.[4] Such devices have great merit, as they obtain data with a reproducible technique, do not fatigue, and will set off an alarm if a preset alarm limit is violated. They provide an intermediate level of monitoring between manual sphygmomanometric and invasive arterial pressure determination. Measurements from the arterial catheter are continuous but, as with other invasive techniques, can be associated with complications. Fortunately, the incidence of serious complications is extremely low (less than 0.01 percent); the description of radial artery cannulation as a ''low-risk high-benefit method of patient monitoring that deserves wide clincal use'' appears to be accurate.[5] Arterial tonometers use a force transducer to measure intraluminal arterial blood pressure externally. The principle of the tonometric method is based on the relationship of arterial pressure to the displacement of a force-sensing transducer located over a superficial artery. Advantages of the method include noninvasive, atraumatic, nonocclusive, and continuous monitoring of arterial blood pressure. Present-day tonometer sensors are relatively sophisticated devices using well defined algorithms to detect lateral and vertical displacement with reasonable fidelity.

Respiratory Rate

One of the earliest responses to a decrease in PaO_2 or a rise in $PaCO_2$ is an increase in respiratory rate. The normal range is 10 to 16/min, and a rate over 20/min should be viewed as abnormal, particularly if an upward trend continues. Rates over 30/min indicate severe respiratory distress. A sudden increase in respiratory rate may be the first detectable sign of sepsis or a pulmonary embolization. It should be considered that the method used for determining respiratory rate can have a considerable impact on the derived value; for example, if respirations are counted for 10 seconds and multiplied by 6 to obtain a rate/min, any counting error is also multiplied by six.

Recently, large intravenous carbohydrate loads administered as a part of total parenteral nutrition have been shown to increase $\dot{V}CO_2$ markedly and require a much higher minute ventilation to excrete the excess carbon dioxide[6] (Fig. 11-1). This abnormality can be a significant physiologic stress, especially to the patient with chronic obstructive pulmonary disease (COPD) who is already hypercapnic. Thus, overfeeding may make weaning impossible and be manifested by tachypnea and dyspnea when

Table 11–4. Selected Variables: Their Units, Formulas, and Normal Values

Abbreviation	Variable name	Formula	Normal values	Unit
MAP	Mean arterial pressure	MAP = diastolic + $\frac{1}{3}$ pulse pressure	85–95	mmHg
CVP	Central venous pressure	Direct measurement	0–10	cm H_2O
Hgb	Hemoglobin concentration	Direct measurement	12–15	g/dl
MPAP	Mean pulmonary arterial pressure	Direct measurement	10–18	mmHg
WP	Pulmonary arterial wedge pressure	Direct measurement	2–12	mmHg
CI	Cardiac index	Cardiac output/B.S.A.	2.5–3.5	L/min/M^2
LVSW	Left ventrical stroke work	LVSW = S1 × MAP × 0.0144	44–68	kgM/M^2
LCW	Left cardiac work	LCW = C1 × MAP × 0.0144	3–3.5	kgM/M^2
SVR	Systemic vascular resistance	SVR = 80 (MAP − CVP)/CI	1200–1800	dynes·sec/$cm^5 \cdot M^2$
PVR	Pulmonary vascular resistance	PVR = 80 (MPAP − WP)/CI	150–250	dynes·sec/$cm^5 \cdot M^2$
HR	Heart rate	Direct measurement	65–80	beats/min
Temp	Temperature	Direct measurement	98–98.6; 37	°F; °C
O_2	O_2 availability	O_2 avail = CI × CaO_2 × 10	500–700	ml/min/M^2
$\dot{V}O_2$	O_2 consumption	$\dot{V}O_2 = CI \times (CaO_2 - C\bar{v}O_2) \times 10$	180–200	ml/min/M^2
O_2 ext	O_2 extraction	$O_2\ ext = \frac{(CaO_2 - C\bar{v}O_2)}{CaO_2}$	0.2–0.3	
V_D/V_T	Dead space/tidal ventilation	$V_D/V_T = \frac{P_ACO_2 - P_ECO_2}{P_ACO_2}$ or $\frac{PaCO_2 - P_ECO_2}{PaCO_2}$	0.30	
POsm	Plasma osmolality	Direct measurement	279–295	mOsm/kg
P_AO_2	Alveolar oxygen tension	$P_AO_2 = (P_B - 47)\ F_IO_2 - \frac{PaCO_2}{R}$	5–20	mmHg
$\dot{Q}s/\dot{Q}t$	Physiological shunt	$\dot{Q}s/\dot{Q}t = \frac{C\acute{c}O_2 - CaO_2}{C\acute{c}O_2 - C\bar{v}O_2}$	3–5	percent

the patient breathes spontaneously through a T tube. Two alternatives are available: (1) decrease the caloric load, and (2) use fat emulsions as a source of nonprotein calories, because they are associated with lesser degrees of CO_2 production than isocaloric amounts of glucose.[7]

Chest Inspection and Auscultation

Observation of chest movement often provides a general assessment of ventilatory adequacy. Asymmetric movement of the chest or asymmetric breath sounds indicate unequal ven-

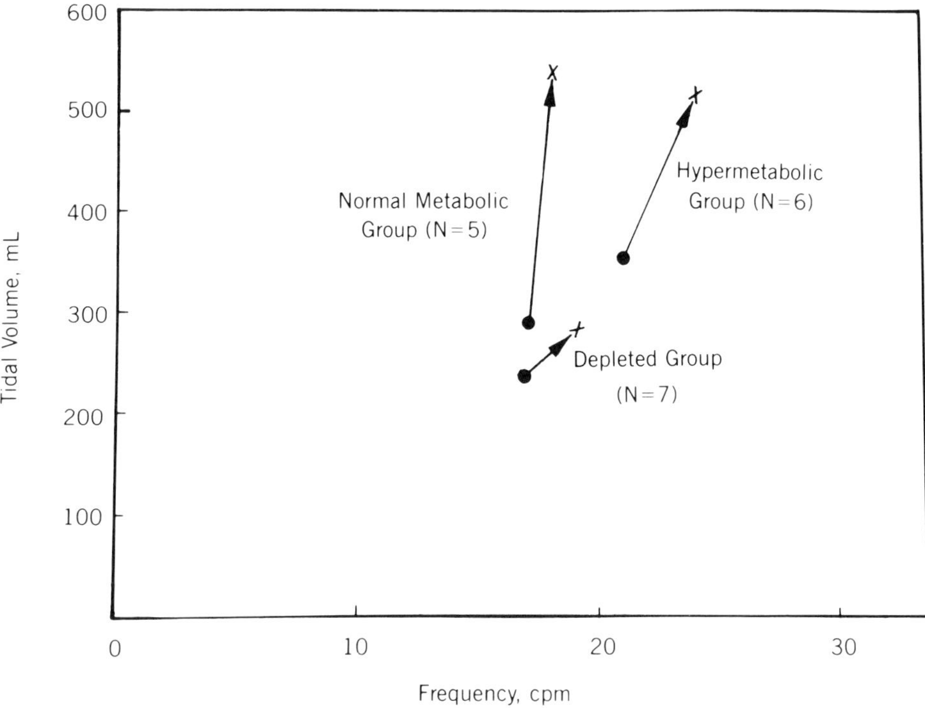

Fig. 11-1. Gas exchange before and during (X) total parenteral nutrition. (From Askanazi et al.,[6] with permission.

tilation associated with abnormalities such as right mainstem bronchial intubation, atelectasis, or pneumothorax. Dyssynchronous motion of the chest and abdomen is also an indicator of diaphragmatic fatigue[8] (Fig. 11-2).

Crackles, wheezes, and dullness to percussion are usually late signs of pulmonary disease. Nevertheless, physical examination is important in detecting preoperative chronic pulmonary disease, failure of ventilation, and airway obstruction. Auscultation may also permit detection of an inadequately inflated cuff on an endotracheal or tracheostomy tube. The intermittent and subjective nature of inspection and auscultation suggest that some form of objective continuous monitoring is helpful in assessing and identifying changes in respiratory and hemodynamic status (see Pulse Oximetry and Capnography).

Body Weight

An accurate record of daily weight is often the most important indicator of fluid balance. Patients receiving only intravenous fluids usually lose 0.3 to 0.5 kg (0.6 to 1.1 lb) per day. If weight loss is greater than this amount, it is excessive. Unless a patient is receiving substantial intravenous or enteral alimentation, stable weight or a weight gain indicates retention of water. Unfortunately, accurate and reproducible weight measurement is often difficult to achieve.

Radiologic Examination

The chest radiograph may reflect late changes. However, it is very useful in following the treatment of respiratory failure. As positive end-ex-

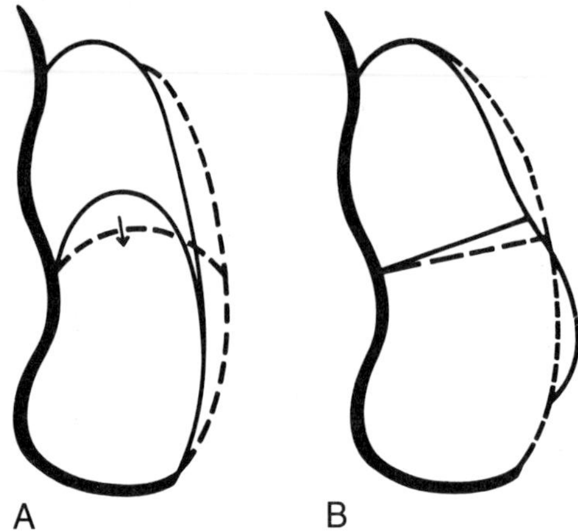

Fig. 11-2. During normal inspiration the diaphragm descends (**A**), and the thorax and abdomen move outward synchronously. On expiration, the chest and abdomen move inward synchronously. With asynchronous breathing (**B**), outward movement of the abdomen occurs during expiration. Asynchronous breathing probably results from an inefficient position of the diaphragm plus maximal use of accessory muscles of respiration. (From Bone,[8] with permission.)

piratory pressure (PEEP) is applied to patients with the adult respiratory distress syndrome (ARDS), the chest radiograph may assist in the evaluation of localized hyperinflation associated with unequal lung damage. It is also useful in detecting certain complications (e.g., atelectasis, pneumonia, right mainstem bronchial intubation, and pulmonary barotrauma).[9,10]

The radiograph should be examined meticulously to ascertain the position of an artificial airway. The tube may move in and out of a main bronchus with respiration and flexion or with extension of the neck. It has been shown that an endotracheal tube will move an average of 1.9 cm toward the carina with flexion from a neutral position and a similar distance away from the carina with extension. In some patients, the endotracheal tube can move considerably further.[11] Thus, when viewing a radiograph for endotracheal tube position, the position of the neck should be considered as indicated by the chin.

An especially important use of chest radiography is to detect pneumothorax from trauma, venous catheterization, or localized lung hyperinflation. The recognition of a pneumothorax depends on the visualization of air separating the visceral and parietal pleurae. A thin white line representing visceral pleura and a peripheral lucent space devoid of lung structures are usually seen. When only supine films are available for interpretation, the diagnosis may be more difficult. Two findings on a supine film that should raise a suspicion of pneumothorax are (1) an abrupt curvilinear change in density projected over the upper quadrant of the abdomen, with increased radiolucency over the upper quadrant; and (2) a deep lateral costophrenic angle on the involved side.[9,10] Either finding should prompt a follow-up cross-table lateral or decubitus film to confirm the diagnosis of pneumothorax.

Electrocardiogram

Visual systems for detection of dysrhythmias are an integral part of most monitoring systems. Computer programs are now available that provide more accuracy and consistency than human observers can provide. Rhythm disturbances are usually late manifestations of respiratory problems and should not be relied on to detect early changes. Approximately 10 percent of patients receiving postoperative care have serious dysrhythmias, about one-half of which are attributable to undetected respiratory complications.[12]

Laboratory Examination

Renal Function

Renal failure complicating respiratory failure leads to a precipitous increase in mortality. Among 400-plus critically ill patients, Sweet et al.[13] reported a mortality of 32 percent with respiratory failure alone, 44 percent with renal failure alone, and 65 percent with combined renal and respiratory failure (see Ch. 14). A significant increase in the requirement for PEEP was found in patients with combined renal-respiratory failure compared with those with respiratory failure alone. Alterations in renal hemodynamic and tubular functions occur in association with respiratory failure as a result of hypoxemia, acidosis, mechanical ventilation, and PEEP. Decreased urine output, decreased sodium excretion, and increased antidiuretic hormone secretion have been associated with mechanical ventilation and PEEP. Other factors implicated in the pathogenesis of renal failure are hypovolemia, hypotension, sepsis, and nephrotoxic drugs.

Renal failure in the critically ill patient can be classified into four types: prerenal azotemia, oliguric acute tubular necrosis, nonoliguric acute tubular necrosis, and obstructive uropathy. Patients with respiratory failure and prerenal azotemia have the greatest mortality compared with those with the other categories of renal failure despite a lower mean serum creatinine level.[13] Because respiratory failure combined with renal failure is associated with increased mortality, factors known to predispose to renal failure should be eliminated prophylactically or treated aggressively as they are detected.

Urine output provides a good estimate of the adequacy of renal perfusion, and urine specific gravity reflects renal concentrating ability. Serum creatinine and blood urea nitrogen (BUN) levels are traditionally used to monitor renal function; however, other less frequently used tests may also be useful. An early sign of relative hypovolemia may be a falling urine sodium concentration and/or a rising urine osmolality. Urine sodium of less than 10 to 20 mEq/L or urine osmolality greater than 600 mOsm/L suggests hypovolemia.

Hematocrit and Hemoglobin

The hematocrit is a static measurement and is affected by gains or losses of red blood cells and plasma volume. After hemorrhage associated with trauma, the hematocrit gradually falls. This change results from transcapillary refilling of the plasma volume by extracellular fluid and reflects a compensatory reaction to, rather than a direct measure of, blood loss. Compensation requires time. Blood loss is replaced by interstitial water at an initial rate of 1 ml/min. With severe hemorrhage, transcapillary refilling is more rapid. Serial hematocrit determinations at maximum 4-hour intervals should be performed on blood samples from patients with suspected hemorrhage.[14] Serial hemoglobin measurements are needed to calculate the oxygen content of the blood wth the following formula:

$$CaO_2 = 1.39 \times \text{Hb} \times \%\ \text{saturation} + 0.003 \times PaO_2 \qquad (1)$$

The hematocrit value for optimal oxygen delivery is disputed.[15] For example, active changes in coronary arterial dilatation occur in response to changes in hematocrit. At normal blood pressure, maximum myocardial oxygen consumption ($M\dot{V}O_2$) is achieved over a wide range of hematocrit values (20 to 60 percent), and the optimal hematocrit is the same for the heart and the rest of the body.[14] However, during hemorrhagic hypotension, changes in hematocrit over a much narrower range adversely affect $M\dot{V}O_2$. Here, the optimum hematocrit for the coronary circulation is lower.

Arterial Blood Gas Analysis

Arterial blood gas partial pressures are determined by the composition of alveolar gas and the efficiency of gas transfer between the alveoli and pulmonary capillary blood. Alveolar gas partial pressures depend on the mixture of inspired gas, ventilation and blood flow in the lungs, the matching of ventilation and perfusion ($\dot{V}/\dot{Q}$), and the composition of mixed venous blood gases. Because $S\bar{v}O_2$ usually varies with cardiac output, significant arterial hypoxemia can result from shunting of venous blood with a low PO_2 through the pulmonary circulation. Failure to recognize this nonpulmonary cause of arterial hypoxemia may cause a clinician to ascribe a falling PaO_2 falsely to deteriorating pulmonary function.

Pulmonary abnormalities which may result

in hypoxemia, alone or in combination, include diffusion block, $\dot{V}/\dot{Q}$ inequality, intrapulmonary shunting, and hypoventilation. Diffusion abnormalities lead to hypoxemia if pulmonary end-capillary blood fails to equilibrate fully with alveolar gas. Such conditions are probably a very uncommon cause of hypoxemia except in patients with chronic lung disease during exercise or exposure to a decreased P_{IO_2} at high altitude.[17–19]

Although bulk oxygen is carried in combination with hemoglobin, delivery to tissue depends on its partial pressure in the blood, which also reflects the amount of oxygen available to be delivered from hemoglobin. A drop in PaO_2 without a change in $PaCO_2$ suggests that blood oxygenation is deteriorating despite constant alveolar ventilation. In the acutely ill patient, this finding usually is attributable to $\dot{V}/\dot{Q}$ imbalance or intrapulmonary shunting. An important feature of shunting is that hypoxemia cannot be abolished by the administration of 100 percent oxygen because shunted blood totally bypasses ventilated alveoli. A shunt usually does not result in a raised $PaCO_2$ because the chemoreceptors sense any elevation in $PaCO_2$ and reflexly induce an increase of ventilation.

When patients hypoventilate while breathing ambient air, hypoxemia results from an increase in P_ACO_2. Calculation of the alveolar oxygen partial pressure and determination of the alveolar-arterial oxygen partial pressure difference, $P(A\text{-}a)O_2$, permit separation of hypoventilation from other causes of hypoxemia. With hypoventilation, the $P(A\text{-}a)O_2$ oxygen gradient is normal; with other causes of hypoxemia, it is increased. The alveolar oxygen partial pressure can be estimated from the following abbreviated formula which is adequate for clinical purposes:

$$P_AO_2 = P_IO_2 - \frac{PaCO_2}{R} \qquad (2)$$

P_IO_2 is equal to the barometric pressure (P_B) minus the water vapor pressure (47 mmHg at 37°C) multiplied by the F_IO_2. The respiratory quotient (R) is approximately 0.8 in the steady-state resting condition. It is assumed to be 0.8 in respiratory failure, although this assumption is not always valid.

The correction for R varies depending on the fraction of inspired oxygen (F_IO_2), as can be seen from the nonsimplified alveolar air equation:

$$P_AO_2 = F_IO_2(P_B - 47) - P_ACO_2\left(F_IO_2 + \frac{1 - F_IO_2}{R}\right) \qquad (3)$$

Although this equation appears formidable, if $PaCO_2$ is used rather than P_ACO_2, and 100 percent oxygen is inhaled, solution of the equation is simply the difference between inspired PO_2 and $PaCO_2$. For clinical purposes, it is important to appreciate the small but definite error if P_AO_2 is calculated using the abbreviated formula [Eq (2)] at different F_IO_2 values.

The arterial oxygen partial pressure divided by the alveolar oxygen partial pressure is called the a/A ratio and is relatively stable with a varying F_IO_2. Thus it is a useful index of changes in lung function when the F_IO_2 is changed. The normal a/A ratio is greater than 0.75. The ratio can also be used to predict the new PaO_2 that results from a change in inspired oxygen concentration.[20]

Another nonpulmonary factor that can significantly affect gas exchange is the level of CO_2 production ($\dot{V}CO_2$). The $\dot{V}CO_2$ is determined by the metabolic rate and the substrate(s) used as fuel. It varies from 70 to 100 percent of the O_2 consumption ($\dot{V}O_2$) as the fuel is switched from fat to carbohydrate. When caloric input exceeds metabolic needs, excess calories are converted to fat, further increasing $\dot{V}CO_2$. Hospitalized patients receiving parenteral hyperalimentation can increase their $\dot{V}CO_2$ as much as 50 percent.[7] To excrete this excess CO_2, an increased minute ventilation is needed (Fig. 11–1), which might be impossible in a patient with COPD or cause failure to wean from mechanical ventilation.

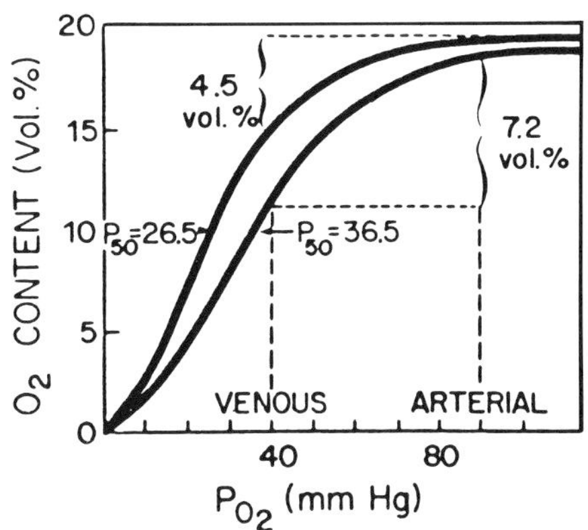

Fig. 11-3. The shape of the oxyhemoglobin dissociation curve results in 90 percent hemoglobin saturation at a PaO_2 of 60 mmHg. At a PO_2 of 60 mmHg, approximately 90 percent of total oxygen content found at a PO_2 of 100 mmHg is persent in the blood. The position of the oxyhemoglobin dissociation curve is expressed as the P_{50}. The P_{50} is the PO_2 at which hemoglobin is 50 percent saturated. The left curve represents normal cells with a P_{50} of 26.5. The right curve has a P_{50} of 36.5. The arterial oxygen tension displayed is 90 mmHg, almost complete saturation. The mixed venous oxygen tension is 40 mmHg. The left curve is capable of releasing an oxygen content of 4.5 ml/dl. The right curve, however, is capable of releasing 7.2 ml/dl, a 60 percent increase in the amount of oxygen available to the tissues. It is apparent that the right-shifted curve, with its property of enhanced unloading of oxygen at the tissue-capillary level, is much more advantageous at this saturation. (From Murphy et al.,[21] with permission.)

Monitoring P_{50} (PO_2 at 50 percent oxyhemoglobin saturation) may also be helpful in assessing oxygen delivery. As shown in Figure 11-3, a right-shifted curve (e.g., higher percent oxyhemoglobin saturation) assists in delivery of oxygen to tissues. The significance of shifts of the oxyhemoglobin curve on overall tissue oxygenation remains a topic of active investigation. Rightward shifts are commonly seen in conditions associated with decreased oxygen delivery (e.g., anemia and chronic hypoxemia).[21]

Beneficial effects of decreased oxygen affinity are difficult to demonstrate experimentally. Increased mortality and decreased oxygen consumption and cardiac output have been associated with a low P_{50} in experimental studies. These findings are of clinical significance to patients receiving large transfusions of stored blood or others who develop respiratory alkalemia or metabolic alkalosis, a resultant leftward shift of the oxyhemoglobin dissociation curve and decreased P_{50}. As these patients are more likely to have limited cardiac reserve because of acute illness, they are at least able to compensate by an increase in cardiac output or a shift in blood flow to tissues using high extraction ratios to meet required oxygen demands. Organs such as the heart and brain are particularly vulnerable.

Marked changes in PaO_2 in critically ill patients that may be missed by intermittent sampling occur during the administration of drugs, suctioning, and changes in body position. Continuous monitoring of PaO_2 by electrodes in the femoral, radial, and brachial arteries as well as the PO_2 in mixed venous blood in the pulmonary artery has been reported.[22] Obviously, these techniques have the same problems as other invasive techniques, and further experience is needed. Clinical trials are underway to determine if continuous invasive PaO_2 monitoring techniques are applicable and accurate in the ICU setting.[23]

Pulse Oximetry

This technique employs the transmittance of red (660-nm) and infrared (IR) (940-nm) light through any pulsatile tissue to which a transducer probe can be attached.[24] Most commonly used are the fingers and toes, but the ears, nose, palm of the hand (infants), and other sites have been employed.

The principles of operation are simple.[25] Oxyhemoglobin and reduced hemoglobin absorb and transmit incident light differently. The probe contains two light-emitting diodes, which alternately emit the red and infrared wavelengths, and a photodetector. Transmission of both wavelengths through the skin, tissues, and venous blood is constant. With each arterial pulsation, however, oxygenated blood enters the

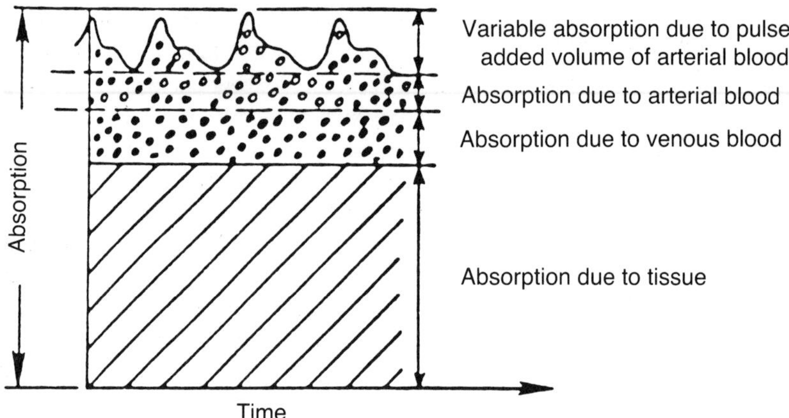

Fig. 11-4. Light transmitted through a tissue site is partially absorbed by each constituent. For a given site, the absorption is constant except for that due to the added volume of arterial blood. (Courtesy Ohmeda, Boulder, CO: A Division of the BOC Group, Inc.)

tissue, changing the absorption/transmittance characteristics. A microprocessor continually compares the amplitude ratio of the red and infrared signals detected by the photodiode at the time of systole and uses this to calculate and provide a digital display of the percent saturation of hemoglobin in arterial blood (i.e., that blood added during systole) (Fig. 11–4).

Since hemoglobin is normally fully saturated with oxygen at a PaO_2 of approximately 150 mmHg, pulse oximetry is of no use in discriminating hyperoxic conditions (PaO_2 greater than 150 mmHg) (Fig. 11–3). It serves as a very useful early warning of impending and progressive hypoxic conditions (PaO_2 less than 60 mmHg), since a nearly linear relationship exists between PaO_2 and oxygen saturation at and below this level (Fig. 11–3).

Problems with pulse oximetry techniques include a falloff in accuracy below a SaO_2 of 80 percent, susceptibility to motion artifact, loss of pulsation in low-flow states such as shock, vasoconstriction in response to cold temperatures, and backscatter from ambient light.[25] Since pulse oximetry is continuous, however, it eliminates the problem of the intermittent nature of ABG analysis. Because only two wavelengths of light transmittance are incorporated into commercially available pulse oximeters, significant errors may be introduced when hemoglobin with different peak absorption characteristics are present (e.g., methemoglobinemia).[26]

Pulse oximeters appear to function optimally when the probe is applied to a finger without nailpolish with the light-emitting portion of the probe over the nail and the light-detecting side directly opposite, completely covered by the flesh of the fingertip. This arrangement limits interference of ambient light by allowing more complete contact beween the detector portion of the sensor and finger. In environments in which bright ambient light is present, the probes are readily shielded by covering them with a towel or one of the opaque foil packets used for alcohol swabs.

In addition to data reflecting hemoglobin saturation, the pulse oximeter may also be used to provide useful hemodynamic monitoring information. A blood pressure cuff on the same arm as the pulse oximeter can be inflated to quickly obtain a systolic blood pressure. The reading occurs at the cuff pressure at which the pulse oximeter first loses the pulse.[27] This method is exactly the opposite of the, perhaps more familiar, return to flow technique. The pulse oximeter can also provide insight into fluid status. Some data suggest that the pulse oximeter derived pulse waveform variations correlate

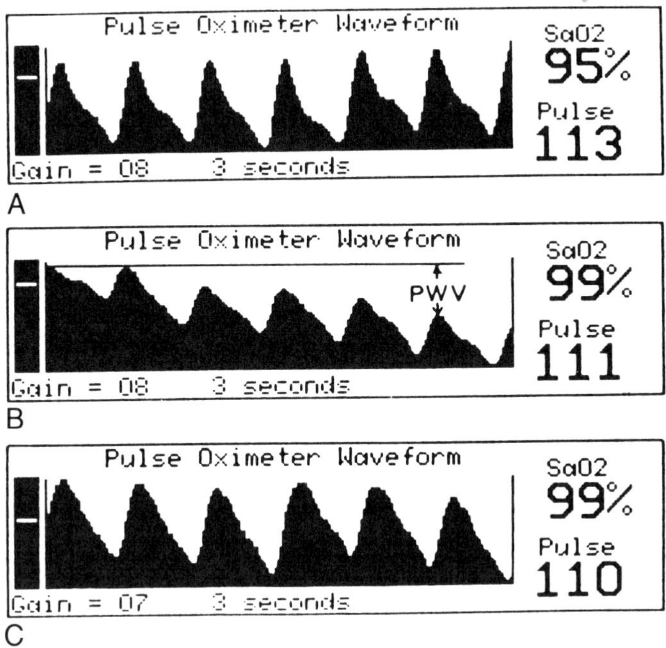

Fig. 11-5. Pulse oximeter waveform representation. (**A**) Patient arrival in operating room: central venous pressure (CVP) = 8 mmHg. Little variation is seen in the waveform with positive-pressure ventilation. (**B**) After third space and blood loss; CVP = 4 to 5 mmHg. Pulse waveform varies with respiration. Method for measuring pulse waveform variation (PWV) is shown. (**C**) After fluid resuscitation, CVP = 8 mmHg. Pulse waveform no longer shows significant variation with respiration. (From Partridge,[28] with permission.)

with systolic pressure variations observed during the respiratory cycle in hypovolemic patients[28] (Fig. 11-5). Improvement in outcome as a result of earlier detection of hypoxemia is suggested in several recent publications[29–32] but has been disputed by others.[33]

Capnography

Capnography refers to the measurement of CO_2 in respired gas. A number of technologies (i.e., IR absorption, mass spectrometry, and Raman scattering) are available for clinical use. The IR absorption method is most commonly used. Because CO_2 absorbs IR light at 4.26 μm, the appropriate IR light source and detector combination can be used to detect the amount of IR absorption and hence CO_2 concentration in a gas sample. Measurements may be made by either mainstream (IR source and detector attached to the airway) or sidestream (gas is sampled at the airway through a catheter and analysis is done by an instrument located at the bedside) devices. If only CO_2 values are displayed, the technique is referred to as capnometry. Capnography is the measurement of CO_2 and the display of the CO_2 partial pressure or concentration over time by a capnograph (Fig. 11-6).[34]

Normally, there is a fairly predictable relationship between the peak exhaled or end-tidal CO_2 ($ETCO_2$) and the $PaCO_2$. In healthy subjects with normal lungs, the $PaCO_2$ is 4 to 6 mmHg higher than the $PETCO_2$.[35] Patients with COPD and other derangements associated with increased dead space (e.g., pulmonary embolism) have an increased $\dot{V}/\dot{Q}$ and therefore an increased $P(a\text{-}ET)CO_2$ gradient. In fact, it may be considerably larger[36] (e.g., greater than 10

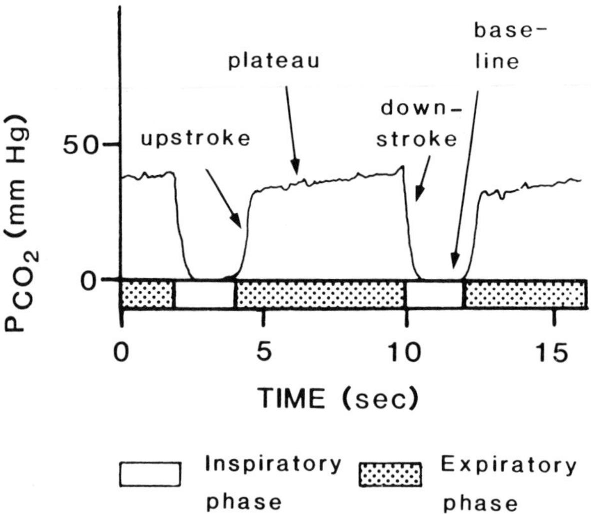

Fig. 11-6. Typical capnogram and its phases. (From Van Genderingen et al.,[34] with permission.)

mmHg). This difference occurs because the exhaled gas from the alveolar deadspace, which contains little or no CO_2, dilutes the CO_2-containing gas from the normally ventilated and perfused alveoli. This gradient may be virtually abolished by examining the peak $ETCO_2$ occurring after a maximal expiration in cooperative patients.[36] Once the $P(a\text{-}ET)CO_2$ gradient has been established by comparing blood gas PCO_2 to capnometer values, it tends to be relatively constant over time in the absence of significant hemodynamic or respiratory pattern changes.[37] However, when knowledge of the precise $PaCO_2$ is important, a capnometer does not substitute for an ABG measurement. It does serve as a useful trend monitor.

The patient treated with intermittent mandatory ventilation (IMV) presents an opportunity to observe the effect of tidal volume, and mechanical and spontaneous ventilation on the $P(a\text{-}ET)CO_2$ gradient. These variables create a heterogeneous set of $\dot{V}/\dot{Q}$ conditions in the face of a stable $PaCO_2$. The result is large breath to breath variations in $PETCO_2$ values (Fig. 11–7). The conclusion of a study by Weinger and Brimm[38] was that monitoring the maximal observed $PETCO_2$, independent of the breathing pattern, was the most clinically useful indicator of $PaCO_2$ in postcardiotomy patients receiving IMV. These observations probably are applicable to all patients. Observations regarding ventilator breathing circuit function and patient also are aided by capnography[34] (Fig. 11-8).

The application of capnography to assess ventilation and circulation during cardiac arrest is gaining acceptance.[39] Because circulatory arrest creates total dead space, if ventilation is continued, $ETCO_2$ rapidly disappears (Figs. 11-9 and 11-10). Restoration of circulation (cardiopulmonary resuscitation) improves but does not return $\dot{V}/\dot{Q}$ abnormalities to normal. Carbon dioxide reappears in the expired gas, but at a low level, usually less than 20 mmHg. Restoration of spontaneous circulation is characterized by an abrupt increase in exhaled PCO_2 (Fig. 11-10). An abrupt increase in the $ETCO_2$ under conditions of reasonably constant ventilation thus provides the earliest evidence of successful resuscitation. Accordingly, precordial compressions need not be interrupted in order to confirm that spontaneous circulation has been restored.[39]

The use of $PETCO_2$ to monitor resuscitation is predicated on maintaining a constant minute ventilation so that changes in $PETCO_2$ result

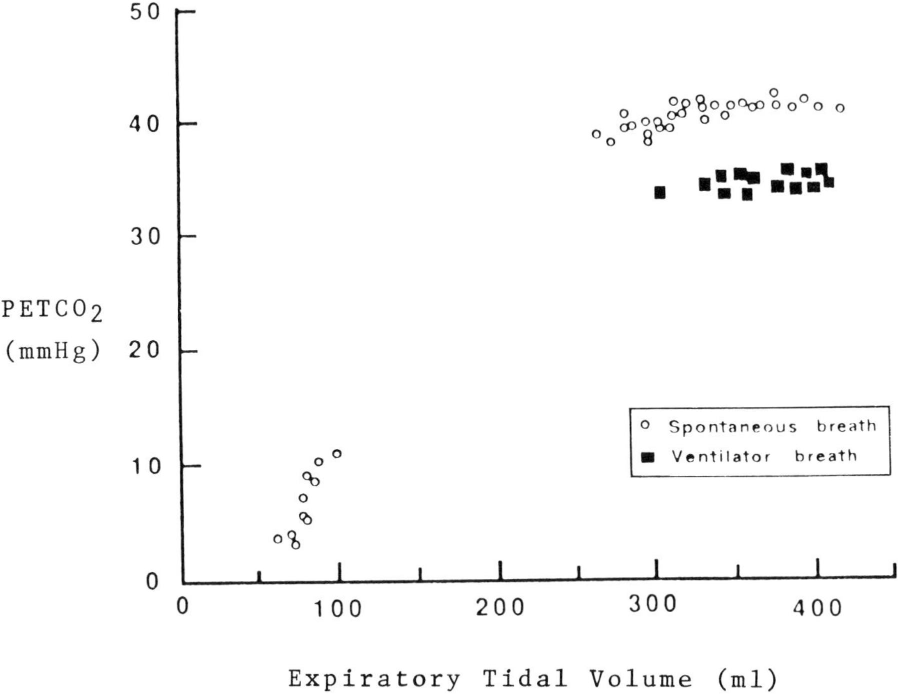

Fig. 11-7. The end-tidal carbon dioxide tension ($PETCO_2$) versus expiratory tidal volume is presented for one representative subject. The graph demonstrates the two classes of spontaneous breaths, as well as the fact that the $PETCO_2$ for spontaneous breaths with moderate tidal volumes is generally greater than that for ventilator breaths. (From Weinger and Brimm,[38] with permission.)

from changes in circulation and not ventilation. Leiplin et al.[40] described a case in which $ETCO_2$ failed to improve as expected during resuscitation: a patient with the lowest $PETCO_2$ at time of closed cardiac compression. Relief of cardiac tamponade improved cardiac output, and the $PETCO_2$ increased. It is tempting to speculate that the adequacy of cardiopulmonary resuscitation and alternate associated diagnoses (e.g., cardiac tamponade, pneumothorax, hypovolemia, and resuscitator fatigue) might all be easier to identify using capnography/capnometry during cardiac resuscitations.

Capnography is also possible for patients who are not intubated.[41] Using a gas-sampling (sidestream) analyzer, a sampling catheter placed in or near the nose can be used to give a reasonable estimate of respiratory rate and an indication of ventilation. Although close agreement between intubated and nasal capnography have been reported, in general, this technique requires close observation and even coaching of the patient to breathe through his nose. Nasal capnography is subject to much larger $P(a\text{-}ET)CO_2$ discrepancies because of variable degrees of mouth breathing, partially or completely obstructed nares at the sampling site, and entrainment of diluting ambient or co-administered air and oxygen, respectively.

Continuous airway CO_2 monitoring is often the best and quickest way to make many diagnoses (Table 11–5). Already emerging standards in the operating room suggest that capnography, along with pulse oximetry, will become routine for the intubated patient in other areas of the hospital as well.

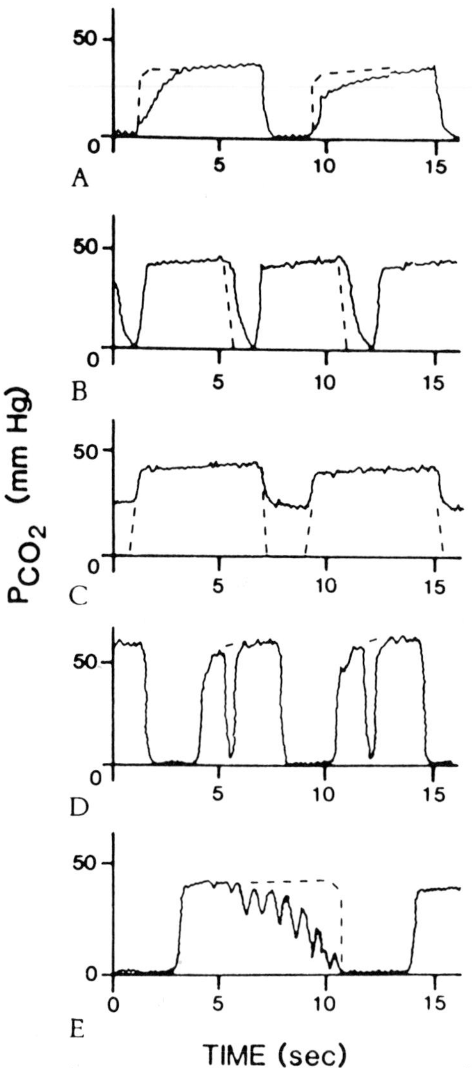

Fig. 11-8. Characteristic abnormal waveforms (continuous line) superimposed on a normal waveform (dotted line). (**A**) Increased airway resistance caused by bronchospasm or a kinked endotracheal tube. (**B**) Incompetent inspiratory valve, where part of the expired air flows back into the inspiratory limb and is inspired with the next inspiration. (**C**) Incompetent expiratory valve, where expired air is reinspired through the expiratory limb or insufficient fresh gas flow during use of a Mapleson D type circuit. (**D**) Patient taking breaths and overriding mechanical ventilation. (**E**) Cardiogenic oscillations caused by the rhythmic increase and decrease in intrathoracic volume with each cardiac cycle. (From Van Genderingen et al.,[34] with permission.)

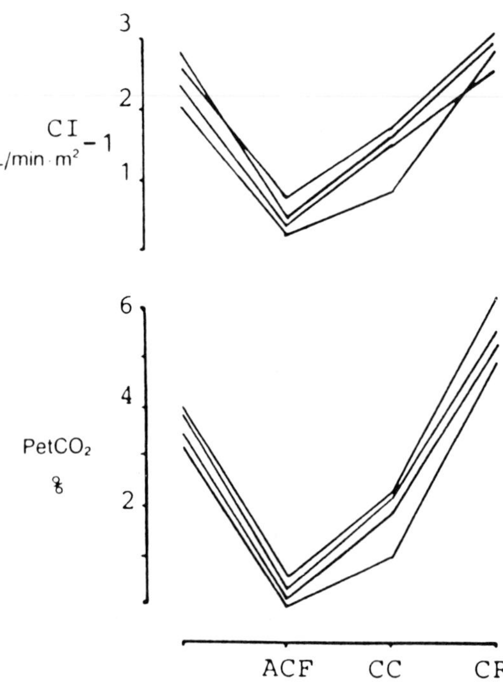

Fig. 11-9. Cardiac index (CI) and $PETCO_2$ in four patients. Baseline values (ACF, acute circulatory failure; CC, closed cardiac compression; CR, circulation) restored after direct-current defibrillation or pericardial decompressions. (From Falk,[39] with permission.)

Transcutaneous Gas Analysis

Another approach that has proved to be effective in infants with respiratory failure is transcutaneous gas analysis. Warming the skin beneath an appropriate electrode causes blood flow to the skin to increase out of proportion to its need in order to eliminate heat. Thus capillary gas tensions are minimally affected by tissue metabolism. Under most circumstances, transcutaneous values in infants accurately reflect ABG tensions.[42,43] Situations associated with changes in oxygen delivery to the skin (changes in cardiac output, blood volume, hematocrit, and acid-base status) may cause considerable differences between directly measured ABG and transcutaneous values.[44,45] In fact, in some adults monitored continuously with an intra-

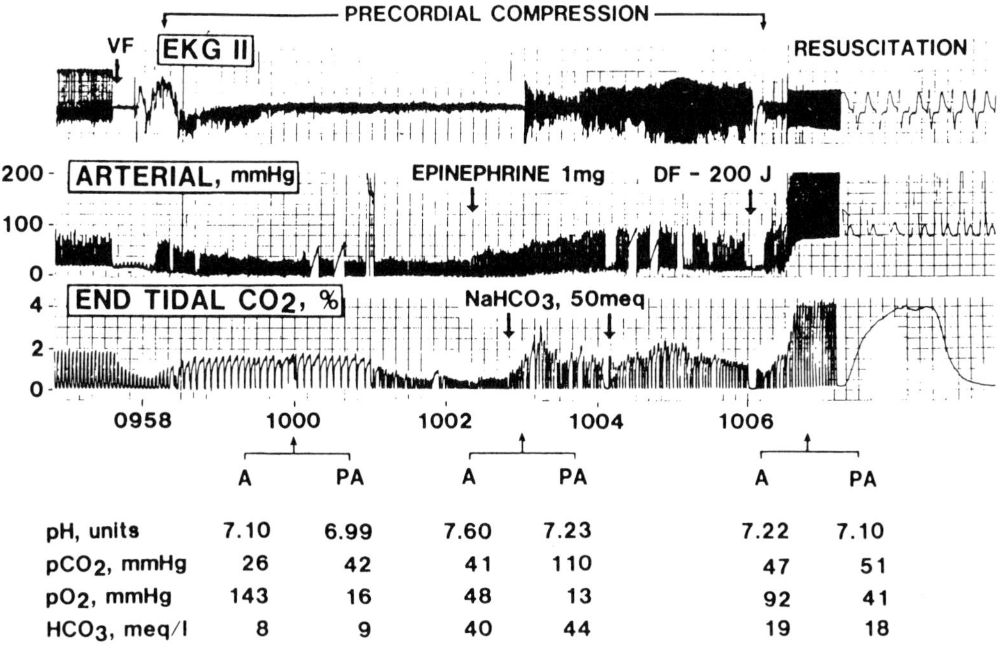

Fig. 11-10. Serial changes in the $ETCO_2$, arterial (A), and mixed venous (PA) blood gases in a representative patient before and immediately after cardiac arrest, during precordial compression, and after defibrillation (DF) and resuscitation. The transient increase in the $ETCO_2$ after the administration of sodium bicarbonate ($NaHCO_3$) is also demonstrated. The original tracing has been modified because of space limitations. (From Falk et al.,[39] with permission.)

Table 11–5. Diagnostic Uses of Capnography

Appropriate endotracheal tube ETT placement
ETT misplacement
ETT displacement
Ventilator disconnect
Endotracheal tube obstruction
Respiratory rate
Changes in respiratory pattern
Changes in exhalation
Hypoventilation
Hyperventilation
Return of spontaneous circulation during CPR

CPR, cardiopulmonary resuscitation; ETT, endotrachael tube.

arterial electrode, transcutaneous PO_2 correlated better with changes in blood pressure than did PaO_2.

In patients with leukocytosis and thromobocytosis, spurious hypoxemia can occur in arterial or mixed venous blood due to consumption of oxygen by leukocytes and platelets before laboratory analysis. With extreme leukocytosis, this decrease in PO_2 can be as much as 72 mmHg within the first 2 mintues after the blood is drawn. Spurious hypoxemia is prevented by the addition of potassium cyanide and blunted by placing the blood sample in ice. Because these patients often have respiratory complications, spurious hypoxemia must be differentiated from true hypoxemia to avoid unnecessary diagnostic and therapeutic intervention.

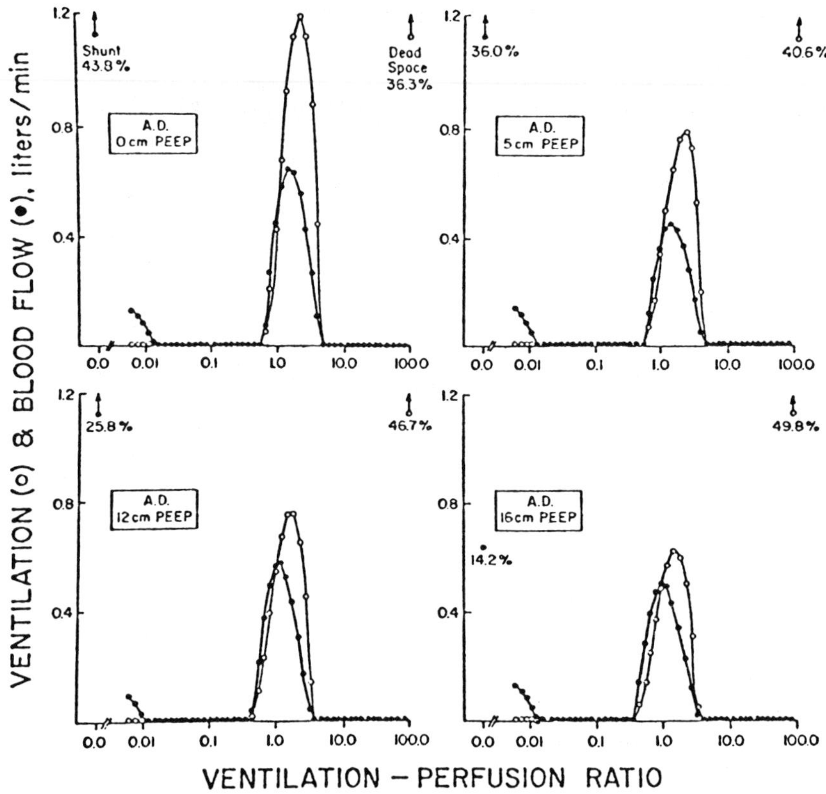

Fig. 11-11. Ventilation-perfusion distribution in a patient with adult respiratory distress syndrome. The blood flow is divided between well-ventilated and shunt lung units. (From Dantzker,[47] with permission.)

The most elegant evaluation of ventilation and perfusion relationships is that developed by Wagner et al.[46] who studied gas exchange with a multiple gas elimination technique. With this method, the distribution of blood flow and ventilation is related to the ($\dot{V}/\dot{Q}$) (Fig. 11-11).[47] True shunt is quantified and separated from units with low $\dot{V}/\dot{Q}$ ratios. Despite its complexity, this multicompartmental model of the lung has added insights not available from the traditional three-compartment analysis of Riley and Cournand (Fig. 11-12). However, it has found little use in critical care units, except as a research tool.

Mass Spectrometry

A mass spectrometer is an instrument that determines components and measures component concentrations of a substance. The type of mass spectrometer most commonly used to measure gases is the magnetic sector mass spectrometer.[48] Gases (oxygen, carbon dioxide, and nitrogen) are converted into a beam of ionic particles by the spectrometer, passed into a magnetic field, and deflected to a collector plate according to their charge and ionic weight. The deposited ions give up an electrical charge and establish a current proportional to the number of ions in the sample. Assuming collectors are present for all ions formed from the sample, the mass spectrometer measures the concentration of each gas in the sample. Inspired and expired oxygen are best measured by the mass spectrometer because most other techniques of gas analysis have a slower response time. For computer-based calculations, a response time of 90 percent in 200 msec is adequate. Most

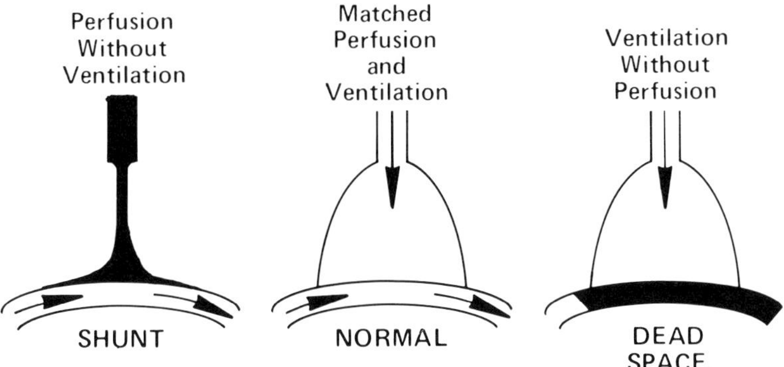

Fig. 11-12. Hypoxemia in the adult respiratory distress syndrome (ARDS) results from intrapulmonary shunting. Shunting results from perfused but unventilated alveoli, as shown on the left. In ARDS many alveoli are also ventilated but not perfused, resulting in an increased physiological dead space, as seen on the right. Both shunt and physiological dead space may exceed 50 percent in severe ARDS. (From Bone,[8] with permission.)

mass spectrometers and carbon dioxide analyzers and some oxygen polarographs fulfill this requirement.

If a number of beds are to be monitored, the mass spectrometer may be cost-effective because a single unit can be multiplexed to several beds. This advantage must be reconciled against the inevitable equipment breakdown where all of the monitored beds lose this monitor at the same time. Potential disadvantages to many institutions are the size of the mass spectrometer, its high initial cost, and the technical inability to measure carbon monoxide. In general, many of the claimed capabilities of the respiratory mass spectrometer in the ICU have not yet been substantiated. Literature describing the intensive care unit applications of mass spectrometry note that it is best viewed as a research tool with potential clinical usefulness.

Intra-arterial Monitoring

Intra-arterial monitoring is usually accomplished by cannulation of the radial artery. Adequate collateral circulation should be ensured when arterial cannulation is performed. Before radial cannulation, an Allen test should be performed to ensure adequacy of collateral circulation. With the Allen test, the hand is blanched by firm pressure on the radial and ulnar arteries. A well-developed collateral circulation exists if release of the ulnar artery is accompanied by suffusion of the hand wihin 5 seconds, particularly the skin around the base of the thumb, although this interpretation has been questioned more recently.[5]

Pressure transducers used in monitoring arterial pressure in the past have been identified as a source of nosocomial bacteremia. Bacteremia resulted from faulty sterilization of the transducer dome. Some transducers incorporate a disposable diaphragm to isolate the sterile fluid chamber from the proximal portion of the dome, which is attached to a nonsterile transducer. Despite a decreased infection risk with transducers utilizing disposable domes, nosocomial bacteremia still has been reported. The current trend is to use completely disposable transducers.

Regular procedures are necessary to evaluate the accuracy of the pressure-measuring system in use. The transducer should be placed as close to the patient as possible, and air bubbles should be assiduously eliminated from the system. Long extension tubes increase resonant frequency and artifactually amplify systolic pressure, while trapped air bubbles ''damp'' the system and record an erroneously low systolic pressure.[49] If any of the factors altering frequency response or damping are present, the mean arterial pressure valve is least sensitive to their influence.

Tidal Volume, Expired Minute Volume, and Peak Negative Pressure

In addition to spirometry, a waterless volume displacement spirometer and a variety of electronic spirometers are readily available. Also, dry gas meters are available to measure exhaled volumes. Two of the most practical and useful instruments for clinical work are the Wright and Dräger respirometers.

Low tidal volumes associated with tachypnea increase dead space ventilation and decrease alveolar ventilation. The product of rate and tidal volume is minute volume, a useful measure of total ventilation. High minute ventilation suggests severe hypocarbia or increased dead space and respiratory work which may lead to exhaustion. A tidal volume greater than 5 ml/kg and a vital capacity greater than 10 ml/kg may be useful guidelines for predicting successful weaning from mechanical ventilation. Measurement of minute volume and maximum inspiratory pressure are also employed. Sahn and Lakshminarayan[50] showed that a resting minute volume of less than 10 L and the ability to double the resting minute volume on command predicts success in weaning. A peak "negative" inspiratory pressure lower than -20 cm H_2O is also used.

Physiologic Dead Space

Physiologic dead space is the portion of tidal volume that does not participate in gas exchange. In healthy adult subjects, the physiologic dead space is approximately 150 ml at rest (about 20 to 30 percent of each tidal volume). This value represents the anatomical dead space from the mouth, pharynx, larynx, trachea, bronchi, and bronchioles as well as the contribution of any alveoli that are overventilated with

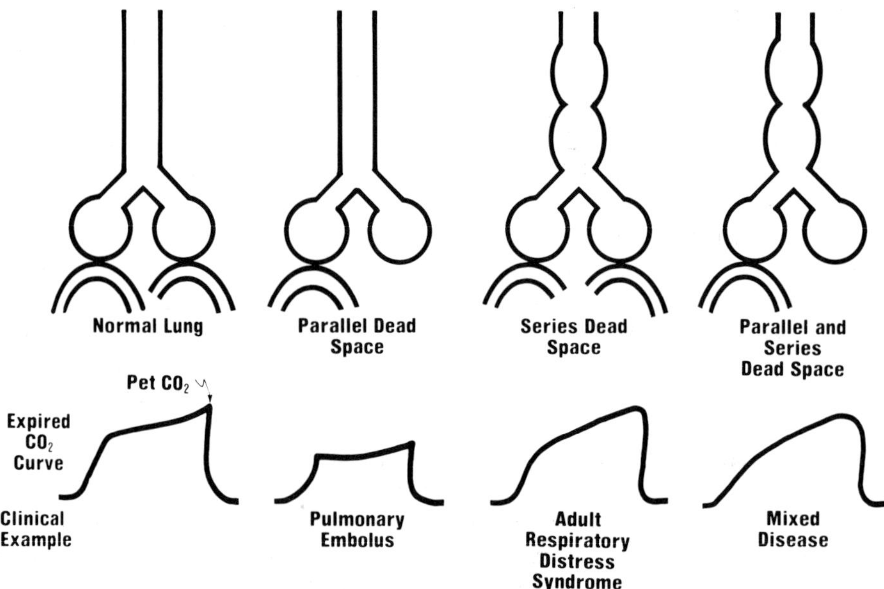

Fig. 11-13. Physiological dead space can be increased by diseases causing ventilation that exceeds perfusion. Graphic representation of diseases producing increased dead space and the resulting expired carbon dioxide curve is shown. (From Bone,[53] with permission.)

respect to perfusion. Positive-pressure ventilation alone can increase dead space.[51] With respiratory failure, the physiologic dead space is increased because of continued ventilation of alveoli with either absent or decreased perfusion.[52,53] Varieties of dead space and the expired CO_2 curve resulting from series and parallel dead space are shown in Figure 11-13. The ratio of dead space to tidal volume (VD/VT) can be calculated by measuring the alveolar and mixed expired CO_2 tension ($PECO_2$) by the Bohr equation (Table 11-4):

$$\frac{V_D}{V_T} = \frac{P_ACO_2 - PECO_2}{P_ACO_2} \quad (4)$$

The Enghoff modification of the Bohr equation is often used clinically:

$$\frac{V_D}{V_T} = \frac{PaCO_2 - PECO_2}{PaCO_2} \quad (5)$$

If the end tidal PCO_2 ($PETCO_2$) is substituted for the $PaCO_2$, anatomic dead space can be calculated, requiring only expired air (arterial blood sampling is eliminated). Changes of physiologic dead space during respiratory failure from the ARDS show a striking relationship to survival[52] (Fig. 11-14).

The breathing circuit to collect exhaled gas is used at the patient's bedside. Calculations are made with measured $PaCO_2$ or $PETCO_2$ and a sample of exhaled gas. This method is applicable to both mechanically ventilated and spontaneously breathing patients. Correction should be made for dead space caused by expansion of the tubing in the mechanically ventilated patient. In the spontaneously breathing patient, the exhaled gas can be collected from a mouthpiece through a one-way valve into a Douglas bag or other suitable apparatus to measure the mixed expired CO_2. Because a spontaneously breathing patient may not breathe with consistent tidal volumes, collection must be continued for 3 to 4 minutes.

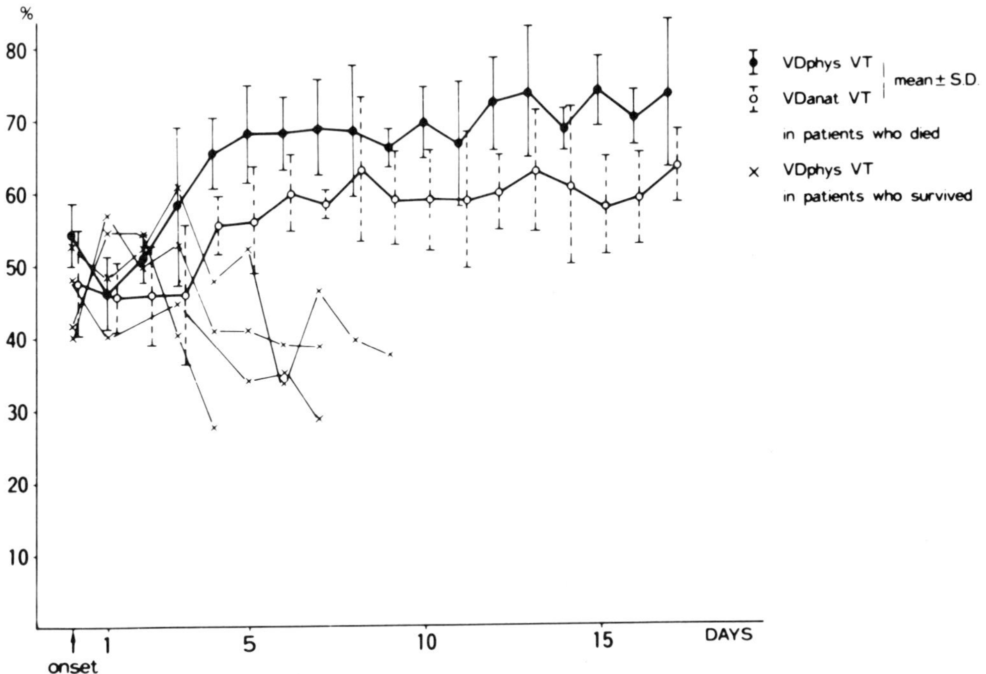

Fig. 11-14. The time course of change in physiological dead space (VD/f) and anatomical dead space (VD anat) to tidal volume (VT) ratios in patients with ARDS. (From Shimada et al.,[52] with permission.)

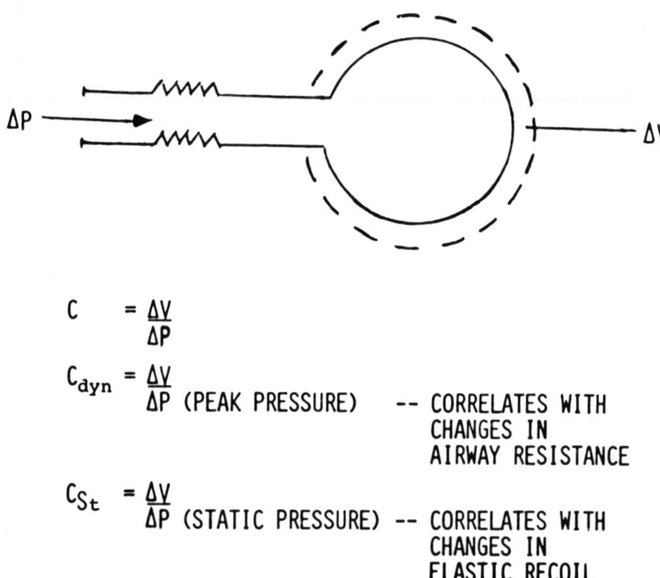

Fig. 11-15. Mechanical analog of the lung. Pressure at the mouth is dissipated in overcoming airway resistance and elastic recoil of the lung and chest wall. (From Bone,[54] with permission.)

Respiratory Mechanics

Volume change per unit of pressure change is compliance, a useful measure of the elastic properties of a body. The compliance of the normal lung is about 100 ml/cm H_2O. If the pressure dial on a ventilator is followed, a rapid rise of airway pressure with a peak at the end of inspiration is noted, followed by a rapid fall to the resting or baseline pressure. This peak pressure is required to overcome the elastic properties of the lung and chest wall and the flow-restrictive properties of the airway (Figs. 11-15 and 11-16).[54] The volume delivered by the ventilator divided by the peak pressure is called dynamic characteristic.[3] It is not correct to call this value dynamic compliance because it is actually an impedance measurement and includes compliance and resistance components. If the outflow limb of the ventilator circuit is occluded momentarily by pinching the tubing to control the expiratory valve opening (or dialing in "expiratory retard" or "inspiratory hold"), the pressure reading will show a momentary plateau, during which time no air is flowing. Normal compliance of the lung and chest wall in the mechnically ventilated patient is about 70 ml/cm H_2O. When the static compliance of the lung and chest wall is less than 25 ml/cm H_2O, as in severe respiratory failure, difficuties in weaning are common because of the high work of breathing.[55–57]

The term *chest wall* includes all structures outside the lungs that move during breathing. Pressure usually is measured from the ventilator anaeroid gauge, which is sufficiently accurate for clinical purposes if the pressure tubing is connected to the proximal airway. The plateau pressure (Pplat) divided by the VT represents the combined static compliance of the lungs and chest wall. If one ventilates the lungs at various tidal volumes and records the peak and Pplat for each volume, dynamic and static curves can be quickly graphed; the former correlates with airway resistance, and the latter is a measure of lung stiffness (Fig. 11-17). The method is outlined in Table 11–16.

These measurements can be made at one volume and followed numerically. A simpler method plots static and dynamic pressures

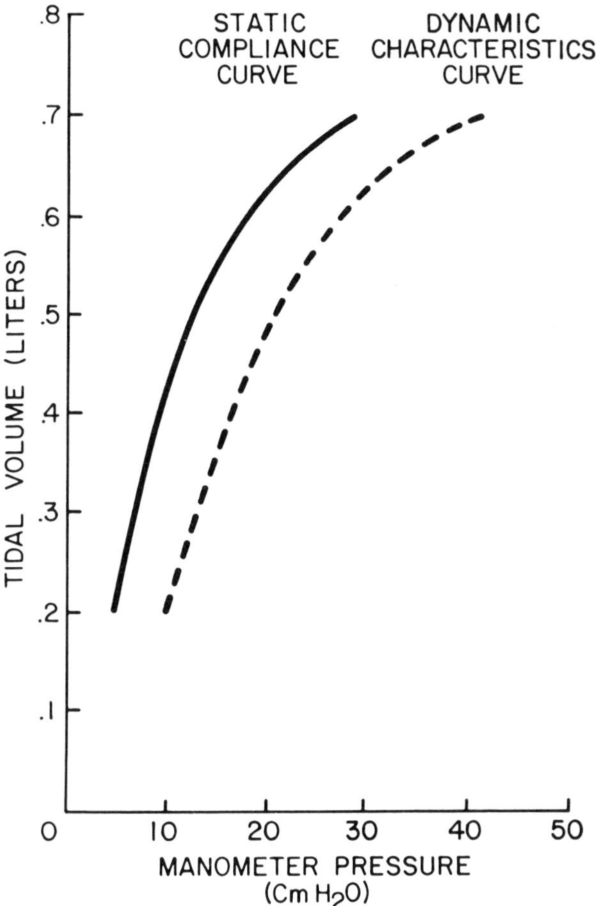

Fig. 11-16. Pressure-volume measurements at various tidal volumes. These measurements are made from many breaths and differ from the compliance measurements made in the pulmonary function laboratory, which are measured during a single breath. (From Bone,[54] with permission.)

graphically at a constant VT, a useful and faster monitoring tool. At higher tidal volumes and/or PEEP, decreasing static compliance often heralds lung hyperinflation. The decrease in static compliance is most pronounced when large tidal volumes are combined with PEEP (Fig. 11-18).

More information is available from inspection of the graphic measurement of the curves at multiple volumes. Figure 11-19 indicates that conditions that increase airway resistance and shift the dynamic curve to the right and flatten it (higher pressure per volume increase). Those conditions producing increased lung or chest wall stiffness flatten and shift both the static and dynamic curves to the right.[3] If the patient is hypoxemic and the compliance curves unchanged, pulmonary embolization should be suspected.

Two errors in these measurements are possible with unrelaxed respiratory muscles. If the patient is resisting mechanical ventilation, the total pressure developed by the ventilator will be greater than that required to inflate the lungs of the relaxed patient. Also, if the patient is actively inspiring, the pressure developed by the ventilator will be less than the total pressure required.

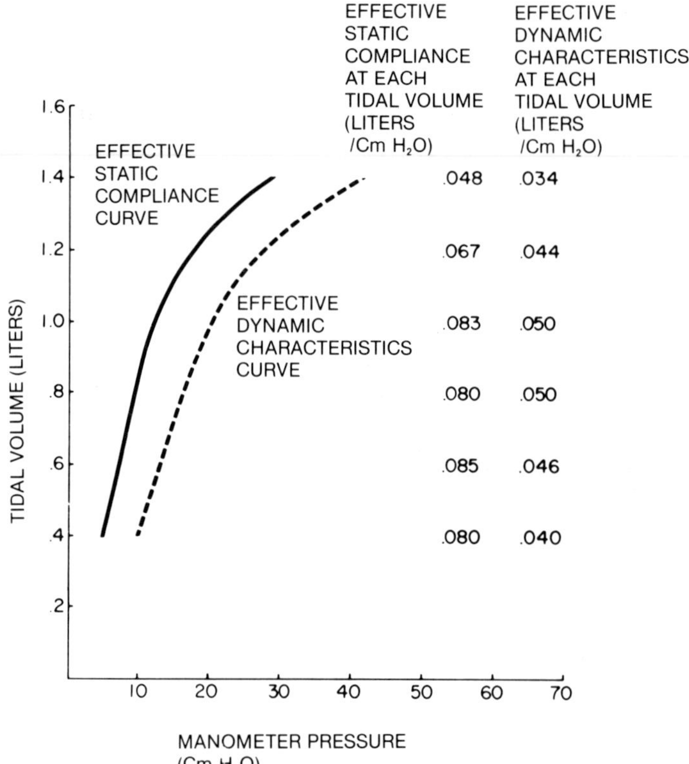

Fig. 11-17. Pressure-volume curves with static compliance and dynamic characteristics calculated at each tidal volume. (From Bone,[54] with permission.)

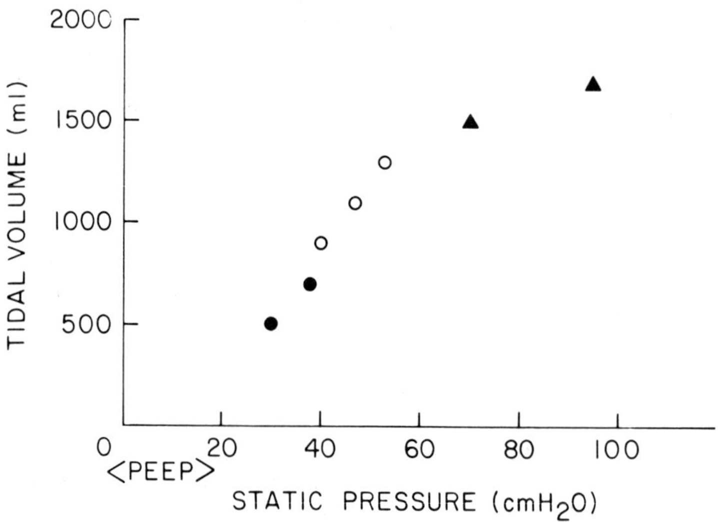

Fig. 11-18. Static pressure-volume relationship of the lungs and thorax. Each observation represents the inflation hold manometer pressure of the ventilator on the horizontal axis, which relates to the tidal volume indicated on the vertical axis. Static compliance = tidal volume/inflation hold pressure − PEEP. In this example, PEEP is 10 cm H_2O. (From Bone,[54] with permission.)

Table 11–6. Determinations of Static Compliance and Dynamic Characteristics

1. Explain the procedure to the patient if he/she is awake.
2. Ensure adequate tracheal tube cuff inflation during the procedure to prevent leaks.
3. Set maximal expiratory retard (if available); otherwise, after each delivered VT, cross-clamp the exhalation tube until a pressure plateau is seen.
4. Select a series of VT settings to be used (e.g., 7, 10, 13, and 16 ml/kg body weight, or 400, 600, 800, 1,000 ml).
5. For each breath, record:
   a. Spirometer volume
   b. Peak airway pressure
   c. Plateau pressure
   When PEEP is used, the value must be substracted from peak and plateau pressures before charting.

Static compliance

$$= \frac{\text{spirometer volume} - \text{tube expansion volume}}{\text{Pplat} - \text{PEEP}} \quad (6)$$

6. Repeat this step for each volume setting selected.
7. If at any setting the pressure increases markedly, do *not* go to larger volumes as pulmonary barotauma may result.
8. Remove expiratory retard.
9. Readjust cuff pressure
10. Carry out a complete ventilator check.
11. Chart data on graph (six such charts can be printed on an 8 × 11-inch sheet).

Factors which are important clinically in respiratory failure produce mechanical changes in lung function that can be detected by the above measurements. The advantage of the method cited is that it requires no special equipment, takes only a few minutes, and can be done routinely by the respiratory therapist. The serial curves give warning of decreasing compliance and help differentiate airway from parenchymal disease. Furthermore, when the compliance decreases, hyperinflation (or barotrauma) may be present. The difference between peak (Pp) and static pressure (Pst) is the pressure required to overcome flow resistance. If flow is measured, airway resistance (RAW) can be calculated:

$$\text{RAW} = \frac{\text{Pp} - \text{Pst}}{\dot{V}} \quad (7)$$

Flow is measured at end-inspiration at the time of peak pressure.[54] From Figure 11–20:

$$\text{RAW} = (40 - 20)/2 = 10 \text{ cm } H_2O/L/sec$$

Alternatively, RAW can be calculated at other points during inspiration. For example, the flow at 0.5 L/sec is corrected for static compliance (Cst), which equals the VT divided by the Pst minus PEEP. Thus:

$$\text{Cst} = \frac{500}{20\text{–}10} = 50 \text{ ml/cm } H_2O$$

Assuming a constant Cst, the pressure at a volume of 200 ml is 4 cm H_2O. The RAW at 0.5 L/sec flow can then be calculated:

$$\text{RAW} = \frac{20 - \text{PEEP} - \text{Pst}}{\dot{V}} = \frac{20 - 10 - 4}{0.5} = 12 \text{ cm } H_2O/L/sec$$

In healthy subjects, RAW ranges between 2 and 3 cm H_2O/L/sec. When measured at flow rates of 1 L/sec, approximately 10 percent of the calculated RAW is due to turbulence. With bronchospasm or airway inflammation, RAW may be 10 times that seen in healthy individuals.

HEMODYNAMIC MONITORING

The major purposes of hemodynamic monitoring are (1) to determine the magnitude of pulmonary congestion and peripheral hypoperfusion, (2) to assess left ventricular pump performance, and (3) to determine the magnitude of the vascular resistance. Several terms are important in understanding hemodynamic monitoring:

Preload—the filling pressure or volume in the ventricle at end-diastole

Afterload—the impedance against which the heart works

Contractility—intrinsic muscle power that allows the heart to increase the extent and force of shortening independent of the Starling mechanism

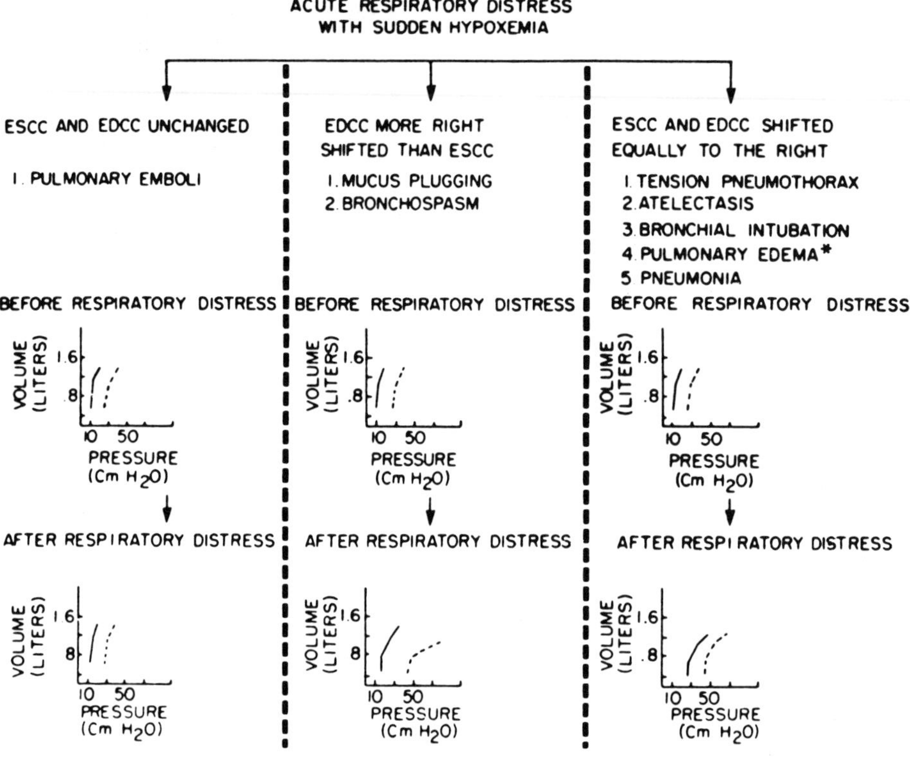

Fig. 11-19. Acute respiratory distress with sudden hypoxemia. ESCC is effective static compliance curve. EDCC is effective dynamic characteristics curve. (From Bone,[54] with permission.)

The most important measurement is the relationship between these factors. Because the heart is a dynamic pump, it must vary the stroke volume with the volume it receives. The degree that the myocardial cell is stretched during diastole (perload) is related to the force developed during systole. Starling's law states that increased myocardial fiber stretching during diastole is associated with increased shortening in systole. Preload (filling pressure) cannot be measured directly in the left ventricle, but it can be measured by a catheter wedged in a small pulmonary artery. This measurement is called the pulmonary artery occlusion pressure (PAOP). Central venous pressure (CVP) is frequently an unacceptable measure of left ventricular preload because of damping of left-sided pressures by variable resistance in the pulmonary circuit and the interposition of the right ventricle, tricuspid, and pulmonary valves downstream from the central venous catheter. An increased PAOP (even within the normal range) in the patient with respiratory failure can be harmful because it induces a large flux of water and solute across the damaged pulmonary capillary. Thus even though "normal," PAOP should be monitored.

Afterload is determined by the volume of blood ejected from the left ventricle and is related to the compliance and total cross-sectional area into which the volume is ejected. The clinical measurement of afterload is the systemic vascular resistance (SVR), the formula for which is shown in Table 11–4.

Contractility is the intrinsic property that enables the heart to increase its force of shortening, independent of preload and afterload. It is assumed that an increase in contractility has oc-

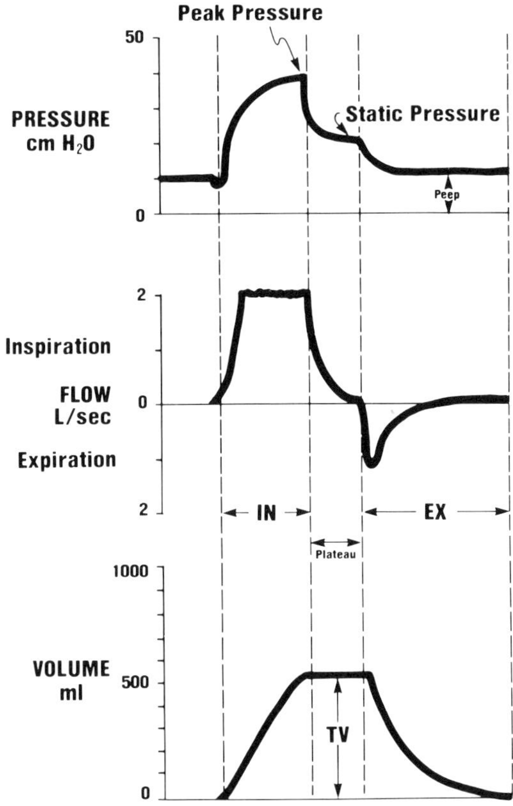

Fig. 11-20. Monitoring pressure, flow, and volume in a patient requiring mechanical ventilation. (From Bone,[54] with permission.)

curred when the stroke volume increases at the same or lesser preload and the same or greater afterload.

A Starling curve provides a graphic presentation of ventricular performance in terms of stroke work and preload. The Starling curve permits a mapping of ventricular performance with time and provides an indication of the optimal preload resulting in optimal cardiac output and stroke work.

Afterload reduction by pharmacologic means is useful in patients with high systemic vascular resistance and decreased forward flow not attributable to hypovolemia or myocardial ischemia. Stroke volume often increases with afterload reduction, so that little or no reduction in arterial pressure may occur.

Techniques of Pulmonary Artery Catheterization

The first balloon flotation catheter contained two lumens. The central lumen measured intravascular pressures through a fluid-filled system connected to a pressure transducer, and the other was used to inflate or deflate a balloon at the catheter tip. When inflated, the balloon acts like a sail to "flow-direct" the catheter tip through the right atrium and ventricle, and into the pulmonary artery. The inflated balloon also surrounds the catheter tip, such that injury to the vessels and heart is less likely and the incidence of catheter-induced dysrhythmias is reduced.

The balloon-flotation catheters are 5 or 7 Fr. double-lumen and triple-lumen (for CVP and pulmonary artery pressure measurements), or 7.5 Fr. triple- or quadruple-lumen, thermodilution cardiac output types. Monitoring equipment includes strain-gauge pressure transducers, connecting tubing and three-way stopcocks, electrocardiogram (ECG) monitor, pressure recorder, the heparinized saline (1,000 U/100 ml). A fluoroscope may facilitate passage of the catheter but usually is not necessary.

The catheter is inserted into the antecubital vein through a variety of commercially available introducer kits. The external jugular vein can be catheterized if a J-wire is used to facilitate introduction.[58] The subclavian, internal jugular, and femoral veins are most frequently used. The femoral vein is easily cannulated and anatomically provides the most direct access to the pulmonary artery. When the antecubital fossa is used, the patient is supine with the arm abducted 90 degrees. The catheter is advanced centrally about 35 to 40 cm from the right antecubital fossa and 45 to 50 cm from the left antecubital fossa. The left antecubital fossa is preferred because of the unidirectional arc construction of the catheter. When respiratory fluctuations are seen in the pressure recording, intrathoracic positioning is indicated. The balloon is fully inflated during passage through the right heart. If multiple ectopic beats are seen, the balloon is deflated and the catheter pulled

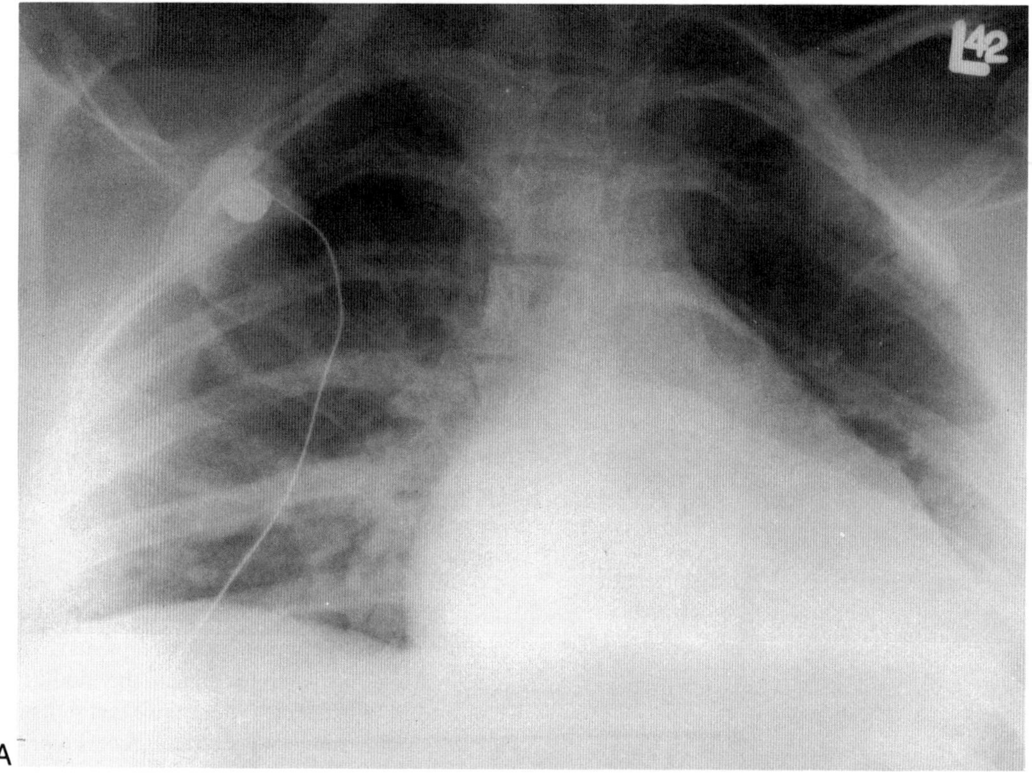

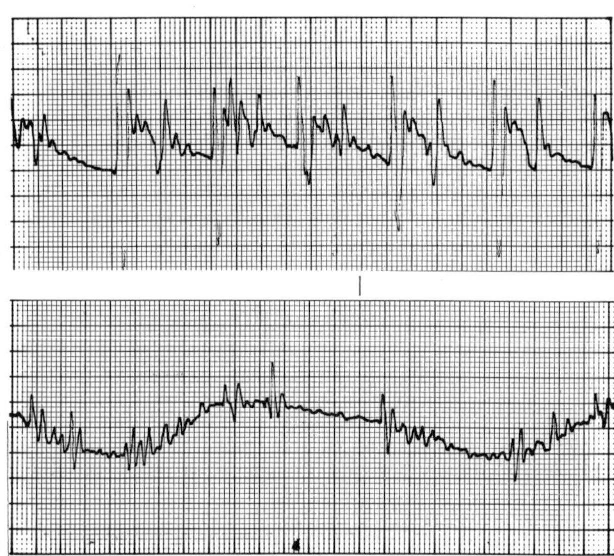

Fig. 11-21. **(A)** Pulmonary infarction. Chest roentgenogram of a patient before insertion of a pulmonary artery catheter. **(B)** Pressure readings from the pulmonary artery catheter. Upper tracing is the pulmonary artery pressure. The lower tracing is similar to one obtained from a pulmonary capillary wedge pressure from the same patient, resulting from peripheral wedging of the catheter with the balloon in the noninflated position. **(C)** An iatrogenic pulmonary infarction resulting from peripheral wedging of a pulmonary artery catheter. Careful attention to the pressure readings in B shows that a wedge reading when the balloon of the catheter was in the noninflated position could have prevented this complication. (From Bone,[53] with permission.) (*Figure continues.*)

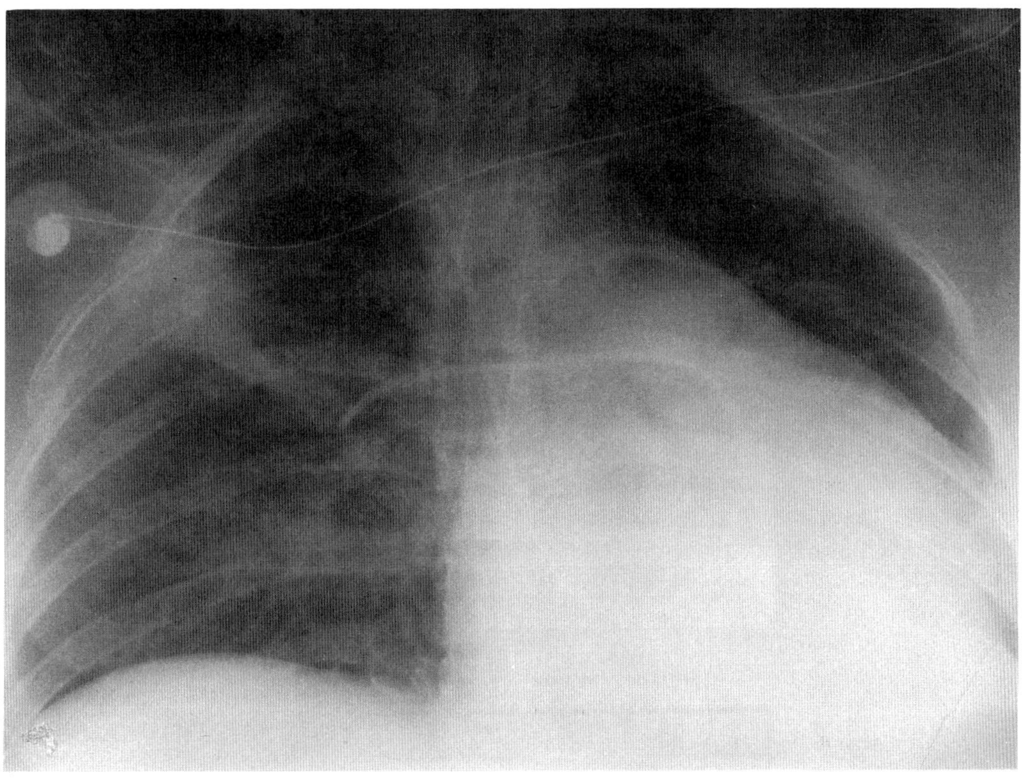

Fig. 11-21 *(Continued)*. **(C)**

back. Otherwise, it is advanced until a PAOP tracing is obtained (similar to a CVP trace).

Proper positioning of the catheter is confirmed if (1) the PAOP is lower than the pulmonary artery pressure (PAP); (2) the change to PAP configuration consistently occurs upon deflation of the balloon; (3) the PAOP waveform is characteristic; and (4) "arterialized" (pulmonary venous) blood can be obtained when the catheter is in the wedged position. A portable chest radiograph should be obtained at completion of the procedure to ensure that the tip of the catheter lies in the main pulmonary artery. Accurate reference to zero (atmospheric) pressure is important. This level is arbitrarily taken in the middle of the chest or a point 5 cm below the sternal angle (angle of Lewis). All subsequent readings should be made at the same reference point. A constant heparin-saline flush of 2 to 3 ml/hr is maintained (0.9 percent saline with 100 to 200 U heparin/100 ml).

The balloon should never be left inflated after measurement of the PAOP. At body temperature, the catheter softens and the transcardiac loop shortens and permits distal catheter migration. This complication is detected and continuously monitored for by continuously transducing and displaying the waveform from the distal (pulmonary artery) lumen of the catheter. If this tracing assumes a damped or wedged waveform, the catheter should be withdrawn sufficiently so that a full 1.5 ml is required to inflate the balloon and again obtain a PAOP waveform. Failure to recognize spontaneous catheter wedging may result in pulmonary infarction (Fig. 11-21) or worse—pulmonary artery perforation.[59]

Rupture of the pulmonary artery is most commonly produced by overinflation of the balloon in a distal vessel. This problem is limited by not using fluid as the inflation medium, never inflating the balloon beyond the recommended amount, and continuously monitoring the PAP waveform during balloon inflation. Stopping balloon inflation as soon as the pressure waveform changes from a PAP tracing to a PAOP tracing, or whenever resistance is encountered is essential. Balloon rupture is also caused by overinflation of the balloon and reuse of the catheter after gas sterilization. For this reason, each catheter should be used only once. Cardiac tamponade results from perforation of the right ventricle by the catheter tip, as may occur with advancement of the catheter with the balloon uninflated. Thus, the catheter should be advanced only when the balloon is inflated.

Catheter kinking or knotting usually is due to insertion of an excessive length of the catheter too rapidly. This problem is avoided by not advancing the catheter beyond a distance where ventricular entrance is anticipated.

Septic phlebitis is minimized by percutaneous versus cutdown insertion and rigid adherence to a sterile protocol during insertion, suturing of the catheter to prevent movement in and out of the skin insertion site, and removal as soon as possible (i.e., within 3 days of insertion). The use of sterile sleeves to protect the catheter has been helpful to decrease catheter contamination and make postplacement catheter manipulations less likely to contaminate the catheter. In one prospective study, 29 of 153 pulmonary artery catheter tips had a positive bacteriologic culture.

Catheter malfunction occurs in up to 24 percent of insertions and maintenance and includes balloon rupture, thermistor malfunction, and luminal obstruction—the incidence of problems being related directly to the duration of the catheterization. Avoiding technical sources of error is important in hemodynamic monitoring. Equipment failure is minimized if the electronic monitors are checked before insertion of the catheter and preventive maintenance of equipment is performed frequently by medical bioengineering personnel. Despite the variety of systems for intravascular monitoring, each employs a closed fluid system interconnected to a pressure transducer that converts a mechanical signal to an electrical one. The fluid pathway must be inspected for air bubbles that dampen the signal. Pressure waveform damping can also be caused by clotting at the catheter tip, loose connections, excessive or asymmetric balloon inflation, catheter tip impingement on a vessel wall, and peripheral placement of the catheter. Abrupt changes in airway and pleural pressure can alter pressure readings from the pulmonary artery catheter strikingly. Pressure readings

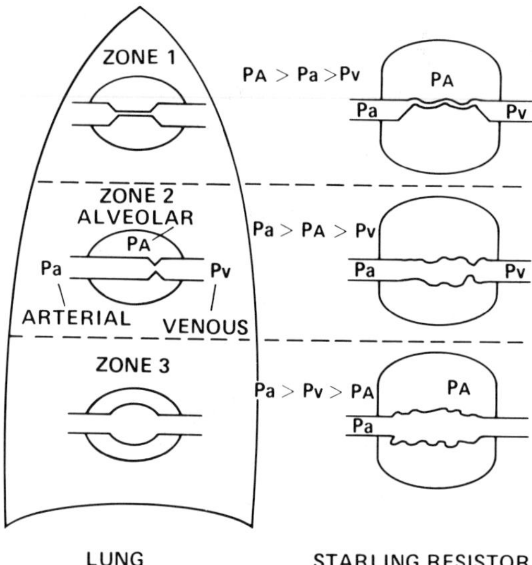

Fig. 11-22. The pulmonary capillary bed has flow characteristics of a Starling resistor, which consists of a length of flaccid collapsible tubing passing through a rigid chamber. In the Starling resistor, when chamber pressure (PA) exceeds the downstream pressure (Pv), flow is independent of downstream pressure. However, when downstream pressure exceeds the chamber pressure, flow is determined by the upstream-downstream difference. The alveolar pressure is the same throughout the lung. The pulmonary artery pressure (Pa) increases down the lung. Zone 1 exists when alveolar pressure exceeds pulmonary arterial pressure and no blood flow occurs. This might occur when the pulmonary arterial pressure is decreased, as in hypovolemia, or when alveolar pressure is increased, as with the application of PEEP. Zone 1 functions as alveolar dead space. In zone 2, pulmonary arterial pressure increases and exceeds alveolar pressure. In zone 2, blood flow is determined by the difference between arterial and alveolar pressures. In zone 3, blood flow is determined by the arteriovenous pressure difference. (From Bone,[61] with permission.)

should be made at end-expiration to reduce respiratory waveform artifact.

The determination of cardiac filling pressures in patients treated with PEEP is often difficult.[60] If the catheter tip is in the base of the lung (West zone 3) (Fig. 11-22), the PAOP reflects left atrial pressure accurately.[61] Because the catheter is flow-directed, one anticipates that it will usually go toward the lung base. Increased alveolar pressure (with PEEP) or decreased pulmonary venous pressure associated with hypovolemia may "convert" a zone 3 area to a zone 1 or 2, and the pressure recorded is not truly indicative of that in the left atrium. If artifactual pressure transduction is suspected, guides to assessment include (1) identification of a, c, or v waves in the wedge pressure tracing, which if present indicate left atrial rather than alveolar pressure, and (2) obtaining a cross-table lateral chest film to determine the location of the catheter tip in relation to the left atrium. If the artifacts persist despite the fact that the catheter tip is properly located in the posterior, lower half of the lung, a fluid challenge may be administered in cases of suspected hypovolemia, or the PEEP level may be decreased transiently (but not removed) if high levels are required. Total discontinuation of PEEP can be dangerous; furthermore, it does not provide an accurate estimation of PAOP because of the acute hemodynamic fluctuations generated by the sudden change in airway pressure.[60]

Physiologic Shunt and Oxygen Delivery

One useful index of ventilation-perfusion inequality is the physiologic shunt (also called venous admixture or wasted blood flow). The shunt equation can be used in the following form:

$$\frac{\dot{Q}sp}{\dot{Q}t} = \frac{C\acute{c}O_2 - CaO_2}{C\acute{c}O_2 - C\bar{v}O_2} \qquad (8)$$

Where $\dot{Q}sp$ refers to the physiologic shunt, $\dot{Q}t$ to the total lung blood flow, and $C\acute{c}O_2$, CaO_2, and $C\bar{v}O_2$ to, respectively, the oxygen content of ideal pulmonary capillary, arterial, and mixed venous blood.[62] The normal value is less than 5 percent. If a physiologic shunt is determined on other than a F_IO_2 of 1.0, hypoxemia due to $\dot{V}/\dot{Q}$ inequality contributes to the calculated shunt. "True" shunt is determined during 100 percent oxygen breathing, and overestimation may result if inadequate time is given to completely wash out poorly ventilated alveoli.[60] PO_2 electrodes may underestimate the true PO_2 at high levels when compared to blood tonometered with 100 percent O_2.[63] The magnitude of the physiological shunt is related to cardiac output. A decrease in flow or cardiac output often (but not always) decreases the shunt. Conversely, an increased cardiac output resulting from volume expansion or pharmacologic intervention increases the shunt in septic shock. Thus, the magnitude of the shunt should be interpreted in relationship to cardiac output. The arteriovenous oxygen difference is often estimated, rather than measured, in the critically ill patient. This "shortcut" may lead to considerable inaccuracy in estimating the physiologic shunt. A clinical example of the detemination of maximal oxygen delivery follows.

A 24-year-old woman with ARDS secondary to thrombotic thrombocytopenic purpura requires PEEP. The initial hemodynamic profile is outlined in Table 11–7. The optimum level of PEEP is 10 cm H_2O because it is associated with the best tissue oxygen delivery of 933 ml O_2/min. Necessary calculations at 10 cm PEEP are

$$\text{Tissue delivery of oxygen} = \text{cardiac output} \times CaO_2 \qquad (9)$$

$$\begin{aligned} CaO_2 &= \text{Hb (g)} \times 1.39 \text{ ml } O_2/\text{g Hb} \times SO_2 + (0.003 \times PaO_2) \\ &= 16.1 \text{ ml } O_2/100 \text{ ml blood} \end{aligned}$$

$$\begin{aligned} CO \times CaO_2 &= \frac{5{,}800 \text{ ml/min} \times 16.1 \text{ ml } O_2}{100 \text{ ml blood}} \\ &= 933 \text{ ml } O_2/\text{min} \end{aligned}$$

Table 11–7. Hemodynamic Profile for "Optimum" PEEP

Measurement	Unit	PEEP 5 cm H_2O	PEEP 10 cm H_2O	PEEP 15 cm H_2O
Blood pressure	mmHg	140/80	132/80	112/82
Pulse	/min	100	90	103
Wedge pressure	mmHg	10	13	15
Pulmonary artery pressure	mmHg	45/22	37/17	51/15
Cardiac output	L/min	5.9	5.8	4
Blood gases				
pH	—	7.3	7.39	7.32
$PaCO_2$	mmHg	28	38	32
PaO_2	mmHg	50	80	55
Sat	percent	85	95	82
Hemoglobin	g	12	12	12
Urine	ml/hr	50	50	30
Oxygen delivery	ml O_2/min	847	933	544

where Hb is hemoglobin. The mixed venous oxygen tension ($P\bar{v}O_2$) has gained popularity as an index of tissue oxygenation, a trend facilitated by the relative ease with which $P\bar{v}O_2$ measurements can be made from the pulmonary artery catheter (Fig. 11–23). Blood drawn from a central venous catheter is not a mixed specimen: a pulmonary artery catheter sample is necessary. At best, the $P\bar{v}O_2$ reflects a weighted mean of tissue oxygenation because of variable flow rates and extraction in different organs. A $P\bar{v}O_2$ of less than 30 mmHg is a sign of severe tissue hypoxia. We usually determine the $P\bar{v}O_2$ together with the PaO_2 when a pulmonary artery catheter is in place; we recently showed that $P\bar{v}O_2$ is an accurate assessment of the tissue oxygen in patients with hemorrhagic and hypoxic shock but is falsely high in those with endotoxin shock because of peripheral arteriovenous shunting. Others have shown that the $P\bar{v}O_2$ at which blood lactate increases is different for patients with anemia and hypoxic hypoxia. Similar findings have been noted by Vaughn and Puri.[64]

When the patient is in a basal state with a constant oxygen consumption, cardiac output is inversely related to the $CaO_2 - C\bar{v}O_2$, as shown by the Fick equation:

$$\frac{O_2 \text{ consumption}}{\text{cardiac output}} = CaO_2 - C\bar{v}O_2 \quad (10)$$

Simultaneous measurement of PaO_2, $P\bar{v}O_2$, cardiac output, and hemoglobin permits calculation of oxygen consumption. Danek et al.[65] showed that as oxygen delivery decreases in patients with ARDS treated with PEEP, a decrease in oxygen consumption results that may not be reflected by $P\bar{v}O_2$ or even $CaO_2 - C\bar{v}O_2$.

CARDIAC OUTPUT

Cardiac output is usually calculated by one of three methods: (1) Fick, (2) indicator dye dilution, and (3) thermodilution. The Fick method involves measurement of oxygen consumption and arterial-venous oxygen content difference. With the indicator dye dilution method, a dye of known concentration and volume is injected into the blood. The concentration of the dye is then measured at a "downstream" site. The thermodilution method employs injec-

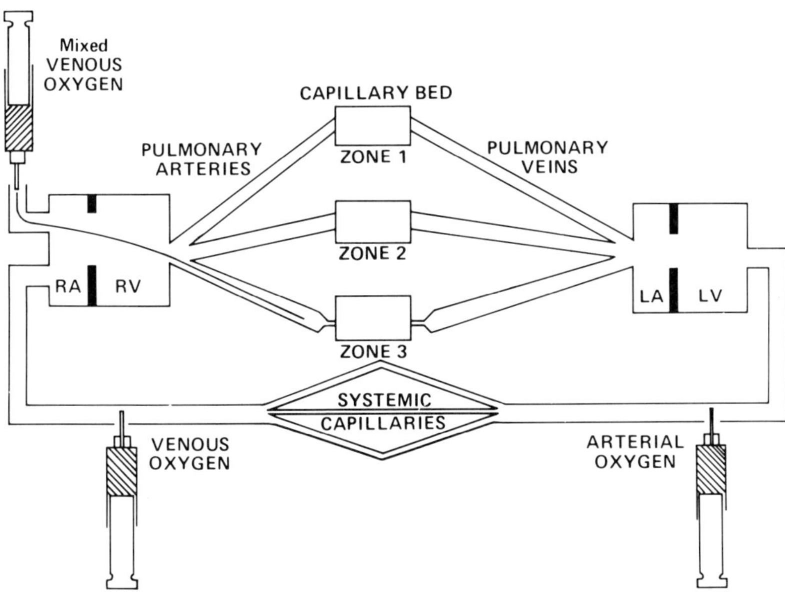

Fig. 11-23. Oxygen determinations can be obtained from the arterial, peripheral venous, or mixed venous blood. Arterial blood provides essential information about lung function. In certain circumstances, the PaO_2 might increase but be accompanied by a deterioration in oxygen delivery to tissue. For example, the application of PEEP in a relatively hypovolemic patient with ARDS might increase PaO_2 but depress cardiac output. In this situation, the arterial-mixed venous oxygen content difference increases, reflecting decreased cardiac output. Peripheral venous oxygen measurements are unreliable because they do not reflect changes from vital organs. $P\bar{v}O_2$ gives important information about decreased oxygenation despite improvement of arterial oxygenation A $P\bar{v}O_2$ of less than 30 mmHg suggests critical impairment of oxygen delivery. $P\bar{v}O_2$ is obtained from the pulmonary artery, as shown in this example. Also, the flow-directed pulmonary artery catheter is more likely to locate in better perfused lung regions (zone 2 or 3). In the supine patient zone 3 is posterior and in the upright patient it is inferior.

tion of a solution of known temperature into the right atrium or superior vena cava. Change in blood temperature is measured in the pulmonary artery by a thermistor near the tip of the thermodilution catheter; the change in resistance across a Wheatstone bridge is converted into liters per minute by a cardiac output computer.

In patients with severe respiratory failure, improvement in tissue oxygenation may require PEEP. Because oxygen delivery is the product of cardiac output and arterial oxygen content, the cardiac output or some index of changes of cardiac output should be followed as the PEEP is changed. Several studies have shown that even when PaO_2 increases, significant reduction in cardiac output can result from PEEP in combination with mechanical ventilation. If cardiac output falls, the patient may be hypovolemic and cardiac filling pressure too low to be maintained in the presence of PEEP. In this case, intravascular volume repletion is indicated. Alternatively, the patient may have primary cardiac dysfunction and require inotropic agents.

On-Line Mechanics

The respiratory system behaves mechanically as a pump with flow-resistive and volume-elastic components connected in series. According to Newton's third law of motion, opposing forces must be overcome to produce a volume change. Any increase of pressure at the mouth causes a flow of gas through the airways, which exhibit resistance to flow. The pressure not used to overcome airway resistance is dissipated by the volume-elastic component (lungs and chest wall) that is capable of deformation and volume change. The total pressure applied must overcome elastic forces (1/C) to produce a volume change (V), resistive forces (R) to produce flow ($\dot{V}$), and inertial forces (I) to produce acceleration ($\ddot{V}$). These components are combined to form the equation of motion for the respiratory system:

$$P = (1/C \times V) + (R \times \dot{V}) + (I \times \ddot{V}) \quad (11)$$

Changes caused by inertia (I) are small and, for clinical use, can be ignored.

Elucidation of the mechanical function of the lung requires the continuous recording of pressure and flow during the respiratory cycle.[66,67] Flow is usually measured by a pneumotachograph, which senses the differential pressure across a resistance in most cases. Inspiratory and expiratory pneumotachographs are a part of some single-patient monitoring systems, as in the Siemens 900C ventilator. With in-line pneumotachographs, expired volume measurements that include volume expended by compression in and expansion of the ventilator circuit are less of a problem. However, incorporation of pneumotachographs into the ventilator system introduces an entirely new set of problems, ranging from incorrect information because of mucus plugging of the pneumotachograph to problems of calibration changes caused by varying gas concentration. Because of problems with constant measurements using the Fleish pneumotachograph, other flow-measuring devices have been developed, including the variable-orifice flowmeter, ultrasonic flowmeter, and turbulent flowmeter. These flowmeters are currently undergoing clinical trials, and their accuracy and durability are still to be determined.

The pneumotachograph must be frequently calibrated to avoid error, usually with a 1- to 3-L syringe in line with a standard spirometer. Because pneumotachographs are sensitive to temperature, humidity, and flow, they should be calibrated under clinical conditions for reliable results. Flow rates should be linear over a range of 0 to 3 L/sec for mechanically ventilated patients. Some patients with respiratory failure may have expiratory flow rates exceeding 5 L/sec; appropriate pneumotachographs should be used in those patients.[55] In automated systems, airway pressure is measured by reliable strain gauges that provide a linear electrical output spanning a range of 0 to 200 cm H_2O.

A Fleish pneumotachograph with pressure- and gas-sampling lines leading to a gas analyzer computer permits simultaneous measurement of inspired and expired gases and mechanics (Fig. 11–24).

To measure lung compliance rather than lung and chest wall compliance, transpulmonary pressure must be determined. Respiratory pressure fluctuations reflected by an esophageal balloon or from the proximal port of a thermodilution Swan-Ganz catheter or a central venous catheter can be used for this purpose. Esophageal balloons are now available that attach to standard nasogastric tubes. If an esophageal balloon is used, a differential pressure transducer is needed to measure intrapleural pressure relative to mouth pressure. Lung plus chest wall compliance measured from airway pressure of the ventilated patient is affected by muscle contractions. The direct measurement of lung compliance thus adds both specificity and resolution.

Static compliance curves plotted in the pulmonary physiology laboratory are measured on a static deflation from total lung capacity. The plot of static transpulmonary pressure against lung volume is curvilinear; compliance is equal to the slope of the curve at a particular point. Unless functional residual capacity is measured and the compliance curve plotted at multiple volumes on deflation from a single breath, static compliance determinations in the ICU are not equivalent to those obtained in the pulmonary function laboratory. In the ICU, the lung volume usually is unknown, and a decrease in compliance can result from a true increase in elastic recoil (pulmonary edema) or the same elastic recoil exerted on a small volume (atelectasis).

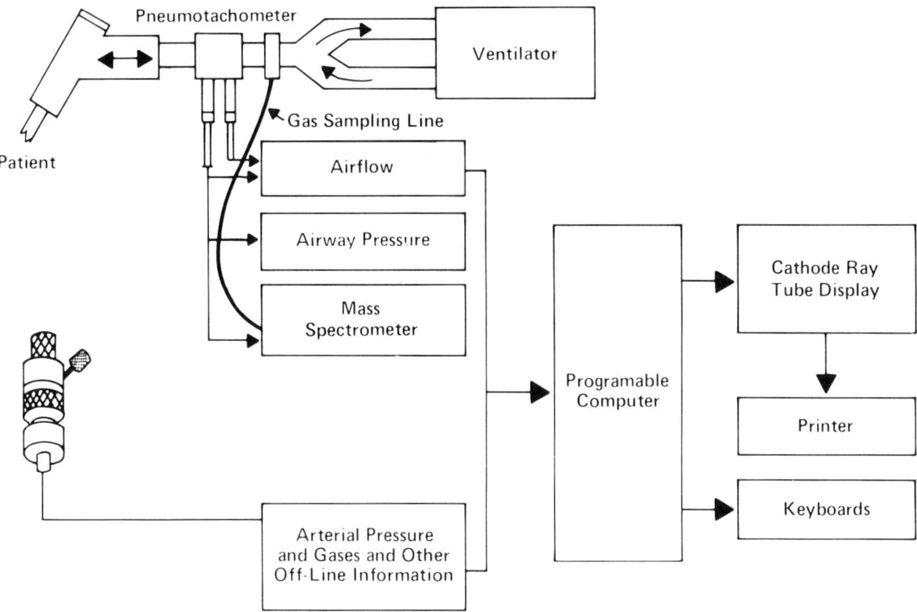

Fig. 11-24. Respiratory monitoring system. Air flow, pressure, and gas concentrations are measured simultaneously. Calculations are made by a computer using these signals and off-line information. (From Bone,[53] with permission.)

Regardless of the mechanism of decrease in compliance, the knowledge that it is decreased is important and should not be ignored because of the lack of knowledge of absolute lung volume before and after the development of atelectasis or pulmonary edema.[3]

DEVELOPMENT OF NEW MONITORING TECHNIQUES

Special scrutiny should be applied to two areas when assessing the potential value of new monitoring techniques. The first question to be asked is: Can the technique provide the information it claims in a reliable manner under usual clinical conditions? If a method is proved in the technical sense, we must still ask: Of what value to patient management are the data produced?

Few convincing data are available to answer these questions with regard to newer, more sophisticated respiratory monitoring methods. Economic considerations demand that resources not be devoted to gathering useless information, although some redundant information is valuable for detecting errors. Possibly the most serious danger of adopting monitoring techniques uncritically is to drown clinicians in a flood of numbers. The presentation of more data than can be assimilated can contribute to incorrect clinical decisions. This factor is too often ignored when assessing the value of new measurements.

Computers have the potential for alleviating some of these problems.[67] They can perform much of the tedious work of analyzing large amounts of data, reducing them to a form useful for making decisions. For example, they can produce summaries that list only aberrant values, reduce long lists of numbers to graphic form, or display only data considered relevant according to predetermined criteria. Even though the availability of inexpensive, powerful microcomputers makes such applications feasible, little has been done toward determining how they can best perform such clerical functions. Thus far, most effort has been devoted to overcoming difficulties assocated with on-line data acquisition and to solving various technical problems. As the quantitative data generated in the ICU increase, it will become increasingly important to have machines do what machines can do best in order to spare people for tasks requiring uniquely human abilities.

WHAT BIOLOGIC VARIABLES SHOULD BE MONITORED?

The generally accepted therapeutic goal of maintaining biologic variables in the normal range is being questioned. For example, the blood pressure and cardiac output can be restored to normal values after shock in most patients, yet many still die. Survivors often show supernormal values, reflecting their stress response to a critical illness and the subsequent metabolic and circulatory adjustment. Bland et al.[68] monitored the 20 most common variables in a series of 113 critically ill patients. For arterial pressure, heart rate, CVP, and cardiac output, normal values were restored in 75 percent of survivors and 76 percent of nonsurvivors. Bland and co-workers suggest that we may not have the correct therapeutic goals or that we may not be monitoring the correct variables. The ability of commonly monitored variables (e.g., vital signs, heart rate, and hemoglobin) to predict outcome was poor. Perfusion-related variables that express the interrelationship of O_2 transport to red blood cell volume and flow correlated best as predictors of outcome. Perfusion-related variables reflecting the maldistribution of systemic circulation should receive at least as much attention as variables reflecting maldistribution of the pulmonary circulation in future research.

REFERENCES

1. Robin ED: The cult of the Swan-Ganz catheter: overuse and abuse of pulmonary flow catheters. Ann Intern Med 103:445, 1985
2. Zwillich CW, Pierson DJ, Creach CE, et al: Complications of assisted ventilation. Am J Med 57:161, 1974
3. Bone RC: Diagnosis of causes for acute respiratory distress by pressure-volume curves. Chest 70:740, 1976
4. Gravenstein JS, Paulus DA: Clinical Monitoring Practice. JB Lippincott, Philadelphia, 1987, p. 62
5. Slogoff S, Keats AS, Arlund BS: On the safety of radial artery cannulation. Anesthesiology 54:42, 1983
6. Askanazi J, Rosenbaum SH, Hyman AL, et al: Respiratory changes induced by the large glucose loads of parenteral nutrition. JAMA 243:1444, 1980
7. Askanazi J, Norderstrom J, Rosenbaum SH, et al: Nutrition for the patients with respiratory failure: glucose vs. fat. Anesthesiology 54:373, 1981
8. Bone RC: Treatment of respiratory failure due to advanced obstructive lung disease. Arch Intern Med 140:1018, 1980
9. Gordon R: The deep sulcus sign. Radiology 136:25, 1980
10. Rhea JT, Sonnenberg EV, McLoud TC: Basilar pneumothorax in the supine adult. Radiology 133:593, 1979
11. Conrardy PA, Goodman LR, Lainge F, et al: Alteration of endotracheal tube position: flexion and extension of the neck. Crit Care Med 4:8, 1976
12. Osborne JJ, Raison CA, Beaumont JD, et al: Respiratory causes of ''sudden unexplained arrhythmia'' in post-thoracotomy patients. Surgery 69:24, 1971
13. Sweet SJ, Glenney JP, Fitzibbons JP, et al: Effect of acute renal failure and respiratory failure in the surgical intensive care unit. Am J Surg 141:492, 1981
14. Skillman JJ, Awwad HK, Moore FD: Plasma protein kinetics of the early transcapillary refill after hemorrhage in man. Surg Gynecol Obstet 123:983, 1967
15. Carpenter RL, Cullen BF: Hematologic and immune function. p. 78. In Brown DL (ed): Risk and Outcome in Anesthesia. JB Lippincott, Philadelphia, 1988
16. Ian EM, Heldman JJ, Chen SS: Coronary hemodynamics and oxygen utilization after hematocrit variations in hemorrhage. Am J Physiol 243:H325, 1980
17. West JB, Wagner PD: Pulmonary gas exchange.

p. 1. In West JB (ed): Bioengineering Aspects of the Lung. Marcel Dekker, New York, 1977
18. Wagner PD: Diffusion and chemical reaction in pulmonary gas exchange. Physiol Rev 57:257, 1977
19. Wagner PD, West JB: Effects of diffusion impairment on O_2 and CO_2 time courses in pulmonary capillaries. J Appl Physiol 33:62, 1972
20. Gilbert F, Keightley JF: The arterial/alveolar oxygen tension ratio: an index of gas exchange applicable to varying inspired concentrations. Am Rev Respir Dis 109:142, 1974
21. Murphy EM, Bone RC, Diederich DA, et al: The oxyhemoglobin dissociation curve in type a and type b chronic obstructive disease. Lung 154:299, 1978
22. Goecbenjan G: Continuous measurement of arterial PO_2—significance and indications in intensive care. Biotel Patient Monit 6:51, 1979
23. Shapiro BA, Cane RD, Chomka CM, et al: Preliminary evaluation of an intra-arterial blood gas system in dogs and humans. Crit Care Med 17:455, 1989
24. Pologe JA: Pulse oximetry: technical aspects of machine design. Int Anesthesiol Clin 25:137, 1987
25. Kelleher JF: Pulse oximetry. J Clin Monit 5:37, 1989
26. Eisenkraft JB: Pulse oximeter desaturation due to methemoglobinemia. Anesthesiology 68:279, 1988
27. Korbon GA, Wills MH, D'Lauro F, et al: Systolic blood pressure measurement: doppler vs. pulse oximeter. Anesthesiology 67:A188, 1987
28. Partridge BL: Use of pulse oximetry as a noninvasive indicator of intravascular volume status. J Clin Monit 3:263, 1987
29. Caplan RA, Ward RJ, Posner K, et al: Unexpected cardiac arrest during spinal anesthesia: a closed claims analysis. Anesthesiology 68:5, 1988
30. Keats A: Anesthesia mortality—a new mechanism (editorial). Anesthesiology 68:2, 1988
31. Coté CJ, Goldstein EA, Coté MA, et al: A single blind study of pulse oximetry in children. Anesthesiology 68:184, 1988
32. Eichorn JH: Prevention of intraoperative anesthesia accidents and related severe injury through safety monitoring. Anesthesiology 70:572, 1989
33. Orkin FK: Practice standards: the Midas Touch or the emperor's new clothes (editorial). Anesthesiology 70:567, 1989
34. Van Genderingen HR, Gravenstein N, Van der Aa JJ, et al: Computer assisted capnogram analysis. J Clin Monit 3:194, 1987
35. Nunn JH, Hill DWL: Respiratory dead space and arterial to end-tidal CO_2 tension difference in anesthetized man. J Appl Physiol 15:383, 1960
36. Tulov PP, Walsh PM: Measurement of alveolar carbon dioxide tension at maximal expiration as an estimate of arterial carbon dioxide tension in patients with airway obstruction. Am Rev Respir Dis 102:921, 1970
37. Whitesell R, Asiddao C, Gollman D, et al: Relationship between arterial and peak expired carbon dioxide pressure during anesthesia and factors influencing the difference. Anesth Analg 60:508, 1981
38. Weinger MB, Brimm JE: End-tidal carbon dioxide as a measure of arterial carbon dioxide during intermittent mandatory ventilation. J Clin Monit 3:73, 1987
39. Falk JL, Rackow EC, Weil MH: End-tidal carbon dioxide concentration during cardiopulmonary resuscitation. N Engl J Med 318:607, 1988
40. Leiplin MG, Vasilyev AV, Bildinov DA, et al: End-tidal carbon dioxide as a noninvasive monitor of circulatory status during cardiopulmonary resuscitation: a preliminary clinical study. Crit Care Med 15:958, 1987
41. Bowe EA, Boysen PG, Broome JA, et al: Accurate determination of end-tidal carbon dioxide during administration of oxygen by nasal cannulae. J Clin Monit 6:105, 1989
42. Peabody JL, Willis MM, Gregory GA, et al: Clinical limitations and advantages of transcutaneous oxygen electrodes. Acta Anesth Scand [Suppl] 68:76, 1978
43. Versmold HT, Linderkamp O, Holzmann M, et al: Limits of $tcPO_2$ monitoring in sick neonates: relation to blood pressure, blood volume, peripheral blood flow and acid base status. Acta Anaesth Scand [Suppl] 68:88, 1978
44. Tremper KK, Waxman K, Bowman R, et al: Transcutaneous oxygen monitoring during arrest and CPR. Crit Care Med 8:377, 1980
45. Tremper KK, Waxman K, Shoemaker WC: Effects of hypoxia and shock on transcutaneous PO_2 values in dogs. Crit Care Med 7:526, 1979
46. Wagner PD, Saltzman HA, West JB: Measurement of continuous distributions of ventilation-perfusion ratios: theory. J Appl Physiol 36:588, 1974
47. Dantzker DR: Gas exchange in the adult respiratory distress syndrome. Clin Chest Med 3:59, 1982

48. Gravenstein JS, Paulus DA: Clinical Monitoring Practice. JB Lippincott, Philadelphia, 1987, p 173
49. Rothe CF, Kim KC: Measuring systolic arterial blood pressure: possible errors from extension tubes or disposable transducer domes. Crit Care Med 8:683, 1980
50. Sahn SA, Lakshminarayan S: Bedside criteria for discontinuation of mechanical ventilation. Chest 63:1002, 1973
51. Suwa K, Hedley-White J, Bendixen HH: Circulation and physiological dead space changes on controlled ventilation of dogs. J Appl Physiol 231:1855, 1966
52. Shimada Y, Yoshiga I, Tamala K, et al: Evaluation of the progress and prognosis of acute respiratory distress syndrome: simple physiologic measurement. Chest 76:180, 1979
53. Bone RC: Monitoring patients in acute respiratory failure. Respir Care 27:700, 1982
54. Bone RC: Monitoring respiratory function in the patient with adult respiratory distress syndrome. p. 140. In Decker BC (ed): Adult Respiratory Distress Syndrome. Seminars in Respiratory Medicine. Vol. 2. Georg Thieme Verlag, Stuttgart, 1981
55. Fallat RJ: Bedside testing and intensive care monitoring of pulmonary function. In Standards and Controversies in Pulmonary Function Testing. California Thoracic Society Annual Postgraduate Course, Jan 1980
56. Luterman A, Horovitz JH, Carrico PC, et al: Withdrawal from positive end-expiratory pressure. Surgery 83:328, 1978
57. Newell JC, Shah DM, Dutton RE, et al: Pulmonary pressure-volume relationships in traumatized patients. J Surg Res 26:114, 1979
58. Fitzpatrick GF: Pulmonary artery catheterization with balloon flotation (Swan-Ganz) catheter. p. 65. In Salem TJV, Cutler BS, Wheeler HB (eds): Atlas of Bedside Procedures. Little, Brown, Boston, 1979
59. Foote GA, Schabel I, Hodges M: Pulmonary complications of the flow-directed balloon-tipped catheter. N Engl J Med 290:927, 1974
60. Downs JB, Douglas ME: Assessment of cardiac filling pressure occurring in continuous positive pressure ventilation. Crit Care Med 8:285, 1980
61. Bone RC: The treatment of severe hypoxemia due to the adult respiratory distress syndrome. Arch Intern Med 140:85, 1980
62. Jordan E, Eveleigh MC, Gurdijon F, et al: Venous admixture in human septic shock: comparative effects of blood volume expansion, dopamine infusion, and isoproterenol infusion on mismatching of ventilation and pulmonary blood flow in peritonitis. Circulation 60:155, 1979
63. Dantazker D: Abnormalities of oxygen transfer. p. 1. In Bone RC (ed): Pulmonary Disease Reviews. Vol. 1. John Wiley & Sons, New York, 1980
64. Vaughn S, Puri VK: Cardiac output charges and continuous mixed venous oxygen saturation measurement in the critically ill. Crit Care Med 16:495, 1988
65. Danek SI, Lynch JP, Weg JG, et al: The dependence of oxygen uptake on oxygen delivery in the adult respiratory distress syndrome. Am Rev Respir Dis 22:387, 1980
66. Turney SZ, McAslan TC, Cowley RA: The continuous measurement of pulmonary gas exchange and mechanics. Ann Thorac Surg 13:229, 1973
67. Wald A, Jason D, Murphy TW, et al: A computer system for respiratory parameters. Comput Biomed Res 2:411, 1969
68. Bland R, Shoemaker WC: Probability of survival as a prognostic and severity of illness score in critically ill surgical patients. Crit Care Med 13:91, 1985

12

Complications of Ventilatory Support

Orlando G. Florete, Jr.
Gary W. Gammage

Ventilatory support is one of the most conspicuous aspects of modern critical care, and complications of this therapy are frequently ubiquitous. Techniques that involve positive rather than negative airway pressure may result in pulmonary barotrauma, cardiovascular depression, and detrimental effects on other organ systems. Such therapy usually requires translaryngeal intubation of the trachea or tracheotomy, both of which have inherent complications. Complexity of the equipment and procedures often leads to significant complications. Finally, social, psychological, and ethical considerations have blurred the distinction between prolonging productive life and retarding the inevitable and agonizing process of dying.

PULMONARY BAROTRAUMA

Pulmonary barotrauma is pressure injury to the lungs that results in extra-alveolar air. Its incidence in mechanically ventilated patients has been reported to be as infrequent as 0.5 percent by Cullen and Caldera,[1] to as high as 39 percent.[2] Although barotrauma is commonly thought to result from pleural rupture of surface blebs, Macklin and Macklin[3] found that such rupture rarely occurs. Instead, when alveoli are overdistended, gas ruptures from their bases, dissects along the perivascular sheathes to the hilum and then to the mediastinum. From there, it can spread in many directions. Rupture of the thin mediastinal pleura produces a pneumothorax. Gas can dissect along tissue planes into the neck, producing subcutaneous emphysema, or into the retroperitoneum and peritoneum along the aorta and esophagus.

When gas is detectable radiographically in the perivascular sheathes, it is termed *pulmonary interstitial emphysema* (PIE). Radiographic evidence of PIE or pneumomediastinum, or physical signs of subcutaneous emphysema, are often thought to be associated with increased risk to the ventilated patient. However, Downs and Chapman[2] reported that although subcutaneous emphysema occurred in 39 percent of their patients, only 7 percent had pneumothorax.

The incidence of pulmonary barotrauma correlates with peak inspiratory pressure (PIP). The magnitude of PIP is more important than the duration of pressure, and barotrauma is rare when PIP is less than 25 mmHg.[7] However, high PIP must also cause alveolar overdistension. The latter is most likely with large tidal volume ventilation[8] or when a normal tidal volume is distributed to fewer alveoli, as may occur with mainstem bronchial intubation[9] or severe atelectasis.[3] Pulmonary barotrauma is more likely to occur with lower airway pressure when the chest is open than when the lungs are confined within the thorax.[7]

The role of positive end-expiratory pressure (PEEP) or continuous positive airway pressure (CPAP) is controversial. A correlation between the level of PEEP and the incidence of pulmonary barotrauma has been noted, but higher levels of PEEP usually are associated with a higher PIP. Decreased intravascular volume and a concomitant decrease in perivascular tissue pressure may also predispose a patient to pulmonary barotrauma because of the increased pressure gradient between the alveoli and the perivascular space.[10] Other predisposing factors include diseases that destroy lung tissue, such as chronic obstructive pulmonary disease (COPD), asthma, and necrotizing pneumonia.

Diagnosis

Early diagnosis of pulmonary barotrauma is essential. Pulmonary interstitial emphysema often is the first manifestation in mechanically ventilated adults. If PIE is detected, early preventative measures may avoid a pneumothorax. Once a simple pneumothorax develops, it may rapidly become a tension pneumothorax if the patient is mechanically ventilated. If a ventilated patient becomes restless, and especially if radiographic evidence of extra-alveolar air is present a pneumothorax should be considered. Should the pneumothorax be large, absent breath sounds and hyperresonance on the affected side are often noted. If it is under tension, mediastinal and tracheal shift, distended neck veins, and hypotension are frequent occurrences (Table 12-1). When the patient is hemodynamically stable, the diagnosis can be confirmed with an upright chest radiograph to reveal a pleural line at the apex. If the patient is hypotensive, a tension pneumothorax should be suspected and pleural pressure should be relieved with a 14-gauge intravenous catheter inserted into the pleural cavity at the second intercostal space in the mid-clavicular line, followed immediately by tube thoracotomy. Catheter insertion is an emergency technique and is indicated only as a temporizing measure until a chest tube tray can be obtained.

Table 12–1. Diagnosis of Pneumothorax

Precursors
Pulmonary interstitial emphysema
Subcutaneous emphysema
Mediastinal emphysema
Signs
Pleural line on radiograph
Restlessness
Large pneumothorax
Decreased breath sounds
Hyperresonance
Tension pneumothorax
Deviated trachea and mediastinum
Distended neck veins
Hypotension
Cardiovascular collapse

Prevention

Any measure to decrease airway pressure theoretically should decrease the incidence of pulmonary barotrauma (Table 12-2). Most ventilators have a pressure relief valve and high pressure alarms. These valves should be initially set to open at 60 mmHg, then subsequently adjusted 15 percent above the patient's PIP. PIP, PEEP, and tidal volumes should be monitored, recorded, and limited to the lowest levels necessary to provide satisfactory ventilation. Monitoring of PIP is especially important when manual inflations are delivered during suctioning procedures. Spontaneous ventilation should be encouraged whenever possible, since it lowers airway pressure requirements. Ventilatory modes, such as synchronized intermittent mandatory ventilation (SIMV), which permit spontaneous ventilation, are preferable in this respect to controlled mechanical ventilation (CMV). Clinicians should attempt to reduce coughing, straining, and fighting against the ventilator. However, muscle paralysis should only be used after extensive attempts to adjust the ventilator to the patient's needs have failed, and then only with sedation. Inverse I:E ratio ventilation (IRV) often permits the same tidal volume to be delivered with lower PIP.

Some patients are at particular risk for pulmonary barotrauma, including those with air trapping due to COPD, asthma or mucus plugging.

Table 12–2. Prevention and Limitation of Pulmonary Barotrauma

1. Use the ventilator to minimize airway pressure.
   A. Set pressure relief valves properly.
   B. Limit peak inspiratory pressure:
      1 Limit tidal volume
      2 Maximize spontaneous ventilation (SIMV, CPAP)
      3. Acute pressure-release ventilation
      4. High frequency ventilation
      5. Inverse I:E ratio
2. Minimize coughing and straining against the ventilator.
3. Ensure independent lung ventilation via double lumen tube.
4. Extracorporeal membrane CO_2 elimination.
5. Use low-resistance breathing circuits and valves.

Compensatory hyperinflation of some lung regions due to atelectasis or infiltrates in other areas renders them more susceptible. Fiberoptic bronchoscopy can retard exhalation and produce inadvertent PEEP; thus pulmonary barotrauma may occur when the endotracheal tube is not much larger than the bronchoscope. The largest possible endotracheal tube should be used for this procedure, and a chest radiograph should be obtained after it is completed. Cardiopulmonary resuscitation (CPR), especially during simultaneous chest compressions and lung inflations, results in airway pressures of 90 to 100 cm H_2O or more. This synergistic effect may explain the frequent occurrence of pulmonary barotrauma after CPR.

Treatment

Once a pneumothorax develops, continued efforts to minimize PIP are indicated. If the pneumothorax produces cardiopulmonary compromise, chest tube insertion is indicated. The tube should be placed under water seal. Suction usually is not necessary. When the patient is transported, the chest tube should remain under the water seal; under no circumstances should it be clamped. The container should remain below the level of the chest to avoid the possibility of water infusion into the pleural cavity. Underwater seal should be maintained until there is no evidence of air leak for at least 24 hours. Critically ill patients may develop loculated pneumothoraces requiring several drainage tubes on the same side of the chest. Frequently, the air leak will not resolve until positive-pressure ventilation is discontinued.

Bronchopleural fistula occasionally develops in some critically ill patients, especially those requiring mechanical ventilation for severe pneumonia. If the patient requires high PIP and PEEP, the air leak may be difficult to manage. Attempts have been made to apply CPAP to the chest tube to limit the loss of gas through the leak.[12] Whenever possible, the PIP should be minimized. If the disease is unilateral, a double lumen endotracheal tube can be inserted and the diseased lung ventilated at very low airway pressures, perhaps with high-frequency ventilation (HFV), while the less diseased lung receives higher pressure. However, even with this method, the prognosis is dismal. In some patients, veno-veno extracorporeal membrane elimination of carbon dioxide has been combined with low pressure, low-frequency ventilation, and oxygenation.

NONPULMONARY EFFECTS OF POSITIVE AIRWAY PRESSURE

Cardiovascular System

The goal of ventilatory support is to normalize carbon dioxide elimination, arterial oxygenation, and oxygen delivery. During normal spontaneous ventilation, airway pressure is atmospheric or subatmospheric. Conversely, with mechanical ventilatory support, airway pressure is increased during part or all of the ventilatory cycle. Positive airway pressure can decrease cardiac output and oxygen delivery. Therefore, it is extremely important to consider the hemodynamic consequences of mechanical ventilation.

Many of the hemodynamic consequences of mechanical ventilation, PEEP, and CPAP result from positive airway pressure transmitted to the pleural space, the heart, and great vessels within the chest. The greater the transmitted pressure, the greater the effect. Constant positive pressures will have a greater effect than the same pressures applied intermittently as in sCPAP versus sPEEP[13] or PEEP + CMV versus PEEP + IMV.[14] If pulmonary compliance is low, less pressure is thought to be transmitted through the lungs to the cardiovascular system, although this traditional view has been challenged recently. Extrapolation of experimental results from healthy anesthetized animals to sick humans with decreased lung compliance must be viewed cautiously. In general, however, reductions of thorax compliance, which tend to reduce lung expansion, appear to minimize pressure transmission, whereas the higher compliance seen with emphysema is associated with increased transmission of pressure and a greater incidence of detrimental cardiovascular effects.

Clinical and experimental studies demonstrate numerous hemodynamic effects of positive airway pressure[15–17] (Table 12-3). Positive pleural pressure decreases venous return and right ventricular (RV) preload, decreases left ventricular (LV) afterload, and may decrease LV compliance.[18–21] The ultimate result of the simultaneous decrease in preload and afterload will depend on the intravascular volume and ventricular function. If intravascular volume is normal or low, the decrease in preload will decrease cardiac output. If vascular volume is elevated and ventricular function is depressed, then the decreased preload and LV afterload may increase cardiac output.[22]

Some evidence in animal studies suggests that either reflex neural mechanisms or humoral products resulting from positive-pressure lung inflation may depress cardiac output.[23,24] The humoral product has not been identified, and the clinical importance of either of these postulated mechanisms is in doubt. Endocardial ischemia leading to depressed cardiac output has been demonstrated in some animal studies, but the clinical relevance of this observation also is uncertain.

Table 12–3. Hemodynamic Effects of Positive Airway Pressure

Decreased right venticular preload
Increased right ventricular afterload
Decreased left ventricular compliance
Decreased left ventricular afterload
Depressed contractility of one or both ventricles
Humoral or reflex neuronal depressant effects
Endocardial ischemia

Other Organs

Most investigations into the potentially adverse effects of positive-pressure ventilation have focused on cardiopulmonary interactions. In recent years, however, interest with respect to other organ systems has increased. This subject is discussed in Chapter 5 but is of sufficient importance to be included here as well. The interplay of several factors affecting renal, hepatic, and splanchnic functions are shown in Figure 12-1.

Kidneys

Positive-pressure ventilation causes a reduction in urine output and retention of salt and water by means of several interactive mechanisms. An increase of intrapleural pressure (Ppl) during a mechanical breath decreases venous return to the heart and depresses cardiac output, as a result of which the sympathetic nervous system is activated.[25] Catecholamines constrict the adrenergically innervated afferent renal arterioles, reducing renal blood flow and causing its redistribution from cortical to juxtamedullary nephrons. The glomerular filtration rate (GFR) and urinary sodium excretion are thereby reduced.[26] The decrease in renal blood flow and sodium delivery to the macula densa, coupled with increased renal sympathetic activity, stimulate the renin-angiotensin-aldosterone system.[27–29] Activation of this system causes additional renal vasoconstriction, further reduction in GFR, and increased sodium and water retention.

Plasma arginine vasopressin is also increased, due either to baroreceptor discharge following a decrease of transmural aortic pressure during positive-pressure ventilation or to the response of left atrial (LA) stretch receptors to a decrease

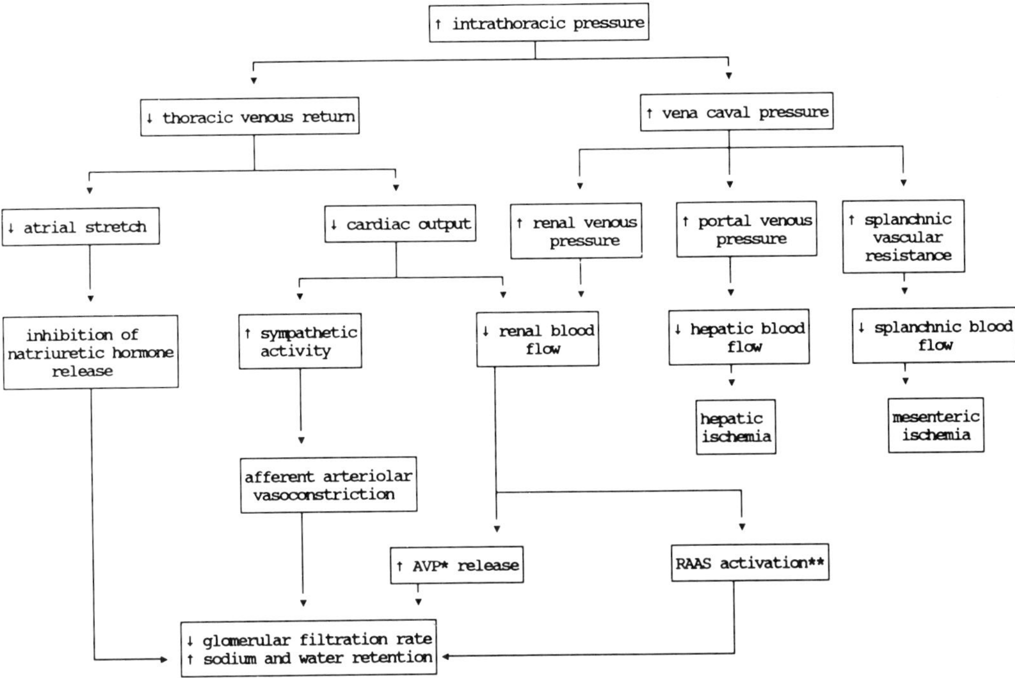

Fig. 12-1. Effects of mechanical ventilation on the kidneys, liver, and gut. *, arginine vasopressin; **, renin-angiotensin-aldosterone system.

in thoracic blood volume.[30,31] Arginine vasopressin acts both as a vasoconstrictor and an antidiuretic agent. It promotes distal tubular reabsorption of water and decreases water clearance. The reduction in the LA stretch may also cause inhibition of atrial natriuretic hormone release. Atrial natriuretic hormone normally antagonizes the effects of vasopressin and the renin-angiotensin-aldosterone system. Its inhibition further exacerbates the already existing reductions in renal blood flow, GFR, and sodium excretion. Finally, an increase in inferior vena caval and renal vein pressures may decrease renal cortical blood flow and increase juxtamedullary blood flow. The net effect of these interacting mechanisms is salt and water retention with decreased urine output.

Liver

During mechanical ventilation, diaphragmatic descent may increase intra-abdominal, hepatic, and portal vein pressures, with a resultant decrease of venous outflow.[32,33] In the presence of reduced cardiac output and mean arterial pressure, a reduction in portal vein flow renders the liver more susceptible to ischemia. Hedley-Whyte et al.[34] found an increase in mean serum bilirubin to more than 3.5 mg/dl in 32 percent of patients with no prior liver disease who received positive-pressure ventilation for the treatment of acute respiratory failure. Seventy-seven percent of patients showed some evidence of hepatic dysfunction. Positive-pressure ventilation also increases resistance to bile flow through the choledochoduodenal junction as a result of vascular engorgement of the mucosal lining of the intramural bile ducts. The vascular engorgement also results from increased resistance to hepatic venous outflow.[35]

Splanchnic Blood Flow

Elevation of inferior vena caval pressure during mechanical ventilation increases splanchnic resistance and decreases mesenteric blood flow.

This combination may predispose to gastric and intestinal ischemia and sometimes contributes to upper gastrointestinal (GI) bleeding.

Central Nervous System

Intracranial hypertension can be aggravated by mechanical ventilation when elevated Ppl impedes venous drainage from the head and increases intracranial blood volume.[36] A reduction in mean arterial pressure and elevation of intracranial pressure (ICP) will reduce cerebral perfusion pressure and cerebral blood flow.[37] Tracheal suctioning also is associated with increases in ICP. Increased ICP stimulates the release of arginine vasopressin, contributing to the adverse renal effects of mechanical ventilation.[31] Even in the absence of increased ICP, high airway pressures are thought by some investigators to result in decreased mental acuity, which returns to normal following weaning from ventilatory support. The mechanism has not been elucidated.

AIRWAY MANAGEMENT

Many complications of ventilatory support are related to airway management. Except in specific types and limited numbers of patients who may benefit from a CPAP mask, positive-pressure airway support necessitates tracheal intubation with oral or nasal translaryngeal tubes or tracheotomy. Some problems are common to all modes of tracheal intubation, while others are specific. They can be classified according to time of onset, that is, during intubation, during maintenance, or after extubation.[38] Those that are ubiquitous include technical difficulties during insertion, tracheal mucosal damage from the tube cuff, inadequate humidification of inspired gas, tracheal contamination and infection, aphonia, tube obstruction, tube malposition, and inadvertent extubation.

General Problems

Difficulties During Insertion

Translaryngeal tracheal intubation usually is rapid, simple, and atraumatic in experienced hands. However congenital and acquired anatomic abnormalities of the upper airway can make the technique difficult or impossible (Table 12-4). Trauma to all structures of the upper airway may occur during intubation.

Tracheotomy is a surgical procedure with a reported mortality rate that varies from 0.9 to 5.0 percent.[39] Increased mortality rates generally are reported in earlier literature in which "slash" tracheotomies were commonly done rapidly in emergencies, without airway control and without proper operating conditions. Recent reports emphasize low mortality when the airway first is controlled by translaryngeal intubation and the operation is carefully performed by trained surgeons under elective conditions.

Tracheal Mucosal Damage

The presence of an inflated cuff against the tracheal mucosa causes tracheal mucosal damage, regardless of the type of tube used.[40] The amount of damage is related to cuff pressure, duration of exposure, and the presence of severe

Table 12–4. The Difficult Airway

1. Edema
2. Upper airway trauma
3. Short thick neck
4. Protruding maxillary incisors
5. Temporomandibular joint range of motion less than 40 mm (2 finger breadths)
6. Cervical range of motion from flexion to extension less than 90 to 165 degrees, respectively
7. High-arched palate with narrow mouth
8. High anterior larynx (mandible to thyroid notch less than 3 finger breadths)
9. Base of tongue large enough to obscure view of the uvula and tonsillar pillars
10. Trachea shifted away from midline, or fixed and immobile
11. Tumor of the airway
12. History of difficult intubation
13. Previous tracheotomy or prolonged intubation

(From Gammage,[127] with permission.)

respiratory failure or infected secretions.[41] Low-volume high-pressure cuffs are the primary culprits. Damage is allegedly reduced by high volume cuffs which allow sealing of the airway with a lower pressure. If cuff pressure is below the perfusion pressure in the capillaries of the tracheal mucosa (about 25 to 30 mmHg), blood flow continues and ischemic mucosal damage is minimized.

Pressure in the cuff is kept to a minimum by inserting just enough air to prevent a leak at PIP (minimum occlusive volume technique). The increased compliance of high volume cuffs is thought to make them safer, because the addition of a small amount of air above the minimally occlusive volume causes a minimal rise in cuff pressure. However, such small increments are difficult to regulate, and too much air inadvertently injected changes the characteristics of the cuff to those of high-pressure types. Wall thickness of the cuff also is important. Thin-walled cuffs prevent the formation of longitudinal ridges, which may lead to aspiration and to uneven pressure on the tracheal wall.[42]

Although mucosal damage increases with time, the damage begins early. After only two hours, superficial loss of ciliated epithelium is present. Ulceration and inflammation extend to involve the perichondrion and eventually, the tracheal cartilages. Mucosal damage contributes to the sore throat experienced by many patients. Because the ciliated epithelium is damaged, mucociliary clearance is inhibited. Extensive tracheal damage can lead to tracheomalacia if the cartilage is destroyed or to tracheal stenosis if the inflammation heals as a contracted scar.

Tracheal stenosis is particularly dangerous because it usually presents acutely months after extubation. It develops slowly as the inflammation heals into a contracted scar. Symptoms will not develop until the lumen is narrowed to about 5-mm diameter. An asymptomatic lesion suddenly can become symptomatic with a small amount of airway edema during an acute respiratory tract infection.

Avoidance of tracheal injury at the cuff site is best achieved by proper inflation technique. Various types of valves have been designed to regulate pressure within the tracheal tube cuffs. The Lanz cuff prevents excessive pressure until the inner latex balloon touches the outer balloon. Unfortunately, such cuffs are only effective when low PIP is used during mechanical ventilation. Attempts to decrease tracheal damage by intermittent cuff deflation were popular during the early 1970s but have had little or no application since the introduction of high-volume, low-pressure cuffs.

Humidification

When an artificial airway is inserted, humidification provided by the natural upper airway is lost. Normally, inspired gases are warmed to body temperature and are 100 percent humidified before they reach the carina. The tracheal tube exposes the lower airways to cold dry gas. Mucosal damage and drying of secretions result. Lack of humidification can lead to airway obstruction because ciliary clearance is inhibited and the normal thin, watery mucus becomes thick and tenacious. In the past, tracheotomy tubes had to be removed and cleaned on a regular basis to prevent obstruction by inspissated secretions, but this procedure rarely is necessary if inspired gases are adequately humidified.

Infection

Artificial airways bypass the antibacterial defenses of the upper airway. Normally, no bacteria are present below the glottis, but insertion of a tracheal tube predisposes to contamination of the lower airways within 24 hours of intubation. Bacterial contamination of the lower airways is eight times more common with a tracheotomy than with translaryngeal tracheal intubation.[44]

Aphonia

Inability to communicate verbally may be a severe psychologic strain for a critically ill patient. Attempts to talk with a tracheal tube between the vocal cords will increase laryngeal trauma[45] and should be discouraged. Other attempts at communication, such as writing and pointing to letters or pictures on a communication board, often are less than adequate.

Talking tracheotomy tubes are available commercially. A separate cannula attached to the tube can be attached to a gas source and a constant flow of gas directed up through the cords to enable vocalization. This technique, of course, is more difficult with an endotracheal tube passing between the cords, but attempts to use speaking endotracheal tubes have been reported.[46] The artificial larynx, a box held against the throat which transmits a buzzing sound to the oral pharynx, is another possible solution, but to date satisfactory verbal communication in intubated patients remains an elusive goal.

Malposition and Unplanned Extubation

Tracheal tubes can be malpositioned into a mainstem bronchus, usually the right, or into the esophagus. Fresh tracheotomy tubes may be displaced from the trachea. Severe mediastinal emphysema, hypoventilation, and arterial hypoxemia occur within minutes if the tube inadvertently is placed anterior to the trachea in the pretracheal fascia. During translaryngeal intubation the endoscopist should see the tube pass between the cords and advance it until the top of the cuff is 1 or 2 cm below them. In this position, it is possible to palpate the inflated cuff at the suprasternal notch.

If direct visualization is not optimal, the distance marks on the endotracheal tube can be used as a rough guide to proper depth of insertion (Fig. 12-2). The tube is numbered in cm from

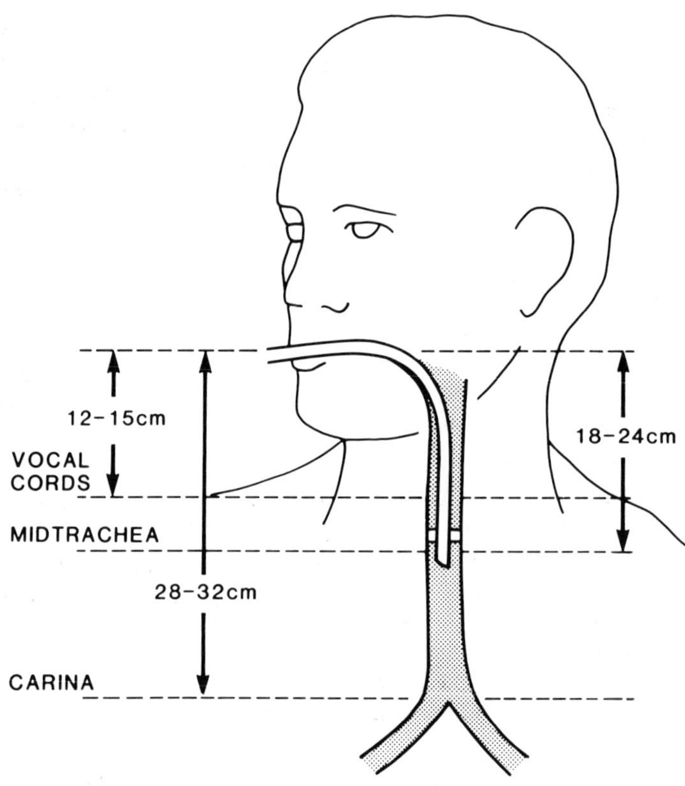

Fig. 12-2. Malposition of the endotracheal tube can be suspected from the depth of insertion. In an average adult, the 18- to 24-cm mark will show at the incisors when the tip of the tube is midway between the vocal cords and the carina. (From Gammage,[127] with permission.)

the tip. In most adults, from the teeth to midtrachea is 18 to 24 cm.[47] Usually the 20- or 22-cm mark is at the teeth if the tube is at the proper depth. For nasal intubation, 4 to 5 cm is added such that the 25- or 26-cm mark shows at the entrance of the tube into the nostril. Immediately after insertion, tube position must be verified by auscultation of bilateral breath sounds (best done in the axillae to minimize transmitted breath sounds) and by chest radiograph. The only foolproof way of ensuring correct placement of a tracheal tube is direct visualization.

Even a properly inserted tube can migrate as a result of poor taping, traction by ventilator hoses, turning of the patient, unsecured restraint of the patient's hands, or changes in head position. With flexion and extension of the neck, the tip of the tube, following the chin, moves toward and away from the carina, respectively. The tube also moves away from the carina with lateral motion of the neck (Fig. 12-3). In a radiographic study of intubated patients, average tube movement was 3.8 cm from full extension to full flexion, but the tube can move as much as 6.4 cm.[48] The neck is neutral if the chin is over the fifth or sixth cervical vertebrae, extended if the chin is above C4, and flexed if the chin is below C7.

From 8.5 to 13 percent of intubated critically ill patients may suffer unplanned (accidental) extubation. Replacement of a tracheal tube requires skilled personnel who are readily at hand. Replacement of a fresh tracheotomy tube can be extremely difficult but is easier if the surgeon has left traction sutures in the tracheal wall.[51] If any difficulty is encountered during replacement of a tube in a fresh tracheostomy stoma, the patient should be translaryngeally intubated quickly. A gentle and controlled exploration of the wound can follow. Optimally, the tube cuff should be below the cricoid cartilage and above the sternal notch. Should stenosis occur, a sternal split will not be necessary for surgical correction. Stenosis at the cricoid level is not easily corrected and may require permanent tracheotomy. Once a tracheostomy stoma has matured, replacement of the tube is simple and is one of the primary advantages of a tracheotomy. Accidental extubation is minimized by careful nursing practice, including secure taping of the tube, routine use of hand restraints in poorly compliant patients, and care in turning and moving intubated patients.

Specific Problems

Translaryngeal Intubation

Problems specifically related to translaryngeal intubation result from trauma to the upper airway and larynx, while those associated exclusively

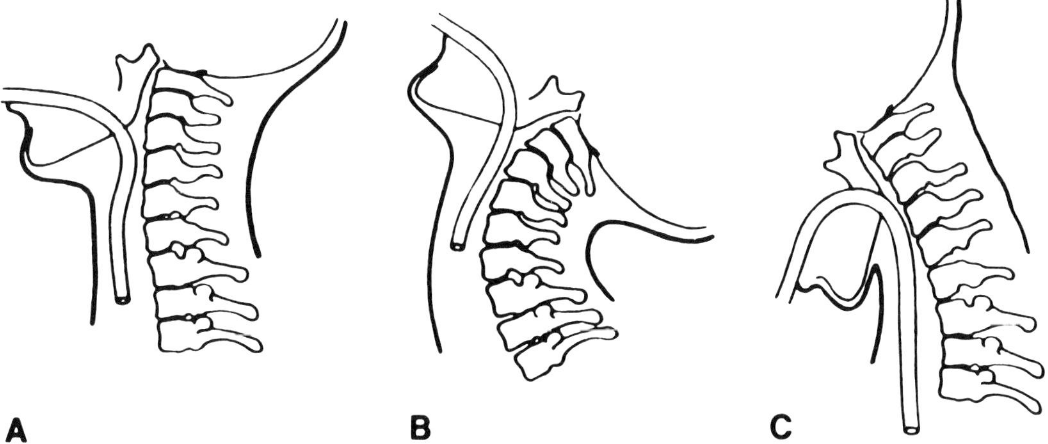

Fig. 12-3. The tip of the endotracheal tube follows the chin (**A**) and moves away from the carina with extension of the neck (**B**) and toward the carina with flexion (**C**) of the neck. (From Conrardy et al.,[48] with permission.)

to tracheotomy result mostly from the surgical procedure and the stoma. Almost every structure cephalad of the diaphragm has been injured during insertion of tracheal tubes.[38]

During nasal intubation, bleeding is common and can be excessive. Nasal intubation should be avoided in patients with a coagulopathy. Bleeding is thought to be minimized with topical vasoconstrictors, although this view has been challenged, and by small, well-lubricated tubes inserted gently. Extensive bleeding may be controlled by withdrawing the endotracheal tube to the bleeding site and inflating the cuff to produce a tamponade effect. The patient then may be intubated orally. Nasal intubation induces a transient bacteremia,[52] which should be considered in patients needing antibiotic prophylaxis for subacute bacterial endocarditis. The turbinates and adenoids can be damaged during insertion of a nasal tube, leading to obstruction. Gentle pressure is important. If undue resistance is encountered, accompanied by no breath sounds, the tube may be dissecting submucosally along the posterior oral pharynx.[53]

Oral insertion of an endotracheal tube can lead to damage of the lips, teeth, gums, tongue, oral pharynx, esophagus, and larynx.[38] Careful technique and proper patient cooperation, pharmacologically induced if necessary, is appropriate. If teeth are avulsed or chipped, the pieces should be retrieved prior to aspiration, or by means of a bronchoscope if aspiration already has occurred.

The larynx sometimes is damaged during tube insertion, or after it is in place. During insertion, the arytenoid cartilages may be dislocated and the vocal cords traumatized. Following intubation, ulceration and inflammation of the vocal cords and subglottic area can occur. Ulceration is more severe with larger tubes, in women (because of smaller glottic openings), and with friction caused by movement of the larynx along the tube. Movement results not only from traction of the ventilator tubing and neck, but also from attempts to talk and even from respiratory movement of the larynx.

Ulceration and inflammation can progress to granuloma formation, leading to chronic hoarseness after extubation. Granuloma formation is not related to the duration of intubation, but does appear to be related to tube material. The incidence is less than 1 percent with polyvinyl chloride tubes. Other causes of chronic hoarseness include severe ulceration of the vocal cords, leading to a persistent glottic chink, vocal cord fibrosis, nerve damage, cricoarytenoid arthritis, dislocated arytenoid cartilages, and vocal cord polyps. Hoarseness after extubation is present in 71 to 86 percent of patients intubated for 5 days, but is persistent beyond 3 months in only 0.7 percent.[45] Chronic hoarseness does appear to be related to the duration of intubation.

Laryngeal complications other than hoarseness and granuloma formation, also can occur after the tube is removed. Acute airway obstruction, due to glottic or subglottic edema, is possible. This problem occurs equally after prolonged and short-term intubation. The protective glottic mechanisms are incompetent immediately following extubation.[54] To protect against aspiration, the patient should not be allowed to eat or drink for at least 8 hours and possibly as long as 24 hours after extubation. Laryngeal or subglottic stenosis can develop more than 5 months after intubation. Rarely is the diagnosis made in less than 3 months. Scar tissue forming with healing of ulcerated and inflamed tissue can lead to fusion of the cords or circumferential narrowing of the subglottic area.[45,55]

Advantages claimed for nasal intubation include patient comfort, secure tube fixation, and reduced laryngeal damage because of the generally smaller size and straighter angle of the tube through the glottis (Table 12-5). Disadvantages of nasal insertion include nasal bleeding and trauma, transient bacteremia, cuff rupture on the turbinates during insertion, submucosal dissection, and sinusitis or otitis media from obstruction of the sinus openings or eustachian tubes. The latter problems should be considered as sources of infection in critically ill patients who are nasally intubated.[56]

Tracheotomy

Significant problems occurring during performance of a tracheotomy include pneumothorax, pneumomediastinum, subcutaneous emphy-

Table 12–5. Oral versus Nasal Intubation

Variables	Oral	Nasal
Ease of procedure	Apneic patient	Awake breathing patient
Nasal bleeding	No	Yes
Sinusitis	No	Yes
Patient comfort	Less	More
Need for bite block	Yes	No
Oral hygiene	Difficult	Easy
Accidental extubation	More likely	Less likely
Tube size	Larger, shorter	Smaller, longer
Suctioning	Easier	More difficult
Laryngeal damage	More	Less
Contraindications	Mandibular fractures	Nasal CSF leak
		Nasal sinusitis
		Nasal fracture

(From Gammage,[127] with permission.)

sema, hemorrhage, and loss of the airway. Better results are seen during controlled, elective procedures.[57] After the tracheotomy is performed, a 0.5 to 4.5 percent incidence of massive hemorrhage is reported from erosion of the tube into nearby major vessels, usually the brachiocephalic artery.[58] This complication, which frequently is fatal, is often heralded by hemoptysis. A pulsating tracheotomy tube provides the earliest warning.[49] Minor bleeding usually occurs at the stoma site.

Later, the stoma commonly becomes infected, and an increase of lower airway infection occurs with tracheotomy as compared to translaryngeal tracheal tubes.[44] Perhaps causally related to this increase in infection is an increase in the aspiration of oral secretions in patients with a tracheotomy versus those with tracheal tubes. Tracheoesophageal fistula (TEF) can result acutely from a surgical incision through the back wall of the trachea and into the esophagus. More commonly, it follows from posterior erosion of the tube through the trachea and into the esophagus.[49] This problem usually presents 2 to 4 weeks after the tracheotomy tube has been in place.

Table 12–6. Translaryngeal Intubation versus Tracheotomy

Variables	Tracheotomy	Endotracheal
Surgical procedure required	Yes	No
Permanent airway	Yes	No
Reintubation requirements, skilled personnel		
First 24 to 48 hours	Yes	Yes
After 48 hours	No	Yes
Sedation, relaxants		
First 24 to 47 hours	Yes	Yes
After 48 hours	No	Yes
Accidental extubation	Less	More
Upper airway trauma	Less	More
Laryngeal damage	Less	More
Sinusitis	No	Yes (with nasal tube)
Oral hygiene	Easy	Difficult (with oral tube)
Tube size	Wider, shorter	Narrower, longer
Flow resistance	Less	More
Suctioning	Easy	More difficult
Massive hemorrhage	Yes, rare	No
Mainstem intubation	Uncommon	Common
Stomal complications	Yes	No
Airway infections	Perhaps more	Perhaps less
Patient comfort	Perhaps better	Perhaps less
Speech	Possible	Impossible

(From Gammage,[127] with permission.)

After decannulation, tracheal stenosis may occur either at the cuff site, similar to a translaryngeal tracheal tube, or more frequently at the stoma site. A 40 to 60 percent decrease in diameter occurs in about one-fourth of patients with tracheal stenosis, but clinical symptoms appear in only 1 to 2 percent (some reports as high as 8 percent).[45] Tracheal stenosis at the stoma may be delayed in presentation and sudden in onset, similar to stenosis at the cuff site. Some surgeons believe that stomal tracheal stenosis is related to the type of opening made in the trachea, more common when a piece of trachea is excised.

In a prospective randomized study, Stauffer concluded that the early complications of tracheotomy were more severe than those of translaryngeal tracheal intubation; that patient discomfort and suctioning were rarely a problem with the latter; and that long-term laryngeal damage was rare. Because some patients tolerated tracheal intubation for 22 days without serious complications, they suggested that tracheotomy should not be performed routinely, simply because an arbitrary time period had elapsed. Nearly all translaryngeally intubated patients who came to autopsy had posterior glottic ulcers, and laryngeal damage was more severe in tracheotomy patients who had prolonged versus short-term prior translaryngeal intubation. Although tracheotomy had serious complications, it does provide a more secure airway with less laryngeal damage (Table 12-6).

OXYGEN TOXICITY

Exposure to high partial pressures of inspired oxygen causes pulmonary cellular disruption and damage. Pulmonary oxygen toxicity did not become a clinically relevant problem until high-flow oxygen delivery systems were developed and mechanical ventilators were used for extended periods of time. Although oxygen toxicity can affect many parts of the body, including the CNS, retina, hematopoietic, endocrine, and respiratory systems, the following discussion deals exclusively with the pulmonary effects of oxygen toxicity.

Oxygen Free Radicals

Oxygen generates two species of free radicals, superoxide (O_2^-) and activated hydroxyl radical (OH^-). The hydroxyl radical is unstable and may not play an important role in the development of oxygen toxicity. However, superoxide radicals can be very destructive and probably are responsible for the biochemical alterations causing the morphologic changes observed with hyperoxic lung injury.[59–61]

Free oxygen radicals attack the polyunsaturated fatty acid side chains of membrane lipids causing lipid perioxidation. The generated lipid peroxides inhibit vital cellular enzymes. Decomposition of these lipid peroxides produces products that are damaging to proteins and membranes. Free radicals also cause direct nucleic acid damage and protein sulfhydryl oxidation, which leads to intracellular enzyme inactivation.

The body has normal defense mechanisms against the toxic effects of oxygen radicals. These include cellular oxidative enzymes such as superoxide desmutase, catalase, cytochrome oxidase, perioxidases, sulfhydryl compounds like glutathione, and nonspecific free radical scavengers including α-tocopherol (vitamin E) and ascorbic acid (vitamin C). These antioxidant defenses protect the body from oxygen toxicity at ambient oxygen concentration, but they are overwhelmed if high levels of inspired oxygen are used.

Hyperoxic lung injury depends on the partial pressure of inspired oxygen and the duration of exposure. Increased oxygen leads directly to an elevation of reactive oxygen species within the lungs and may damage the alveolar epithelium directly.[62,63] Continued hyperoxia induces alveolar macrophages to release factors that attract and stimulate polymorphonuclear leukocytes which release toxic products that increase lung permeability and produce more oxygen radicals.[64,65]

Morphologic Changes

In experimental animals, morphologic changes are observed within 24 to 48 hours of exposure to 100 percent oxygen. These include development of interstitial, perivascular, and intra-alveolar edema, and the influx of polymorphonuclear leukocytes.[66,67] By 72 hours, sloughing and eventual loss of type I alveolar pneumocytes occurs. Type II alveolar cells hypertrophy and proliferate but show signs of mitochondrial swelling and membrane damage. These changes are associated with an altered production of surfactant. Direct perioxidation of surfactant lipids also contributes to the increase in surface tension and the tendency for alveolar collapse to occur. Alveolar septa becomes thickened with increased fibrous tissue, progressing to pulmonary fibrosis.

Functional Impairment

The functional outcome of these structural changes includes absorption atelectasis, impairment of pulmonary gas exchange, and increase in pulmonary venous admixture. The resultant hypoxemia may be treated with increased concentrations of oxygen, thus aggravating the injury. Oxygen irritates the trachea, causing tracheobronchitis. It also inhibits ciliary motility and mucus clearance. Human subjects first complain of cough and chest tightness when exposed to high oxygen, usually after 6 to 30 hours of exposure. After 48 to 60 hours, reductions in forced vital capacity, diffusing capacity and static compliance are observed.[68,69]

The upper limit of oxygen that can be administered safely is uncertain. It has been taught that 45 to 50 percent oxygen may be administered for days without adverse effect. Certainly this concentration does not result in the gross structural changes culminating in pulmonary fibrosis. However, this "safe" concentration may cause more subtle abnormalities such as absorption atelectasis in poorly ventilated, but normally perfused, alveoli. Register et al.[70] compared two equivalent groups of postoperative patients, one ventilated with 50 percent oxygen and the other ventilated with 23 to 24 percent oxygen. They reported that patients ventilated with 50 percent oxygen had a lower PaO_2 when they subsequently breathed room air compared with patients who were ventilated initially with 23 to 24 percent oxygen (Fig. 12-4).

No known therapy exists to prevent, delay, or reverse the changes of oxygen toxicity. Protection against injury in experimental animals has been achieved by intravenous administration

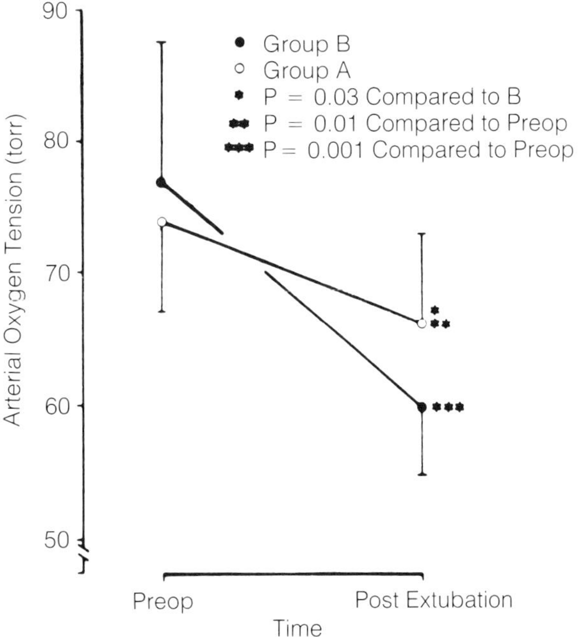

Fig. 12-4. Preoperative PaO_2 was similar for patients in groups A (○) and B (●) while they breathed room air. Postoperatively, PaO_2 fell in both groups. Patients who received 50 percent oxygen had a significantly lower PaO_2 than did those in group A while breathing room air after extubation. (From Register et al.,[70] with permission.)

of superoxide desmutase and catalase.[71] However, the key to prevention is avoidance. Oxygen therapy not only may exacerbate the initial pulmonary problem, but also can produce permanent changes in pulmonary function. If possible, the use of more than 50 percent oxygen should be avoided to reduce the likelihood or hyperoxic lung damage.

NOSOCOMIAL INFECTION

Predisposing Factors

Nosocomial infection of the upper and lower respiratory tracts occurs frequently in patients requiring mechanical ventilation. Infection may involve the paranasal sinuses, pharynx, tracheobronchial tree, or the lung parenchyma. Several factors interact to increase the susceptibility of a critically ill patient. Protective defenses of the airways and lungs are impaired during stress, injury, or disease. Hypoxia, hyperoxia, and pulmonary edema interfere with macrophage function. The mucociliary escalator, is adversely affected by mucosal pressure from the endotracheal tube cuff so that secretions cannot be mobilized and expectorated. Tracheal intubation bypasses the normal cleansing and filtering mechanisms of the oronasal cavity, allowing direct access of organisms to the lower airways. The empirical and prophylactic use of broad spectrum antibiotics promotes overgrowth of opportunistic and pathogenic organisms.

In critically ill patients, the normal bacterial flora of the oropharynx are replaced quickly by enteric gram-negative bacilli, with the degree of colonization paralleling the severity of the disease.[72–75] All patients with endotracheal or tracheotomy tubes acquire gram-negative bacilli as well as anaerobic organisms in their trachea (which is normally sterile) by the third day, nearly half of them having two or more organisms. Colonization increases the likelihood of pneumonia nearly 10-fold compared with noncolonized but similarly ill patients.[74] Leakage of small amounts of oropharyngeal secretions around cuff tubes provides a route for transmission of organisms. Aspiration of even small amounts of oropharyngeal secretions (0.01 ml) may promote colonization of the lower respiratory tract.

Increased adherence of gram-negative bacilli to the airway mucosa occurs in severely ill patients.[76–78] Gram-negative bacteria produce a polysaccharide substance, glycocalyx, which promotes adhesion and biofilm formation. Normally, gram-negative bacteria do not adhere well to the oropharyngeal mucosa because of fibronectin which is present on the epithelial cell surface. During stress, reduced levels of fibronectin allows glycocalyx-producing organisms, such as *Pseudomonas, Staphylococcus,* and *Acinetobacter* to attach readily to the oropharyngeal and tracheal mucosa. The polysaccharide-produced biofilm also adheres to the surface of polyvinylchloride endotracheal tube within 24 hours after intubation. It protects the bacteria from antibiotics and host immune defense mechanisms.[78] Adhesive colonization of the tube and subsequent dislodgement of the biofilm aggravated by suctioning provides a continuous source of bacteria causing a higher incidence of infection.

Contamination of respiratory therapy equipment, such as humidifiers[79] and tubing,[80] is associated with outbreaks of nosocomial infection. Tracheal tube contamination also may result from bacteria-laden pooled condensate in the ventilator circuit.[81] Cross-contamination between patients occurs because of breaks in sterile tracheal suctioning technique.[82] Transfer of bacteria on the hands of unit personnel is the primary mechanism for the spread of infection from patient to patient.[83] Aerosol therapy provides an additional source of contamination, as bacteria breed and are transported in water droplets. The most dangerous droplets are 1 to 2 μm in diameter, since they can bypass normal pulmonary defense mechanisms and reach the smaller bronchioles and alveoli.

The route of intubation may influence the incidence of infection. Direct contamination of the lower respiratory tract through a tracheostomy stoma contributes to the increased incidence of nosocomial infection in patients with tracheotomy compared with translaryngeally intubated patients. One study reported a 6 percent incidence of bacteremia associated with nasotracheal intubation and a zero incidence associated with oral intubation.[84]

Sinusitis

Another reported hazard of nasotracheal intubation is sinusitis, with a reported incidence of 2 to 5 percent.[85–89] The maxillary sinus is the most consistently involved, usually with gram-negative polymicrobial infections. Susceptibility to sinusitis is increased by prolonged intubation of the stomach and trachea through the nares, air-fluid levels in the sinuses, penetrating craniofacial injury, bleeding into the sinuses, and corticosteroid administration.

Nasotracheal intubation causes mucosal irritation and edema of the nasal passages. Tracheal and nasogastric tubes often obstruct the normal drainage of the sinuses allowing the normal sinus flora to proliferate and become pathogenic. Blood and secretions in the sinuses provide a culture medium for bacterial growth. Sinus drainage is inhibited by prolonged immobility in the supine position. Sputum and sinus cultures commonly have identical organisms. A sinus infection may progress to more serious infections including pansinusitis, meningitis, encephalitis, or sepsis.[89–91]

The diagnosis of sinusitis may be difficult because of the lack of clinical signs in a patient too sick to complain or unable to verbalize his complaints because of the endotracheal tube. Sinus films and possibly computed tomographic (CT) scan of the sinuses should be obtained. Treatment includes topical decongestants, aspiration of an infected hematoma or opacified sinus, and specific antibiotics for cultured organisms. Nasal tubes should be replaced with oral tubes as soon as possible. Sinus irrigation or open sinusotomy may be required if medical therapy fails.

Otitis Media

An infrequently reported complication of tracheal intubation and mechanical ventilation is middle ear infection.[50,92,93] However, the incidence is as high as 30 percent. *Pseudomonas, Klebsiella,* and *Enterobacter* account for the majority of the organisms isolated. Reflux of bacteria into the eustachian tubes, or local infection at the eustachian tube orifice with contiguous spread into the middle ear cavity, may cause otitis media during ventilatory support. Treatment consists of tympanocentesis and culture specific antibiotic therapy.

Pneumonia

The most devastating infectious complication of mechanical ventilation is bronchopulmonary bacterial infection, which is associated with high morbidity and mortality.[94–101] Nosocomial pneumonia is the second-most common nosocomial infection, but has the highest fatality rate. Gram-negative nosocomial pneumonia mortality ranges between 20 and 70 percent.[97,99] The high mortality rate may reflect inaccurate or delayed diagnosis, as well as altered patient immune defenses, rather than inadequate therapy. Patients receiving continuous ventilatory support are twenty-one times more likely to develop nosocomial pneumonia.[100]

Other risk factors include the type and duration of surgery, steroid and immunosuppressive therapy, duration of intubation and tracheotomy, and reintubation. The most common etiologic agents are the gram-negative bacilli (*Enterobacter and Pseudomonas* species).[101] *Staphylococcus aureus, Acinetobacter,* anaerobic bacteria, and streptococci also cause nosocomial pneumonia. Less commonly, *Legionella,* fungi, cytomegalovirus, and *Pneumocystis carinii* are implicated.

Three major sources of organisms are responsible: contamination of the oropharynx from the hospital environment, with subsequent aspiration; inhalation of organisms from contaminated

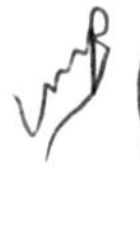

inhalation therapy equipment; and direct introduction of pathogens through tracheotomy or endotracheal tubes. In addition, bacteremia from an infected intravascular catheter and the genitourinary or GI tracts may also cause nosocomial lung infection.

Diagnosis

The diagnosis of nosocomial pneumonia is difficult because of its variable clinical presentation. Noninfectious pathologic changes such as interstitial pulmonary edema, atelectasis, contusion, or embolization may produce pulmonary infiltrates radiographically indistinguishable from infectious infiltrates. Sputum cultures, transthoracic needle aspiration, and protected specimen brushes have been used, but none have been entirely satisfactory in establishing the diagnosis. Blood cultures may not be very helpful, since only 6 percent of patients with nosocomial pneumonia have secondary bacteremia.[101]

Specimens obtained bronchoscopically, using a plugged-telescopic-catheter brush, are considered most accurate in diagnosis.[96,102] Bronchoalveolar lavage is used with increasing frequency, especially in patients treated with high-pressure ventilation in whom transbronchial biopsy may be dangerous.[103] When the involved lung area is inaccessible by bronchoscopy, percutaneous needle aspiration may be performed, but the complication rate is high. If the diagnosis in a severely ill patient remains obscure, open lung biopsy may be considered. The procedure requires general anesthesia, and thoracotomy tube placement. Because of its associated morbidity, open biopsy is considered to be a last option for diagnosis.[104,105]

Treatment

Empirical antibiotic therapy should be started in critically ill patients while culture and sensitivity results are pending. Modification of the treatment regimen is indicated once the etiologic agent is identified and sensitivity data are obtained. Combination drug therapy rather than single drug therapy is favored in the treatment of nosocomial pneumonia to provide optimal coverage for all potential pathogens. Supportive therapy includes proper pulmonary toilet, although the efficacy of such therapy is open to question, adequate hydration and nutrition, drainage of pleural effusions, and good nursing care.

Prevention

Several measures potentially can decrease infection and cross contamination in mechanically ventilated patients. Careful handwashing by hospital personnel between patients is the most important factor. Scrupulous aseptic technique is necessary, especially when one suctions the trachea or handles respiratory therapy equipment. Patients should be properly positioned to avoid aspiration, especially during feeding. Nasotracheal intubation or nasogastric tube insertion should be avoided if possible. Condensate in the circuit tubing should be drained away from the patient and never emptied back into the humidifier reservoir.

Surveillance culture of tracheal secretions may enable the physician to predict changes in the tracheal flora and facilitate the selection of appropriate antimicrobial therapy. However, prophylactic antibiotics should not be employed, since they will facilitate the selection and acquisition of resistant bacteria.

MALNUTRITION

Adequate nutritional support can be overlooked in critically ill, ventilated patients. Up to 50 percent of surgical patients have some form of protein or caloric malnutrition, and the incidence increases when the patient is mechanically ventilated.[106] Nutrition is neglected because the patient is unable to eat or to express hunger, and other more immediate problems take precedence. Malnourished patients have more postoperative complications, including a higher mortality. Driver et al.[106] retrospectively studied 26 mechanically ventilated patients with respiratory failure. In almost all cases, the patients received inadequate amounts of protein, calories, and vitamins.

Malnutrition affects nearly all aspects of respiratory function and leads to reduced surfactant production with increased tendency to alveolar collapse.[107,108] Malnourished patients develop emphysematous changes, with a reduction in lung elasticity,[109] and a decrease in lung protein and fatty acid synthesis.[110,111] Malnutrition predisposes to pulmonary infection because of a reduction of bacterial clearance in the lungs and decreased levels of secretory IgA.[112,113] It is also associated with lower minute ventilation, vital capacity, inspiratory flow, and hypoxic and hypercapnic ventilatory drives.[114–117] The administration of protein to semi-starved subjects leads to a significant enhancement of hypercapnic drive within hours.[117]

Muscular atrophy due to malnutrition and prolonged mechanical ventilation may lead to respiratory muscle fatigue, and failure to wean. During semi-starvation, body weight and diaphragmatic muscle mass fall concurrently, but muscle strength decreases more than muscle mass, and the diaphragm may develop pathologic changes in cellular structure.[118] Nutritional repletion results in improvement in inspiratory muscle strength within 2 weeks.[119] Improved nutritional status has been associated with successful weaning from mechanical ventilation. Bassili and Deitel[120] reviewed 47 medical and surgical patients requiring prolonged mechanical ventilation. Only 54 percent of the group that received 400 cal/day were successfully weaned compared with 93 percent of the group who received 2,000 to 3,000 cal/day.

An increased awareness of the nutritional problems in patients receiving mechanical ventilation is necessary. Adequate nutritional support should be a multidisciplinary team effort. Proper nutritional support requires adequate calories based on measurement of energy requirements, as well as appropriate amounts of protein, fat, vitamins, and minerals. The nutritional status should be monitored by physical examination and biochemical measurements. Adequate support presumably will avoid some serious iatrogenic complications. Nevertheless, no convincing evidence shows that outcome (intact survival) is improved by proper attention to nutritional requirements, despite the seeming logic of such an assumption.

EQUIPMENT FAILURE

There is a paucity of literature dealing specifically with morbidity and mortality resulting from ventilator and respiratory equipment failure in the intensive care unit (ICU). Much of the available data concern anesthetized patients in the operating room, where conditions and equipment are substantially different. The breathing circuit accounts for nearly 40 percent of all reported problems.[121] Failures of electrical circuits, mechanical devices, and controls/indicators/alarms are responsible for the next most commonly reported problems, each accounting for 14 percent of the total.

Disconnections

The most serious (and frequent) equipment problem occurring during mechanical ventilation is accidental disconnection of the breathing circuit.[122,123] This problem is most likely to result in injury when it is compounded by other accidents, equipment failure, or human error. A disturbing report published by Cooper et al.[123] in 1983, indicated the responses of nine critical care physicians who were asked about the frequency of disconnections (Table 12–7). Four of the nine were unable to answer because the event was so frequent as to be considered routine.

Presently, no solid data is available on the incidence of accidental disconnection in the ICU, but Cooper et al. reported that 7.5 percent (27 of 359) of the incidents of equipment failure or human error during anesthesia in the operating room were due to circuit disconnections. Seventy-five percent of the disconnections occurred

Table 12–7. Result of an Interview of Critical Care Physicians on the Frequency of Accidental Ventilator Disconnections

Interview no.	No. of ICU beds	Average no. of patients ventilated per day	Frequency of accidental disconnections
1	32 (+ nominal 5 transitional beds)	10	17–20/day
2	66 (+ transitional unit)	46	Too frequent to estimate
3	72 transitional beds	2	Unable to estimate because of its "routine" occurrence
4	142	40	14/week
5	20	10	21/week minor; 1/week major
6	56	28	Too numerous to count; 30% of patients disconnect repeatedly
7	28 (+ 16 transitional beds)	10	20/week
8	49	30	Very frequent; routine part of care
9	13	2	14/week

(From Cooper et al.,[123] with permission.)

between the tracheal tube and either the elbow connector or the Y-piece. Several factors make it likely that breathing circuit disconnections are even more frequent in the ICU than in the operating room. Patients in the ICU are more mobile and can disconnect themselves by moving in the bed. Humidifiers, a constant part of the breathing circuit in the ICU, produce condensation in the tubing. This condensation makes tubing and connections wet and less secure. The condensations may also pool in dependent portions of the tubing, adding enough weight and traction to loosen connections. Finally, "one-on-one" continuous care is seldom available in the ICU as it is in the operating room.

Miscellaneous

Other problems include excessive gas pressure if "pop-off" valves fail, leading to decreased cardiac output and blood pressure or pneumothorax.[124] The circuit may become obstructed due to water, secretions, faulty valves, kinked tubing, or improper assembly. Bacterial or viral contamination can occur. Major leaks in the circuit may prevent adequate ventilation.

Alarms

Most critical care ventilators now incorporate alarm systems to warn of disconnections or excessive airway pressure. If properly set and functioning, these alarms will detect dangerous conditions promptly, before injury has occurred. They can be disabled by turning them off, activating a delay switch, disconnecting them, or setting the limits outside the useful range being monitored. The disconnect (low-pressure) alarm is commonly turned off during tracheal suctioning, and if it is not reactivated at the end of the procedure, a disconnection may go unrecognized until severe cardiovascular changes activate one of the hemodynamic monitor alarms.

Malfunction and misuse of ventilator alarm

systems is a common problem.[49,123] Current alarm systems exhibit high false-positive rates, and the sounds of one alarm are not easily differentiated from another. False alarms may be caused by improper settings or calibration, and/or malfunction. When properly used, current alarms rarely miss true disconnections or increase in airway pressure. False alarms, however, decrease staff responsiveness to alarm conditions, causing the alarm to be either ignored or disabled. A common factor in fatal outcomes from disconnection is the absence of or intentional disabling of an alarm.

Zwillich et al.[49] reviewed 314 consecutive patients during 354 episodes of assisted ventilation in a 5-month period. They identified complications attributable to ventilator operation on 103 occasions. Mechanical failure of the ventilator occurred six times (5.9 percent), alarm failure 13 times (3.7 percent), and overheating of inspired air seven times (6.8 percent). The ventilator alarm was found in the off position without a nurse in attendance 32 times (9.0 percent), and inadequate nebulization or humidification was noted 45 times (43.7 percent). They reported no mortality as a direct result of these events and concluded that survival was unaffected by ventilator malfunction. They also felt the prospective design of their study may have increased awareness of potential equipment problems and decreased both the incidence and the consequences of these problems.

In a retrospective study, Abramson et al.[125] reviewed the incidence of adverse occurrences in their ICU over a 5-year period. There were 145 incidents, 37 percent of which were attributed to equipment malfunction and 30 percent of which involved the misuse of equipment. Mortality was 41 percent for those with adverse occurrences versus 21 percent for all ICU patients. Fifty-nine percent of equipment malfunction and misuse involved respiratory equipment, and equipment malfunction resulted in patient injury in 48 percent of cases. Table 12–8 lists the respiratory equipment involved in the adverse incidents.

Prevention

Prevention of equipment-related complications requires that physicians, nurses, and respiratory therapists be familiar with ventilators and other support equipment. Alarm systems and pressure monitors should help prevent the hazards associated with ventilator failure. However, the alarm system does not always identify the nature and cause of the problem, and does not eliminate the requirement for constant, vigilant attendance of trained personnel. Policies must be developed to help ensure that alarms are reactivated if they must be turned off at any time. Routine preventive maintenance and inspection of equipment are mandatory. In instances in which a ventilator malfunctions or a problem cannot be identified, the ventilator

Table 12–8. Reported Adverse Incidents Involving Respiratory Equipment

	No. of incidents		
Type of equipment	Malfunction	Human error	Total
Mechanical ventilators	9	6	15
Ventilator tubing	12	3	15
Ventilator alarms	7	2	9
Airway control	2	4	6
Continuous positive airway pressure system	0	3	3
Manual resuscitator	1	1	2
Oxygen blenders	1	1	2
Miscellaneous	2	3	5
Total	34	23	57

(From Abramson et al.,[125] with permission.)

and entire breathing circuit should be replaced. Finally, a good hospital risk-management program, including incident reporting and review, may increase the awareness of the staff, reduce the incidence of preventable injuries, and improve patient outcome.

PSYCHOLOGICAL, ETHICAL, AND SOCIETAL CONSIDERATIONS

Ventilatory support contributes to the survival of critically ill patients with reversible injury and illness. Unfortunately, it also prolongs the survival of patients who are hopelessly or terminally ill. Before the modern era of mechanical ventilation, when brain death occurred and ventilation ceased, the patient unequivocally was dead. Now, with ventilatory support, the body can be maintained long after the brain is dead, blurring the distinction between life and death. On the positive side, such care allows organ harvesting and donation, but introduces ethical and societal conflicts.

The prolongation of "existence" comes at a great cost both financially and psychologically to patients, their families, and the ICU personnel. When and whether to "pull the plug" remains as controversial as ever.[126] These concerns are discussed in detail in Chapter 13.

REFERENCES

1. Cullen DJ, Caldera DL: The incidence of ventilator-induced pulmonary barotrauma in critically ill patients. Anesthesiology 50:185, 1979
2. Downs JB, Chapman RL: The incidence of ventilator-induced pulmonary barotrauma in critically ill patients. Anesthesiology 50:185, 1979
3. Macklin TM, Macklin CC: Malignant interstitial emphysema of the lungs and mediastinum as an important occult complication in many respiratory diseases and other conditions: an interpretation of the clinical literature in the light of laboratory experiment. Medicine (Baltimore) 23:281, 1944
4. Hilman KM: Pneumoperitoneum—a review. Crit Care Med 10:476, 1982
5. Kumar A, Pontoppidan H, Falde KT, et al: Pulmonary barotrauma during mechanical ventilation. Crit Care Med 1:181, 1973
6. Petersen GW, Baier H: Incidence of pulmonary barotrauma in a medical ICU. Crit Care Med 11:67, 1983
7. Hillman K: Pulmonary barotrauma. Clin Anesthesiol 3:877, 1985
8. Hilman KM: Severe coughing and pneumoperitoneum. Br Med J 285:1085, 1982
9. Rohling BM, Webb R, Schlobohm RM: Ventilator related extra-alveolar air in adults. Radiology 121:25, 1976
10. Lenaghan R, Silva YJ, Walt AJ: Haemodynamic alterations associated with expansion rupture of the lung. Arch Surg 99:339, 1969
11. Killen DA, Goven WG: Spontaneous Pneumothorax. Little, Brown, Boston, 1968, p. 45
12. Downs JB, Chapman RL: Treatment of bronchopleural fistula during continuous positive pressure ventilation. Chest 69:363, 1976
13. Sturgeon CL, Douglas ME, Downs JB, et al: PEEP and CPAP: cardiopulmonary effects during spontaneous ventilation. Anesth Analg 56:633, 1977
14. Kirby RR, Perry JC, Calderwood HW, et al: Cardiorespiratory effects of high positive end-expiratory pressure. Anesthesiology 43:533, 1975
15. Pick RA, Handler JB, Murata GH, et al: The cardiovascular effects of positive end-expiratory pressure. Chest 82:345, 1982
16. Dorinsky PM, Whitcomb ME: The effect of PEEP on cardiac output. Chest 84:210, 1983
17. Smith PK, Tyson GS, Hammon JW, et al: Cardiovascular effects of ventilation with positive expiratory airway pressure. Ann Surg 195:121, 1982
18. Qvist J, Mygind T, Crottogini A, et al: Cardiovascular adjustments to pulmonary vascular injury in dogs. Anesthesiology 68:341, 1988
19. Robotham JL, Lixfeld W, Holland L, et al: The effects of positive end-expiratory pressure on right and left ventricular performance. Am Rev Respir Dis 121:677, 1980
20. Abel JG, Salerno TA, Panos A, et al: Cardiovascular effects of positive pressure ventilation in humans. Ann Thorac Surg 43:198, 1987
21. McGregor M: Pulsus paradoxus. N Engl J Med 301:480, 1979

22. Mathru M, Rao TLK, El-Etr AA, et al: Hemodynamic response to changes in ventilatory patterns in patients with normal and poor left ventricular reserve. Crit Care Med 10:423, 1982
23. Manny J, Patten MT, Liebman PR, et al: The association of lung distention, PEEP and biventricular failure. Ann Surg 187:151, 1978
24. Patten MT, Liebman PR, Hechtman HB: Humorally mediated decreases in cardiac output associated with positive end-expiratory pressure. Microvasc Res 13:137, 1977
25. Hall SV, Steinman TI: Alterations in renal function during acute respiratory failure. Int Anesth Clin 14:179, 1976
26. Moore ES, Galvez MB, Patin JB, et al: Effects of positive pressure ventilation on intrarenal blood flow in infant primates. Pediatr Res 8:792, 1974
27. Annat G, Viale JP, Bui Xuan B, et al: Effect of PEEP ventilation of renal function, plasma renin, aldosterone, neurophysins and urinary ADH, and prostaglandins. Anesthesiology 58:136, 1983
28. Marquez JM, Douglas ME, Downs JB, et al: Renal function and cardiovascular responses during positive airway pressure. Anesthesiology 50:393, 1979
29. Laver MB: Dr. Starling and the "ventilator kidney" (editorial). Anesthesiology 50:383, 1979
30. Hammer M, Viquerat CE, Suter P, et al: Urinary antidiuretic hormone excretion during mechanical ventilation and weaning in man. Anesthesiology 52:395, 1980
31. Bark H, LeRoith C, Nyska M, et al: Elevations in plasma ADH levels during PEEP ventilation in the dog: mechanisms involved. Am J Physiol 239:E474, 1980
32. Johnson EE, Hedley-Whyte J: Continuous positive pressure ventilation and portal flow in dogs with pulmonary edema. J Appl Physiol 33:385, 1972
33. Bonnet F, Richard C, Blaser P, et al: Changes in hepatic flow induced by continuous positive pressure ventilation in critically ill patients. Crit Care Med 10:703, 1982
34. Hedley-Whyte J, Burgess GE III, Feeley TW, et al: Effect of pattern of ventilation on hepatitic, renal, and splanchnic function. p. 27. In Applied Physiology of Respiratory Care. Little, Brown, Boston, 1976
35. Johnson EE, Hedley-Whyte J: Continuous positive pressure ventilation and choledochoduodenal flow resistance. J Appl Physiol 39:937, 1975
36. Shapiro HM, Marshall LF: Intracranial pressure responses to PEEP in head injured patients. J Trauma 18:254, 1978
37. Huseby JS, Pavlin ES, Butler J: Effects of positive end-expiratory pressure on intracranial pressure in dogs. J Appl Physiol 44:25, 1978
38. Blanc VF, Tremblay NAG: The complications of tracheal intubation: a new classification with a review of the literature. Anesth Analg 53:202, 1974
39. Selecky PA: Tracheostomy: a review of present day indications, complications, and care. Heart Lung 3:272, 1974
40. Lindholm CE, Grenvik A: Tracheal tube and cuff problems. Int Anesthesiol Clin 20:103, 1982
41. Kastanos N, Miro RE, Perez AM, et al: Laryngotracheal injury due to endotracheal intubation: incidence, evolution, and predisposing factors. A prospective long-term study. Crit Care Med 11:362, 1983
42. Bernhard WN, Cottrell JE, Sivakumaran C, et al: Adjustment of intracuff pressure to prevent aspiration. Anesthesiology 50:363, 1979
43. Shapiro BA, Harrison RA, Kacmarek RM, et al: Clinical Application of Respiratory Care. 3rd Ed. Year Book Medical Publishers, Chicago, 1985, pp. 90 and 242
44. El-Naggar M, Sadagopan S, Levine H, et al: Factors influencing choice between tracheostomy and prolonged translaryngeal intubation in acute respiratory failure: a prospective study. Anesth Analg 55:195, 1976
45. Bishop MJ, Weymuller EA, Fink BR: Laryngeal effects of prolonged intubation. Anesth Analg 63:335, 1984
46. Walsh JJ, Rho DS: A speaking endotracheal tube. Anesthesiology 63:703, 1985
47. Natanson C, Shelhamer JH, Parrillo JE: Intubation of the trachea in the critical care setting. JAMA 253:1160, 1985
48. Conrardy PA, Goodman LR, Lainge F, et al: Alteration of endotracheal tube position: flexion and extension of the neck. Crit Care Med 4:8, 1976
49. Zwillich CW, Pierson DJ, Creagh CE, et al: Complications of assisted ventilation. Am J Med 57:165, 1974
50. Stauffer JL, Olson DE, Petty TL: Complications and consequences of endotracheal intubation

and tracheostomy: a prospective study of 150 critically ill adult patients. Am J Med 70:65, 1981
51. Chew JY, Cantrell RW: Tracheostomy: complications and their management. Arch Otolaryngol 96:538, 1972
52. Berry FA, Blankenbaker WL, Ball CG: A comparison of bacteremia occurring with nasotracheal and orotracheal intubation. Anesth Analg 52:873, 1973
53. Stoelting RK: Endotracheal intubation. p. 523. In Miller RD (ed): Anesthesia. 2nd Ed. Churchill Livingstone, New York, 1986
54. Burgess GE III, Cooper JR, Marino RJ, et al: Laryngeal competence after tracheal extubation. Anesthesiology 51:73, 1979
55. Hawkins DB: Glottic and subglottic stenosis from endotracheal intubation. Laryngoscope 87:339, 1977
56. Deutschman CS, Wilton P, Sinow J, et al: Paranasal sinusitis associated with nasotracheal intubation: a frequently unrecognized and treatable source of sepsis. Crit Care Med 14:111, 1986
57. Dayal VS, El Masri W: Tracheostomy in intensive care setting. Laryngoscope 96:58, 1986
58. Timmis HH: Tracheostomy: an overview of implications, management, and morbidity. Adv Surg 7:199, 1973
59. Butler JA, Rhodes ML: Oxygen toxicity. J Ind State Med Assoc 587, 1980
60. Mustafa MG, Tierney DF: Biochemical and metabolic changes in the lung with oxygen, ozone, and nitrogen dioxide toxicity. Am Rev Respir Dis 118:1061, 1978
61. Winter PH, Smith G: The toxicity of oxygen. Anesthesiology 37:210, 1972
62. Freeman BA, Crapo JD: Hyperoxia increases oxygen radical production in rat lungs and lung mitochondria. J Biol Chem 256:10986, 1981
63. Matalon S, Egan EA: Effects of 100 percent oxygen breathing on permeability of alveolar epithelium to solute. J Appl Physiol 50:859, 1981
64. Crapo JD, Barry BE, Foscue HA, et al: Structural and biochemical changes in rat lungs occurring during exposure to lethal and adaptive doses of oxygen. Am Rev Respir Dis 122:123, 1980
65. Harada RN, Bowman CM, Fox RB, et al: Alveolar macrophage secretions: initiators of inflammation in pulmonary oxygen toxicity? Chest 581:52, 1982
66. Havgaard N: Cellular mechanisms of oxygen toxicity. Physiol Rev 48:311, 1968
67. Clark JM, Lambertson CJ: Pulmonary oxygen toxicity: a review. Pharmacol Rev 23:37, 1971
68. Welch BE, Morgan TE, Clammon HG: Time concentration effects in relation to oxygen toxicity in man. Fed Proc 22:1053, 1963
69. Caldwell PRB, Lee WL, Schildnaut HS, et al: Changes in lung volumes, diffusing capacity, and blood gases in men breathing oxygen. J Appl Physiol 21:1477, 1966
70. Register SD, Downs JB, Stock C, et al: Is 50 percent oxygen harmful? Crit Care Med 15:598, 1987
71. Turrens JF, Crapo JD, Freeman BA: Protection against oxygen toxicity by intravenous injection of liposome entrapped catalase and superoxide desmutase. J Clin Invest 73:87, 1984
72. Bryant LR, Trinkle JK, Mobin-Uddin K, et al: Bacterial colonization profile with tracheal intubation and mechanical ventilation. Arch Surg 104:647, 1972
73. Schwartz SN, Dowling JN, Benkovic C, et al: Sources of gram negative bacilli colonizing the trachea of intubated patients. J Infect Dis 138:227, 1978
74. Johanson WG Jr, Pierce AK, Sanford JP, et al: Nosocomial respiratory infection with gram negative bacilli: the significance of colonization of the respiratory tract. Ann Intern Med 77:701, 1972
75. Aass AS: Complications of tracheostomy and long term intubation. A follow-up study. Acta Anaesthesiol Scand 19:127, 1975
76. Woods DE, Straus DC, Johanson WG Jr, et al: Role of fibronectin in the prevention of adherence of *Pseudomonas aeruginosa* to buccal cells. J Infect Dis 143:784, 1981
77. Johanson WG Jr, Woods DE, Chaudruni T, et al: Association of respiratory tract colonization with adherence of gram-negative bacilli to epithelial cells. J Infect Dis 139:667, 1979
78. Sottile FD, Marrie TJ, Prough DS, et al: Nosocomial pulmonary infection: possible etiologic significance of bacterial adhesion to endotracheal tubes. Crit Care Med 14:265, 1986
79. Reinarz JA, Pierce AK, Mays BB, et al: The potential role of inhalation therapy equipment in nosocomial pulmonary infection. J Clin Invest 44:831, 1965
80. Phillips F, Spenser P: *Pseudomonas aeruginosa* cross infection. Lancet 2:1325, 1965

81. Cravens DE, Goularte TA, Make BJ: Contaminated condensate in mechanical ventilation circuits. Am Rev Respir Dis 129:625, 1984
82. Sutter VL, Hurst V, Grossman M, et al: Source and significance of *Pseudomonas aeruginosa* in sputum. Patients requiring tracheal suction. JAMA 197:132, 1968
83. Steere AC, Mallison GF: Hand-washing practices for the prevention of nosocomial infections. Ann Intern Med 83:638, 1975
84. Dinner M, Tjeuw M, Artusio JF: Bacteremia as a complication of nasotracheal intubation. Anesth Analg 66:460, 1987
85. Gallagher TJ, Civetta JM: Acute maxillary sinusitis complicating nasotracheal intubation: a case report. Anesth Analg 55:885, 1976
86. Grindlinger GA, Niehoff J, Hughes SL, et al: Acute paranasal sinusitis related to nasotracheal intubation of head injured patients. Crit Care Med 15:214, 1987
87. Arens JF, Lejeune FE Jr, Weber DR: Maxillary sinusitis: a complication of nasotracheal intubation. Anesthesiology 40:415, 1974
88. Caplan ES, Hoyt NJ: Nosocomial sinusitis. JAMA 247:839, 1982
89. O'Reilly MJ, Reddick EJ, Black W, et al: Sepsis from sinusitis in nasotracheally intubated patients. Am J Surg 147:601, 1984
90. Morgan PP, Morrison WV: Complications of frontal and ethmoidal sinusitis. Laryngoscope 90:661, 1980
91. Remmier D, Boler R: Intracranial complication of frontal sinusitis. Laryngoscope 90:1814, 1980
92. Balkany TJ, Berman SA, Simmons MA, et al: Middle ear effusion in neonates. Laryngoscope 88:398, 1978
93. Lucks D, Consiglio A, Stankiewicz J: Incidence and microbiological etiology of middle ear effusion complicating endotracheal intubation and mechanical ventilation. J Infect Dis 157:368, 1988
94. Tobin MJ, Grenvik A: Nosocomial lung infection and its diagnosis. Crit Care Med 12:191, 1984
95. Andrews CP, Coalson JJ, Smith JD, et al: Diagnosis of nosocomial bacterial pneumonia in acute diffuse lung injury. Chest 80:254, 1981
96. Podnos JD, Toews GB, Pierce AK: Nosocomial pneumonia in patients in intensive care units. West J Med 143:672, 1985
97. Shires GT, Dineem P: Sepsis following burns, trauma, and intra-abdominal infection. Arch Intern Med 142:2012, 1982
98. Hessem MT, Kaye D: Nosocomial pneumonia. Crit Care Clin 4:245, 1988
99. Craig CP, Connelly S: Effect of intensive care unit nosocomial pneumonia on duration of stay and mortality. Am J Infect Control 12:233, 1984
100. Hooton TM, Haley RW, Culver DH, et al: The joint associations of multiple risk factors with the occurrence of nosocomial infection. Am J Med 70:960, 1981
101. Centers for Disease Control: Nosocomial infection surveillance 1984. MMWR 35:17SS, 1986
102. Wimberley NW, Bass JB, Boyd BW, et al: Use of a bronchoscopic protected catheter brush for the diagnosis of pulmonary infections. Chest 81:556, 1982
103. Stover DE, Zaman MB, Hojdu S, et al: Bronchoalveolar lavage in the diagnosis of pulmonary infiltrates in the immunosuppressed host. Ann Intern Med 101:1, 1984
104. Rossiter SJ, Miller DC, Churg AM, et al: Open lung biopsy in the immunosuppressed patient: is it really beneficial? J Thorac Cardiovasc Surg 77:338, 1979
105. Leight GS Jr, Michaelis LL: Open lung biopsy for the diagnosis of acute diffuse pulmonary infiltrates in the immunosuppressed patient. Chest 73:477, 1978
106. Driver AG, Lebrun M: Iatrogenic malnutrition in patients receiving ventilatory support. JAMA 244:2195, 1980
107. Garbagni K, Cappo F, Gassini B, et al: Effects of lipid loading and fasting on pulmonary surfactant. Respiration 25:458, 1968
108. D'Amour SR, Clerh L, Massaro D: Food deprivation and surfactants in adult rats. J Appl Physiol 55:1413, 1983
109. Sahebjami H, Vasallo CL, Wirman JA: Lung mechanics and ultrastructure in prolonged starvation. Am Rev Respir Dis 117:77, 1978
110. Gacad G, Dickie K, Massaro D: Protein synthesis in lung: influence of starvation on amino acid incorporation into protein. J Appl Physiol 33:381, 1972
111. Gross I, Rooney SA, Warshaw JB: The inhibition of enzymes related to pulmonary fatty acid and synthesis by dietary deprivation in rats. Biochem Biophys Res Commun 64:59, 1975
112. Green GM, Kass EH: Factors influencing the

clearance of bacteria by the lung. J Clin Invest 43:769, 1964
113. Green GM, Jakab GS, Low RB, et al: Defense mechanisms of the respiratory membrane. Am Rev Respir Dis 115:479, 1977
114. Doekel RC, Zwillich CW, Scoggin CH, et al: Clinical semi-starvation: depression of the hypoxic ventilatory response. N Engl J Med 295:358, 1978
115. Zwillich CW, Sahn SA, Weil JV: Effects of hypermetabolism on ventilation and chemosensitivity. J Clin Invest 60:900, 1977
116. Branson RD, Hurst JM: Nutrition and respiratory function: food for thought (editorial). Respir Care 33:89, 1988
117. Weissman C, Askanazi J, Rosenbaum S, et al: Amino acids and respiration. Ann Intern Med 98:41, 1983
118. Arora NS, Rochester DF: Respiratory muscle strength and maximal voluntary ventilation in undernourished patients. Am Rev Respir Dis 126:5, 1982
119. Kelsen SG: The effects of undernutrition on the respiratory muscles. Clin Chest Med 7:101, 1986
120. Bassili HR, Deitel M: Effect of nutritional support on weaning patients off mechanical ventilators. JPEN J Parenter Enteral Nutr 5:151, 1981
121. Feeley TW, Bancroft ML: Problems with mechanical ventilators. Int Anesth Clin 20:83, 1982
122. Gross B: Non-slipping, nonkinking airway connections for respiratory care. Anesthesiology 34:571, 1971
123. Cooper JB, Couvillon LA Jr, Little AD: Accidental System Disconnection. Interim Report to the Food and Drug Administration. Arthur D. Little, Cambridge MA, 1983, p. 1
124. Dinnick DP: Hazards of respiratory circuits. Ann R Coll Surg Engl 52:349, 1973
125. Abramson NS, Wald KS, Grenvik AN, et al: Adverse occurrences in intensive care units. JAMA 244:1582, 1980
126. Schneiderman LJ, Spragg RG: Ethical decisions in discontinuing mechanical ventilation (editorial). N Engl J Med 318:984, 1988
127. Gammage GW: Airway management. p. 197. In Civetta JM, Taylor RW, Kirby RR (eds): Critical Care. JB Lippincott, Philadelphia, 1988

13

Medicolegal Considerations

S. David Register

IRREVERSIBLE CENTRAL NERVOUS SYSTEM INJURY WITH BRAIN DEATH

During the late 1950s, several techniques were introduced which revolutionized the practice of medicine: mouth-to-mouth ventilation, closed-chest cardiac massage, and electrical termination of ventricular fibrillation.[1–3] Widespread clinical application of these techniques resulted in a significant number of ventilator-dependent patients in whom cardiac function had been restored following irreversible ischemic injury of the central nervous system.[4] In 1968, the Ad Hoc Committee of the Havard Medical School published their report, *A Definition of Irreversible Coma*. The stated purpose of this report, now known as *The Harvard Criteria for Brain Death,* was ''to define irreversible coma as a new criterion for death.''[5] This report was necessary because (1) improvements in resuscitative and supportive therapy had yielded a substantial number of patients who were comatose with no discernible central nervous system activity, and (2) an increasing number of organs were needed for transplantation.[5]

In the decade that followed, a series of studies[6–12] established criteria that predicted ''inevitable somatic or bodily death'' among ventilator-dependent, irreversibly comatose patients. The realization that somatic death inevitably follows brain death hastened the acceptance of this new definition of death by the lay public, the legal profession, and the medical profession. Following the example of the Kansas legislature, several states enacted statutory definitions of death allowing the application of the brain death concept as an alternative means of declaring death. In these states, the concept of brain death was challenged in the courts a number of times in appeals to homicide convictions; most of these cases involved removal of organs from the brain-dead person for transplantation. In each and every case, the courts upheld the brain death concept as defined by the Harvard Ad Hoc Committee. In a landmark case, *Commonwealth v. Golston,*[4] the Massachusetts Court accepted the Harvard Ad Hoc Committee's definition of death despite the lack of statutory definition of death in that state. In 1978, the Kansas Supreme Court reviewed and upheld the Kansas Brain Death Statute.[13] Significantly, the Court expressly recognized the need to maintain mechanical ventilation and cardiovascular support following the pronouncement of brain death in order to allow subsequent removal of transplantable organs.

Medically and legally, patients meeting the strict criteria for brain death are not ''imminently terminal''; they are already ''dead.'' Therefore, discontinuation of mechanical ventilation, known to the lay public as ''turning off the respirator'' or ''pulling the plug,'' has become common practice by physicians in cases that meet the strict criteria of brain death; this practice is medically, legally, and ethically justified and accepted. In some cases of brain death, however, ''life-supportive therapy,'' such as mechanical ventilation, may be continued for medical reasons (maintenance of somatic viabil-

Table 13-1. Discontinuation of Mechanical Ventilation and Other Life-Support Measures: Controversial Issues

Mentally incompetent nonterminal patient
Mentally competent terminal patient
Mentally competent, nonterminal patient
Mentally incompetent terminal patient
Patients of questionable mental competency
Minors

ity until organ harvest can be arranged) or for humanitarian reasons (to provide family members additional time to adjust to the inevitability of death). During the past two decades, most legislative and judicial decisions regarding mechanical ventilation and other life-support therapy have not involved brain-dead patients. Instead, six other categories of patients have generated legal and ethical controversy (Table 13–1). These groups are discussed in detail.

LIFE-SUPPORT DECISIONS

Mentally Incompetent Nonterminal Patients

Most patients categorized as mentally incompetent nonterminal have irreversible central nervous system (CNS) disease or injury but are not medically, legally, or ethically brain dead. This category includes, but is not limited to, patients with mental retardation, organic brain syndrome, Alzheimer's disease, cerebrovascular accidents, and hypoxic encephalopathy sustained during cardiopulmonary arrest. Prior to 1975, these cases were dealt with quietly and individually by the physician, family, and hospital "ethics committee," but rarely by the courts.[4]

In the Matter of Karen Quinlan

On April 15, 1975, 22-year-old Karen Ann Quinlan entered a "comatose" state following the alleged ingestion of both tranquilizers and ethanol. She clearly did not meet the criteria for brain death, but in September 1975, her father-by-adoption, Joseph Quinlan, requested that her ventilator support be discontinued and that she be allowed to die. The physicians and hospital administrators responsible for her care refused to comply with this request. Mr. Quinlan then filed suit requesting authority as her legal guardian to remove ventilator support. The story was widely publicized by *Time* magazine, alerting the world to the realization that mechanical ventilation and other means of life support sometimes created moral and ethical questions more difficult to answer than the medical ones.

Superior Court Judge Robert Muir, Jr. refused Mr. Quinlan's request.[14] Because Karen was not brain dead, public and medical opinion generally supported this decision. However, some members of the lay public, the media, and the legal and medical professions criticized the ruling. In so doing, they overlooked two important facts that were not widely publicized by the media. First, and most importantly, Karen clearly did not meet published brain-death criteria. Her electroencephalogram (EEG) was not isoelectric, and she responded to pain with weak movement. Therefore, it was irrelevant that New Jersey was one of the first states in the United States to have adopted a statutory definition of brain death. For the court and for Karen's physicians, discontinuation of mechanical ventilation would have been a deliberate action intended to produce death in a nonterminal patient based on a "quality of life" judgment. Second, the decision to discontinue mechanical ventilation was (and is) more difficult than the decision to withhold such therapy before it is initiated.[15] This distinction, which is often impossible to define logically, morally, or ethically, has been accepted by some courts but rejected by others.

Mr. Quinlan's lawyers did not claim that Karen was brain dead but that she should, nevertheless, be allowed to die. They justified their action by claiming:

1. *"Medical science holds no hope for Miss Quinlan's recovery."* By this they did not mean that bodily death or brain death was imminent, but rather that Karen was not expected to regain normal cerebral function; subjectively, she would have a poor quality of life.

2. *"Miss Quinlan would want the respirator turned off."* This concept of "substituted judgment" was to become the basis for legal debate in numerous other cases involving the withdrawal or withholding of live-saving medical therapy from incompetent patients.

3. *"Doctors have no legal obligation to keep Miss Quinlan alive."* Judge Muir disagreed, stating "that a patient placed in the care of a doctor expects that the doctor 'will do all within his power to favor life against death.' " The statement ignored the moral and ethical obligation felt by Karen's physicians to avoid her death.

4. *"The wishes of the parents of an incompetent patient should be paramount in a doctor's life or death decision."* Judge Muir disagreed. (This argument had been used in 1973 in the U.S. Supreme Court decision *Roe v. Wade* allowing abortion on demand and would later be resurrected in legal debate regarding infanticide.)

5. *"The constitutional right of privacy should allow parents or guardians to make the decision that an incompetent child's life should no longer be prolonged."* Judge Muir, however, believed that previous legal right-to-privacy cases concerned the right to maintain a particular lifestyle, not the right to die.

6. *"Freedom of religion should allow Miss Quinlan, a Roman Catholic, to die."*

7. *"The beauty and meaning of Karen's life was over and she should be allowed to die."* Mr. Quinlan's attorneys argued that quality of life is more important than the sanctity of life. The belief that there is "life unworthy of life"[16] was responsible for the Nazi holocaust and the more recent widespread acceptance of involuntary, active euthanasia in the Netherlands. This highly controversial issue is now the center of legal debate which still rages in American courts today.

Judge Muir's 44-page ruling stated that judicial conscience and morality indicated that the treating physician was handling Karen's case properly. He noted, despite the fact that the victim is on the threshold of death, no humanitarian motives can justify, under common law, taking life. Judge Muir labeled as "semantics" the debate regarding whether discontinuation of mechanical ventilation was an act of commission or omission, since either would result in deliberate death and, thus, constitute legal homicide. He stated that "there is no constitutional right to die that can be asserted by a parent for his incompetent adult child."

Mr. Quinlan's lawyers appealed this decision. Like the lower court, the New Jersey Supreme Court agreed that Karen was not brain dead and was not imminently terminal; nevertheless, it reversed the lower court's decision. The Court specified a three-tiered procedure for decision-making in such cases:

> Upon the concurrence of the guardian and family of Karen, should the responsible attending physicians conclude that there is no reasonable possibility of Karen's ever emerging from her present comatose condition to a cognitive, sapient state and that the life-support apparatus now being administered to Karen should be discontinued, they shall consult with the hospital Ethics Committee or like body of the institution in which Karen is then hospitalized. If that consultative body agrees that there is no reasonable possibility of Karen's ever emerging from her comatose condition to a cognitive, sapient state, the present life-support system may be withdrawn and said action shall be without any civil or criminal liability therefore on the part of any participant, whether guardian, physician, hospital or others.

The Court also ruled that "the state's interest contra weakens and the individual's right to privacy grows as the degree of bodily invasion increases and the prognosis dims." Thus a quality-of-life decision was allowed by creating the legal doctrine of "substituted judgment," declaring that Karen's right to refuse treatment required that her guardian "render their best judgment . . as to whether she would exercise it in these circumstances." Before entering her comatose state, Karen had verbally expressed on at least one occasion that she would choose not to live if confined to a ventilator.[17]

Mechanical ventilatory support was subsequently discontinued. To everyone's surprise, she breathed spontaneously and remained in her baseline state of unconsciousness until 1986. Her failure to die when mechanical ventilation was discontinued clearly demonstrated that the issues involved ethical decisions separate and distinct from those reported by the Harvard Ad Hoc Committee.

The widely publicized *Quinlan* decision fueled an already heated legal and ethical debate regarding the relative importance of the sanctity of life versus the quality of life. Only 2 years earlier, *Roe v. Wade,* the most controversial United States Supreme Court decision of modern times, had legalized abortion on demand.[18] Dr. C. Everett Koop, a well-known pediatric surgeon and recent United States Surgeon General, predicted 10 natural consequences of this decision. Several were relevant to the Quinlan case and to the question of discontinuation of life support in general, including the processes of depersonalization and dehumanization. He stated that "liberty leads to license" and that "the right to die leads to the right to kill in mercy."[19] The significance of these predictions has become more apparent as a result of legal decisions in the 15 years that have elapsed since the *Roe v. Wade* decision.

> Over the last ten years, there has been a dramatic shift in the courts' attitude toward incompetent persons in need of life-sustaining medical care. Whereas formerly there was a presumption to treat and preserve life, since *Quinlan,* in 1976, the courts have instead focused on "preserving" the incompetent patients's "right" to choose to withhold consent to medical treatment through application of the "substituted judgment doctrine."

It should be noted, however, that "substituted judgment" is always exercised in favor of withdrawal of needed medical treatment, nutrition, and hydration.[20] During the late 1970s, the substituted judgment doctrine gained support from individuals who feared that rejection of this doctrine would always require treatment if a life of any sentence can be even briefly prolonged.

In re Eichner

Brother Joseph Fox was an 83-year-old priest who was ventilator-dependent and in a persistent vegetative state as a result of an intraoperative cardiac arrest. Several years before the cardiac arrest, Brother Fox had participated in a formal, careful discussion of the Quinlan case and had expressed his opinion that he would not want extraordinary treatment, such as mechanical ventilation, were he in similar circumstances. He had verbally reaffirmed that personal opinion several months before his cardiac arrest.

Father Philip Eichner, the director of Fox's religious order, petitioned the courts for permission to discontinue Fox's mechanical ventilation. The New York Court of Appeals approved the petition because "Brother Fox made the decision for himself." The court emphasized that Fox had "carefully reflected on the subject, expressed his views and concluded not to have his life prolonged by medical means if there were no hope of recovery" and that Fox had made "solemn pronouncements and not casual remarks . . . at some social gathering."[21] His statements were interpreted legally as oral imputed consent for withdrawal of life-support therapy under the substituted judgment doctrine. However, the written opinion of the Court went far beyond the doctrine of "substituted judgment" and into the doctrine of life unworthy of life[16]:

> As a matter of established fact, such a patient has no health and, in the true sense, no life for the State to protect. . . . Indeed, with *Roe[v. Wade]* in mind, it is appropriate to note that the State's interest in preservation of the life of the fetus would appear greater than any possible interest the State may have in maintaining the life of a terminally ill comatose patient . . . [whose] claim to personhood is certainly no greater than that of a fetus.[21]

As is so often the case, this decision contrasted with a more recent one in which a Texas District Court ruled that a single isolated statement made by an incompetent patient, while still competent, that she did not want to be maintained on life-support equipment was insufficient evidence to allow substituted judgment to terminate nasogastric feeding; her isolated remark was not adequate oral imputed consent for death by dehydration and starvation.[22]

In re Conroy

A New Jersey court defined the "best interest" method of decision-making for incompetent patients even more elaborately than the *Quinlan* Court's substituted judgment tests. Claire Conroy was an 83-year-old nursing home patient with severe organic brain syndrome. The trial court granted her guardian's request for termination of nasogastric feedings, but the decision was reversed by the Appellate Court.[23] The ruling by the Appellate Court judge is noteworthy:

> The trial judge . . . authorized euthanasia. . . . If the trial judge's order had been enforced, Conroy would not have died as the result of an existing medical condition, but rather she would have died, and painfully so, as the result of a new and independent condition: dehydration and starvation. Thus she would have been actively killed by independent means. . . .

However, the New Jersey Supreme Court reversed the Appellate Court's decision. While acknowledging that the subjective substituted judgment test was meaningless for a patient who had never competently expressed a desire regarding life or death, the Court authorized termination of treatment under either of two "best interest" tests: (1) the "limited objective" test, where there is some trustworthy indication of what the patient would have wanted and the burdens of life with treatment outweigh its benefits; and (2) the "pure objective" test, where there is no such indication, but the burdens markedly outweigh the benefits.

According to the Court, the final decision in such cases was the responsibility of the New Jersey Ombudsman for the Institutionalized Elderly, whose involvement in such matters had already been mandated by state statute. The importance of the Ombudsman was emphasized:

> Because of the particularly vulnerable nature of incompetent patients [aged 60 or more] in nursing homes, the Ombudsman must scrutinize all decisions to withhold or withdraw life-sustaining medical treatment from them.

In re Grant

By a narrow margin (5–4), the Washington Supreme Court ruled in *In re Grant* that a guardian was authorized to approve and direct the future withholding of mechanical (ventilation) or other life-sustaining procedures from her incompetent daughter with an incurable progressively degenerative neurologic disease resulting in mental retardation and loss of voluntary muscle control. The court decided that "in the absence of countervailing state interests, a person has the right to have life-sustaining treatment withheld where he or she (1) is in an advanced stage of a terminal incurable illness, and (2) is suffering severe and permanent mental and physical deterioration."

In the case of an incompetent patient, the benefits and burdens of treatment are to be decided by the guardian, immediate family, and physician to determine whether medical treatment should be withheld. The dissenting opinion expressed concern about the majority's distinction between treatment that merely prolongs death and that which results in some measure of recovery. "The fact that her functioning is limited does not mean that it is in her best interest to die. I object to the majority's obvious judgment that Barbara's life is not of value. . . . The court is imposing its own morality on the public in extending a legislative act."[24]

University Health Services, Ins v. Robert Piazzi et al.

Piazzi was a widely publicized case of first impression from a Georgia Superior Court in 1986. Donna Piazzi had become comatose and then brain dead during her second trimester of pregnancy. David Hadden's claim that he was the father of the unborn child was not disputed by Robert Piazzi, Donna's husband. Robert Piazzi requested that mechanical ventilation and other life-support therapy be discontinued. Hadden requested that life-support therapy be continued, since the baby was "quickened" but not yet viable. The Division of Family and Children Services of the Department of Human Resources of the State of Georgia contended that the case involved purely medical decisions and that the 1973 *Roe v. Wade* deprived the Georgia Court of legal jurisdiction in this case. Two previous Georgia Supreme Court cases had demonstrated the State's interest in preservation of life or potential life, and that public policy favored maintenance of every reasonable possible chance for life. Therefore, the Superior Court ordered that life-support systems be maintained; as a result, the infant was born alive.[25]

Rasmussen v. Fleming

A case of first impression in Arizona, concerned a Public Fiduciary's request for broad, unreviewable authority to refuse medical treatment (including mechanical ventilation), food, and fluids for any incompetent or incapacitated patient under his jurisdiction.[26] Mildred Rasmussen was a nursing home patient in a persistent vegetative state who was not terminally ill. The county Public Fiduciary petitioned an Arizona trial court for appointment as Rasmussen's guardian for the purpose of refusing medical treatment and discontinuation of nasogastric feedings. The court appointed the Public Fiduciary as *guardian without restriction.* The Arizona Court of Appeals held that life-sustaining treatment (including artificially provided hydration and nutrition) may be withdrawn from an incompetent person if it is determined by the attending physician and two other physicians that the patient is "comatose and there is no reasonable possiblity that he will return to a cognitive sapient state." The guardian ad litem petitioned the Arizona Supreme Court for review. In an Objection to the Petition for Review, the Public Fiduciary asked that "the holding of the Court of Appeals be expended to apply to all patients in a chronic vegetative state or otherwise incompetent or incapacitated." The Arizona Supreme Court ruled that Arizona law gives the court the authority to appoint guardians for incompetent persons and that such guardians have the authority to refuse medical treatment, including artificially provided nutrition and hydration, for all incapacitated persons under their care. When patients have not previously expressed their medical preferences, the court ruled that medical decisions should be guided by the best interest standard.

In re Peter

Another widely publicized New Jersey Supreme Court decision involving decision-making for incompetent, nonterminal patients was rendered in 1987.[27] Hilda Peter was a 65-year-old nursing home patient in a persistent vegetative state following cardiopulmonary resuscitation. Prior to her neurologic impairment, Peter had given durable power of attorney to Ebeirhard Johanning, a close friend with whom she lived. Mr. Johanning, having been appointed legal guardian with certain legal restrictions regarding medical care, sought the Ombudman's acquiescence in the removal of the nasogastric feeding tube which was sustaining Peter's life. After investigation, the Ombudsman concluded that: "Though she is vegetative without any hope of recovery, her physical condition is quite good. She could survive for many years, possibly decades. As long as the precise and careful nursing care that she now receives is maintained, she can continue in this state for an indeterminate length of time."

Announcing his findings before a press conference, the Ombudsman concluded that the decision *In re Conroy* prevented him from authorizing removal of Peter's feeding tube because of her long life expectancy. Johanning appealed the Ombudsman's decision to the New Jersey Supreme Court. The Court ruled that not all of the tests described in *In re Conroy* applied to Peter. Conroy had been awake and able to interact with her environment to a limited extent, while Peter was in a persistent vegetative state. The Court also ruled that the 1-year life-expectancy test and the objective and limited-objective tests used in *Conroy* did not apply. Life expectancy is unimportant when a patient is in a persistent vegetative state.[27]

In re Jobes

This opinion was reemphasized by another 1987 ruling.[28] Jobes was a 31-year-old woman in a persistent vegetative state as the result of an intraoperative hypoxic and/or ischemic episode following a motor vehicle accident. The hospital refused to grant her husband's and parents' request to withdraw a feeding jejunostomy tube, her only means of hydration and nourishment. Although Jobes had not left clear and convincing evidence of her beliefs and desires regarding life and death, the Court ruled that treatment decisions, including determining whether or not a feeding tube should be removed, may be made by a surrogate decision-maker. In the case of nonhospitalized or non-elderly patients, the Court specified that statements are required from two neurologists and the patient's attending physician that the patient is in a persistently vegetative state before the decision-maker is allowed to implement the decision to withdraw or withhold medical therapy.

Discrimination Against the Handicapped

Many of those who advocate withdrawal or withholding of medical therapy from incompetent patients with a poor quality of life support their philosophical position by pointing out that patients have the right to refuse therapy. Courts generally have recognized the right of a mentally competent adult to refuse medical treatment. Until recently, however, this right was not absolute. Courts also have recognized that the state's interests in preserving life, preventing suicide, protecting innocent third parties, and maintaining the ethical integrity of the medical profession often outweigh the patient's asserted constitutional right to privacy and common law right to bodily self-determination.[29]

Many competent patients with poor quality of life (by societal standards) give informed consent for and receive aggressive medical therapy, and only rarely does a competent patient refuse food and water. Therefore, withholding hydration, nutrition, mechanical ventilation, and other medical therapy from mentally incompetent patients has been held to represent illegal discrimination against the handicapped, especially in cases involving nonterminal patients. Section 504 of the United States Rehabilitation Act of 1973 specifically defines and protects handicapped individuals against discrimination in employment, education, and health services. The United States Supreme Court, in their 1987 ruling in *School Board of Nassau County, Florida v. Arline,* supported the intention of the Rehabilitation Act of 1973 to protect handicapped individuals form discrimination in health care; in fact, this ruling expanded Congress's definition of "handicapped" to include those with contagious diseases; thus opening the door for the protection of persons with acquired immunodeficiency syndrome (AIDS) against discrimination in health care. The Court did not address the question of whether Section 504 protects persons who are carriers of an infectious disease but who do not have a physical impairment (such as individuals with the human immunosuppressive virus (HIV) who do not yet have AIDS-related complex). The Court expressly declined to determine "whether a carrier of a contagious disease such as AIDS could be considered to have a physical impairment, or whether such a person could be considered, a handicapped person as defined by the Act, solely on the basis of contagiousness.[30]

Others advocate that withholding therapy from nonterminal, incompetent patients is necessary because the average age of our population is increasing and medical costs have become burdensome to society. While all are in agreement that rising medical costs must be contained, clinicians and courts using cost containment as an excuse for withholding needed medical therapy from nonterminal patients should ponder the annual expenditures of Americans for nonessentials such as pets ($10 billion), tobacco products ($31.8 billion), alcoholic beverages ($53.5 billion), and illegal drugs ($100 billion).[31]

According to Dr. Leo Alexander, the U.S. medical consultant at the Nuremberg Trials, "[w]hatever proportions these crimes finally assumed . . . the beginnings at first were merely a subtle shift in emphasis in the basic attitude of the physicians . . . toward the nonrehabilitable sick."[32] Euthanasia had gained acceptance in substantial sectors of the German society and medical profession long before Hitler assumed power in 1933. Organized medicine collaborated on a wide scale in the mass extermination of the chronically ill in order to avoid useless expense to society. In fact, Hitler's authorization of mass extermination was not so much a command but an extension of the authority of physicians. The eradication of terminally ill patients quickly deteriorated into the eradication of nonterminal physically and/or mentally impaired individuals and, finally, deteriorated even further into the extermination of racially, socially, and ideologically unwanted individuals.

This expansion of criteria was not forced upon the doctors by the Nazi regime, but evolved according to its own dynamics within the medical profession. In fact, the liberalization of indications for euthanasia actually became most wanton after Hitler had officially ended the euthanasia project in 1941.[33] On the basis of his experiences, Dr. Alexander[32] stated,

> The case therefore that I should like to make is that American medicine must realize where it stands in its fundamental premises. There can be no doubt that in a subtle way the Hegelian premise of "what is useful is right" has infected society including the medical portion of society. Physicians must return to their older premises, which were the emotional foundation and driving force of an amazingly successful quest to increase powers of healing and which are bound to carry them still farther if they are not held down to earth by the pernicious attitudes of an overdue practical realism.

Although increasingly condoned by American courts, the act of withholding or withdrawing food, water, and medical therapy from the nonterminal patient with permanent neurologic deficit is medically and ethically quite different than the withholding or withdrawal of life support therapy from the brain-dead patient. Deliberate failure to provide medical therapy for these incompetent nonterminal patients based on quality-of-life judgments is involuntary euthanasia, an increasingly common practice in Europe.[34]

Dr. P. Schepens, a Belgian physician and General Secretary of the World Federation of Doctors Who Respect Human Life, writes:

> You and I, we have escaped the abortion trap. We are alive and well. But we all know that some day we will die. The probability that it might be at the hands of a physician, by virtue of a medical decision, is one that is increasing every day. For the first time Europe, and in particular the Netherlands, is ahead of the United States in medical matters, particularly in the area of euthanasia.

The Netherlands, with a population of more than 14 million, has an annual mortality of approximately 125,000. According to official death registration figures, approximately 3,000 persons are killed each year by doctors upon their proper request. However, experts estimate that, in reality, as many as 18,000 to 20,000 people are killed by euthanasia in the Netherlands each year. Thus, more than 15 percent of deaths in the Netherlands may be "euthanasia," with most of these deaths by euthanasia being "involuntary," that is, without patient consent.[34]

According to the Dutch Penal Codes, euthanasia is still a criminal offense. However, during the past 15 years, Dutch courts have steadily expanded the circumstances in which a doctor may avoid prosecution if he kills. In 1984, the Supreme Court of the Netherlands decided a case which was the first and only decision by a court of final appeal in which assisted euthanasia has been held to be privileged conduct in certain defined situations.[35] "The Royal Dutch Medical Association had endorsed 'euthanasia on demand,' if performed by physicians, not only for competent adults but also even for minors without parental consent."[33]

Numerous other recent court cases, both state and federal, have dealt with the issue of discontinuation of "artificial" hydration and nutrition (intravenous, nasogastric, jejunal). Varied rulings have been handed down, even by courts in the same state reviewing similar cases. Many courts have held that the provision of hydration and nutrition to a patient is medical care, which can be denied on the basis of the patient's right to refuse medical therapy. Other courts have argued that food and water are basic human needs, not medical therapy.[36]

It is apparent that physicians are increasingly basing decisions regarding the withholding or withdrawal of medical therapy (including food and water) from incompetent patients who are not terminally ill on nonmedical quality-of-life factors: recent court decisions have increasingly refuted the sanctity of life doctrine long held in the United States. For example, a Philadelphia physician had his medical licenses restored just 6 months after revocation for his guilty plea to the murder of his terminally ill mother-in-law by lethal injection. He was sentenced to 2 years' probation, 400 hours of community service, and a $10,000 fine.[37]

Two California physicians were criminally prosecuted for termination of intravenous fluids of a patient who was brain damaged but not brain dead. However, the prosecution was dismissed because the court held that cessation of life-support measures (the intravenous fluids) represented a withdrawal or omission of further treatment rather than an affirmative act. The California court ruled that medical provision of nutrition and hydration is more similar to other medical procedures than to typical human ways of providing nutrition and hydration; therefore, their benefits and burdens were to be evaluated in the same manner as any other medical procedure." Similarly, a Delaware court authorized a no code order, no antibiotics for infection, and no reimplantation of a feeding tube for a nonterminal, comatose patient.[38]

Mentally Competent Terminal Patients

Each year, thousands of lucid, mentally competent American adults learn that they are imminently terminal. Difficult legal and ethical decisions regarding mechanical ventilation and other forms of life-support therapy for these patients must be made. Not infrequently, judicial involvement has been requested in such cases, either by the patients or by the health-care providers.

In re Farrell

Thirty-seven-year-old Kathleen Farrell began experiencing symptoms of amyotrophic lateral sclerosis in 1982. By 1986, she was paralyzed and confined to bed, requiring home mechanical ventilation and round-the-clock nursing care. Her husband requested legal authority to disconnect the ventilator with judicial assurance that neither he nor his assistants would incur any civil or criminal liability. Kathleen, who was mentally competent, testified to the court in a special session held at her home that she wished to discontinue mechanical ventilator therapy and die. The trial court granted Mr. Farrell's request but stayed the order pending appellate review.

Although Kathleen died while still receiving ventilator therapy, the New Jersey Supreme Court agreed to hear the case because of its importance and because of the inevitability of similar cases in the future. The Court reaffirmed the common-law right that

> Every human being of adult years and sound mind has a right to determine what shall be done with his own body. . . . Nevertheless the right to refuse life-sustaining medical treatment is not absolute. The state has at least four potentially countervailing interests in sustaining a person's life: preserving life, prevent-

ing suicide, safeguarding the integrity of the medical profession, and protecting innocent third parties.

These interests were individually addressed by the Court. The Court ruled that the state's interest in preserving life gives way to the right of a mentally competent patient to "direct . . . the course of his own life." Quoting *In re Conroy,* the court stated that:

> Declining life-sustaining medical treatment may not properly be viewed as an attempt to commit suicide. Refusing medical intervention merely allows the disease to take its natural course; if death were to eventually occur, it would be the result, primarily of the underlying disease, and not the result of a self-inflicted injury.

The Court also noted that health care providers are bound by certain ethical criteria and that the patient has no right to compel a health-care provider to violate generally accepted professional standards. Finally, the Court noted that Kathleen's minor children would be cared for even in her absence.[39]

The *Farrell* Court provided guidelines to be applied when life-sustaining treatment is refused by a patient. First, the patient must be competent and properly informed about the prognosis, the alternative treatments available, and the risks involved in the withdrawal of life-sustaining treatment. Second, it must be determined that the choice was made by the patient voluntarily and without coercion. Third, the patient's right to choose to disconnect the life-sustaining apparatus must be balanced against the four potentially countervailing state interests.[40]

In the Matter of Beverly Requina

Beverly Requina was a mentally competent 55-year-old woman with amyotrophic lateral sclerosis who was quadriplegic and unable to speak. The Appellate Division of the Superior Court of New Jersey affirmed a lower court decision requiring that a hospital must comply with a mentally competent, terminally ill patient's refusal of artificial feeding and that it may not transfer the patient to another care facility without express consent.[41]

In re Jane Doe

In a similar case, a Philadelphia trial court ruled that a competent but paralyzed patient with amyotrophic lateral sclerosis could refuse life-sustaining treatment. The court ruled that the patient's common-law right of self-determination and constitutional right to privacy in refusing or discontinuing medical treatment outweighed any countervailing state interests. In making this determination, the court reviewed six specified criteria, assuring that the patient was competent and was voluntarily refusing life-support therapy.[42]

Acquired Immunodeficiency Virus

By mid-1988, approximately 1.5 million people in the United States were infected with HIV; 40,000 people had, thus far, developed AIDS or AIDS-related complex, and about 25,000 had died. By 1991, it is estimated that there will be about 179,000 people dying from AIDS; it will be the leading cause of death among people between the ages of 25 and 40. The medical costs will be significant: more than $8.5 billion in 1991 alone, excluding public or private disability expenditures.[43] More money will be needed for treating AIDS than for any other category of diseased patients.[43]

Although AIDS may result in a progressive dementia, most patients with AIDS are mentally competent for the majority of their terminal phase. Therefore, physicians have a legal obligation to obtain informed consent for any and all nonemergent medical therapy, including tracheal intubation and mechanical ventilatory support. As the disease progresses, many of these patients refuse additional medical therapy, thereby hastening the process of dying.[43] Some seek more active means. Males between the ages of 20 and 59 with AIDS are 36 times more likely to commit suicide than are males of the same age without AIDS.[44] Derek Humphrey, executive director for the Hemlock Society, reports that many AIDS patients call the Society for help in committing suicide and report that their doctors are willing to help them.[37]

According to a recent publication of the American Academy of Medical Ethics:[43]

> A multiplicity of factors thus point to the prospect that the AIDS epidemic may lead to sanctioned euthanasia: the economic and social costs of caring for those with the virus; the deadly, infectious, progressive and particularly ugly nature of the disease; the socially undesired and stigmatized population affected. . . . Those who tend to regard AIDS as a disease made in Heaven to punish moral reprobates should thus consider an alternative proposition: Namely, the AIDS may create a greater evil yet by short-circuiting opposition to sanctioned euthanasia, and thereby opening the floodgates of a hell on earth.

Mentally Competent NonTerminal Patients

Rodas v. ErkenBrack

In 1987, the first known American request for court authorization of active euthanasia by the administration of a lethal injection or overdose for a person with disabilities, was dismissed in Colorado.[45] A Colorado district court, in *In re Rodas,*[46] had previously ruled that Hector Rodas, a mentally competent adult who was not imminently terminal, had the right to refuse all medical therapy, including food and fluids provided by gastrostomy tube. Rodas was quadriplegic and "locked in" as a result of brainstem injury resulting from basilar artery occlusion secondary to intravenous drug abuse. Wishing to die, Rodas refused gastrostomy fluids and feedings. Although he was not terminal, the Court declared that Rodas had the right to refuse medication, food, and hydration. In addition, the Court specifically forbade his transfer to another care facility without his expressed consent. Even though Rodas's *stated motive was to cause his own death,* the Court concluded that termination of therapy *did not constitute suicide* on the part of Rodas or assisted suicide on the part of Hilltop Rehabilitation Hospital.[46]

Eight days later, *Rodas v. ErkenBrack* was filed by the American Civil Liberties Union (ACLU) seeking a lethal injection or drug overdose for Rodas.[45] Because the Fourteenth Amendment provides that no state shall deprive any person of life, liberty or property, without due process of law; nor deny to any person . . . the equal protection of the laws,[47] those who seek legalization of assisted suicide must argue that there exist other constitutional rights which circumvent Fourteenth Amendment protection. Therefore, the ACLU attorneys argued that Rodas had a constitutional right to receive "medicinal agents" that would cause his death based on the right to privacy, the right to autonomy and the right to refuse medical treatment.[48]

Countervailing state's interests were ignored by this filing. Also ignored was the fact that the Constitution contains within it a priority of rights to be applied when they cannot be reconciled, and that the right to life has a priority over the right to liberty.[48] Eventually, the case was dismissed because Rodas denied having requested the assistance of the ACLU or anyone else in shortening his life with "medicinal agents." Rodas eventually died in February of 1987 as a result of court-sanctioned, medically assisted, self-imposed dehydration and starvation.[49]

Bouvia v. Superior Court

The most widely publicized case involving sanctioned assisted suicide was that of Elizabeth Bouvia, a competent 26-year-old woman with a nonterminal disease, cerebral palsy, who petitioned the court for the right to die by starvation in a California hospital. Bouvia recently had experienced a number of major life crises, including divorce, persistent unemployment, withdrawal from a graduate program in social work, and parental rejection.[50] By the time she won her court battle to receive hospital assistance in starving herself to death, she had changed her mind and decided she wanted to continue living.[51] However, the decision of the court will have legal repercussions for many years.

While the decision of the appellate court eventually turned primarily on the right of a patient to refuse medical care, many disabled people were distressed by the court's implicit assumption that death represented an appropriate and acceptable solution to the problems posed by a severe disability.[52] Distressing to many others is the concurring opinion by Judge Compton asserting a right of patients to die with the assistance of the medical profession. His opinion goes far beyond any other official pronouncement on the question of sanctioned assisted suicide in the United States[50]:

> This state and the medical profession instead of frustrating her desire [to commit suicide], should be attempting to relieve her suffering by permitting and in fact assisting her to die with ease and dignity. . . . The right to die is an integral part of our right to control our own destinies so long as the rights of others are not affected. That right should . . . include the ability to enlist assistance from others, including the medical profession, in making death as painless and quick as possible.

This is the only public endorsement by a U.S. judge of the right to engage the assistance of others in ending one's life.[53] Noteworthy is the fact that approximately one-half the American states have statutes specifically criminalizing the acts of assisting, advising, or encouraging suicide.[50] In the remaining jurisdictions, assisting or inciting a suicide may well be criminal homicide if death ensues.[53]

American courts have begun to accept nonmedical, quality-of-life judgments as acceptable defense for deaths resulting from the withholding of medical therapy from disabled but nonterminal patients. Many of the recent court decisions regarding withdrawal or withholding of "medical therapy," including food and water, have dealt with patients in this category, that is, patients with physical and/or mental deficiencies who are not imminently terminal. According to the National Legal Center for the Medically Dependent and Disabled, in 1987 requests for withdrawal of treatment began "to shift from removing burdensome treatments, so that an incurable disease might run its natural course, toward removing food and fluids from people with disabilities and even toward active intervention to end life by lethal injection or overdose."[53]

Several state Supreme Court decisions during 1987 contained dissents that vigorously voiced concern and uneasiness about how the courts' majority opinions devalued the lives of persons with disabilities. The majority opinions were viewed as threats to the health care rights of older persons and persons with disabilities because these decisions expanded the class of people for whom treatment, food, and fluids may be terminated to include persons with disabilities who are not terminally ill.[53] The potential importance of this trend is highlighted by the 1987 estimate that approximately 15 percent of the total population has some general physical disability.[54]

Mentally Incompetent Terminal Patients

The substituted judgment doctrine popularized by the *Quinlan* Court often has been applied to allow withholding or withdrawal of life-prolonging therapy from patients who are imminently terminal and are no longer mentally competent. Ironically, this doctrine even has been applied to patients who were never mentally competent and, therefore, never had an opportunity to express their beliefs and desires regarding matters such as these.

Superintendent of Belchertown State School v. Saikewicz

Joseph Saikewicz was a profoundly retarded 67-year-old man with leukemia. Although chemotherapy offered a 30 to 50 percent chance of 2- to 13-month remission, the court waived the relatively objective best interest standard and applied the substituted judgment doctrine, thereby allowing therapy to be withheld.[55]

In re Storar

John Storar had terminal bladder cancer. His mother requested that blood transfusions be discontinued so that he might be allowed to die. The New York court rejected the substituted judgment doctrine, since Storar had been profoundly retarded throughout life. It held that applying the doctrine in a case such as this was equivalent to asking: "If it snowed all summer, would it then be winter?" Because the transfusions did not cause excessive pain, as had been claimed by Storar's mother, and because they improved his level of function, the court refused to order the termination of therapy. However, Storar died before the legal controversy could be resolved.[56]

The frighteningly rapid appearance of American court rulings on both active and passive euthanasia suggests that America is following in the footsteps of the Netherlands. Although euthanasia is still a criminal offense in the Netherlands, physicians are rarely prosecuted.[57]

> [E]ven without any formal legislation, euthanasia is generally accepted and practiced by many physicians. It is likewise admitted as current practice by many hospital boards and administrators, nursing personnel, Health Ministry officials, and even by judicial and political authorities. What has not as yet been codified in law, has been accepted as common practice. Euthanasia is ardently demanded by an active minority of the population, while the majority is at a loss what to make of it and remains relatively silent. Only the active pro-life groups are sounding the alarm and strive to propagate the fact that in this way the Netherlands is paving the way for a new holocaust of "undesirable" persons.[34]

Patients of Questional Mental Competence

Even more problematic for physicians than the mentally incompetent patients are the patients of questionable mental competency. Often, a patient's mental competency is not questioned until his expressed choice is not in agreement with the physician's recommendation. However, the legal presumption is that a patient is competent to make medical treatment decisions until proved otherwise.

Mental illness, the inability to perform certain functions, and/or the refusal of medical recommendations do not necessarily provide legal proof of mental incompetence. For example, in *In re Milton* (1987), the Supreme Court of Ohio ruled that a 53-year-old inpatient at a mental hospital could refuse potentially life-saving gynecologic surgery on religious grounds. The patient had not been declared legally incompetent and the Court found her reasons for refusal of medical therapy distinguishable from her psychotic delusions.[59]

In *In re Quackenbush,*[29] the refusal of a 72-year-old man to allow life-saving surgical amputation of his gangrenous feet was upheld by the court. The *Quackenbush* court cited from the *Quinlan* ruling:

> The State's interest contra weakens and the individual's right of privacy grows as the degree of bodily invasion increases and the prognosis dims. Ultimately, there comes a point at which the individual's rights overcome the State interest.

The *Quackenbush* court explicitly noted the contrast between Mr. Quackenbush and a young patient who could be returned to excellent health by a minimally invasive procedure such as a blood transfusion. Thus, the patient's age, quality of life, and degree of bodily invasion were the important factors in the *Quackenbush* court's decision.

There are numerous other examples of the courts' inconsistency regarding withdrawal or withholding of medical therapy for patients of questionable mental competency. The ruling in *State Department of Human Services v. Northern* suggests that an otherwise competent patient may be declared incompetent so that previously refused life-saving therapy may be given.[60] However, "inherent in the requirement of informed consent for treatment is the recognition that a competent patient has a right to choose to forego treatment. Legal recognition of this right to refuse is based on the common law right to bodily integrity, which underlies the informed consent doctrine. It may also be based on the constitutional right to privacy, which protects an individual's right to make his or her own decisions about fundamental personal matters. This right to privacy has been held to extend to a person's decisions about medical treatment.''[16]

However, the courts have previously recognized several interests which may override a patient's right to refuse life-saving medical therapy. The President's Commission for the Study of Ethical Problems in Medicine and Biomedical and Behavioral Research suggested that the determination of mental competence is best made by the patient's family, physician, and hospital ethics committee without routine adjudication.[61]

Minors

Roe v. Wade

Without question, the U.S. Supreme Court's 1973 *Roe v. Wade* decision was the most controversial judicial ruling of modern times.[18] With what Justice Byron White referred to as raw judicial power, the U.S. Supreme Court struck down legislative restrictions on abortion in every state. As noted by then President Ronald Reagan, ''Our nationwide policy of abortion-on-demand through all nine months of pregnancy was neither voted for by our people nor enacted by our legislators—not a single state had such unrestricted abortion before the Supreme Court decreed it to be national policy in 1973. . . . Make no mistake, abortion-on-demand is not a right granted by the Constitution.[62]

President Reagan also noted that ''we cannot diminish the value of one category of human life—the unborn—without diminishing the value of all human life.'' One of the previously mentioned predicted ''natural consequences'' of the *Roe V. Wade* decision was that abortion would lead to infanticide.[19] Indeed, the same year an article in the *New England Journal of Medicine* reported that 14 percent of the deaths in a special care nursery of the Yale-New Haven Hospital were the result of withholding treatment.[63]

In 1974, the International Correspondence Society of Obstetricians and Gynecologists surveyed obstetricians to learn how they dealt with live births in abortions. A Philadelphia physician wrote:[18]

> At the time of delivery it has been our policy to wrap the fetus in a towel. The fetus is then moved to another room, while our attention is turned to the care of the gravida. She is examined to determine whether placental expulsion has occurred and the extent of vaginal bleeding. Once we are sure her condition is stable, the fetus is evaluated. Almost invariably all signs of life have ceased.

Ironically, some states have statutes requiring the abortionist to make every effort to resuscitate the baby being aborted; however, such is not the usual practice. Dr. Mary Ellen Avery, Professor of Pediatrics at Harvard University and Physician-in-Chief of Boston's Children's Hospital, suggested that the physician should make the decision regarding institution of medical therapy when an attempted abortion results in the live birth of a child of sufficient birthweight to have a chance for survival.

Much more common than infants who survive abortions are infants with congenital birth defects; approximately 3 percent of live births are associated with major congenital defects.[54] These people, too, have become a target for some in our society, raising important legal questions. Immediately following *Roe v. Wade, Time* magazine reported a quotation by Nobel laureate, Dr. James D. Watson, co-discoverer of DNA, which originally was published by the American Medical Association:

> If a child were not declared alive until three days after birth, then all parents could be allowed the choice only a few are given under the present system. The doctor could allow the child to die if the parents so choose and save a lot of misery and suffering. I believe this view is the only rational, compassionate attitude to have.

Justice Blackmun, in the *Roe v. Wade* decision, stated that the Supreme Court "need not resolve the question of when life beings." Legally speaking, it is unclear when the "fetus" or "product of conception" becomes a "person" or "human being" with the inalienable rights guaranteed by the Constitution of the United States and the Fourteenth Amendment.

The controversy surrounding *Roe v. Wade* polarized Americans into Pro-choice and Pro-life factions and led to raging debate, as well as repeated episodes of violence, including the bombing of abortion clinics. By the late 1980s, it had become the most significant domestic political concern. In July 1989, the U.S. Supreme Court, in a retreat from its 1973 decision, gave states the right to impose significant restrictions on abortion. By a 5 to 4 ruling, the Justices upheld a Missouri law which barred public employees from performing abortions not necessary to save a woman's life, barred the use of public buildings for performing abortions (even if no public funds were used), and required physicians to perform tests to determine if fetuses past 20 weeks gestation were viable. The Court stopped short of overturning *Roe v. Wade*, but most observers on both sides feel that such a decision will be forthcoming, perhaps during the 1990 term.

The decision to withhold medical treatment from a child is even more complicated than the decision to withhold medical treatment from an incompetent adult because the rights of the parents must also be considered. In general, parents have a legal right to make fundamental decisions regarding their children. According to the U.S. Supreme Court, "it is cardinal with us that the custody, care, and nurture of the child reside first with the parents, whose primary function and freedom include preparation for obligations that the state can neither supply nor hinder." Meanwhile, however, the legal standard to be upheld is that of serving the child's best interests. One court has ruled that the child "belongs" to his parents, but also to his state. The fact that the child belongs to the state imposes on the state many duties. Chief among them is the duty to protect the child's right to live and grow up with a sound mind in a sound body and to brook no interference with that right by any person or organization.[64]

Parental refusal of medical treatments has not always been overruled by the courts. In *In re Seiferth,* the court refused to overrule the parents and order surgical repair of cleft lip for a 15-year-old because the condition was not emergent.[65] In *In re Green,* the court upheld the parent's refusal of splenectomy for their child with sickle cell anemia, since the underlying disease would still be fatal.[66]

However, in most cases involving life-threatening conditions, such as blood transfusions for children of Jehovah's Witnesses, the courts have ordered needed medical treatment despite parental objections. In *Custody of a Minor,*[67] a Massachusetts court ordered resumption of chemotherapy treatments for Chad Green, a minor with acute lymphocytic leukemia, whose treatments had been terminated by his parents. The court also prohibited further treatments with laetrile, megadose vitamins A and C, folic acid, and enzyme enemas which had already resulted in chronic cyanide poisoning, hypervitaminosis, and possible colon injury. Courts have even overruled a father's refusal for tonsillectomy and adenoidectomy for his children and a mother's refusal of medical and dental care for her child with cavities, dental fractures, and an umbilical hernia.

During the 1970s and 1980s, many disabled infants have been denied necessary medical therapy because of coexisting disabilities. Nonmedical factors are increasingly considered in the life-or-death equation. For example, a survey of pediatricians published in 1977 indicated that parental willingness to care for a child with disabilities was a major factor in deciding on the aggressiveness of medical treatment.[33] In 1982, Surgeon General Koop[69] wrote:

> Semantics have made infanticide palatable by never referring to the practice by that word, but by using such euphemisms as "selection." "Starving a child to death" becomes "allowing him to die." Although infanticide is not talked about even in professional circles, the

> euphemisms are. It is all illegal, but the law has turned its back. The day will come when the argument will be as it was for abortion: "Let's legalize what is already happening." Then what is legal is right. Attention will then be turned to the next class of individuals that might be exterminated without too loud an outcry.

Lifton[69] pointed out that the Nazi program of euthanasia "began with newborns, then proceeded to children up to the ages of 3 and 4 and soon to older ones. Eventually, the killing included all ages. The key question in this 'medical decision' was the patient's ability to work."

Baby Doe

By the early 1980s, an estimated 5,000 American babies were denied life-saving medical therapy each year. Many naively assumed that all of these cases involved the withholding of futile medical therapy from infants in the final stages of death; often however, this was not the case.[54] In 1982, the Baby Doe Case of Bloomington, Indiana focused national attention on the issue of withholding life-saving medical therapy from infants because of coexisting disabilities, inspiring much medical, legal, and ethical debate. Because he had Down's syndrome, Baby Doe's parents refused surgical correction of his tracheoesophageal fistula. Although neither the underlying syndrome (trisomy 21) or the tracheoesophageal fistula would necessarily have been fatal during infancy, the court upheld the parents' refusal of life-saving medical and surgical therapy. The family and physicians were given judicial permission to allow the infant to die by starvation.[70]

In response to the Baby Doe decision, President Reagan[63] wrote:

> The death of that tiny infant tore at the hearts of all Americans because the child was undeniably a live human being—one lying helpless before the eyes of the doctors and the eyes of the nation. The real issue for the courts was not whether Baby Doe was a human being. The real issue was whether to protect the life of a human being who had Down's Syndrome, who would be mentally handicapped, but who needed a routine surgical procedure to unblock his esophagus and allow him to eat. A doctor testified to the presiding judge that, even with his physical problem corrected, Baby Doe would have a "non-existent" possibility for "a minimally adequate quality of life"—in other words, that retardation was the equivalent of a crime deserving the death penalty. The judge let Baby Doe starve and die, and the Indiana Supreme Court sanctioned his decision.

In his well-known treatise, *The Slide to Auschwitz,* Dr. Koop quoted a statement by Millard Everett: "No child [should] be admitted into the society of the living who would be certain to suffer any social handicap—for example, any physical or mental defect that would prevent marriage or would make others tolerate his company only from the sense of mercy."[71]

Dr. Koop[71] further noted that:

> We are rapidly moving from the state of mind where destruction of life is advocated for children who are considered to be socially useless or have non-meaningful lives to a place where we are willing to destroy a child because he is socially disturbing. . . . Destructiveness eventually is turned on the destroyer and self-destruction is the result. If you do not believe me, look at Nazi Germany. My concern is that the next time around the destruction will be greater before the ultimate self-destruction brings an end to the holocaust.

In response to the Baby Doe case, President Reagan directed the Department of Justice and the Department of Health and Human Services (DHHS) to apply civil rights regulations to protect handicapped neonates. Richard Schweiker, then Secretary of the DHHS, was instructed to notify hospitals and health care providers that Section 504 of the 1973 Rehabilitation Act forbids recipients of federal funds from withholding from handicapped citizens, simply because they are handicapped, any benefits or services that would ordinarily be provided to persons without handicaps. The DHHS Office for Civil Rights issued a "Notice to Health Care Providers" in May, 1982 informing hospital administrators that their hospitals risked losing federal funds if they allowed nourishment or medical treatment to be withheld from handicapped infants. The notice stated that: "It is unlawful . . . to withhold from a handicapped infant nutritional sustenance or medical or surgical treatment required to correct a life-threatening condition if: (1) the withholding is based on the fact that the infant is handicapped; and (2) the handicap does not render the treatment or nutritional sustenance medically contraindicated."[72]

Although well-received and praised by many, the DHHS notice was considered offensive and/or unnecessary by many professional and medical organizations. The American Hospital Association formally denied that hospitals had previously been guilty of discrimination and promised to assure that such simplistic solutions to complex situations involving health care delivery are avoided. The American Academy of Pediatrics claimed that the DHHS's effort "to solve this complex problem through strict interpretation and enforcement of the letter of Section 504 may have the unintended effect of requiring treatment that is not in the best interest of handicapped children."[73]

In March 1983, the DHHS issued a rule requiring hospitals receiving federal funds to post signs in delivery suites, neonatal intensive care units (ICUs), nurseries, and pediatric wards warning that "discriminatory failure to feed and care for handicapped infants in this facility is prohibited by federal law. Failure to feed and care for infants may also violate the criminal and civil laws of your state." A toll-free 24-hour hotline allowed violations to be reported directly to the DHHS. Hotline calls resulted in a number of investigative teams being sent to hospitals around the country.

Meanwhile, the American Academy of Pediatrics, the National Association of Children's Hospitals and Related Institutions, and Children's Hospital National Medical Center filed court suit challenging the DHHS rule. One month after its issuance, the U.S. District Court for the District of Columbia declared the DHHS rule invalid for several reasons, including failure of the DHHS to give advance notice of the rule.

Baby Doe II

In July 1983, the DHHS issued a revised set of regulations (the "Baby Doe II Rule") with the mandatory 60-day advance notice period. The required notices were smaller in size and only needed to be posted so as to be visible to medical and nursing staff. Prompted by the criticism of the American Academy of Pediatrics, the Baby Doe II Rule stressed that Section 504 applies only "when non-medical consideration, such as subjective judgments that an unrelated handicap makes a person's life not worth living, are interjected in the decision-making process." Infants for whom care would be futile were exempted from the regulations. The new rule also called for the establishment of Infant Care Review Committees (ICRCs). Thus, violations of Section 504 would be reported first to the hospital ICRC, then the state Child Protective Services Agency, and, finally, to the DHHS hotline, if necessary.

Baby Jane Doe

Baby Jane Doe was born with multiple congenital anomalies, including microcephaly, hydrocephalus, and spina bifida. She was transferred to University Hospital of the State University of New York at Stony Brook for corrective surgery but her parents refused their consent allegedly because of the baby's congenital anomalies. Therefore, an attorney filed suit in New York State Court seeking the appointment of a guardian ad litem and a court order allowing the corrective surgery. The State Court granted the requests, but the Appellate Court reversed both decisions; the New York Supreme Court affirmed the Appellate Court's decision.[70]

Meanwhile, the DHHS had received an anonymous complaint of discrimination that Baby Jane Doe was being denied medical care because of her physical handicaps, thus violating Section 504 of the Rehabilitation Act. The hospital refused requests by the U.S. Surgeon General and the DHHS for access to Baby Jane Doe's medical records. The federal goverment, therefore, filed suit against the hospital in the Eastern District of New York. The District Court ruled that the nontreatment of Baby Jane Doe did not violate Section 504 of the Rehabilitation Act. The Court also refused to require the hospital to disclose Baby Jane Doe's medical records. In February 1984, the Court of Appeals for the Second Circuit upheld the District Court's decision that Section 504 does not apply to treatment decisions involving critically ill newborns.

One month later, the American Medical Association and five other organizations filed suit against the DHHS and Secretary Margaret Heckler challenging the Baby Doe II Rule. In May 1984, the U.S. District Court for the Southern District of New York struck down the Baby Doe II Rule, ruling it to be "invalid, unlawful, and without statutory authority."

Public outcry resulting from the Baby Doe and Baby Jane Doe cases resulted in House and Senate bills from the 98th Congress of the United States seeking to protect handicapped children. On October 9, 1984, President Reagan signed into law the Child Abuse Prevention and Treatment and Adoption Reform Act Amendments, which mandate physicians to provide medically indicated treatment (including hydration, nutrition, and medication) to children with disabilities except when the child is chronically and irreversibly comatose or when the provision of such treatment would merely prolong dying or be virtually futile and inhumane.[74]

After President Reagan signed the Act into law in October, 1984, the DHHS issued final regulations to implement the Child Abuse Amendments and guidelines for the establishment of hospital Infant Care Review Committees. The exemption for treatment which would "merely prolong dying" referred to cases in which death will occur" in the near future" and not to more lingering deaths, such as Tay-Sachs Disease. The exemption for treatment which would be "virtually futile" and "under the circumstances inhumane" referred to cases where treatment involves significant suffering "for an infant highly unlikely to survive." Failure of a state to adhere to the regulations may result in loss of federal child abuse funds.

Medically, legally, and ethically, however, the debate continues. In 1987, a Massachusetts probate court enjoined a hospital from denying mechanical ventilation to an infant with disabilities. The same year a federal district court in Oklahoma denied a motion to dismiss claims for violations of constitutional rights filed on behalf of infants born with myelomeningocele and their parents. The suit was brought by Carlton Johnson, a child born with myelomeningocele who survived despite being denied treatment, advocacy groups, and parents of children with myelomeningocele. It alleged that 24 children died during a 5-year period at Oklahoma Children's Memorial Hospital as a result of physicians' recommendations that treatment be denied based on an evaluation of nonmedical factors, including family finances, projected intellectual capacity, projected ability to walk, geographical location, and political and fiscal matters.

The district court denied a motion to dismiss the plaintiffs' claims that their constitutional rights had been violated, but did dismiss plaintiffs' claims for violation of Section 504 of the Rehabilitation Act of 1973 and for engaging in human experimentation without providing necessary safeguards or obtaining consent.[53]

In re D.H. involved an infant with multiple severe disabilities who was hospitalized for severe pneumonia. Despite vehement objection by the child's mother, the hospital medical staff entered a "no ventilation" order on the chart. The hospital then refused the mother's demand that the order be removed and that her child receive all necessary medical care. Following legal petition by the mother, a Massachusetts probate court enjoined the defendants from entering the order based on its conclusions that "the defendant is committing or threatens to commit . . . irreparable injury to the plaintiff."[53]

Equally alarming is the ruling by a California Court of Appeals in 1982 suggesting that parents could be held liable for damages to their children who were born with handicaps rather than aborted. Two years later, the California Supreme Court agreed that it was no longer state policy that all life was worth living. A North Carolina Court of Appeals took a similar stance in the same year. In 1986 the Colorado Court of Appeals stated: "we are unwilling to say as a matter of law that life even with the most severe and debilitating of impairments is always preferable to non-existence (death)."[54]

The newest legally sanctioned threat to the unborn child, particularly those without disabilities, is the transplantation of fetal tissue (endocrine glands, kidneys, bone marrow, skin, nervous tissue) to adults. Fetal tissues must be obtained from mid-pregnancy (elective late-term abortions). Because of the growing controversy, National Institute of Health researchers were recently denied permission to treat patients with fetal tissue implants until legal and ethical issues can be studied.[75] Legislation has been proposed to ban the sale of body parts and prevent women from designating recipients of fetal tissue.[76]

SEEKING JUDICIAL RULING

Decision-making on behalf of incompetent patients is made even more difficult by the courts' inability to agree amongst themselves which cases need judicial involvement. In *Quinlan,* the New Jersey Supreme Court ruled that:

> We consider that a practice of applying to a court to confirm such decisions would generally be inappropriate, not only because that would be a gratuitous encroachment on the medical profession's field of competence, but because it would be impossibly cumbersome.

Instead, the *Quinlan* Court recommended oversight by hospital ethics committees with judicial review in unusual or exceptionally complicated cases.[14]

The *Saikewicz* Court strongly disagreed, stating[29]:

> We take a dim view of any attempt to shift ultimate decision-making responsibilty away from a duly established court of proper jurisdiction to any committee, panel, or group, ad hoc or permanent. Thus, we reject the approach adopted by the New Jersey Supreme Court in the *Quinlan* case of entrusting the decision whether to continue artificial life support to the patient's guardian, family, attending doctors and hospital "ethics committee.". . . We do not view the judicial resolution of this most difficult and awesome question—whether potentially life-prolonging treatment should be withheld from a person incapable of making his own decision—as constituting a "gratuitous encroachment" on the domain of medical expertise.

The *Saikewicz* ruling has been criticized for being unclear: Did the decision mean that a court presented with such a case should not delegate the resolution to others, or that all non-treatment decisions involving incompetent patients should be made by the courts? Most people initially interpreted the ruling as requiring routine adjudication.

However, *Matter of Dinnerstein* served as clarification of the *Saikewicz* ruling. Shirley Dinnerstein was a 67-year-old woman in a permanent vegetative state. Her family and physician sought court approval to enter a "Do Not Resuscitate" order into her chart. The court ruled that such an order could be entered into her chart without judicial approval and specifically referred to the confusion created by the *Saikewicz* ruling. *Saikewicz* was interpreted as applying only to treatments that could be "administered for the purpose and with some reasonable expectation of effecting a permanent or temporary cure of or relief from the illness or condition being treated." The *Dinnerstein* ruling stated: " 'Prolongation of life,' as used in the *Saikewicz* case, does not mean a mere suspension of the act of dying, but contemplates, at the very least, a remission of symptoms enabling a return towards a normal, functioning, integrated existence.''[77]

A Massachusetts Appellate Court's ruling, *Matter of Spring,* that judicial approval was unnecessary before discontinuing dialysis treatments for an incompetent 78-year-old patient was overruled by the Massachusetts Supreme Court. The latter body agreed with the termination of dialysis in this case (although by now the patient had already died from an unrelated cause), but disapproved of delegating decision-making power to the family and physician, and declared: ''When a court is properly presented with the legal question whether treatment may be withheld, it must decide that question and not delegate it to some private person or group.''[78]

Although the Massachusetts Supreme Court provided a long list of factors for physicians to consider, it failed to specify which factors were sufficient to make prior judicial approval unnecessary. Other states' courts also have made it difficult for physicians to determine when prior judicial approval is needed before termination of some form of medical therapy. For example, in *In re Eichner,* the previously discussed case of Brother Fox, the New York intermediate court directed an elaborate judicial process requiring a minimum of four to six physicians, five attorneys, and a judge before allowing discontinuation of the ventilator. Eichner, the guardian of Fox who sought to have the ventilator discontinued, referred to this elaborate process as ''a lawyer's paradise, not to mention a doctor's bonanza.''[79]

The New York Court of Appeals upheld the decision allowing discontinuation of mechanical ventilation (after the patient was already dead), but rejected the intermediate court's proposed procedures. Instead, this Court decided that:

> Neither the common law nor existing statutes require persons generally to seek prior court assessment of conduct which may subject them to civil and criminal liability. If it is desirable to enlarge the role of the courts in cases involving discontinuance of life-sustaining treatment for incompetents by establishing a mandatory procedure of successive approval by physicians, hospital personnel, relatives, and the courts, the change should come from the legislature.

Because of disagreements in the state court opinions, the President's Commission for the Study of Ethical Problems in Medicine and Biomedical and Behavioral Research recommended the approach suggested in *Quinlan,* that is, decisions made by the physicians and families with review by hospital ethics committees. The Commission noted that litigation is costly, creates long delays, and can seriously strain the relationships between the parties by forcing them into adversarial roles.[61] It remains to be seen if the state courts and legislatures will adopt the Commission's recommendation.

NATURAL DEATH ACTS AND LIVING WILLS

The 1976 California Natural Death Act was the first statute to explicitly authorize an individual to direct, in advance, that life-saving treatment be withdrawn when death is imminent.[80] The act specifically required that an individual must wait at least 14 days from the date that the terminal illness is made known before execution of the document. However, as of 1978, approximately one-half the individuals to whom the act was potentially applicable were comatose before the 14-day waiting period had elapsed and, therefore, could not benefit from it.

By 1987, 38 states and the District of Columbia had Natural Death Acts designed to give legal validation to living wills, that is, to provide a means through which individuals may provide written documentation of their wishes and desires regarding life-supportive therapy should they subsequently become mentally incompetent while terminally ill. The scope of the legislation and the requirements vary from state to state.[35,53,54] As an example, Florida's ''Right to Decline Life-Prolonging Procedures''[81] holds that any competent adult with a terminal illness can, at any time, direct the withdrawal or withholding of life-prolonging procedures. If the individual is physically unable to sign a written statement, the declaration may be given orally. The declarant is responsible for notification of his or her physician of the declaration; if the declarant is unable to give notification, any individual may give notification. The written or oral declaration must be made part of the patient's directive or transfer care of the patient to another physician who is willing to comply with the directive. Unfortunately, what constitutes a terminal illness is not defined.

Originally, living wills were not intended as legally binding documents. The legal power these documents have now attained was recently highlighted by the decision of the Supreme Court of Florida in *John F. Kennedy Memorial Hospital v. Bludworth*. The lower court had ruled that the living will created by a competent person who had later become permanently vegetative could be implemented only by a court order authorizing a court-appointed guardian to consent to nontreatment. The Supreme Court of Florida, recognizing that avoidance of litigation was a major purpose of living wills, ruled that family and physician can agree to withdraw life-sustaining treatments from a permanently vegetative patient without judicial review. The Court directed that the patient's living will be strongly considered in the decision-making process.

The Natural Death Acts of most states do not authorize withdrawal of life-sustaining therapy in patients who are not terminal. In most states, directives to withdraw or withhold life-sustaining treatment come into effect only when the patient's death is imminent, such that treatment would merely prolong or interrupt the process of dying. Thus, the physician who uses a living will to justify withdrawing or withholding life-sustaining treatment from a nonterminal patient with physical and/or mental disability is going beyond the legal (and ethical) boundaries of the Natural Death Acts of most states.[72] In the future, one may expect additional living will legislation and judicial rulings equating the permanently impaired state of consciousness with a terminal condition. This trend will be heatedly protested by those who believe that life is sacred and that there is no life unworthy of life.[21]

In ten states, the living will legislation provides for a hierarchy of surrogate decisionmakers when no living will has been executed.[53] By 1986, 13 states had living will legislation granting proxy decision-making provisions.[33] In addition, all 50 states and the District of Columbia now have statutes authorizing "durable power of attorney," that is, powers of attorney that remain in effect even if the person becomes mentally incompetent. With increasing frequency, these durable power of attorney statutes are being used by private individuals to appoint relatives or friends to make proxy health care decisions should they become incompetent.[53] In 1985, four states had living will laws with proxy provisions for minors.[33]

Some living will statutes specifically state that the implementation of a living will does not constitute suicide, but rather the withdrawal or withholding of futile medical therapy from a terminally ill patient.[82] However, living will requests that medication be administered in quantities sufficient to alleviate suffering, even at the expense of hastening death, are already common. As the scope of living wills continues to increase, and as they become increasingly binding, physicians may find a widening of the chasm between that which is legal and that which the physician believes to be ethical and moral.

A well-organized "vocal minority" is working to secure the "right to die" on demand by lethal injection or overdose. A 1987 California Initiative Statue, euphemistically entitled, "The Humane and Dignified Death Act,"[83] failed to gather the support needed to be put to public vote in November of 1988. The Initiative, which drew national attention as the "Right to Die Act," stated that the

> fundamental right of adult persons to control decisions relating to the rendering of their own medical care, stems from the right of privacy. . . . This includes the decision to have life-sustaining procedures withheld or withdrawn, or, if suffering from a terminally ill condition or being in an irreversibly incompetent state,

> which can cause loss of patient dignity and unnecessary pain and suffering, to have administered "aid-in-dying." . . . "Aid-in-dying" means any medical procedure that will terminate the life of the qualified patient swiftly, painlessly, and humanely. . . . The withholding or withdrawal of the life-sustaining procedures from, or administered aid-in-dying to, a qualified patient in accordance with this title shall not, for any purpose, constitute a suicide. . . .

As of 1987, 22 of the 38 jurisdictions with living will legislation specifically had excluded the provision of nutrition and hydration from the types of life-sustaining procedures that may be withheld or withdrawn pursuant to such declarations. The other sixteen states and the District of Columbia have living will legislation that either equates food and fluids to medical treatment (which can be withdrawn or withheld) or is silent on the matter.[53] Proposed U.S. House of Representative Bill 3109 would prohibit any federally funded health-care facility from withholding hydration and nutrition from a patient if it would result in the patient's death.[37]

Living wills are increasingly being advocated as a means of decreasing the costs of health care for our aging society. It has been suggested that living will forms should be distributed throughout the Veterans Administration Hospitals, so that the "no hope veterans" could be permitted to die, eliminating overcrowding and saving the federal government $2 billion annually.[84] A former head of the Health Care Financing Administration stated that over one-fifth of Medicare expenditures are for persons in their last year of life, and that a national system of living wills would have saved the federal government $1.2 billion in fiscal year 1978.[85]

DO NOT RESUSCITATE ORDERS

Cardiopulmonary resuscitation (CPR), which may include tracheal intubation and initiation of mechanical ventilation, is a form of medical therapy and, therefore, may not be indicated under certain circumstances. This conviction was clearly advanced at the first National Conference on Cardiopulmonary Resuscitation and Emergency Cardiac Care in 1974. The same year, the *Journal of the American Medical Association* published the Standards for Cariopulmonary Resuscitation and Emergency Cardiac Care which proposed that decisions not to attempt cardiopulmonary resuscitation be formally documented in the patient's medical records and communicated to all staff involved in the patient's care. CPR was intended for patients with sudden, unexpected "death" but not for those with terminal illness. However, fear of civil and criminal liability often has caused Do Not Resuscitate or No Code orders to be verbally communicated by physicians but not to be entered in the medical record.[4]

In 1976, Rabkin et al.[86] proposed a method by which orders not to resuscitate may be implemented. The report, which referred to an "irreversibly, irreparably ill patient whose death was imminent," suggested that the medical judgment on the appropriateness of an order not to resuscitate should be made by the primary physician after discussion with an ad hoc committee composed of physicians, nurses, and others. The report also recommended obtaining consent for the order from the patient (if competent) or family (if the patient was incompetent). The patient's terminal condition, the recommendation of the ad hoc committee, the patient's (or family's) consent, and a formal Do Not Resuscitate order should then be clearly recorded in the medical record. Since 80 percent of American deaths occur in hospitals and nursing homes, CPR is not legally or ethically indicated in every circumstance.[36]

In 1987, the Washington State Court of Appeals reviewed a case, *Strickland v. Deaconess Hospital,* which resulted because a physician entered a Do Not Resuscitate order into the patient's chart without his consent. At the time, Mr. Strickland was receiving mechanical ventilation for cardiopulmonary failure. He subsequently improved and was discharged from the hospital. After filing suit for the wrongful entry of the DNR order, Strickland died. The Appellate Court ruled that the claim could not be maintained under the Washington Survival Statute because it was personal to Strickland. The sons of a woman whose marriage to Strickland had been invalidated were co-filers of the suit, but were legally not in the class of individuals who could maintain the action in their own right.[53] Nevertheless, the case serves as a reminder that, at the present time, the mentally competent patient legally (and ethically) must not be excluded from decision-making regarding withholding of CPR.

INFORMED CONSENT AND REFUSAL

The requirement of consent from mentally competent patients for medical therapy, including life-support therapy such as mechanical ventilation, is not a new concept in medicine or law. Early court cases involved failure of physicians to obtain consent (which constitutes the intentional tort of battery) or exceeding the scope of the given consent. As a result of the landmark case of *Canterbury v. Spence* in 1972, the concept has shifted from mere "consent" to "informed consent"; that is, a physician who fails to provide the patient with information sufficient to allow a free and fully informed choice may be found liable in negligence for not meeting the professional standard of care.[48]

The requirement for advance disclosure of risks of medical treatment has resulted in considerable legal debate. Most courts have required the plaintiff to prove that adequate disclosure of the risks of the treatment would have caused a "reasonable person" to refuse treatment. However, other courts have ruled that this objective "reasonable person" standard is too rigid and does not allow an individual's subjective beliefs and values to be considered.[17]

In addition to "informed consent," some courts have dealt with the concept of "informed refusal." Under this doctrine, the physician may be found negligent for failing to inform a patient of the risks of not receiving a particular form of medical therapy. For example, the California Supreme Court recently ruled that a physician may be found negligent for failing to inform a patient of the risks of failing to have a Pap smear to test for cervical cancer.[17]

The legal concepts of "informed consent" and "informed refusal" are applicable whenever mechanical ventilatory support is being considered. Patients have a legal right to be fully informed of the risks of accepting and refusing life-support therapy; many times, however, it is not possible to obtain informed consent from critically ill patients. In general, proxy consent (usually from the family) is required for treatment of the critically ill patient who is unable to give informed consent. In medical emergencies, where consent cannot be obtained but failure to treat will have grave consequences, the law waives the requirement for informed consent and considers consent to be implied by the circumstances. There are two other situations in which fully informed consent is not necessary: (1) the patient may consent to therapy while waiving the right to be fully informed ("waiver"), or (2) the physician may withhold information which may be emotionally harmful to the patient ("therapeutic privilege").[17] The concept of therapeutic privilege is not yet well-defined legally.

REFERENCES

1. Zoll P, Linenthal A, Gibson W, et al: Termination of ventricular fibrillation in man by externally applied electric countershock. N Engl J Med 254:727, 1956
2. Safar P: Mouth-to-mouth airway. Anesthesiology 18:904, 1957
3. Kouwenhoven W, Jude J, Knickerbocker G: Closed-chest cardiac massage. JAMA 173:1064, 1960
4. McIntyre KM: Medicolegal aspects of cardiopulmonary resuscitation and emergency cardiac care. p. 277. In McIntyre KM, Lewis AJ (eds): Textbook of Advanced Cardiac Life Support. American Heart Association, Dallas, 1983
5. Beecher H, Adams R, Barger C, et al: A definition of irreversible coma. JAMA 205:85, 1968
6. Ouaknine G, Kosary IZ, Graham J, et al: Laboratory criteria of brain death. J Neurosurg 39:429, 1973

7. Korein J, Maccario M: On the diagnosis of cerebral death; a prospective study of 55 patients to define irreversible coma. Clin Electroencephalogr 2:178, 1971
8. Ibe K: Clinical and pathophysiological aspects of the intravital brain death. Electroencephalogr Clin Neurophysiol 30:272, 1971
9. Becker D, Robert C, Nelson J, et al: An evaluation of the definition of cerebral death. Neurology (NY) 20:459, 1970
10. Plum F, Posner T: Diagnosis of Stupor and Coma. 2nd Ed. FA Davis, Philadelphia, 1972
11. Ingvar DM, Widen L: Mjarndod-Samm anfattning av ett symposium. Lakartidningen 69:3804, 1972
12. Black P. Brain death. N Engl J Med 299:339, 1978
13. Curran W, Hyg S: Settling the medicolegal issues concerning brain-death statutes: matters of legal ethics and judicial precedent. N Engl J Med 299:32, 1978
14. *In the Matter of Karen Quinlan*. 70 NJ 10, 355 A2d 647, 1976
15. Casem NH: Ethical considerations in critical care. Refresher Courses in Anesthesiology. American Society of Anesthesiologists 5:13, 1977
16. Johnson M: Life Unworthy of Life. The Disability Rag. Jan/Feb:24, 1987
17. Rhoden NK: Deciding about treatment in the ICU. In Benesch K, Abramson NS, Grenvik A, et al (eds): Medicolegal Aspects of Critical Care. Aspen Systems, Rockville, MD, 1986
18. *Roe v. Wade* 410 US 113 (1973)
19. Koop CE: The Right to Live; The Right to Die. Tyndale House, Wheaton, 1976
20. Weber S: Substituted Judgment Doctrine: A Critical Analysis, p. 131. (1985) In Bopp J (ed): Issues in Law and Medicine. Vol. 1. National Legal Center for the Medically Dependent and Disabled, Terre Haute, IN, 1987
21. *In re Eichner,* AD2d, 637 E, March 28, 1980, Supreme Court: Appellate Division Second Department
22. *Newman v. William Beaumont Army Medical Center,* No. EP-86-CA-276, W.D. Tex. Oct 30, 1986, reviewed in Nota Bene, Vol. 3. Issues Law Med 3:67, 1987
23. *Matter of Claire Conroy,* 464 A2d 303 NJ App, 1983
24. *In re Grant,* No. 52609–5 (Wash. Sup. Ct., Dec 10, 1987), reviewed in Issues Law Med 3:333, 1988
25. *University Health Services, Inc. v. Robert Piazzi, David Hadden, and the Division of Family and Children Resources of the State of Georgia and Samuel G. Nicholson,* Civil Action file NO. CV86-RCCV-464 Superior Court of Richmond County, State of Georgia, reviewed in Issues Law Med 2:415, 1987
26. *Rasmussen v. Fleming,* 741 P 2d 674 (Ariz 1987), reviewed in Nota Bene, *Rasmussen v. Fleming*. Issues Law Med 3:297, 1987
27. *In re Peter,* 108 NJ 365, 529 A2d 419 (1987), reviewed in Nota Bene, *In re Peter*. Issues Law Med 3:175, 1987
28. *In re Jobes,* 108 NH 394, 529 A2d 434 (1987), reviewed in Nota Bene, *In re Jobes*. Issues Law Med 3:183, 1987
29. *In re Quackenbush,* 156 NJ Super, 282, 283 A2d 785, 1978
30. *School Board of Nassau County, Florida v. Arline*. Issues Law Med 3:334, 1988
31. America on Drugs. U.S. News and World Report p. 48. July 28, 1986
32. Alexander L: Medical science under dictatorship. N Engl J Med 241:39, 1949
33. Shewmon DA: Active voluntary euthanasia: a needless pandora's box. Issues Law Med 3:219, 1987
34. Schepens P: Euthanasia: our own future? Issues Law Med 3:371, 1988
35. Garbesi GC: The law of assisted suicide. Issues Law Med 3:93, 1987
36. Gibson CD: Perimortal initiatives: issues in foregoing life-sustaining treatment, suicide, and assisted suicide. Issues Law Med 3:29, 1987
37. Medical/Legal Briefs. Healing Ethic 1:3, 1988
38. *Severns v. Wilmington Medical Center, Inc.* 421 A2d 1334, Del Superior, 1980
39. *In re Farrell,* reviewed in Nota Bene. Issues Law Med 3:171, 1987
40. *In re Farrell,* reviewed in Issues Law Med 3:333, 1988
41. *In the Matter of Beverly Requena,* reviewed in Nota Bene. Issues Law Med 3:75, 1987
42. *In re Jane Doe,* reviewed in Issues Law Med 3:345, 1988
43. American Academy of Medical Ethics: AIDS and the future. Healing Ethic 2:1, 1988
44. Marzuk PM, Tierner H, Tardiff K, et al: Increased risk of suicide in persons with AIDS. JAMA 259:1333, 1988

45. *Rodas v. ErkenBrack,* reviewed in Nota Bene. Issues Law Med 2:481, 1987
46. *In re Rodas,* reviewed in Issues Law Med 2:471, 1987
47. U.S. Constitution, Amendment XIV, Section 1
48. Bopp J: Is assisted suicide constitutionally protected? Issues Law Med 3:113, 1987
49. *In re Rodas,* reviewed in Issues Law Med 3:333, 1988
50. *Bouvia v. Superior Court,* reviewed in Issues Law Medicine 3:93, 1987
51. *Bouvia v. Superior Court,* reviewed in Issues Law Med 3:219, 1987
52. *Bouvia v. Superior Court,* reviewed in Issues Law Med 3:3, 1987
53. National Legal Center Staff: Medical treatment for older people and people with disabilities: 1987 developments. Issues Law Med 3:333, 1988
54. Wardle LD: Sanctioned assisted suicide: separate but equal treatment for the new illegitimates. Issues Law Med 3:245, 1987
55. *Superintendent of Belchertown State School v. Saikewicz,* Massachusetts Supreme Judicial Court No. 5JC-711, 1977
56. *In re Storar,* 52 NY2d 363, 420, NE2d 64, 1981
57. Guidelines for Euthanasia, Royal Netherlands Society for the Promotion of Medicine and Recovery, Interest Society for Nurses and Nursing Aids (transl. by Walter Lagerwey). Issues Law Med 3:429, 1988
58. Bopp J: Preface. Issues Law Med 3:4, 1988
59. *In re Milton,* reviewed in Nota Bene. Issues Law Med 3:71, 1987
60. *State Department of Human Services v. Northern,* 563 SW2d 197, Tenn, 1978
61. Decision to Forego Life-Sustaining Treatment: Ethical, Medical and Legal Issues in Treatment Decisions. President's Commission for the Study of Ethical Problems in Medicine and Biomedical and Behavioral Research. U.S. Government Printing Office, Washington, D.C., 1983
62. Reagan RW: Abortion and the Conscience of the Nation. Thomas Nelson, Nashville, TN, 1984
63. Duff RS, Campbell AGM: Moral and Ethical Dilemmas in the Special Care Nursery. N Engl J Med 289:890, 1973
64. *John F. Kennedy Memorial Hospital v. Heston,* 48 NJ 576, 279 A2d 670, 1971
65. *In re Seiferth,* 309 NY 80, 127 NE2d 820 (1955)
66. *In re Green,* 12 *Crime and Delinquency* 377 (Child Div. Milwaukee County Ct, Wis 1966)
67. *Custody of a Minor,* 393 NE2d 836 (Mass 1979) and 434 NE2d 601, 607 (Mass 1982)
68. Koop CE: Ethical and Surgical Considerations in the Care of the Newborn with Congenital Abnormalities. p. 89. In Horan D, Delahoyde M (eds): Infanticide and the Handicapped Newborn. Brigham Young University, Provo, UT, 1982
69. German doctors and the final role. New York Times Magazine, Sept 21, 1986
70. Shapiro RS, Fader JE: Critically Ill Infants. In Benesch K, Abramson NS, Grenvik A, Meisel A (eds): Medicolegal Aspects of Critical Care. Aspen Systems, Rockville MD, 1986
71. Koop CE: The slide to Auschwitz. p. 41. In Reagan RW (ed): Abortion and the Conscience of the Nation. Thomas Nelson, Nashville, TN, 1984
72. Register SD: Important Legal Decisions in Critical Care. p. 1657. In Civetta JM, Taylor RW, Kriby RR (eds): Critical Care. JB Lippincott, Philadelphia, 1988
73. Strain E: The American Academy of Pediatrics comments on the "Baby Doe II" regulations. N Engl J Med 309:403, 1983
74. Hahn H: Public policy and disabled infants: a sociopolitical perspective. Issues Law Med 3:3 1987
75. Brave New World Upon Us? Christian Action Council Newsl 12(3): May 15, 1988
76. Sherman: The Selling of Body Parts, reviewed in Healing Ethic 1:3, 1988
77. *In re Dinnerstein,* 380 NE2d 134, Mass App Ct, 1978
78. *Matter of Spring,* 405 NE2d 115, Mass, 1980
79. Kirby RR: Ethics, law, and medicine: termination of life support and mechanical ventilation. p. 293. In Kirby RR, Smith RA, Desautels D (eds): Mechanical Ventilation. Churchill Livingstone, New York, 1985
80. 1976 Cal Stat, Chapter 1439 (Natural Death Act), Sept 30, 1976
81. Life-Prolonging Procedure Act of Florida, Ch 765 FS, 1985
82. Velasquez MG: Defining suicide. Issues Law Med 3:37, 1987
83. The Humane and Dignified Death Act, 5A 87 RF 0048. (personal communication)
84. V.F. Sullivan (Executive Director of American Euthanasia Foundation), letter to the White House. Excerpts read by Joseph Mauro before

the Judiciary Committee of the Maryland White House of Delegates concerning bills HB 764 and SB 596, March 12, 1975. Quoted in Shewmon DA: Active voluntary euthanasia: a needless Pandora's box. Issues Law Med 3:219, 1987
85. R. Derzon (Administrator, Health Care Financing Administration, U.S. Department of Health, Education, and Welfare), Memorandum on Additional Cost-Saving Initiatives, June 4, 1977. Quoted in Shewmon DA: Active voluntary euthanasia: a needless Pandora's box. Issues Law Med 3:219, 1987
86. Rabkin MT, Gillerman G, Rice NR: Orders not to resuscitate. N Engl J Med 295:364, 1976

14

Outcome

Tina E. Banner
Robert R. Kirby

The reputed success or failure of any therapy depends on an analysis of the outcome of treated patients. Analyses may incorporate mortality data, including short- and long-term survival, length of hospitalization, complications, quality of life, and other variables too numerous even to list. Such studies are notoriously difficult to perform, are subject to all sorts of investigational biases and variables, which are nearly impossible to control and are almost always challenged with regard to accuracy, adequacy of the study population, statistical analysis, and the methods employed.

Respiratory care in general and mechanical ventilatory support specifically are among the most difficult clinical entities to evaluate. Use of the term *mechanical ventilation* tends to obscure the fact that ventilators and ventilator techniques are vastly different. There probably is as much difference between high-frequency oscillation (HFO) and intermittent mandatory ventilation (IMV) as there is between conventional intermittent positive-pressure ventilation (IPPV) and spontaneous breathing. Yet HFO, IMV, and IPPV are all referred to generically as mechanical ventilation. Small wonder then, that the effects of therapy are so difficult to assess.

Contributing to this problem is the fact that relatively few "ventilator patients" are afflicted with only respiratory insufficiency. Consider a motor vehicle accident victim with a pulmonary contusion and flail chest, a ruptured spleen, fractured femur, and closed head injury, who 5 days following admission to the hospital develops gram-negative sepsis followed rapidly by disseminated intravascular coagulation (DIC) and renal failure. When the patient dies (as he almost certainly will), who can assess what role his initial respiratory insufficiency played and whether the ventilator support was of any value? Multiple organ failure (MOF) obviously complicates any outcome analysis.

In only two conditions has the role played by respiratory care techniques in improving survival been clearly documented. Before 1952, the mortality of paralytic poliomyelitis was 87 percent. In 1952, an epidemic of polio beset Denmark and, in a 4-month period, 2,722 patients were admitted to the Hospital for Communicable Diseases in Copenhagen.[1] Initial therapy employed a single iron lung and several cuirass ventilators. Twenty-seven of the first 31 patients who required assisted ventilation succumbed within 3 days. Thereafter, therapy was converted to tracheotomy and positive-pressure manual or mechanical ventilation. A subsequent reduction in mortality from 87 percent to 40 percent followed.

Some 20 years later, Gregory and colleagues[2] introduced continuous positive airway pressure (CPAP) for the treatment of hyaline membrane disease (HMD). Before that time, the mortality of infants with HMD who required mechanical ventilation was 80 percent or greater. For infants less than 1,000 g, mortality approached 100 percent. By contrast, survival of the CPAP-treated babies was 70 percent, a result that led to a complete revamping in the subsequent therapy of this and other forms of infantile respiratory failure.

The discerning reader will note that both poliomyelitis and HMD basically are single organ failure disease processes. Clinicians, are therefore faced with a relatively simple management problem compared with that of a patient with MOF. In such circumstances, the role played by the support technique can be evaluated. Although such an evaluation relies on historical controls (always suspect), the conclusions regarding the impact of therapy on survival seem fully justified. We are aware of no other type of respiratory failure to which a similar analysis can be applied with as much precision.

Rather arbitrarily, we have chosen a relatively well-defined period of time, 1960 to the present, over which to evaluate outcome. Our reasons are simple. Before 1960, the major form of respiratory failure for which good information is available was poliomyelitis. The results of therapy in this entity are well known. Also, in 1958, the first respiratory care units for the treatment of disease other than polio were established in North America (Toronto and Baltimore), and their early therapeutic results were published in 1961.[3,4] Finally, the modern approach to mechanical ventilation began during the early 1960s, as did a new era of ventilator design.

ACUTE RESPIRATORY FAILURE

The Early Years: 1960 to 1974

The earliest papers providing useful information on survival were those of Safar et al.[3] and Fairley.[4] Safar's group reported a 2-year study of the ventilatory management of 224 surgical patients with postoperative complications, head injury, burns, and chest injury, of whom 74 (33 percent) died. An additional 267 medical patients also were treated for a variety of conditions, including pulmonary edema, pneumonia, cerebrovascular accident, sepsis, emphysema, and polio. Ninety-six (43 percent) died. Overall mortality was 36 percent. Safar's work is critically important for its historical impact, because it established many of the principles of modern respiratory care and was the forerunner of critical care medicine. However, a detailed evaluation of the specific ventilator techniques and complications was not presented in this early publication.

Fairley's work is of equal importance.[4] He outlined the indications for ventilator support and discussed the use of muscle relaxants as an adjunct to mechanical ventilation. Mortality in the Toronto respiratory unit was approximately 26 percent overall but was 40 percent for surgical patients. However, only 28 patients were reported in the latter group. Both Safar and Fairley emphasized the importance of a centralized area for the treatment of respiratory insufficiency.

In 1969, Asmundsson and Kilburn[5] reported their experience with 239 episodes of respiratory failure in 146 patients with chronic respiratory insufficiency. This report covered a 4-year period from 1963 to 1967. Sixty percent of the patients survived the first episode, and 55 percent were alive after 6 months. However, only 20 percent of these survivors were alive at 30 and 48 months. Their findings suggested that increasing age, decreased weight (below 110 lb), anemia, and edema were associated with a poor prognosis. Pressure-cycled Bird Mark 7 ventilators were used to control ventilation in 64 episodes, assist it in 54, and intermittently assist in the remaining 121. This paper was one of the first to demonstrate the importance of looking at both short- and long-term mortality.

By 1972, the Task Force on Problems, Research, Approaches, and Needs for Respiratory Disease of the National Heart and Lung Institute[6] reported that acute hypoxic respiratory failure occurred in 150,000 patients annually in the United States, with 40,000 (27 percent) deaths resulting. This figure of 150,000 is still quoted almost 20 years later, although the population increase that has occurred during the intervening period would suggest that the current incidence probably is much higher.

Also in 1972, Rogers et al.[7] reviewed their experience in the treatment of 212 patients with respiratory failure with mechanical ventilation from 1965 to 1968 (prior to the establishment of a respiratory care unit). They compared their results with those involving the first 200 patients treated in the unit which opened in 1969. In the first group, 134 patients (63 percent) died. The highest mortality occurred in those patients with associated conditions (uremia, heart disease, tetanus), while the lowest mortality (22 percent) was in postcardiopulmonary bypass patients; 126 of the 134 patients who died were still receiving mechanical ventilation at the time of their demise. In this group, age below 60 was not a factor, but the type of ventilator appeared to be significant. Mortality was 75 percent in those patients treated with pressure-cycled (Bird) ventilators; it was 50 percent when time-cycled ventilators (Emerson, Engström) were employed; and it was 41 percent in those patients treated by both types.

Overall mortality in the second group of 200 patients was reduced to 18 percent. The highest mortality (40 percent) occurred in pneumonia patients. Only 36 percent of those who died were thought to have succumbed from respiratory causes. Here, then, was one of the first suggestions to note that patients die "with" respiratory failure, as well as "of" respiratory failure. A drawback to this paper is that the study groups were different with respect to the causes of respiratory failure. For example, there were fewer postoperative patients in the second group. Also, an increased use of other therapy such as low-flow oxygen, chest physiotherapy, postural drainage, and nasotracheal suctioning was initiated in the second group. These problems notwithstanding, this report confirmed those of Safar et al.[3] and Fairley[4] with respect to the importance of a centralized unit approach to the management of respiratory failure.

Petty et al.[8] reported the results of treatment of 18,077 consecutive patients who received mechanical ventilatory support for the 10-year period from 1964 to 1974. Overall survival was 75 percent and did not change appreciably during the last 5 years of this period. Included were all adult patients admitted to the surgical or medical intensive respiratory care modules at the University of Colorado. No patients were treated "on the wards." The poorest survival occurred in trauma patients (59 percent), those who sustained cerebrocardiovascular catastrophe (57 percent), and miscellaneous causes including cardiac arrest (50 percent). These data suggested, once again, that respiratory failure, per se, was not the proximate cause of death in many patients.

The Later Years: 1975 to the Present

The early studies of respiratory failure outcome and the results of mechanical ventilation were global in nature. They were, to a large extent, concerned with the establishment of centralized respiratory care units and basic principles of care. While they reported mortality, they did not, in many instances, address the actual causes or contributory factors which ultimately resulted in death. Later, as care became more sophisticated and ventilator support escalated, the continued high mortality (19 to 80 percent, with an average of about 50 percent) became a major source of concern. Investigators began to examine closely the specific reasons that patients died.

Multiple Organ Failure

From September 1975 to March 1977, a multi-institutional study was conducted to compare the efficacy of extracorporeal membrane oxygenation (ECMO) to conventional mechanical ventilation for the management of patients with acute respiratory failure.[9] A total of 90 patients (42 ECMO, 48 ventilator) were studied. Mortality in both groups was approximately 90 percent.

An additional 490 patients between the ages of 12 and 65 years did not meet the entry criteria for the ECMO study but were followed, nevertheless, to assess outcome.[10] A striking relationship was noted between death and MOF (Table

14–1). Overall mortality was 66 percent. The contribution of MOF, which had been suggested earlier, was confirmed most impressively in this study. The effect of increasing age also was noteworthy. For 196 patients over 65 years of age, the mortality increased to 81 percent.

The impact of sepsis, which obviously is responsible for MOF in a significant number of patients, was evaluated by Montgomery et al.[11] Mortality was 68 percent in 47 patients with adult respiratory distress syndrome (ARDS) compared with 35 percent in a control group without ARDS. Only 5 of the 32 ARDS deaths (16 percent) were judged to have resulted from irreversible respiratory failure. Of the 22 patients with ARDS who died after 3 days, 16 (73 percent) had probable sepsis syndrome, a sixfold increase compared with the control group.

Bell et al.[12] evaluated the role of MOF and infection in 37 consecutive survivors of ARDS and in 47 nonsurvivors on whom autopsies were performed. The results of their study are summarized in Table 14–2. All patients with bacteremia and a clinically identified site of infection that could be treated survived. By contrast, those with bacteremia and no identifiable source of infection uniformly died. Multiple organ system failure was present in 93 percent of infected patients compared with only 47 percent of those who were not infected.

Cancer

Of even greater apparent significance is the effect of cancer on the mortality of acute respiratory failure. Schuster and Marion[13] reviewed the records of 77 patients with hematologic malignancy admitted to a medical intensive care unit (ICU). Hypotension and acute respiratory failure were the reasons for admission in 75 percent, but shock rather than refractory hypoxemia was the predominant cause of death. Nevertheless, only 4 of 52 patients who required mechanical ventilation survived to hospital discharge.

Table 14-1. Mortality and MOF in Acute Respiratory Failure

Number of systems involved	< 65 Years	> 65 Years
1 (Isolated pulmonary)	40	68
2	54	78
3	72	91
4	84	96
5	100	—

(Data from Bartlett et al.[10])

Table 14-2. Infection and Survival in ARDS

Infection Site	No. of patients	No. of survivors
Pulmonary	20	8
Body cavities/soft tissue	10	4
Disseminated/immunosuppressed	5	0

(Data from Bell et al.[12])

Cox's findings were similar in a multidisciplinary ICU.[14] Ninety-eight patients who required mechanical ventilation for more than 72 hours were studied. Patients with malignancy were compared with those with nonmalignant disease. The combination of malignancy and acute respiratory failure resulted in a 100 percent mortality if the clinical course was complicated by one additional organ system failure. Patients with only respiratory failure had a 40 percent mortality. In contrast to Bartlett's study,[10] age did not appear to be a factor.

These findings were similar to earlier reports by Goldiner et al.[15] and Snow et al.[16] In Goldiner's report,[15] the mortality of patients with Hodgkin's lymphoma and acute respiratory failure was 96 percent. Patients in Snow's study[16] had a slightly better outcome. Of the 180 cancer patients who required mechanical ventilation, 26 percent survived to extubation, while 13 percent and 7 percent, respectively, were alive at 2 and 6 months. Snow et al. commented that long-term survival was poor, but immediate survival was comparable to that of other non-cancer patients with respiratory failure.

Hauser et al.[17] examined the medical records of 40 patients with cancer and 684 patients without cancer admitted to their medical ICU over a 13-month period from 1978 to 1980. Patients with cancer had a 55 percent mortality compared with only 17 percent for those without. The mortality of patients with both cancer and acute respiratory failure was 75 percent, whereas those patients with respiratory failure but no cancer had only a 25 percent mortality. If respiratory failure was characterized as ARDS, the mortality in the cancer patients increased to 86 percent. However, this value was statistically no different from the mortality of patients with cancer but non-ARDS failure (60 percent) or noncancer patients with ARDS (65 percent). They concluded that a decision to apply mechanical ventilation and critical care should not be based on the presence or absence of cancer. This conclusion was opposite that of Schuster and Marion,[13] who viewed the outlook for patients with hematologic malignancy and respiratory failure as uniformly grim.

A shortcoming of Hauser's study was that the long-term mortality rates were not available. Survival was defined as unit discharge in stable condition with a reasonable expectation of hospital discharge. The actual discharge rate, however, was not reported.

CHRONIC OBSTRUCTIVE PULMONARY DISEASE

A vexing problem traditionally viewed as having a particularly bad outcome is the occurrence of acute exacerbation of chronic obstructive pulmonary disease (COPD). However, the results of therapy in this area appear to be better than has been assumed. Hudson[18] reported that from 1968 to 1973, the overall mortality of 914 patients who sustained acute respiratory failure superimposed on their underlying COPD was only 28 percent.[5,19–24]

If mechanical ventilation was necessary, mortality increased to 49 percent. In the two large series reported after 1974,[25,26] the mortality of nonmechanically ventilated patients decreased to 7 percent. Again, however, of the 29 patients reported who were treated with mechanical ventilation, it increased to 30 percent.[19]

Hudson[18] believed that the most important variable associated with increased mortality included the severity of the acute respiratory failure, including a pHa below 7.25; and the development of complications such as nosocomial pneumonia.

Although mechanically ventilated patients had a higher mortality, the precise role of this therapy as a causative factor is difficult to ascertain for several reasons. First, the decision to use a ventilator, as often as not, is purely subjective. Second, ''conservative'' treatment may be continued for too long a period before ventilator therapy is finally begun. Thus, any chance of success with the more aggressive treatment can be lost. Third, patients selected for mechanical ventilator support are often sicker than those for whom such therapy is not used. The more severe nature of the disease rather than the choice of therapy may be responsible for patients' failure to survive.

Hudson's review of the nine reported series (1968 to 1982) involving acute exacerbation of COPD is summarized in Table 14–3.

Table 14-3. Survival in Acute Exacerbations of COPD

Series	Year	Mortality (%)	Ventilated (%)	Mortality in those ventilated (%)
Vandenberg et al.[19]	1968	22	10	50
Asmundsson and Kilburn[5]	1969	32	49	—
Sluiter et al.[20]	1972	34	68	46
Moser et al.[21]	1973	30	—	—
Kettel[22]	1973	26	17	80
Burk and George[23]	1973	26	44	42
Seriff et al.[24]	1973	28	—	—
Bone et al.[25]	1978	7	24	30
Martin et al.[26]	1982	6	—	—

(Data from Hudson.[18])

MECHANICAL VENTILATION

The difficulties in assessing outcome in general already have been discussed. In a book dealing primarily with ventilator strategies in the treatment of respiratory failure, we are interested in two principal issues. First, is the therapy beneficial, and, second, is it harmful? The first subject has been discussed in some detail. The second requires careful evaluation.

The term *mechanical ventilation* covers a wide range of divergent approaches to respiratory care. Such therapy is applied to many conditions which do not represent respiratory failure in the sense that we have discussed in this chapter. Thus, intraoperative and postoperative ventilatory support administered until the depressant effects of anesthetics and muscle relaxant drugs have been reversed are different from the treatment of ARDS.

With respect to respiratory failure (acute or chronic), the following general statements seem reasonable:

1. Mechanical ventilation does not cure any form of respiratory insufficiency.
2. Such therapy can support life until the primary disease process has been corrected (i.e., treatment of pneumonia with antibiotics).
3. No evidence establishes the superiority of any specific mechanical ventilatory technique in terms of reducing mortality.
4. Evidence does support the view that some techniques are associated with fewer adverse effects than others.

The first of these considerations is self-evident. Even the successful reduction of mortality in poliomyelitis so clearly demonstrated by investigators such as Anderson and Ibsen[1] and Engström[27] did not represent a cure or reversal of disease but rather a means to offset the devastating respiratory consequences. In essence, such support is an example of the second statement, except that poliomyelitis, unlike pneumonia, ARDS, drug overdose, Guillain-Barré syndrome, et cetera, is not reversible.

The lack of demonstrated superiority of one ventilatory technique (or, for that matter, a particular ventilator) is discussed in detail in Chapters 7, 8, and 9. This observation does not imply that in a given individual's hands, no difference in performance or perhaps even outcome may be demonstrable. In such a case, however, we are dealing with familiarity, experience, bias, or institutional parochialism rather than an intrinsic or innate advantage of the instrument or method.

Our personal view is that ventilators and ventilatory techniques usually can produce gas exchange satisfactory enough to support life in most patients. Thus we agree with what appears to be the prevalent view that death from refractory hypoxemia is unusual—patients usually die *with* respiratory failure, not *of* it. We suspect that terminal, mechanically ventilated patients are dealt with similarly and that few, if any, discernible differences in techniques are evident. The decision to employ one form of therapy or another perhaps should result from perceived differences in the adverse effects of the approaches in question.

Cardiovascular Depression

Cournand and associates[28] were among the first to describe the adverse effects of IPPV on cardiac output. Transmission of pressure to the pleural space resulted in a reduction of venous return, stroke volume, and cardiac output. When they reduced the inspiratory phase to no more than one-third the total respiratory cycle, this adverse effect was decreased. Later studies showed that this problem was exacerbated by hypovolemia and could be catastrophic.

Early attempts to minimize this phenomenon included the description by Maloney et al.[29] of a "negative" (subambient) pressure applied to the airway during the ventilator exhalation phase. The hope was that transmission of the reduced pressure to the pleural space would enhance venous return. This supposition was never borne out in clinical practice. Assisted (patient-triggered) ventilation (AV) also was thought to be potentially beneficial in this regard, since the initial inspiratory effort would produce a transient decrease of intrapleural pressure (Ppl). Once again, however, careful laboratory and clinical investigations did not substantiate this impression, and cardiovascular function was affected to the same degree with both AV and controlled mechanical ventilation (CMV).

During the early 1970s, Kirby et al.[30,31] and Downs et al.[32] introduced IMV for the treatment of respiratory failure in infants and adults, respectively. Because spontaneous breathing was an integral part of this technique, fewer high-pressure, large tidal volume breaths were delivered by the ventilator. At the same time, spontaneous inspiration was associated with a sustained reduction of Ppl. The result overall was a substantial enhancement of venous return and cardiac output, even when positive end-expiratory pressure (PEEP) was used at high levels.[33,34]

High-frequency ventilation (HFV) also has been reported to have minimal effects on the circulation because of a reduction in tidal volume (VT) and peak airway pressure (PAW).[35,36] In some instances, this observation appears to have been confirmed, but in other studies, no improvement in cardiovascular function can be demonstrated compared with IMV.

Airway pressure release ventilation (APRV) is associated with significant reduction in peak and mean airway pressures compared to all other forms of mechanical ventilation, including IMV. Presumably, such reductions should be beneficial to the circulation, but this possibility has not been tested sufficiently to establish its clinical relevance.

In summary, it is possible to minimize the adverse impact of conventional AV and CMV on cardiovascular function through the use of alternative modes such as IMV and possibly HFV and APRV. If the patient's condition does not otherwise preclude such therapy, its use appears to be indicated. A word of caution is necessary, however. Significant reductions in Ppl during spontaneous breathing can increase left ventricular afterload.[37] In patients with severe left ventricular dysfunction, IMV or any spontaneous breathing technique that uses equipment associated with large "negative" swings in Ppl is potentially detrimental.[38] Therefore, the theoretically beneficial effects of such therapy can be offset by its inapproriate clinical application.

Recently, an ominous cardiovascular complication was reported with HFV.[39] A multi-institutional study was designed to test the efficacy of HFO in reducing the incidence of bronchopulmonary dyplasia (BPD) compared with conventional mechanical ventilation. Originally scheduled to incorporate 1,430 infants, it was terminated prematurely after only 673 infants were enrolled, when it became apparent that BPD occurred equally in the two study groups. Of significance, however, was the fact that grades 3 and 4 intraventricular hemorrhage occurred in 26 percent of the HFO-treated infants versus only 18 percent of the conventionally treated ones ($P = 0.02$). The incidence of periventricular leukomalacia also was much higher in the HFO groups than in the conventional group (12 percent versus 7 percent; $P = 0.05$). The HIFI Study Group postulated that the near-constant mean airway pressure associated with HFO may have restricted venous return to the heart, thereby increasing intracerebral blood pressure, decreasing cerebral blood flow, and increasing the tendency toward intracranial bleeding. (See Ch. 7, p. 210 for further discussion of this study).

Pulmonary Barotrauma

The factors responsible for cardiovascular depression also predispose to pulmonary barotrauma. Therefore, an attempt to reduce the frequency of large, high-pressure tidal volumes is a useful strategy. The overall incidence of barotrauma has been reduced by IMV in both infants and adults.[40] The aforementioned study,[39] which demonstrated a higher incidence of intracranial hemorrhage in infants treated with HFO, also revealed an increase of pneumoperitoneum of pulmonary origin in the HFO-treated babies. However, an earlier report by Carlon et al.[41] reported no difference in barotrauma in adults with ARDS treated with high-frequency jet ventilation (HFJV) and IMV.

Work of Breathing

The work of breathing during mechanical ventilation never received much attention until patients began to breathe spontaneously with IMV. Before that time, it was assumed that such work was minimal to nonexistent with AV or CMV. However, a study by Marini et al.[42] has shown that the total work performed by the patient during AV may be greater than that required for lung-thorax ventilation because of poorly designed circuitry, insensitive triggering mechanisms, and delay in attaining high ventilator gas flows.

Similar increases in work of breathing can occur with IMV because of inadequate demand flow regulators,[43] the use of flow-resistor PEEP valves,[44,45] and poorly designed ventilator circuits.[46] Accordingly, an understanding of the equipment used and its design limitations is essential to minimize the external work of breathing superimposed on that resulting from the disease process.

PEEP/CPAP

Few topics have generated more controversy with respect to outcome than PEEP. There is little dispute that PEEP, when used in appropriately selected patients, increases functional residual capacity (FRC), decreases intrapulmonary shunting, and increases PaO_2. Considerable debate exists as to whether survival is improved, however, and many investigators believe that complications such as cardiovascular depression and barotrauma are increased.

For reasons discussed at the beginning of this chapter, it is unlikely that the survival benefit of PEEP/CPAP can be established in adults with respiratory failure. Thus, one must take a practical approach in evaluating the merits of such therapy. If a patient is hypoxemic, and the hypoxemia cannot be corrected with conservative measures, there seems to be little reason to withhold therapy that will predictably raise the PaO_2. The patient may still die, as is quite obvious from the information already presented. However, in cases with severe hypoxemia, that outcome is almost certain if an intervention with PEEP is not attempted. Thus, arguments as to whether such therapy ultimately is beneficial represent academic snobbery at its worst.

Although described as early as 1912, PEEP burst forth on the medical community in full force following the publications by Ashbaugh et al.[47,48] in 1967 and 1969 and the landmark article by Gregory et al.[2] in 1971. Early work focused primarily on the pulmonary effects of increased airway pressures, but later studies began to examine other areas including methods by which PEEP could be titrated to reach an optimal or best level.[33,49–51] In addition, the importance of maintaining cardiovascular function received increasing attention, together with recommendations as to how best this goal might be achieved.

From their inception, PEEP/CPAP were viewed by many clinicians as having potentially devastating complications. These were thought to be much the same as those associated with mechanical ventilation, although almost no evidence supported these concerns.

Cardiovascular Depression

Numerous studies have confirmed that when used appropriately, PEEP/CPAP are not major cardiovascular depressants.[53,55] When adverse effects do occur,[33,50] they are almost always reversible by aggressive fluid administration and by the correction of hypovolemia (which may be unmasked by PEEP).[33,34,56,57] As with any form of therapy, inappropriate use can be problematic. Thus, the use of high PEEP in patients with severe COPD is contraindicated. Not only will the basic problems not be resolved, but severe complications will probably result.

Pulmonary Barotrauma

Air leaks also are no more frequent in patients treated with PEEP/CPAP.[58,59] One of the problems in the analysis of the specific role played by such therapy is that it is almost always used in conjunction with mechanical ventilation. Thus, the effects of PEEP/CPAP are at least additive, and ascertaining which factor is directly responsible for a pneumothorax or other form of barotrauma is next to impossible.

Work of Breathing

Since most patients treated with PEEP/CPAP, independently or in combination with mechanical ventilation, breathe spontaneously, the work of breathing is important. The same factors previously discussed with respect to breathing with IMV are operative here as well.[43–45] Poor circuit design and improper equipment contribute to most problems. Another factor of importance is that some patients are incapable of maintaining a satisfactory level of spontaneous ventilation. To force them to attempt to do so, even with the best of systems, makes no sense whatsoever from a medical standpoint. Airway pressure release ventilation appears to be useful in such cases.

IATROGENIC COMPLICATIONS

Many of the adverse effects described in the preceding sections can occur even when mechanical ventilatory support and PEEP/CPAP are appropriately managed. Other situations arise, however, in which the management strategy chosen is so obviously wrong that severe, even life-threatening, complications are predictable. In such cases, the therapy is the direct cause of the problem and falls into the category of iatroepidemics described by Robin.[60] A brief description of two such problems follows.

Patent Ductus Arteriosus

Uncomplicated HMD generally is self-limited and resolves, with proper care, in 3 to 5 days. Mechanical ventilation and PEEP are the mainstays of therapy to correct the hypoxemia, which is initiated by surfactant deficiency and atelectasis. Intact survival is the rule (as high as 95 percent in babies above 1,500 g birthweight). A frequently associated complication, however, is patent ductus arteriosus (PDA) with a resultant left-to-right intrapulmonary shunt that may predispose to heart failure.

Failure to monitor the effects of therapy can result in gradual overinflation of the lungs and a marked increase of pulmonary vascular resistance. Right ventricular afterload is increased and as a result, a reversal of shunt flow through the PDA occurs. The effects of this cardiovascular shunt are indistinguishable from that associated with atelectasis so far as oxygenation is concerned. An inexperienced clinician faced with this situation assumes that the progressive hypoxemia that results is a reflection of deteriorating lung function, and responds by increasing the ventilator rate, V_T, and PEEP, singly or in combination. This intervention can do nothing but make the situation worse, ultimately turning a serious but reversible problem into one which results in the patient's death.

It has been suggested that persistent fetal circulation (persistent pulmonary hypertension of the newborn), when it occurs in the manner described, is an entirely iatrogenic complication, not a natural progression of the primary disease process; Gluck holds that HMD that persists for longer than 3 to 5 days is no longer a problem of surfactant deficiency but rather of a PDA that has remained open, almost without exception, because of inappropriate use of positive-pressure ventilatory support (Gluck L: personal communication, 1989). While this viewpoint is no doubt opposed by many neonatologists, we believe it probably is true in a majority of cases.

Inappropriate Equipment Selection

This subject has been addressed earlier, but is so important that it deserves additional emphasis. Several studies over the past few years have delineated specific design flaws of commercially available ventilator equipment. These include (but are not limited to) inadequate sensing devices for AV and IMV[42,43] and high flow-resistant PEEP valves.[44] Such problems could be easily corrected but, for a variety of reasons (known only to themselves), manufacturers frequently have failed to do so.

Clinicians nevertheless continue to use this marginally acceptable equipment, forcing their patients to submit to therapy that is suboptimal at best and dangerous at worst. In view of the fact that the deficiencies have been described, and alternative equipment is available that does not have these limitations, complications that occur during the use of an inferior product must be regarded as iatrogenic. Failure of a treating physician, nurse, or respiratory therapist to be aware of the problems and to correct them, is inexcusable when disease processes with such a high morbidity and mortality are involved.

PREDICTION OF OUTCOME

For several years, attempts have been made to evaluate severity of illness in critical care patients early in the course of therapy in order to predict their eventual outcome. Many reasons have been cited to justify such efforts. Development of an accurate predictive system would allow the allocation of limited resources to those patients with the greatest chance for intact survival and presumably would reduce the cost of medical care. A scientifically validated predictive system would also allow comparison of results among various institutions. Thus, if the predicted survival for a given problem was 50 percent, but one group of investigators consistently achieved a survival of 80 percent, the probability would be great that their approach had significant advantages over those used by other groups. In the absence of objectively derived criteria to assess the severity of illness and the number and types of interventions, however, comparative studies heretofore have been difficult to evaluate.

Historically, the severity of illness was felt to be a major factor in determining the costs of critical care.[61] Yet more careful analysis has revealed that this apparently obvious conclusion is not always true. In a study of 375 patients in a surgical ICU, 110 were admitted for one day and survived.[62] Fourteen other patients died within 24 hours of admission. These patients were the sickest, yet costs generated by their 1-day admission were essentially the same, as for the other 110 patients whose admissions were largely for close observation following surgery. Although these two groups represented 34 percent of total admissions, they were responsible for only 5 percent of the ICU days and 8 percent of the charges.

Any predictive system, including clinical judgment, should distinguish between patients who represent the opposite ends of a severity of illness spectrum. The problem lies with the patients who have an essentially equal chance of survival or death at the time of ICU admission. It is this group, which often is small in number but consumes a disproportionate amount of available resources, that represents the greatest challenges with respect to outcome prediction. Since 1974, a large number and variety of predictive indices have been proposed[63–71] (Table 14-4). None, however, has been completely successful, and each has demonstrated shortcomings.

The major problem attendant to all predictive indices thus far developed is that some variables that determine outcome are either unknown or

Table 14-4. Predictive Indices for ICU Outcome

System/index	Measured variables
Cullen et al.[63]	Quantitation of interventions (therapeutic intervention scoring system, TISS)
Civetta[64]	Organ system diagnosis/complications (complications impact index)
Shoemaker et al.[65]	Cardiorespiratory patterns/oxygen transport
Snyder et al.[66]	Assigned weight to 225 complications (condition index score)
Knaus et al.[67]	34 physiologic variables (APA); readmission health status (CHE)—APACHE
Shoemaker et al.[68]	12 cardiorespiratory parameters; 20 derived calculations
Keene et al.[69]	Original TISS plus additional interventions
Knaus et al.[70]	12 physiologic measurements; age plus preadmission health status—APACHE II
Lemeshow et al.[71]	Multiple logistic regression analysis of 7 variables

are not abnormal at the time of admission.[72] For example, a tension pneumothorax that occurs on the tenth day of ventilator therapy, could not be predicted at admission, yet may lead to the patient's death. All systems have an approximate 15 percent misclassification rate, which is the same value reported for clinical judgment alone.[73,74] Predictive indices appear to quantitate such judgment but do not improve on it.

The preceding discussion has focused on general admissions to medical and surgical ICUs. Respiratory failure was present in many of the patients studied and was a major determinant of outcome. However, it was not evaluated independently. Since MOF so frequently complicates respiratory failure, clear-cut information pertaining to pulmonary problems alone is difficult to obtain. Some factors of importance have already been discussed.[10–17] Fowler and associates[75] recently reported their experience with 88 patients who developed ARDS requiring mechanical ventilation. Fifty-seven patients died, one-half by the 13th day following the onset of treatment. Age, the hospital, race, sex, and the type of ICU were not associated with mortality. Factors associated significantly with mortality included less than 10 percent bands on a peripheral blood smear, persistent acidemia, calculated HCO_3^- less than 20 mEq/L, and blood urea nitrogen (BUN) greater than 65 mg/dl. These relationships again suggest that the patient's overall condition rather than the degree of ARDS, per se, was the important determinant.

In view of the fact that such a precisely derived variable, such as age, cannot be agreed on in terms of its impact on outcome,[5,7,10,14,74] it is highly unlikely that more complex determinants can be systematically evaluated. Clinical judgment will continue to be the mainstay of evaluation and therapy.

FOLLOW-UP

Thus far we have addressed the issues that are important as determinants of whether patients survive or die. Some of the unresolved problems have been discussed. Perhaps the ultimate analysis of outcome, however, is what happens to those patients who survive and are discharged from the hospital. Surprisingly, considering the devastating impact respiratory failure has in the hospital, the outlook for survivors is relatively good.

In a review of 21 publications involving 129 patients with 131 episodes of ARDS, Alberts et al.[76] reported that 83 percent were asymptomatic two months or more after their acute illness. In 80 percent, chest radiographs were normal, with residual infiltrates present in 11 percent. Resting PaO_2 was normal in 74 percent but decreased with exercise in 48 percent. Pulmonary function tests, with the exception of a restrictive defect in some patients, returned toward normal.[77]

With respect to acute exacerbation of COPD, the outlook is considerably better than formerly supposed.[5,8,19–26] In such patients, acute respiratory failure requiring mechanical ventilation appears to be associated with a lower mortality rate than is ARDS. When they are discharged home, their death rate appears to be consistent with the natural progression of their primary disease.

CONCLUSION

The cost of long-term respiratory care in an ICU is high. However, cost savings can be generated without reduction in the qualtiy of care.[78] Whether the results of this care can be ascertained to be cost effective is for others to judge.[79] Overall, however, respiratory care techniques, particularly positive-pressure mechanical ventilation, appear to have been beneficial. When we become as adept at treating sepsis, renal failure, hepatic insufficiency, and central nervous system dysfunction, then the efficacy of ventilatory support, which has often been hidden by the prohibitively high mortality of MOF, should become apparent.

REFERENCES

1. Andersen EW, Ibsen B: The anaesthetic management of patients with poliomyelitis and respiratory paralysis. Br Med J 1:786, 1954

2. Gregory GA, Kitterman JA, Phibbs RH, et al: Treatment of the idiopathic respiratory distress syndrome with continuous positive airway pressure. N Engl J Med 284:1333, 1971
3. Safar P. DeKornfeld TJ, Pearson JW, et al: The intensive care unit: a three year experience at Baltimore City hospitals. Anaesthesia 16:275, 1961
4. Fairley HB: The Toronto general hospital respiratory unit. Anaesthesia 16:267, 1961
5. Asmundsson T, Kilburn KH: Survival of acute respiratory failure: a study of 239 episodes. Ann Intern Med 70:471, 1969
6. Task Force on Problems, Research Approaches, Needs: Respiratory Diseases. DHEW Publication No. (NIH) 73–432, National Heart and Lung Institute, Bethesda, MD, 1972
7. Rogers RM, Weiler C, Ruppenthal B: Impact of the respiratory care unit on survival of patients with acute respiratory failure. Chest 62:94, 1972
8. Petty TL, Lakshminarayan S, Sahn S, et al: Intensive respiratory care unit: review of ten years' experience. JAMA 233:34, 1975
9. Zapol WM, Snider MT, Hill JD, et al: Extracorporeal membrane oxygenation in severe acute respiratory failure: a randomized prospective study. JAMA 242:2193, 1979
10. Bartlett RH, Morris AH, Fairley HB, et al: A prospective study of acute hypoxic respiratory failure. Chest 89:684, 1986
11. Montgomery AB, Stager MA, Carrico CJ, et al: Causes of mortality in patients with the adult respiratory distress syndrome. Am Rev Respir Dis 132:485, 1985
12. Bell RC, Coalson JJ, Smith JD, et al: Multiple organ system failure and infection in adult respiratory distress. Ann Intern Med 99:293, 1983
13. Schuster DP, Marion JM: Precedents for meaningful recovery during treatment in a medical intensive care unit. Am J Med 75:402, 1983
14. Cox SC, Norwood SH, Duncan CA: Acute respiratory failure: mortality associated with underlying disease. Crit Care Med 13:1005, 1985
15. Goldiner P, Pinilla J, Turnbull A: Acute respiratory failure in patients with advanced lymphoma. In Lacher MJ (ed): Hodgkin's Disease. John Wiley & Sons, New York, 1976
16. Snow RM, Miller WC, Rice DL, et al: Respiratory failure in cancer patients. JAMA 241:2039, 1979
17. Hauser MJ, Tabak J, Baier H: Survival of patients with cancer in a medical critical care unit. Arch Intern Med 142:527, 1982
18. Hudson LD: Respiratory failure: etiology and mortality. Respir Care 32:584, 1987
19. Vandenbergh E, van de Woestigne KP, Gyselin A: Conservative treatment of acute respiratory failure in patients with chronic obstructive lung disease. Am Rev Respir Dis 98:60, 1968
20. Sluiter HJ, Blokzyl EJ, Van Dijl W, et al: Conservative and respirator treatment of acute respiratory insufficiency in patients with chronic obstructive pulmonary disease: a reappraisal. Am Rev Respir Dis 105:932, 1972
21. Moser KM, Shibel EM, Beamon AJ: Acute respiratory failure in obstructive lung disease: long term survival after treatment in an intensive care unit. JAMA 225:705, 1973
22. Kettel LH: The management of respiratory failure in chronic obstructive lung disease. Med Clin North Am 57:781, 1973
23. Burk RH, George RB: Acute respiratory failure in chronic obstructive pulmonary disease: immediate and long term prognosis. Arch Intern Med 132:865, 1973
24. Seriff NS, Khan F, Lazo BJ: Acute respiratory failure: current concepts of pathophysiology and management. Med Clin North Am 57:1539, 1973
25. Bone RC, Pierce AK, Johnson RL: Controlled oxygen administration in acute respiratory failure in chronic obstructive pulmonary disease: a reappraisal. Am J Med 65:896, 1978
26. Martin TR, Lewis SW, Albut RK: The prognosis of patients with chronic obstructive pulmonary disease after hospitalization for acute respiratory failure. Chest 82:310, 1982
27. Engström C-G: Treatment of severe cases of respiratory paralysis by the Engström universal respirator. Br Med J 2:666, 1954
28. Cournand A, Motley HL, Werko L, et al: Physiological studies of effects of intermittent positive pressure breathing on cardiac output in man. Am J Physiol 152:162, 1948
29. Maloney J: Importance of negative pressure phase in mechanical respirators. JAMA 152:212, 1953
30. Kirby RR, Robinson EJ, Schulz J, et al: A new pediatric volume ventilator. Anesth Analg 50:533, 1971
31. Kirby RR, Robison E, Schulz J, et al: Continuous-flow ventilation as an alternative to assisted or controlled ventilation in infants. Anesth Analg 51:871, 1972

32. Downs JB, Klein EF Jr, Desautels D, et al: Intermittent mandatory ventilation: a new approach to weaning patients from mechanical ventilation. Chest 64:331, 1973
33. Kirby RR, Downs JB, Civetta JM, et al: High level positive end-expiratory pressure (PEEP) in acute respiratory insufficiency. Chest 67:156, 1975
34. Kirby RR, Perry JC, Calderwood HW, et al: Cardiorespiratory effects of high positive end-expiratory pressure. Anesthesiology 43:533, 1975
35. Sjöstrand U, Eriksson IA: High rates and low volumes in mechanical ventilation—not just a matter of ventilatory frequency. Anesth Analg 16:176, 1980
36. Carlon GC, Ray C Jr, Pierri MK, et al: High-frequency jet ventilation: theoretical considerations and clinical observations. Chest 81:350, 1982
37. Mathru M, Rao TLK, El-Etr AA, et al: Hemodynamic response to changes in ventilatory patterns in patients with normal and poor left ventricular reserve. Crit Care Med 10:423, 1982
38. Kirby RR: Positive airway pressure: system design and clinical application. p. G1. In Shoemaker WC (ed): Critical Care: State of the Art. Society of Critical Care Medicine, Fullerton, CA, 1985
39. HIFI Study Group: High-frequency oscillatory ventilation compared with conventional mechanical ventilation in the treatment of respiratory failure in preterm infants. N Engl J Med 320:88, 1989
40. Kirby RR: Intermittent mandatory ventilation. p. 169. In American Society of Anesthesiologists Refresher Course Lectures. JB Lippincott, Philadelphia, 1979
41. Carlon GC, Howland WS, Ray C, et al: High frequency jet ventilation. Chest 84:551, 1983
42. Marini JJ, Rodriquez RM, Lamb V: The inspiratory workload of patient-initiated mechanical ventilation. Am Rev Respir Dis 134:902, 1986
43. Gibney RTN, Wilson RS, Pontoppidan H: Comparison of work of breathing on high gas flow and demand valve continuous positive airway pressure systems. Chest 82:692, 1982
44. Banner MJ, Lampotang S, Boysen PG, et al: Flow resistance of expiratory positive pressure valve systems. Chest 90:212, 1986
45. Banner MJ, Downs JB, Kirby RR, et al: Effects of expiratory flow resistance on inspiratory work of breathing. Chest 93:795, 1988
46. Downs JB: Mechanical ventilatory therapy. Part II. Curr Rev Respir Ther 11:81, 1981
47. Ashbaugh DG, Bigelow DB, Petty TL, et al: Acute respiratory distress in adults. Lancet 2:7511, 1967
48. Ashbaugh DG, Petty TL, Bigelow DB, et al: Continuous positive-pressure breathing (CPPB) in adult respiratory distress syndrome. J Thorac Cardiovasc Surg 57:31, 1969
49. Downs JB, Klein EF, Modell JH: The effect of incremental PEEP on PaO_2 in patients with respiratory failure. Anesth Analg 52:210, 1973
50. Suter PM, Fairley HB, Isenberg MD: Optimum end-expiratory pressure in patients with acute respiratory failure. N Engl J Med 292:284, 1975
51. Kirby RR: Best PEEP: issues and choices in the selection and monitoring of PEEP levels. Respir Care 33:567, 1988
52. McIntyre RW, Laws AK, Ramachandran PR: Positive expiratory plateau: improved gas exchange during mechanical ventilation. Can Anaesth Soc J 16:477, 1969
53. Kumar A, Falke KJ, Geffin B, et al: Continuous mechanical ventilation in acute respiratory failure. N Engl J Med 283:1430, 1970
54. Sugarman HJ, Rogers RM, Miller LD: Positive end-expiratory pressure (PEEP): indications and physiologic considerations. Chest 62:865, 1972
55. Leftwich EI, Witorsch RJ, Witorsch P: Positive end-expiratory pressure in refractory hypoxemia. Ann Intern Med 79:187, 1973
56. Walkinshaw M, Shoemaker WC: Use of volume loading to obtain preferred levels of PEEP. Crit Care Med 8:81, 1980
57. Qvist J, Pontoppidan H, Wilson RS, et al: Hemodynamic responses to mechanical ventilation with PEEP: the effect of hypervolemia. Anesthesiology 42:45, 1975
58. Kumar A, Pontoppidan H, Falke KJ, et al: Pulmonary barotrauma during mechanical ventilation. Crit Care Med 1:181, 1973
59. Pepe PE, Hudson LD, Carrico CJ: Early application of positive end-expiratory pressure in patients at risk for the adult respiratory distress syndrome. N Engl J Med 311.281, 1984
60. Robin ED: Iatroepidemics: a probe to examine systematic preventable errors in (chest) medicine. Am Rev Respir Dis 135:1152, 1987
61. Civetta JM: The inverse relationship between cost and survival. J Surg Res 14:265, 1973

62. Civetta JM, Hudson-Civetta J, Nelson LD: Costly care: data, problems and proposed remedies. Crit Care Med 14:357, 1986
63. Cullen DJ, Civetta JM, Briggs BA, et al: Therapeutic intervention scoring system: a method for quantitative comparison of patient care. Crit Care Med 2:57, 1974
64. Civetta JM: The ICU milieu: an evaluation of the allocation of a limited resource. Respir Care 21:498, 1974
65. Shoemaker WC, Pierchala BS, Potter C, et al: Prediction of outcome and severity of illness by analysis of the frequency distribution of cardiorespiratory variables. Crit Care Med 5:82, 1977
66. Snyder JV, McGuirk M, Grenvik A, et al: Outcome of intensive care: an application of a predictive model. Crit Care Med 9:598, 1981
67. Knaus WA, Zimmerman JE, Wagner DP et al: APACHE-Acute physiology and chronic health evaluation: a physiologically based classification system. Crit Care Med 9:591, 1981
68. Shoemaker WC, Appel P, Bland R: Use of physiologic monitoring to assist in clinical decisions in critically ill postoperative patients. Am J Surg 146:43, 1983
69. Keene AR, Cullen DJ: Therapeutic intervention scoring system: update 1983. Crit Care Med 11:1, 1983
70. Knaus WA, Draper EA, Wagner DP, et al: APACHE II: A severity of disease classification system. Crit Care Med 13:818, 1985
71. Lemeshow S, Teres D, Pastides H, et al: A method for predicting survival and mortality of ICU patients using objectively derived weights. Crit Care Med 13:519, 1985
72. Kirby RR, Civetta JM: Critical care. p. 184. In Brown DL (ed): Risk and Outcome in Anesthesia. JB Lippincott, Philadelphia, 1988
73. Civetta JM, Caruthers-Banner T: Does clinical judgment correctly allocate surgical intensive care? Crit Care Med 11:236, 1983
74. Rodman G: How accurate is clinical judgment? Crit Care Med 6:127, 1978
75. Fowler AA, Hamman RF, Zerbe GO, et al: Adult respiratory distress syndrome: prognosis after onset. Am Rev Respir Dis 132:472, 1985
76. Alberts WM, Priest GR, Moser KM: The outlook for survivors of ARDS. Chest 84:272, 1983
77. Douglas ME, Downs JB: Pulmonary function following severe acute respiratory failure and high levels of positive end-expiratory pressure. Chest 71:18, 1977
78. Civetta JM, Hudson-Civetta JA: Maintaining quality of care while reducing charges in the ICU. Ann Surg 202:524, 1985
79. Farmer C: Intensive care: how do we measure outcome? p. 511. In Farmer C (ed): Problems in Critical Care. JB Lippincott, Philadelphia, 1989

15

Mechanical Ventilators

Michael J. Banner
Paul Blanch
David A. Desautels

Mechanical ventilators . . . we have often been perplexed about these devices and questions have come readily to our minds: How do they work? How should they work? What should they be able to do? What are the clinical effects, good and bad, that are associated with their use?—and many other questions too.

W.W. Mushin, M.D.

Robert Hooke in 1667 inserted a fireside bellows into the trachea of a dog and kept it alive by regular intermittent inflations. Employed as a mechanical ventilator, the hand-operated bellows was among the first mechanical devices to facilitate the movement of gas in and out of the lungs. In Hooke's era, a carpenter was all that was required to construct a bellows device. Today, a responsible approach essential for the development of a mechanical ventilator is to combine the efforts of experts from various disciplines, such as medicine, physiology, respiratory therapy, mechanical engineering, and computer programming, as well as electronic, pneumatic, and fluidic experts. All too often, however, this approach has been the exception, rather than the rule.

Evolving from a simple hand-operated bellows, modern-day mechanical ventilators are complex microprocessor-operated devices capable of providing a variety of ventilatory modalities. An understanding of modern mechanical ventilators, and the various modalities of mechanical and spontaneous positive-pressure ventilation and related physiologic implications, is imperative for the practice of respiratory care. Thus, the purpose of this chapter parallels the aforementioned questions broached by Dr. Mushin, that is, to provide clinicians with the requisite information on how ventilators work, how they should work, and what they should be able to do.

VENTILATOR CLASSIFICATION

Cycling Mechanisms

Time, volume, pressure, and flow rate are interrelated variables used to describe spontaneous and mechanical positive-pressure ventilation (Table 15–1). The changeover from the mechanical inhalation to the exhalation phase, that is, the process used to cycle the ventilator "OFF," is a means of classifying mechanical ventilators. Time, volume, pressure, or flow-cycling mechanisms are employed on most ventilators.

Table 15–1. Parameters Used to Describe Ventilation

Time
- May be divided into inspiratory (I) and expiratory (E) periods and is expressed in seconds or by the relationship of inspiratory time (T_I) to expiratory time (T_E) expressed as an I:E ratio
- Used to define the number of respiratory cycles within a given period of time

Volume
- A measure of the tidal volume delivered by the ventilator to the patient
- Reflects the volume of gas the patient breathes
- Is usually expressed in milliliters (ml) for tidal volume, and in liters (L) for minute volume

Pressure
- A measure of the impedence to gas-flow rate encountered in the ventilator breathing circuit and the patient's airways and lungs
- Refers to the amount of backpressure generated as a result of airways resistance and lung-thorax compliance
- Is expressed in centimeters of water (cm H_2O), millimeters of mercury (mmHg), or kilopascals (kPa) (1 cm H_2O = 1.36 mmHg, 7.6 mmHg = 1 kPa)

Flow rate
- A measure of the rate at which the gas volume is delivered to the patient
- Refers to the volume change per unit time
- Is expressed as liters per second (L/sec) or liters per minute (L/min)

Time-Cycled

Time-cycled mechanical inhalation is terminated after a preselected inspiratory time elapses. The timing mechanism can be pneumatic (e.g., IMV bird) or electronic (e.g., Hamilton Veolar). The key concept is that the duration of the inhalation phase is controlled by the operator and is not influenced by either the peak inflation pressure (PIP) generated or the patient's lung-thorax compliance (C_{LT}) and airway resistance (R_{AW}). The tidal volume (V_T) delivered is the product of inspiratory time (seconds) and inspiratory flow rate (ml/sec). PIP generated is inversely proportional to C_{LT} and directly proportional to R_{AW} and the V_T delivered (Table 15–2). Thus, when C_{LT} decreases, for example, inspiratory time is unaffected, but PIP increases. Under these conditions, inspiratory flow rate may decrease as a result of increased backpressure; thus, V_T decreases. V_T can be restored to the initial value by increasing either inspiratory time or inspiratory flow rate, or both.

Volume-Cycled

Volume-cycled mechanical inhalation is terminated after a preselected V_T has been ejected from the ventilator, irrespective of the PIP, inspiratory time, and inspiratory flow rate (Table 15–3). A common misconception is that V_T delivered to the patient is always constant, despite increases in PIP, as a result of decreases in C_{LT} and/or increases in R_{AW}. During mechanical inhalation, ejected V_T is distributed in the ventilator breathing circuit tubing and the patient's lungs. The greater the PIP, the greater the fraction of V_T compressed or "left behind" in the breathing circuit and the less volume delivered to the patient (Fig. 15–1). The more compliant the breathing circuit tubing, the more volume that remains in the tubing, and the less volume that is received by the patient. When high PIP are required, noncompliant and nondistensible tubing should be used, and the humidifier should be full to minimize gas compression. Thus, the so-called volume-constant ventilator is a myth. No currently available ventilator delivers constant V_T as alterations in pulmonary mechanics occur.

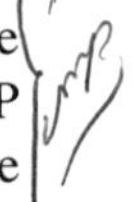

Table 15–2. Time-Cycled Ventilators

Definition: Mechanical inhalation terminates after a preselected inspiratory time (T_I) elapses.

1. $V_T = T_I \times \dot{V}$
   where V_T = tidal volume (ml)
   $\dot{V}_I$ = inspiratory flow rate (ml/sec)
2. $PIP \propto \dfrac{T_I \times \dot{V}_I}{C_{LT}}$
   where PIP = peak inflation pressure (cm H_2O)
   C_{LT} = lung-thorax compliance (ml/cm H_2O)

Example:

Normal adult C_{LT}:

$$10 \text{ cm } H_2O = \frac{(2 \text{ sec}) \times (500 \text{ ml/sec})}{100 \text{ ml/cm } H_2O}$$

Decreased C_{LT}:

$$100 \text{ cm } H_2O = \frac{(2 \text{ sec}) \times (500 \text{ ml/sec})}{10 \text{ ml/cm } H_2O}$$

Table 15–3. Volume-Cycled Ventilator

Definition: Mechanical inhalation terminates after a preselected volume (VT) has been ejected from the ventilator

$$PIP = \frac{V_T}{C_{LT}}$$

where PIP = peak inflation pressure (cm H_2O)
C_{LT} = lung-thorax compliance (ml/cm H_2O)

Example:

Normal adult C_{LT}:

$$10 \text{ cm } H_2O = \frac{1{,}000 \text{ ml}}{100 \text{ ml/cm } H_2O}$$

Decreased C_{LT}:

$$100 \text{ cm } H_2O = \frac{1{,}000 \text{ ml}}{10 \text{ ml/cm } H_2O}$$

Pressure-Cycled

Pressure-cycled mechanical inhalation is terminated when a preselected PIP is achieved within the ventilator breathing circuit, irrespective of the VT, inspiratory time, or inspiratory flow rate. When the preselected PIP is reached, inspiratory flow rate ceases, and the exhalation valve opens to permit passive exhalation. VT delivered and inspiratory time are related directly to CLT and inversely to RAW. VT may be expressed as the product of the change in airway pressure and CLT (Table 15–4). Therefore, with a pressure-cycled ventilator, a decrease in CLT and/or increase in RAW predispose to a decrease in inspiratory time and since VT = inspiratory time × inspiratory flow rate, VT decreases.

Substantial leaks in the breathing circuit tubing or at the airway (e.g., improperly inflated endotracheal tube cuff) preclude generation of the requisite inspiratory cycling pressure. Most of the ventilators formerly used for intermittent positive-pressure breathing therapy were pressure-cycled (e.g., Bird Mark 7).

Flow-Cycled

Flow-cycled mechanical inhalation is terminated when the inspiratory flow rate delivered by the ventilator decreases to a critical value, irrespective of inspiratory time and VT. Flow-cycling is employed by microprocessor-con-

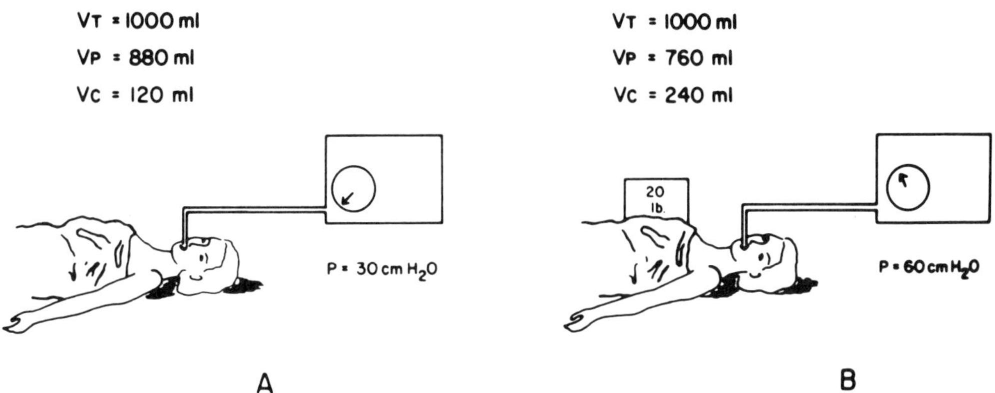

Fig. 15-1. Effect of changing compliance (simulated by a weight on the chest) on patient ventilation. **(A)** Volume-cycled ventilator is set to deliver a tidal volume of 1,000 ml, of which 880 ml reaches the patient and 120 ml is compressed within the ventilator circuit. Note that the peak inflation pressure (P) is 30 cm H_2O. **(B)** A 20-lb weight is placed on the patient's chest to simulate a decrease in CLT. The ventilator again delivers the 1,000-ml tidal volume but, because of the patient's decreased compliance, a pressure of 60 cm H_2O is required and only 760 ml reaches the patient, while 240 ml is compressed or left behind in the breathing-circuit tubing. In this example, the compression factor is 4 ml/cm H_2O; i.e., 4 ml/cm H_2O × 60 cm H_2O = 240 ml. VT, set tidal volume; VP, patient tidal volume; VC, compression volume. (From Kirby et al.,[54] with permission.)

Table 15–4. Pressure-Cycled Ventilators

Definition: Mechanical inhalation terminates when a preselected peak inflation pressure is achieved within the breathing circuit tubing.

$V_T = PIP \times C_{LT}$
where V_T = tidal volume
PIP = peak inflation pressure (cm H_2O)
C_{LT} = lung-thorax compliance (ml/cm H_2O)

Example:
Normal adult C_{LT}:
1,000 ml = 10 cm H_2O × 100 ml/cm H_2O

Decreased C_{LT}:
100 ml = 10 cm H_2O × 10 ml/cm H_2O

trolled mechanical ventilators operating in the pressure support ventilation mode. For example, in the pressure support ventilation mode when the ventilator is patient-triggered "ON" (as in assisted mechanical ventilation), an abrupt increase in airway pressure to the pressure support level and a high peak inspiratory flow rate are delivered immediately to the patient. The inhalation phase continues until the inspiratory flow rate decays to a predetermined percentage of the initial peak value; at this critical value, flow rate ceases (i.e., the ventilator flow cycles "OFF") and the exhalation valve opens, permitting passive exhalation.

Inspiratory Flow Waveforms

Sinusoidal, constant, decelerating, or accelerating inspiratory flow waveforms are available on many newer microprocessor-controlled mechanical ventilators (Fig. 15–2). Whether a particular type of flow waveform can improve the distribution of ventilation, alveolar ventilation-to-perfusion ($\dot{V}_A/\dot{Q}$) matching, and gas exchange is controversial. The discrepancy among some reports relates to a host of confounding variables. In some studies, altering the inspiratory flow waveform may have affected inspiratory time, inhalation to exhalation time ratio (I:E), peak inspiratory flow rate, V_T, and minute ventilation. Using an end-inspiratory pause, some investigators have compared various inspiratory flow waveforms and have found little difference in distribution of ventilation.[1] However, the duration of inspiratory time is increased by the presence of an end-inspiratory pause, which suggests that the duration of inspiratory time is as important in influencing the distribution of ventilation and gas exchange, if not more so, as the type of flow waveform.[2]

Ventilation in mechanical lung models and patients has been studied to evaluate the effects of inspiratory flow waveform on gas distribution by altering the inspiratory flow waveform and by keeping other ventilator variables constant. Several studies of lung models with multiple compartments having different resistances have demonstrated that a decelerating inspiratory flow waveform distributes ventilation more evenly than does other types of waveforms.[3,4] These data may be relevant to treating patients with chronic obstructive pulmonary disease (COPD) who require ventilatory support. Clinical reports suggest similar findings.[5–7] In one investigation in which V_T, inspiratory time, I:E ratio, and ventilator rate were held constant; PIP, $PaCO_2$, dead space-to-tidal volume ratio (V_D/V_T), and alveolar-arterial gradient for oxygen were significantly lower with a decelerating inspiratory flow waveform than with a constant inspiratory flow waveform.[6] However, with the decelerating flow waveform, mean airway pressure was greater, which may predispose a patient to adverse hemodynamic effects.

TECHNIQUES OF MECHANICAL VENTILATION

Mechanical ventilation is indicated if spontaneous ventilation is inadequate (or absent) and a normal $PaCO_2$ and pHa cannot be maintained. Current modes of mechanical ventilation include controlled mechanical ventilation (CMV); CMV with end-expiratory pressure, that is, continuous positive-pressure ventilation (CPPV); assisted ventilation (AV): and assist-control ventilation. These forms of positive-pressure ventilation do not permit normal spontaneous breathing and for CMV require either sedation or neuromuscular paralysis, or both, to blunt spontaneous at-

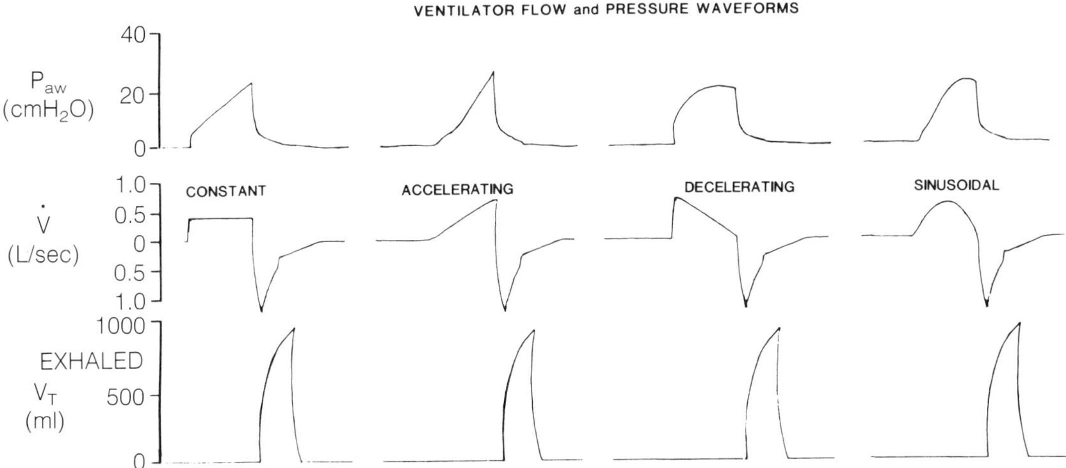

Fig. 15-2. Airway pressure (PAW), flow rate ($\dot{V}$), and tidal volume (VT) are shown for constant, accelerating, decelerating, and sinusoidal inspiratory flow waveforms. Inspiratory time and VT were held constant. PIP was highest with the accelerating waveform and lowest with the decelerating one; however, mean airway pressure was highest with the latter inspiratory flow waveform. (From Banner and Lampotang,[2] with permission.)

tempts to breathe. Intermittent mandatory ventilation (IMV) combined with continuous positive airway pressure (CPAP) and expiratory positive airway pressure (EPAP) or spontaneous positive end-expiratory pressure (PEEP) permits spontaneous and controlled ventilation. Synchronized IMV (SIMV) is a special form of IMV. End-inspiratory pause (EIP) and pressure-limited time-cycled mechanical ventilation may be used during CMV and IMV. Mandatory minute ventilation (MMV), like IMV, permits spontaneous ventilation and, when appropriate, mechanical ventilation is provided. Pressure support ventilation (PSV), like AV, enables the patient to trigger the ventilator "ON" as often as desired. It also allows the patient to determine ventilator rate, inspiratory time, VT, and minute ventilation.

Controlled Mechanical Ventilation

Controlled mechanical ventilation delivers a preselected ventilatory rate, VT, and inspiratory flow rate independent of spontaneous effort on the part of the patient (Fig. 15–3A). The PIP generated varies inversely with CLT and directly with RAW (if the ventilator is volume or time cycled). Indications for CMV include apnea, secondary to central nervous system (CNS) depression (brain or spinal cord trauma or both); drug overdose; or neuromuscular paralysis (either drug-induced or the result of pathology, e.g., Guillain-Barré syndrome, myasthenia gravis, poliomyelitis). Because many patients treated with CMV are sedated, paralyzed, or hyperventilated below their apneic threshold, accidental disconnection or a mechanical malfunction represents a life-threatening situation. Therefore, a "disconnect" or "failure-to-cycle" alarm is crucial.

Continuous Positive-Pressure Ventilation

Continuous positive-pressure ventilation, like CMV, delivers a positive-pressure breath followed by a fall in airway pressure to a previously selected positive-pressure plateau; airway pressure never returns to zero (Fig. 15–3B). This form of ventilation was popularized by Ashbaugh et al.[8] for treatment of adult respiratory

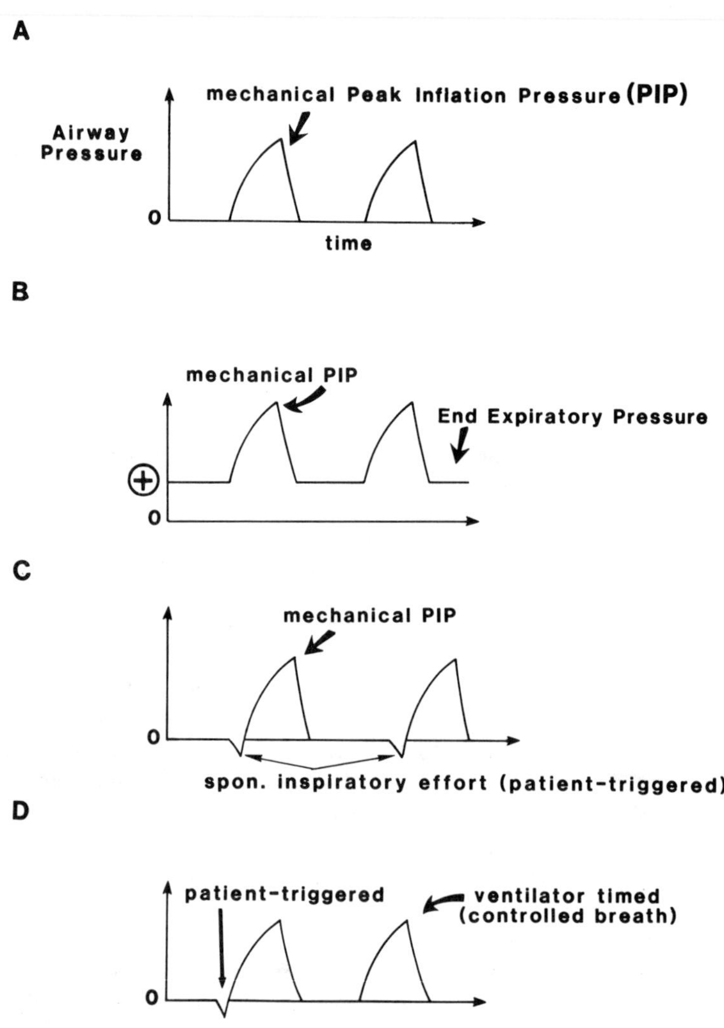

Fig. 15-3. Mechanical ventilatory airway pressure patterns. **(A)** Controlled mechanical ventilation (CMV). Mechanical ventilator rate, tidal volume (V_T), and inspiratory flow rate are present and cannot be affected by the patient's respiratory efforts. **(B)** CMV with end-expiratory pressure or continuous positive-pressure ventilation (CPPV). When mechanical inhalation ends, pressure drops to a set positive-pressure plateau, i.e., the end-expiratory pressure level. **(C)** Assisted mechanical ventilation (AV). Patient-triggered mechanical inhalation; V_T is preset and cannot be affected by the patient. If the patient does not initiate inhalation, the ventilator does not switch "ON." **(D)** Assist-control ventilation. The ventilator may be triggered to mechanical inhalation by the patient's inspiratory efforts or by a timing device, whichever comes first. The patient may trigger the ventilator as often as desired, and the timing device determines the minimum ventilator cycling rate.

distress syndrome (ARDS) to prevent alveolar collapse during the ventilator's expiratory phase, and thereby improve and maintain overall $\dot{V}_A/\dot{Q}$ relationships.

Assisted Ventilation

Assisted ventilation is more appropriately termed patient-triggered positive-pressure ventilation (Fig. 15–3C). If the patient does not initiate a spontaneous breathing effort, the ventilator *will not* deliver a mechanical breath; thus, apnea can be fatal with this mode of ventilation. This technique has been employed as intermittent positive-pressure breathing (IPPB) for short-term delivery of gases and therapeutic aerosols to patients with pulmonary parenchymal or airway disease. It is also used (infrequently now) for support of patients with acute or chronic respiratory failure. Some practitioners also use AV to wean patients from CMV and to promote spontaneous breathing.

Assisted ventilation was more popular during the 1960s than now because it was thought to be more "physiologic" than CMV. The prevalent idea at that time—that AV enhances maintenance of respiratory muscle tone, augmentation of venous return, and more normal pHa and $PaCO_2$—has not proved significant in severe ARDS. Patients treated with AV tend to develop respiratory alkalemia, the deleterious effects of which are listed in Table 15–5, to the same extent as those managed with CMV.

Table 15–5. Physiological Effects of Respiratory Alkalemia (Hypocapnia)

Decreased
Cardiac output
Cerebral blood flow
Coronary blood flow
P_{50} (leftward shift O_2-hemoglobin dissociation curve—decreased oxygen availability)
Serum ionized calcium
Serum potassium
Increased
Airway resistance
Oxygen consumption

The greatest operational difficulty with AV is that many of the assist mechanisms, which trigger the inhalation phase, are unreliable.[9] Response sensitivity must be preset, and as the patient's condition changes, his ability to generate an appropriate effort (usually a decrease in the breathing circuit pressure associated with spontaneous inspiratory effort) varies. The ventilator sensitivity may then be too great (resulting in repetitive cycles or autocycling) or too slight, so that the ventilator fails to cycle.

Assist-Control Ventilation

Assist-control ventilation combines AV and CMV; the ventilator may be triggered by the patient's spontaneous inspiratory efforts or by a timing device, whichever comes first (Fig. 15–3D). The patient may trigger the ventilator "ON" at any time, but the timer determines a minimal preselected rate. Thus, CMV acts as a backup should the patient become apneic or attempt to breathe at a lower rate than that set by the timer.

All the aforementioned modes of mechanical ventilation predispose the patient to ventilator-induced $\dot{V}_A/\dot{Q}$ abnormalities. This untoward effect is related to the maldistribution of ventilation to nondependent lung regions (Fig. 15–4). In the supine, paralyzed individual, a disproportionate amount of V_T is delivered anteriorly to nondependent lung regions with decreased perfusion.[10] Conversely, spontaneous ventilation tends to promote more normal distribution of $\dot{V}_A/\dot{Q}$ and minimizes the ventilator-induced abnormalities (Fig. 15–4). Some studies have demonstrated that V_D increases during mechanical ventilation with or without positive expiratory pressure.[11,12] Downs and Mitchell[11] showed that increases of dead-space ventilation were related to the rate of mechanical cycling regardless of the ventilatory pattern and/or whether positive expiratory pressure was employed.

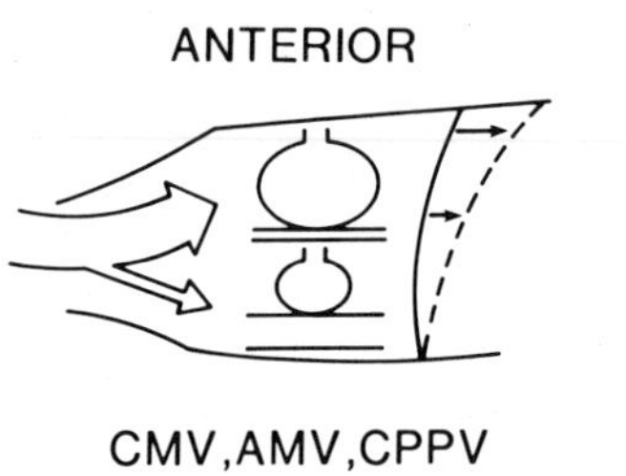

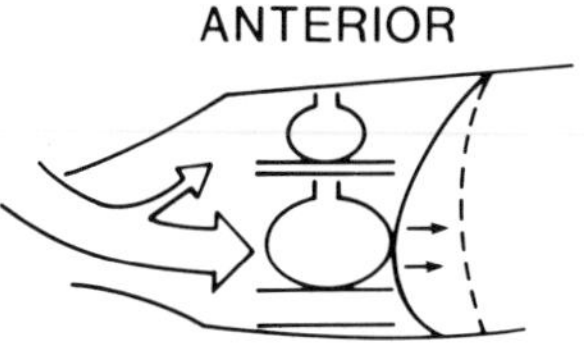

Fig. 15-4. Relationships of alveolar ventilation to perfusion ($\dot{V}A/\dot{Q}$) under various ventilatory conditions. During controlled mechanical ventilation (CMV), assisted ventilation (AV), and continuous positive-pressure ventilation (CPPV), a disproportionate amount of the tidal volume (V_T) is directed anteriorly with passive diaphragmatic displacement. Thus, the ventilator induces new $\dot{V}A/\dot{Q}$ abnormalities: increased $\dot{V}A/\dot{Q}$ in the anterior nondependent areas and decreased $\dot{V}A/\dot{Q}$ (relative shunt) in the posterior perfusion-dependent areas. Spontaneous ventilation, as occurs with intermittent mandatory ventilation (IMV) and continuous positive airway pressure (CPAP) tends to provide better $\dot{V}A/\dot{Q}$ matching. Active contraction of the diaphragm during spontaneous inhalation facilitates the distribution of V_T to posterior areas of the lung. In the relatively low-pressure pulmonary arterial system, blood flow also gravitates to the same areas. Thus, in both posterior and anterior lung regions, normal physiologic $\dot{V}A/\dot{Q}$ matching results.

Intermittent Mandatory Ventilation

Originally proposed by Kirby et al.[13,14] as a method to ventilate infants with hyaline membrane disease (HMD) and by Downs et al.[15] for use with adults, IMV enables the patient to breathe spontaneously with a mechanical inflation provided at preset intervals (Fig. 15–5 and 15–6A). The mechanical ventilatory rate, like CMV, cannot be influenced by the patient. Between sequential mechanical breaths, an unrestricted flow of gas equal to or greater than the patient's peak spontaneous inspiratory demand is provided.

Intermittent mandatory ventilation was introduced initially as a method to wean patients from mechanical ventilation[13–15] by permitting a smooth transition from mechanical ventilation to spontaneous breathing, as the rate of cycling was gradually decreased and spontaneous effort increased. As clinical experience has been accumulated, IMV has evolved as a primary ventilatory technique.

Several physiologic advantages have been proposed for IMV. Spontaneous breathing, with its attendant lower inspiratory intrapleural pressure, and a decreased rate of mechanical cycling combine to lower mean intrapleural pressure below that associated with CMV and AV. Thus, right heart filling pressure and cardiovascular function may be better preserved with IMV than with CMV.[16,17] When IMV is combined with CPAP or EPAP (Fig. 15–6B,C), the cardiopulmonary effects differ substantially from those of CPPV (Fig. 15–7). IMV allows the use of higher levels of CPAP with fewer deleterious effects on venous return and cardiac output.[16,17] In addition, spontaneous breathing with IMV promotes more normal $\dot{V}A/\dot{Q}$ matching than is possible with CMV or AV (Fig. 15–4).

The IMV rate should be titrated to deliver only that support which, in conjunction with spontaneous breathing, maintains normal alveolar ventilation and $PaCO_2$. When used in patients with antecedent pulmonary disease (emphysema, chronic bronchitis), IMV is extremely useful in regulating $PaCO_2$ and pHa compared with either CMV or AV.

Equipment

Sufficient flow rate through the IMV breathing circuit must be provided to satisfy the patient's peak spontaneous inspiratory flow demand. Gas-

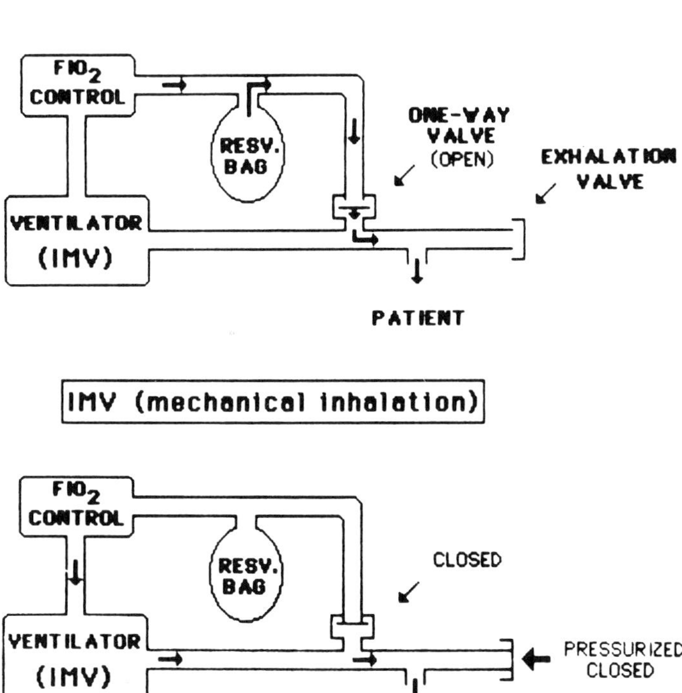

Fig. 15-5. Intermittent mandatory ventilation (IMV) system as originally described by Downs and Kirby. IMV system components: F_{IO_2} control provided by an air-oxygen blender; time- or volume-cycled ventilator for mandatory breaths; demand-flow reservoir for spontaneous breathing (reservoir bag or demand-flow valve); and one-way valve. Requirements for an IMV system: (1) minimal work of breathing during spontaneous ventilation: (a) gas flow sufficient to meet the patient's inspiratory flow demand, (b) low resistance to gas flow throughout the breathing circuit; (2) no rebreathing; (3) full humidification during spontaneous and mechanical ventilation; and (4) facility to provide continuous positive airway pressure (CPAP).

flow rates of two to three times the patient's minute ventilation are usually sufficient. Also, the resistance to gas flow through the IMV system must be minimal during spontaneous breathing (i.e., highly resistant humidifiers and one-way valves, narrow-bore breathing circuit tubing, and right-angled connectors should *not* be used). Systems that cannot provide adequate gas flow on demand increase the patient's work of breathing to intolerably high levels and can result in failure of the technique. No rebreathing should occur with this mode. If the exhalation valve on the expiratory limb of the breathing circuit is only competent (closed) during mechanical inhalation, entrainment of ambient air may occur during spontaneous inhalation, with rebreathing of exhaled gas.

Full humidification of inspired gas during a spontaneous and mechanical inhalation should be provided. Two problems arise with humidifiers used in IMV systems: (1) the capability to humidify gas sufficiently during high-flow rate conditions (up to 60 L/min), which is occasionally necessary to satisfy spontaneous inspiratory demand; and (2) the flow resistance characteristics of the humidifer itself. Poulton and Downs[18]

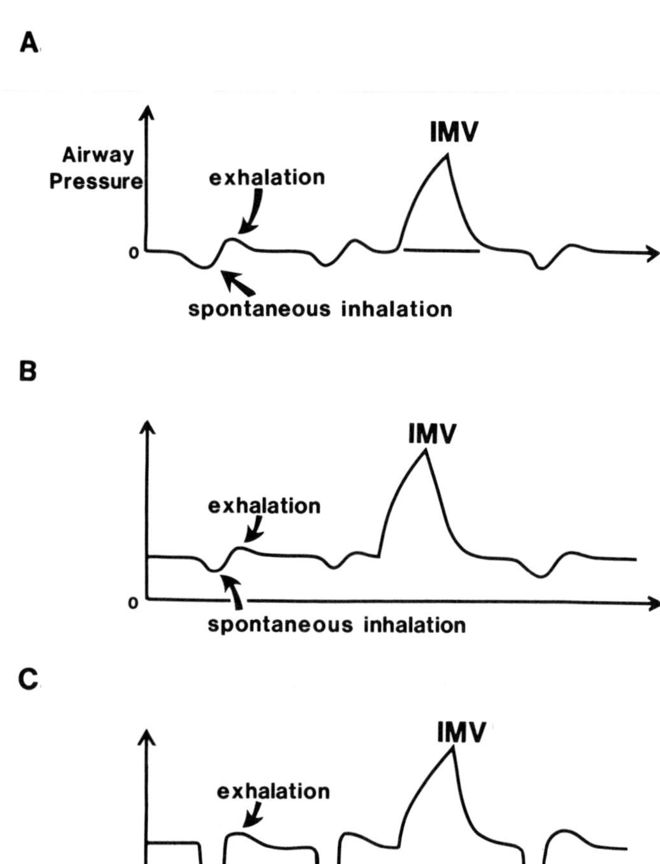

Fig. 15-6. (A) Intermittent mandatory ventilation (IMV) airway pressure patterns. With IMV, the patient is allowed to breathe spontaneously as desired; however, at set intervals, a mechanical inflation is provided (the ventilator rate is the IMV rate). IMV tidal volume is set and cannot be affected by the patient. **(B)** With IMV and continuous positive airway pressure (CPAP), the patient breathes spontaneously with CPAP between IMV breaths. **(C)** With IMV and expiratory positive airway pressure (EPAP) or positive end-expiratory pressure (PEEP), the patient is allowed to breathe spontaneously with PEEP between IMV breaths.

studied several commercially available humidifiers. The Bird heated-wick humidifier delivered acceptable humidity with negligible flow resistance during high-flow conditions. Other humidifiers failed to provide sufficient humidity or imposed excessive resistance to gas flow, either of which precludes their use in an IMV system. High-flow resistance is not a problem during CMV because the ventilator provides essentially all the work of breathing. However, during spontaneous inhalation with IMV, the patient must provide this work.[19]

The IMV system should be capable of pressurizing the inspiratory reservoir to the CPAP level. A continuous-flow or demand-flow system can be used for this purpose. Most commercially available IMV-CPAP systems today are of the latter design. Demand-flow valves should be

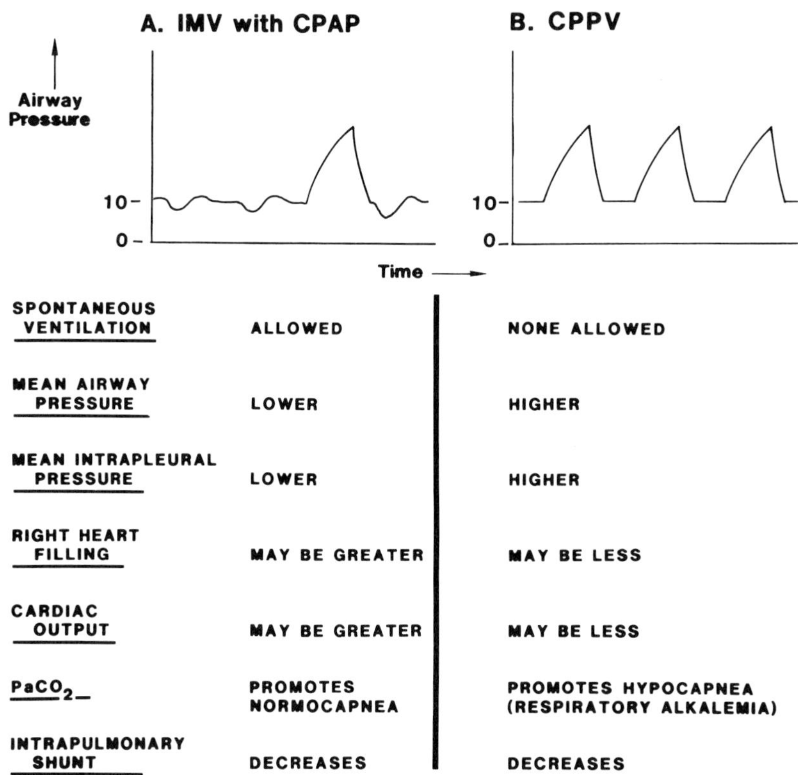

Fig. 15-7. Comparison of the physiological effects of intermittent mandatory ventilation (IMV) with continuous positive airway pressure (CPAP), and controlled mechanical ventilation (CMV) with end-expiratory pressure, or continuous positive-pressure ventilation (CPPV). (The rate of IMV is assumed to be approximately 4 breaths/min compared with the CMV rate of 10 to 16 breaths/min; both have the same end-expiratory pressure.)

capable of providing high inspiratory flow rates (up to 120 L/min) in order to prevent large decreases in airway pressure.

Synchronized Intermittent Mandatory Ventilation

Synchronized intermittent mandatory ventilation, like IMV, allows the patient to breathe spontaneously between mechanical breaths. At regular intervals, the mandatory breath is synchronized to begin with the next spontaneous inhalation (Fig. 15–8) in a manner analogous to AV. This technique was introduced because of concern that a mechanical breath might be superimposed on a spontaneous breath (''breath stacking''), which may predispose to increases of peak inflation, mean airway, and mean intrapleural pressures. Similar fears were expressed if the mechanically delivered volume was added at the peak of spontaneous exhalation.[20]

Subsequently, investigations were conducted to examine the clinical efficacy of SIMV. Shapiro et al.[20] noted that mean pleural pressure ($\overline{Ppl}$) measured with an esophageal balloon was substantially lower with SIMV than with IMV in normal volunteers. However, Hasten et al.[21] compared SIMV with IMV in 25 critically ill patients and found that, although PIP was greater

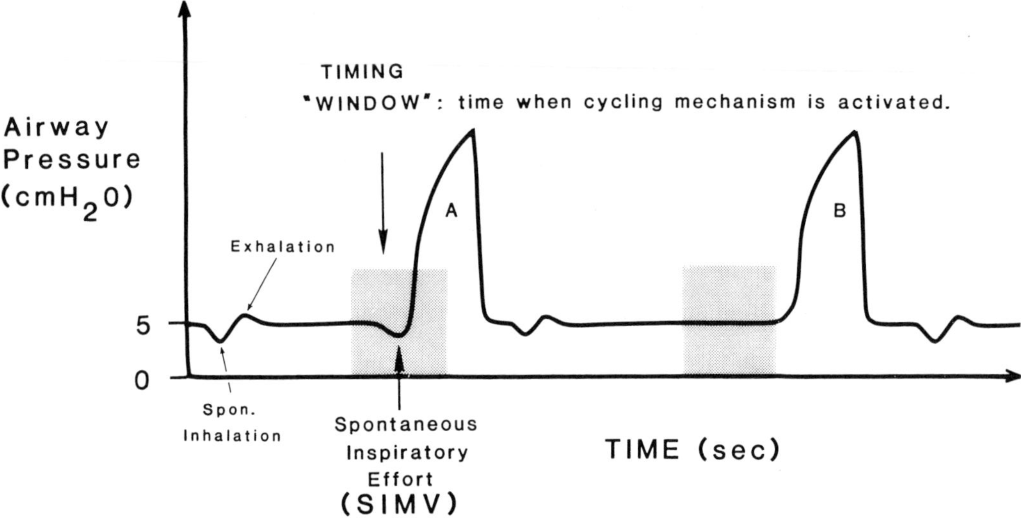

Fig. 15-8. Synchronized intermittent mandatory ventilation (SIMV), like intermittent mandatory ventilation (IMV), allows the patient to breathe spontaneously between ventilator breaths. At set intervals, the ventilator's electrical rate-timing circuit becomes activated and a timing window appears. If the patient initiates a breath in the timing window, the mandatory breath is delivered, *A;* thus, IMV is synchronized to occur with the patient's spontaneous inspiratory effort. If no spontaneous inspiratory effort registers during the timing window, the ventilator delivers the mandatory breath at the end of the timing sequence, *B*. This tracing shows a combination of SIMV with 5 cm H_2O CPAP.

with IMV than with SIMV, cardiovascular variables (blood pressure, cardiac output, stroke volume, central venous pressure, and pulmonary artery pressure) in the two groups did not differ significantly.

In another study, Heenan et al.[22] obtained baseline data from spontaneously breathing, anesthetized dogs that were subsequently near-drowned and ventilated with IMV or SIMV. Again, no differences between the two modes were noted with respect to cardiac output, stroke volume, intrapleural pressure, and intrapulmonary shunting ($\dot{Q}sp/\dot{Q}t$). PIP and mean airway pressure ($\overline{P_{AW}}$) were significantly increased with IMV, and breath stacking occurred but without demonstrable adverse effects. On the basis of these data, SIMV does not seem to offer any physiologic advantage compared with IMV and may be an expensive solution to a problem that has not been shown to exist.

Mandatory Minute Volume

Hewlett and colleagues [23] described a technique called mandatory minute volume (MMV) in which the patient is guaranteed a preselected minute volume, either through spontaneous ventilation or as positive-pressure breaths from the ventilator. If the desired minute volume is breathed spontaneously, no mandatory ventilation is provided by the ventilator. If not, that portion of the preselected minute volume which is not breathed spontaneously is then provided by the ventilator and delivered automatically (Fig. 15–9). Theoretically, weaning with MMV is simplified because the clinician is not required to make periodic adjustments of the ventilator rate as spontaneous ventilation changes.[24] Ventilators that incorporate MMV are the Hamilton Veolar, Bear-5, Ohmeda CPU 1, and the Engström Erica.

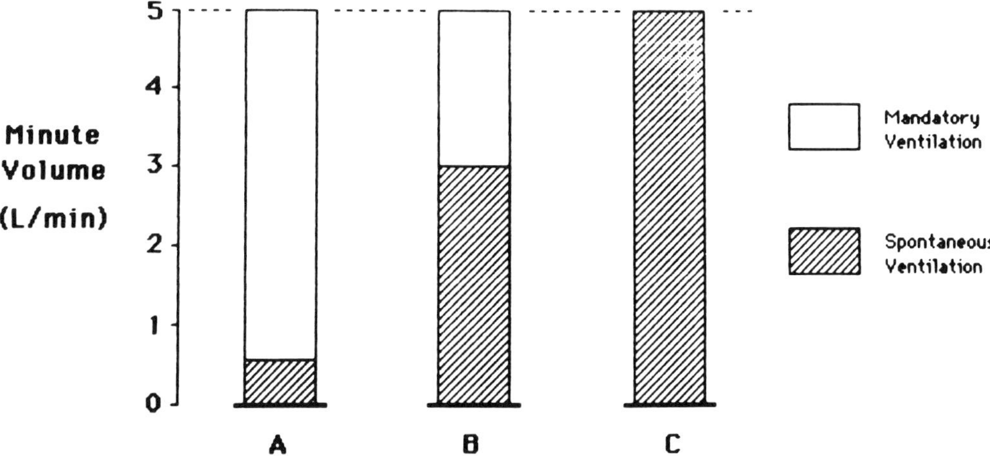

Fig. 15-9. Basic concepts of mandatory minute volume (MMV). In this example, the preselected MMV is 5 L/min. **(A)** The patient's spontaneous ventilation is negligible; as a result, mandatory ventilation from the ventilator provides most of the minute volume. **(B)** The patient's spontaneous ventilation provides a minute volume of 3 L/min, while 2 L/min mandatory ventilation is delivered by the ventilator. **(C)** Since the patient's spontaneous minute volume equals 5 L/min, no mandatory ventilation is provided by the ventilator. When appropriate, the ventilator automatically provides ventilation to maintain the preselected minute volume.

The Hamilton Veolar incorporates PSV in its MMV mode. With every 8 breaths, a microprocessor compares the spontaneous minute volume with the preselected MMV and corrects for any differences between the two by automatically adjusting the level of PSV in increments of approximately 2 cm H_2O.

The Bear 5 uses SIMV in its MMV mode. MMV with the Bear-5 is referred to as *augmented minute ventilation*. The exhaled minute volume is monitored and compared with the preselected MMV. No SIMV breaths are delivered to the patient when the spontaneous minute volume is greater than the preselected MMV. If the spontaneous minute volume falls below the threshold, the ventilator calculates an SIMV rate and supplies an appropriate number of mandatory breaths at a preselected VT to satisfy the MMV requirements.

The Ohmeda CPU-1 combines SIMV also with its MMV mode via a sophisticated monitoring process. Before MMV is initiated, the patient is ventilated with SIMV. Subsequently, when MMV is initiated, a microprocessor reviews the previous ventilation data during SIMV and then automatically adjusts itself to ensure that the spontaneous ventilation and the mandatory ventilation achieves the preselected MMV. Following this initial period, the microprocessor compares the spontaneous minute volume to the preselected MMV every 24 seconds. If the spontaneous minute volume falls below 75 percent of the preselected MMV, the ventilator automatically switches to a set of security values and provides a minute volume (SIMV breaths) equal to 75 percent of that selected.

Mandatory minute ventilation with the Engström Erica is referred to as *extended mandatory minute ventilation*. With this ventilator, the preselected MMV is compared by a microprocessor with the patient's spontaneous minute volume in order to calculate the frequency of the ventilator breaths. The mechanical frequency is continually adjusted so that the sum of the mandatory and spontaneous volumes is equal to the preselected MMV.

Potentially, MMV is a useful ventilatory technique. Because it ensures a minimal level of support, MMV has been advocated for weaning patients from mechanical ventilation. However,

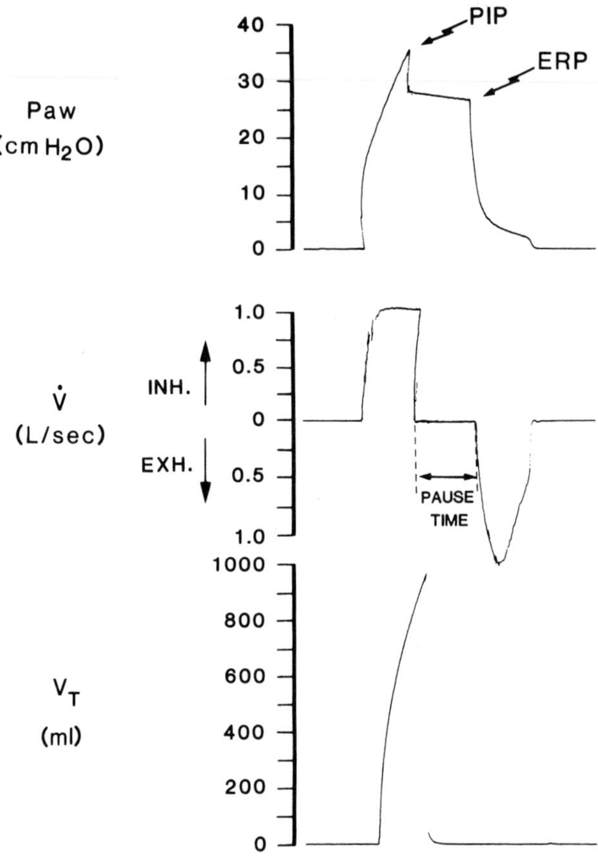

Fig. 15-10. Airway pressure (PAW), flow rate (V̇), and tidal volume (VT) during end-inspiratory pause (EIP). Peak inflation pressure (PIP) is generated (35 cm H_2O), while gas flows from the ventilator. During the pause, no flow is delivered to the patient and airway pressure decreases to the level of the static elastic recoil pressure (ERP) or plateau pressure of the respiratory system (27 cm H_2O). The greater the decrease from PIP to ERP, the greater the airways resistance. After the previously determined pause time, the exhalation valve opens, permitting passive exhalation.

it is not without potential problems. Patients may become tachypneic and breathe with a small VT; under these conditions, the spontaneous minute volume can equal or even exceed the preselected MMV. Consider an adult at a preselected MMV of 8 L/min; if the spontaneous breathing frequency and VT were 40/min and 225 ml, respectively, the spontaneous minute volume would equal 9 L/min, and thus exceed the level of MMV. Although indicated, *no* mechanical ventilation would be provided by the ventilator. Hence, it would be inappropriate to allow this pattern of ventilation to continue, since the patient could become even more tachypneic, and eventually fatigue, followed by deterioration of pulmonary function.

End-Inspiratory Pause

Postinflation hold, end-inspiratory plateau, or *end-inspiratory pause* (EIP)—all terms for the same procedure—represents a period of time after mechanical inhalation when *no flow* is delivered from the ventilator, positive-pressure is maintained in the lungs, and the opening of the exhalation valve is delayed (Fig. 15–10). EIP is considered a part, or extension, of the mechanical inhalation phase because the ventilator does not initiate exhalation until after the EIP time has elapsed. The duration of EIP is designated in seconds, or is expressed as a percentage of the total time of the respiratory cycle.

With EIP, a PIP is generated when VT is delivered to the patient. During the pause time, airway pressure decreases to the static elastic recoil pressure (ERP) or plateau pressure of the respiratory system. PIP and ERP are useful in determining CLT and RAW (Tables 15–6 and 15–7).

End-expiratory pause has been advocated as a method of enhancing distribution of inhaled VT and therefore, of decreasing arterial carbon dioxide tension and VD/VT.[25] This may be explained by the fact that inhalation time is increased during EIP; if inhalation time is long enough to exceed the time constant of slow-filling spaces in the lung, distribution of ventilation is improved. Collateral ventilation and Pendeluft flow, also thought to enhance the distribution of ventilation, occur more readily when time is allowed for pressure to equalize throughout the lung during the EIP. Collateral ventilation occurs when gas enters alveoli through collateral channels; these may be channels in the alveolar walls (Kohn's pores) or communications between the bronchioles and alveoli (Lambert's canals). Pendeluft flow occurs when, during the EIP, surplus volume from fast-filling spaces redistributes and flows to slow-filling spaces. Gas flow between different regions of the lung is caused by instantaneous pressure gradients resulting from inequalities of time constants among these regions.

Table 15–6. Calculation of Compliance and Airways Resistance

Definition: End-inspiratory pause may be used to differentiate dynamic (CDYN) (L/cm H_2O) from static lung-thorax compliance (CST) (L/cm H_2O) and to determine airways resistance (RAW) (cm H_2O/L/sec).

1. CDYN = VT/PIP − baseline airway pressure
   where VT = exhaled tidal volume (L)
   PIP = peak inflation pressure (cm H_2O)
   Baseline airway pressure = atmospheric pressure, or the continuous positive airway pressure (CPAP) (cm H_2O) level

   Example[a]:
   CDYN = 1 L/35 cm H_2O − 0 cm H_2O
   = 0.028 L/cm H_2O

2. CST = VT/ERP − baseline airway pressure
   where ERP = static elastic recoil pressure of the respiratory system (cm H_2O)

   Example[a]:
   CST = 1 L/27 cm H_2O − 0 cm H_2O
   = 0.037 L/cm H_2O

3. RAW = PIP − ERP/V̇I
   where V̇I = inspiratory flow rate (L/sec)

   Example[a]:
   RAW = 35 cm H_2O − 27 cm H_2O/1 L/sec
   = 8 cm H_2O/L/sec

[a] See Figure 15–10.

Table 15–7. Factors Affecting Peak Inflation Pressure

Definition: Elastic and resistive components of the peak inflation pressure (PIP) can be estimated using end-inspiratory pause. Factors affecting PIP may be represented mathematically as follows:

PIP α (VT/CST) + (RAW + V̇I)
where VT = exhaled tidal volume (L)
CST = static lung-thorax compliance (L/cm H_2O)
RAW = airways resistance (cm H_2O/L/sec)
V̇I = inspiratory flow rate (L/sec)

Example[a]:
PIP = (1 L/0.037 L/cm H_2O) + (8 cm H_2O/L/sec × 1 L/sec)
= 27 cm H_2O + 8 cm H_2O
= 35 cm H_2O

[a] See Figure 15–10.

Pressure-Limited, Time-Cycled Mechanical Ventilation

With this technique, a pressure limit is applied by presetting an overpressure governor to limit the PIP to a selected value. Once the pressure limit is reached, airway pressure is held at that level until the ventilator time-cycles "OFF" (mechanical inhalation terminates when a preselected inspiratory time is reached) (Fig. 15–11). Gas actively flows from the ventilator during the pressure limit or the inspiratory pressure plateau period. This is in contrast to EIP; when flow from the ventilator is interrupted during the hold period, gas is redistributed throughout the ventilator circuit and the patient's airways, and a characteristic decrease in airway pressure from PIP to the elastic recoil or plateau pressure occurs (Fig. 15–10). The decrease in pressure is directly related to RAW.

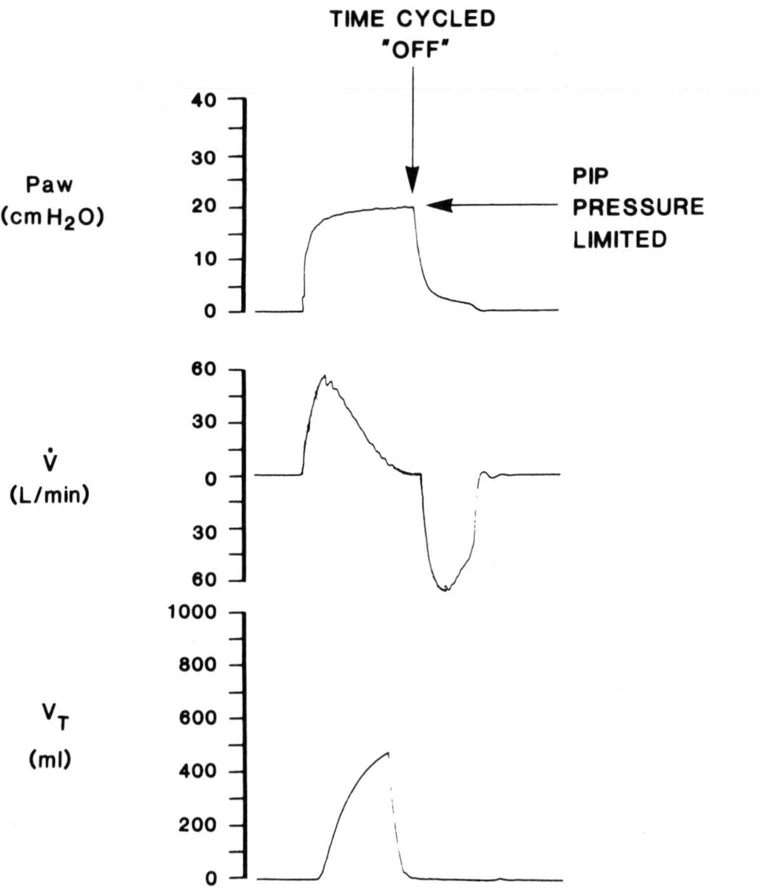

Fig. 15-11. Airway pressure (PAW), flow rate ($\dot{V}$), and tidal volume (VT) during pressure-limited time-cycled ventilation. The PIP is pressure-limited to 20 cm H_2O, and the ventilator time cycles "OFF" after a preselected inspiratory time has elapsed. When the pressure limit is reached, the inspiratory flow waveform decelerates exponentially from approximately 60 to 0 L/min. VT, the integral of inspiratory flow rate and time, is 500 ml.

Pressure-limited time-cycled mechanical ventilation is often used for infants with HMD. Limiting PIP can also reduce the risk of barotrauma. Pressure-limited, time-cycled ventilation has been advocated by Reynolds, who has posited that one factor in the pathogenesis of bronchopulmonary dysplasia is mechanical trauma caused by high airway pressures during mechanical ventilation.[26] In terms of gas exchange, it is suggested that, if alveoli are held open longer with mechanical inhalation, arterial oxygenation and distribution of ventilation may be improved.

Pressure-Support Ventilation

Newer microprocessor-driven mechanical ventilators include PSV that operates in conjunction with their demand flow valve systems. The airway pressure, flow, and lung volume changes during PSV are more akin to AV than to spontaneous positive pressure with CPAP. Work of breathing appears to be decreased by PSV; however, the technique is based on an entirely different concept than CPAP. In the PSV mode, the ventilator is patient-triggered "ON," and continues in the inhalation phase to a preselected

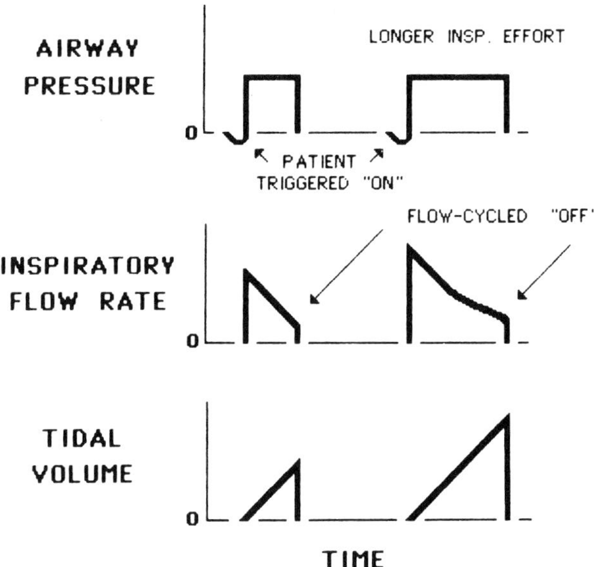

Fig. 15-12. Pressure support. The ventilator is patient-triggered "ON" and, as long as inspiratory effort is maintained, airway pressure stays constant with a variable flow rate of gas from the ventilator. The ventilator cycles "OFF" when the patient's inspiratory flow rate demand decreases to a predetermined percentage of the peak inspiratory flow rate, i.e., the ventilator is flow-cycled "OFF." In the PSV mode, the airway pressure level is preselected, while the patient retains control over inspiratory time and flow rate, tidal and minute volume, and ventilator rate.

positive-pressure limit.[27,28] *As long as the patient's inspiratory effort is maintained, the preselected airway pressure stays constant, with a variable flow of gas from the ventilator.* Inhalation cycles "OFF" when the patient's inspiratory flow demand decreases to a predetermined percentage of the initial peak mechanical inspiratory flow (Fig. 15–12). Thus, the ventilator is *flow-cycled,* following which passive exhalation occurs (Table 15–8). With PSV, the peak inspiratory flow rate, flow waveform, inspiratory time, V_T, $\overline{P_{AW}}$, and airway pressure contour depend on the patient's breathing pattern (Fig. 15–12). V_T is determined by patient effort, lung compliance, R_{AW}, and the level of PSV.

Because PSV augments every breath initiated by the patient, most authorities tend to agree that work of breathing is decreased for patients with decreased lung compliance and/or increased R_{AW}. The technique combines power from the ventilator plus the patient's effort in order to ventilate, a hybrid form of ventilation. MacIntyre contends that PSV is a "pressure assisted" form of ventilation that may be employed to decrease overall effort and work of breathing, and allows the patient to breathe comfortably because the V_T, inspiratory time, and the inspiratory flow rate profile are controlled by the patient.[27,28] Using a mechanical model to mimic patients with compromised pulmonary function, MacIntyre[27] reported that increasing levels of PSV progressively decreased respiratory muscle requirements and work for ventilation. It was shown that a reduction in the ventilatory muscle pressure requirement and the pressure/volume change ratio for each breath resulted when appropriate levels of PSV were employed.

Because PSV is a form of mechanical ventilation, patients treated with it *should not* be considered to be breathing spontaneously. When receiving PSV, with or without CPAP, they may appear to be assuming the full workload of spontaneous ventilation, and arterial blood

Table 15–8. Ventilators Incorporating Pressure Support Ventilation

Ventilator	Cycling Mechanism[a]	Range (cm H_2O)
Hamilton Veolar and Amadeus	Flow-cycled[b]	1–50
Siemens 900C	Flow-cycled[b]	1–100
Bear-5	Flow-cycled[b]	1–72
Puritan-Bennett 7200a	Variable: exhalation after 300 msec may begin when the inspiratory flow rate is ≤5 L/min for 100 msec or if airway pressure exceeds the end-expiratory pressure plus the PSV level by 1.5 cm H_2O for 100 msec.	1–70
Ohmeda CPU-1	Flow-cycled[b]	1–30
Engström Erica	Flow-cycled[b]	1–30
Bird 6400 ST	Flow-cycled[b]	1–50

[a] Refers to the mechanism responsible for the changeover from the inhalation to exhalation phase during pressure support ventilation.

[b] Ventilator flow cycles "OFF" when the inspiratory flow demand decreases to a predetermined percentage of the initial peak mechanical inspiratory flow rate.

gas tensions and pH values can lead the clinician to conclude erroneously that this is the case. Consider a patient who still has unresolved pulmonary abnormalities (decreased FRC and lung compliance). Treatment with PSV of 5 cm H_2O and CPAP of 5 cm H_2O, with a low inspired oxygen concentration, may result in "normal" blood gas values. However, after tracheal extubation, the patient may become dyspneic and hypercapnic while breathing spontaneously (ambient pressure) in the absence of this support. This point was illustrated in a group of patients treated with PSV, whose $PaCO_2$ averaged 40 ± 2 mmHg, following extubation, $PaCO_2$ increased to 47 ± 2 mmHg.[29]

A potential complication of PSV is the sudden inadvertent application of high, unremitting pressure due to a leak in the breathing circuit. For example, when the Puritan-Bennett 7200 ventilator set at a PSV level of 20 cm H_2O is patient-triggered "ON," airway pressure rises abruptly to 20 cm H_2O and is maintained until the inspiratory flow rate decreases to approximately 5 L/min at which time the ventilator flow cycles "OFF." If a leak around the endotracheal tube cuff develops that exceeds 5 L/min, 20 cm H_2O will be maintained throughout the respiratory cycle, that is, inadvertent "CPAP."[30] Under these conditions, a continuous pressure of 20 cm H_2O may predispose to adverse hemodynamic effects, that is, decreased thoracic venous blood inflow, preload, and cardiac output. Some ventilators limit inspiratory time in the PSV mode as a safety precaution so as to prevent the aforementioned scenario; for example, the Hamilton Veolar ventilator limits its inspiratory time to approximately 3 seconds in the PSV mode.

Application

Two approaches are described.[28] The first employs a low PSV level (e.g., 5 to 10 cm H_2O) to assist spontaneous breathing between IMV breaths, and presumably decrease inspiratory work (Fig. 15–13). The rationale cited for using PSV includes poorly designed demand-valve flow systems (low-flow rate on demand, long response time, highly resistant breathing circuit, and a flow-resistor expiratory pressure valve) and endotracheal tube resistance (Fig. 15–14). However, unless the PSV level is set precisely to match the pressure drop needed

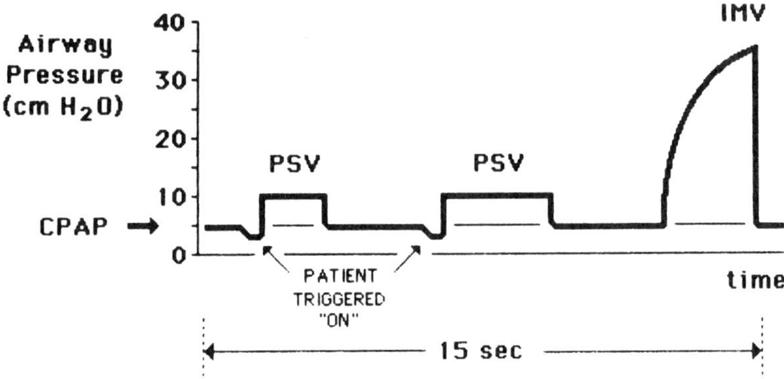

Fig. 15-13. Pressure support ventilation (PSV) used at a low level with continuous positive airway pressure (CPAP) and intermittent mandatory ventilation (IMV). PSV is 5 cm H_2O, CPAP is 5 cm H_2O, and IMV is 4/min. During PSV, the ventilator is patient-triggered "ON," and the PIP increases immediately to 10 cm H_2O (5 cm H_2O greater than CPAP). During the next PSV breath, inspiratory time (determined by the patient) is greater than the previous one, resulting in a greater tidal volume. After 15 seconds elapses, the IMV breath is delivered and a greater PIP is generated.

due to breathing system resistance, positive-pressure ventilation results.[31]

The second approach employs PSV as a stand-alone mechanical ventilatory mode. Here, the level is adjusted to provide the desired tidal and minute volume. Since large variations in tidal and minute volume can occur at a set level of PSV, titration based on volume exchange is sometimes difficult (Fig. 15–5). In this case, capnography is useful in titrating the level of PSV to an appropriate end-tidal PCO_2. When used as a stand-alone technique on some ventila-

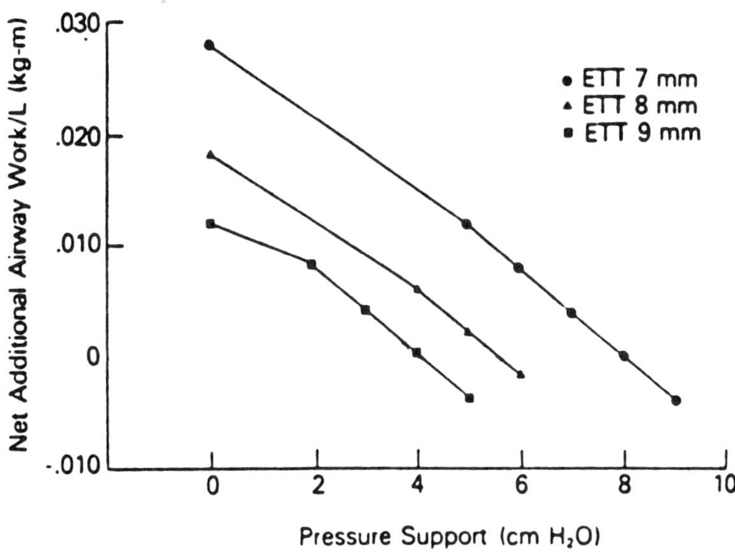

Fig. 15-14. Titration of pressure support with various-sized endotracheal tubes (ETT) and airway work. Note that the narrower the diameter of the endotracheal tube, a greater level of pressure support is required to decrease the net additional work to zero. (From Fiastro et al.,[55] with permission.)

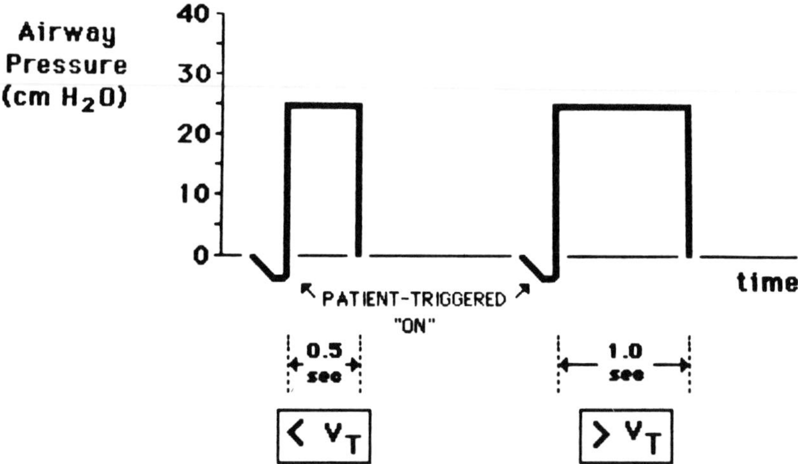

Fig. 15-15. Pressure support ventilation (PSV) used as a stand-alone mechanical ventilatory mode (e.g., PSV level set at 25 cm H_2O). Like assisted mechanical ventilation, the ventilator is patient-triggered "ON," and airway pressure increases abruptly to a pressure plateau of 25 cm H_2O and the inspiratory time is 0.5 seconds (left). On the right, the patient increases his inspiratory time to 1 second for the next PSV breath and, since tidal volume (VT) equals inspiratory time × inspiratory flow rate (not shown), a greater VT is delivered compared with the previous breath. Even though PIP is constant from breath to breath, VT is variable.

tors (except with the Hamilton Veolar, Puritan-Bennett 7200, and Ohmeda CPU-1 ventilators), no safety or backup mechanism to ventilate the patient exists in the event of apnea.

CONTINUOUS POSITIVE AIRWAY PRESSURE AND EXPIRATORY POSITIVE AIRWAY PRESSURE

Continuous positive airway pressure and EPAP are positive-pressure modes used with spontaneous breathing, and can be employed individually or in conjunction with mechanical ventilation (e.g., IMV). With CPAP, both inspiratory and expiratory pressures are positive, although the inspiratory level is less than the expiratory. With EPAP, airway pressure is zero or negative (subambient) during inhalation but increases at the end of exhalation to a predetermined positive-pressure (Fig. 15–16). The level of CPAP or EPAP used is designated by the value measured at end-exhalation. Both are designed to increase expiratory transpulmonary pressure and lung volume (functional residual capacity). Inspiratory and mean airway pressures do not reflect the total alveolar distending pressure at end-exhalation (Fig. 15–17).

Equipment

Continuous-Flow CPAP

A variety of mechanical devices are used to deliver CPAP. A common and convenient method, with or without a ventilator, uses continuous gas-flow rate (usually 15 to 30 L/min at a specified FIO_2), a reservoir bag, one-way valve, humidifier, and an expiratory pressure valve (Fig. 15–18). Both FIO_2 and gas-flow rate are precisely regulated by an air-oxygen blender with a backpressure-compensated flowmeter. The gas is then directed into a 3-L bag that acts as a reservoir for the patient's breathing, and passes through the one-way valve, which opens during spontaneous inhalation and closes during exhalation. During exhalation, when breathing circuit airway pressure is greatest, a compliant reservoir bag distends

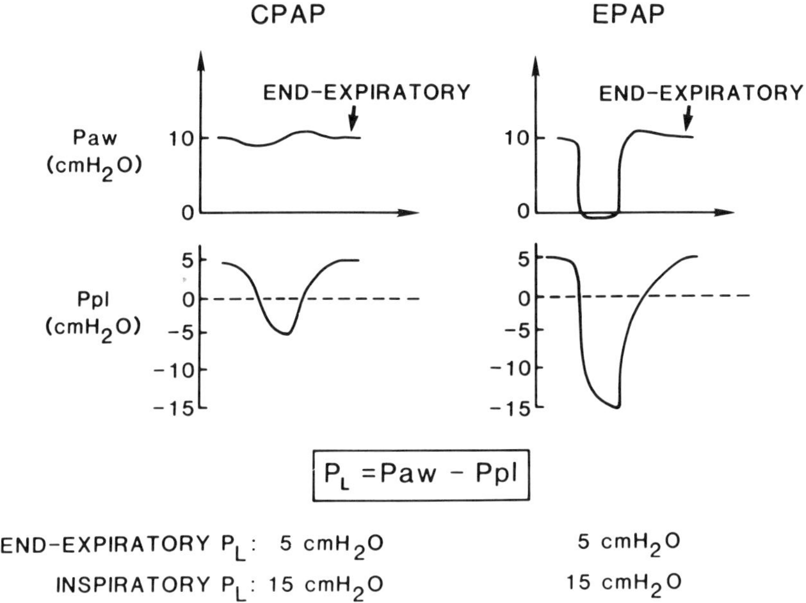

Fig. 15-16. Changes in airway (Paw), intrapleural (Ppl), and transpulmonary pressure (PL) or distending pressure during spontaneous ventilation on continuous positive airway pressure (CPAP) and expiratory positive airway pressure (EPAP). End-expiratory PL (PL = Paw − Ppl) for CPAP and EPAP is 5 cm H_2O (5 cm H_2O = 10 cm H_2O − [+5 cm H_2O]). Inspiratory PL increases to approximately 15 cm H_2O for both modes of spontaneous ventilation (CPAP: 15 cm H_2O = 10 cm H_2O − [−5 cm H_2O]; EPAP: 15 cm H_2O = 0 cm H_2O − [−15 cm H_2O]). Although the changes in PL are the same for both modes of ventilation, changes in Paw and Ppl are greater for EPAP than CPAP when compared at the same end-expiratory airway pressure.

or "balloons" to a larger volume. Expiratory closure of the one-way valve precludes retrograde flow to the reservoir bag and maintains a fairly nondistensible breathing circuit, with only the expiratory pressure valve influencing airway pressure.

The relationship between the rate of gas inflow provided to the breathing system and the rate of the patient's inspiratory flow determines whether the system provides CPAP or EPAP. If the rate of gas inflow is greater than the patient's spontaneous inspiratory flow rate, CPAP results (i.e., airway pressure is positive during inhalation). Conversely, when the rate of inflow to the breathing system is less than the patient's inspiratory flow rate, EPAP results (i.e., airway pressure is zero or subambient during inhalation). The latter situation is associated with increased inspiratory work of breathing (Fig. 15–19).

An increase in work required to breathe against the external load of the breathing system,* in addition to the patient's intrinsic flow-resistive and elastic work of breathing, is associated with a greater decrement in airway pressure, since

$$\text{Work} = \int P_{AW}\, V_T.$$

Because the fundamental goal for treatment of acute respiratory failure is to reduce respiratory work, careful attention is necessary when delivering CPAP in order to minimize fluctuations in airway pressure during spontaneous breath-

* Terminology recommended by Arthur B. Otis, Ph.D, to describe the work performed by the patient which is imposed by the apparatus used to provide CPAP (personal communication, 1988).

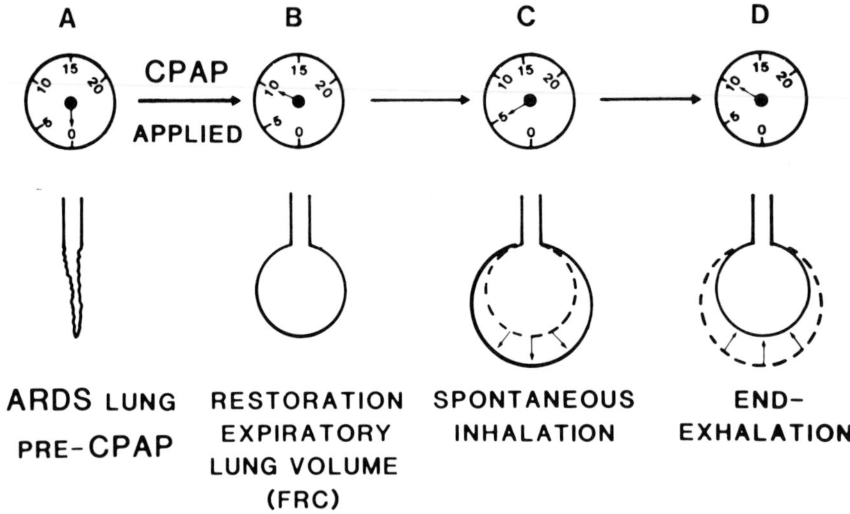

Fig. 15-17. Pressure and volume changes in the lung during spontaneous ventilation with continuous positive airway pressure (CPAP). **(A)** With the acute lung injury, the lung characteristically has reduced functional residual capacity (FRC); airway pressure is zero. **(B)** In this example, CPAP increases the airway pressure to 10 cm H_2O and restores FRC to normal. **(C)** During spontaneous inhalation, airway pressure decreases to 5 cm H_2O, while inspiratory transpulmonary pressure and lung volume increase. **(D)** At end-exhalation, airway pressure returns to 10 cm H_2O, and the lung volume to FRC. (From Banner and Smith,[53] with permission.)

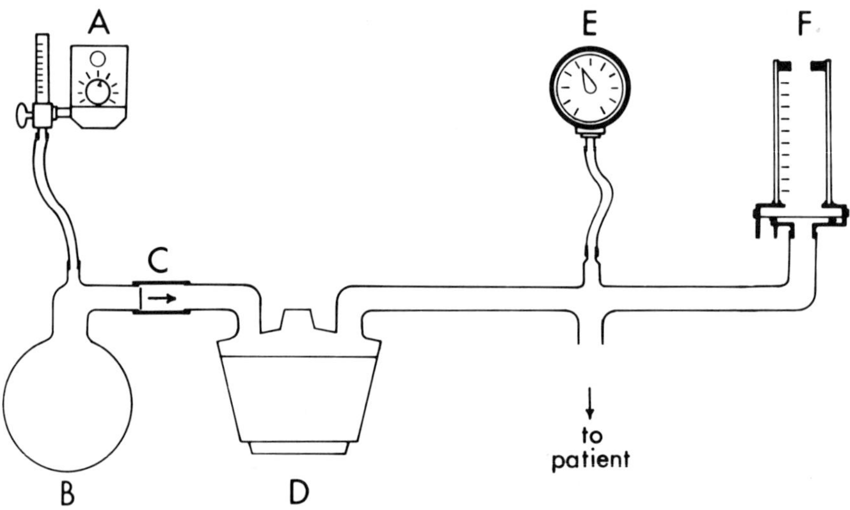

Fig. 15-18. Reservoir bag continuous positive airway pressure (CPAP) system. *A*, air oxygen blender and flowmeter; *B*, 3-L reservoir bag; *C*, one-way valve; *D*, humidifier; *E*, aneroid pressure manometer; and *F*, threshold resistor expiratory pressure valve (Emerson). (From Banner and Smith,[53] with permission.)

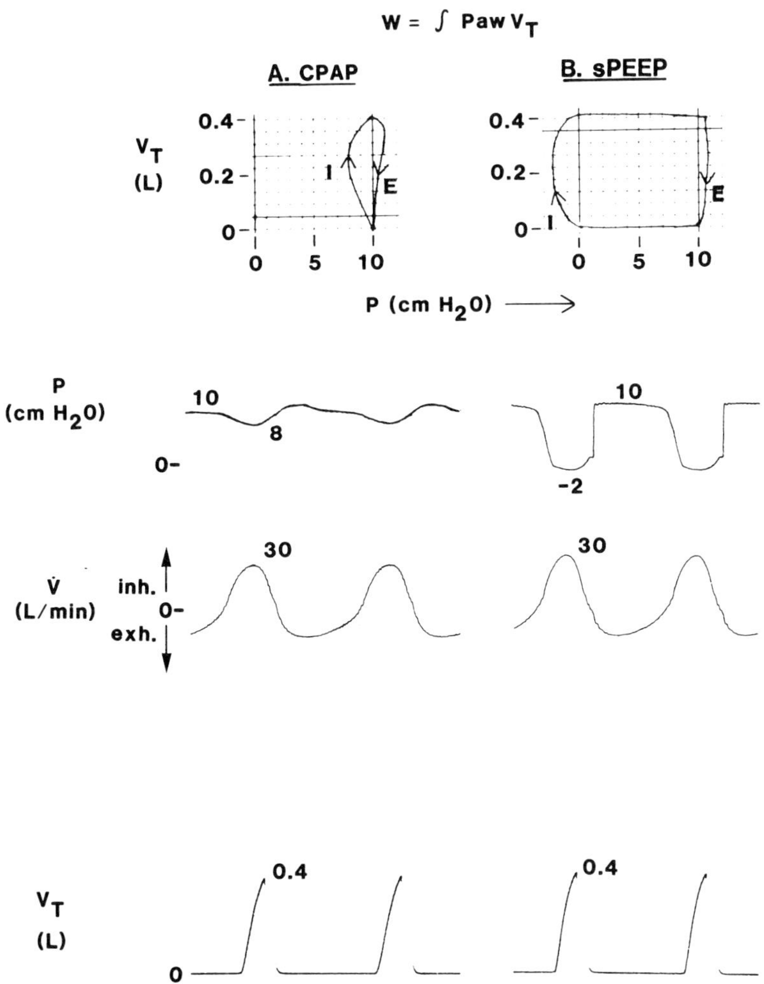

Fig. 15-19. Work (W) required to breathe spontaneously against the external load of the breathing system during continuous positive airway pressure (CPAP) and expiratory positive airway pressure (EPAP) or spontaneous positive end-expiratory pressure (sPEEP) is the integral of the change in airway pressure (PAW) and tidal volume (VT). End-expiratory PAW is 10 cm H_2O and VT and inspiratory flow rate ($\dot{V}$) are equal for both modes of ventilation. During spontaneous inhalation (I) with CPAP, PAW decreases to 8 cm H_2O, and with EPAP or sPEEP, PAW decreases to −2 cm H_2O. During exhalation (E), PAW returns to 10 cm H_2O for both modes. For the same changes in VT, a greater change in PAW occurs during EPAP or sPEEP, resulting in a larger pressure-volume loop. The areas within these loops represent W. For CPAP, W is 0.25 kg/m/min; for EPAP or sPEEP, W is 1.56 k/m/min, a 524 percent increase. (From Banner and Smith,[53] with permission.)

ing. A low-resistive breathing system that supplies high flow rates on demand (usually greater than 60 L/min) during spontaneous inhalation usually meets these requirements and minimizes airway pressure fluctuations.

Demand-Flow CPAP

Demand-flow valves provide CPAP efficiently. These systems were introduced during World War II as a means of increasing altitude

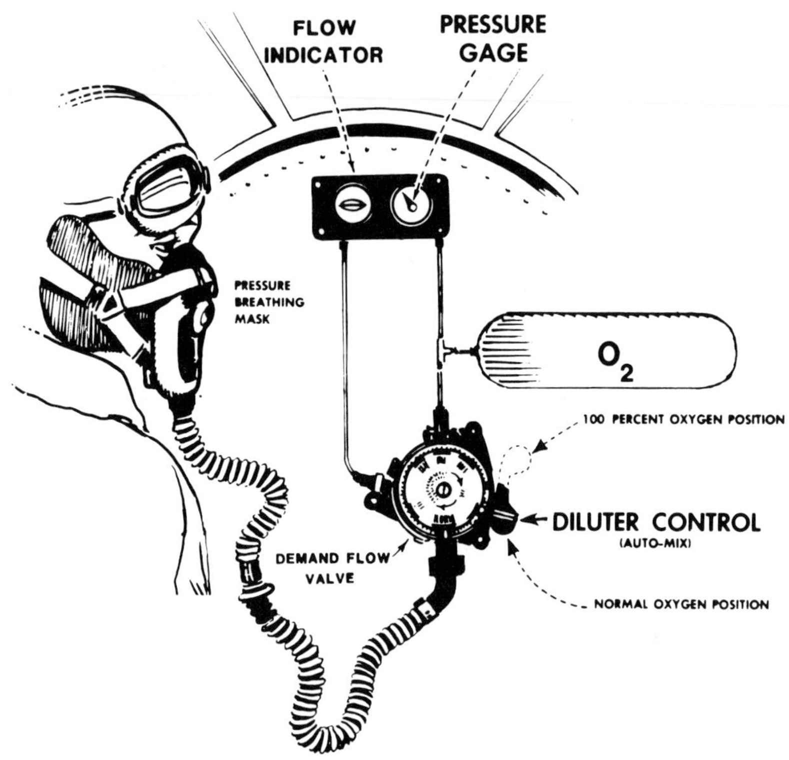

Fig. 15-20. Aviation demand-flow valve (continuous positive airway pressure) system, circa 1944, as used by pilots in World War II. Variable inspiratory flow rate, positive airway pressure (up to about 30 mmHg), and F_{IO_2} were provided using a demand-flow valve attached to a positive-pressure breathing mask. (Modified from Your Body in Flight, Aero Medical Laboratory, Wright Field, Dayton, OH, United States Air Force, 1944.)

tolerance by delivering face mask oxygen under pressure (Fig. 15–20). Some 30 years later, Dr. Forrest M. Bird and Mr. Jack H. Emerson introduced similar devices as alternatives to the continuous-flow reservoir bag apparatus. Demand-flow valves ideally should provide intermittent inspiratory flow rate at a level sufficient to reduce spontaneous inspiratory work and maintain high inspiratory positive airway pressure. The rate of gas flow should accelerate and decelerate automatically in response to the patient's requirements for inspiratory flow rate (Fig. 15–21).

A demand-flow valve CPAP system offers

Fig. 15-21. Example of a commercially available demand flow valve (DFV) CPAP system (IMV Bird) set to provide 10 cm H_2O CPAP. In **(A)** At end-exhalation, the patient's airway pressure (PAW) and the pressure loading the diaphragms of the DFV and expiratory pressure valve are 10 cm H_2O; both valves are closed, and the system is at equilibrium. **(B)** During spontaneous inhalation, PAW decreases to <10 cm H_2O; pressure decreases in the airway pressure sensing line, causing the DFV to open; and gas flow is directed through a Venturi tube, where additional flow is entrained. The greater the inspiratory effort, the greater the opening of the DFV and hence, the greater the flow rate on demand. Since PAW is less than the pressure loading the expiratory pressure valve, the valve is closed. **(C)** At the beginning of exhalation, PAW increases to >10 cm H_2O; this pressure increase is directed along the airway pressure sensing line, causing the DFV to close (cessation of flow rate). Since PAW is slightly greater than the pressure loading the expiratory pressure valve (10 cm H_2O), the valve opens, allowing exhalation. Eventually, the expiratory pressure valve closes when PAW decreases to 10 cm H_2O at end-exhalation, as in (*A*).

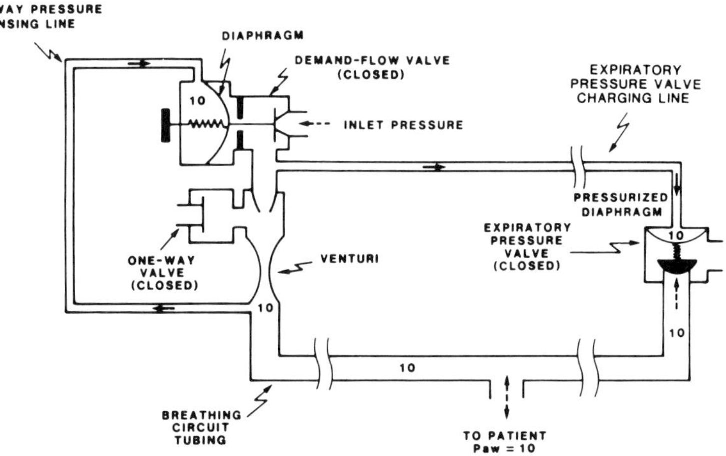

A
END-EXHALATION:
AIRWAY PRESSURE SENSING LINE
DIAPHRAGM
DEMAND-FLOW VALVE (CLOSED)
INLET PRESSURE
EXPIRATORY PRESSURE VALVE CHARGING LINE
10
PRESSURIZED DIAPHRAGM
EXPIRATORY PRESSURE VALVE (CLOSED)
ONE-WAY VALVE (CLOSED)
VENTURI
10
10
10
10
BREATHING CIRCUIT TUBING
TO PATIENT
Paw = 10

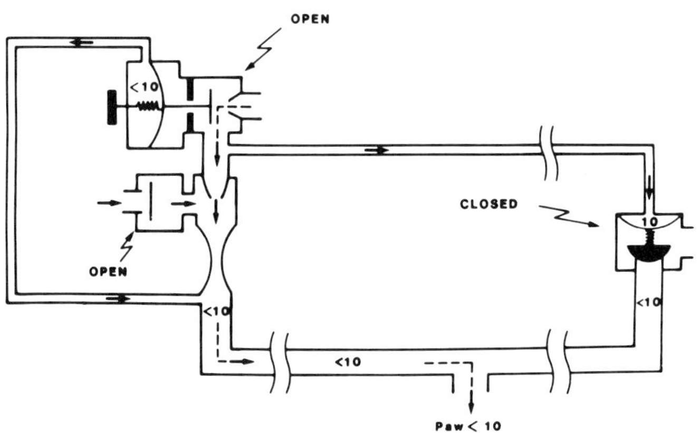

B
SPONTANEOUS INHALATION:
OPEN
<10
CLOSED
10
OPEN
<10
<10
<10
Paw < 10

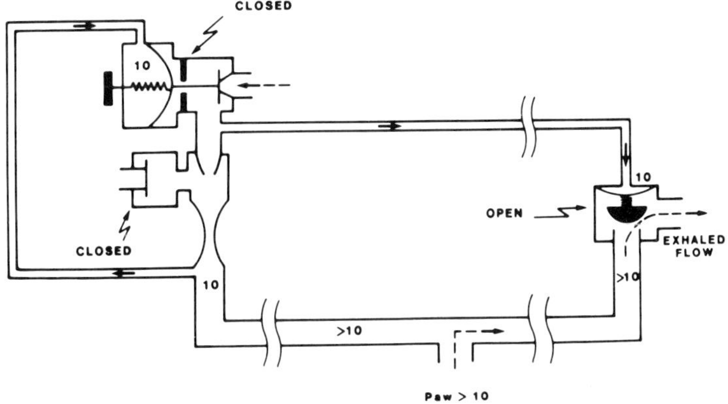

C
BEGINNING EXHALATION:
CLOSED
10
10
OPEN
EXHALED FLOW
CLOSED
10
>10
>10
Paw > 10

two theoretical advantages. First, since both the valve and the breathing circuit are pressurized at the same level, inspiratory effort is negligible. Thus, a decrease of 1 cm H_2O or less below the baseline pressure provides instantaneous gas flow rate at any CPAP level. Second, significant gas loss, inherent in continuous high-flow reservoir bag CPAP systems, does not occur because flow is intermittent and only on demand.

Overall, however, some poorly designed demand-flow valve CPAP systems actually predispose to increased inspiratory work.[32–37] If flow rate output is inadequate, greater inspiratory effort results as the patient struggles to meet his peak inspiratory flow rate requirements. Such demand-flow valves, in combination with highly resistant humidifiers and low-flow air-oxygen blenders, lead to intolerably high resistance to flow and failure of CPAP in an overly stressed and fatigued patient.

Reports involving healthy volunteers,[32,33] lung models,[34,35] and patients[36] demonstrate significant variability in the operational characteristics of commercially available demand-flow CPAP systems. In some of these reports, a continuous flow (60 L/min) reservoir bag system, with a low-resistance threshold resistor expiratory pressure valve (Emerson), required less inspiratory effort, maintained higher inspiratory airway pressure, and was associated with less work of breathing when compared to several demand-flow systems[32,34,36,38] (Fig. 15–22). The desirable characteristics of a demand-flow system are listed in Table 15–9.

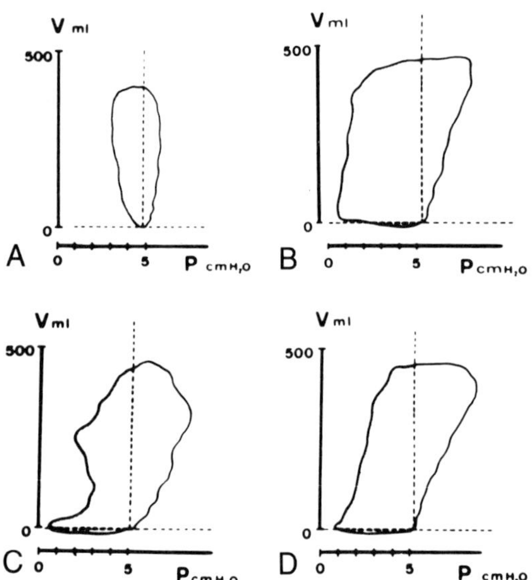

Fig. 15-22. Comparisons in work required to breathe against the external load of CPAP systems (W). W is the integral of airway pressure (P) and tidal volume (V), i.e., the greater the area of the P–V loop, the greater W and vice versa. The end-expiratory pressure was 5 cm H_2O for all CPAP systems. Starting at the bottom, a clockwise movement of the P–V loop occurs during spontaneous breathing. W was less with a continuous-flow system **(A)** and greater with three commercially available demand flow systems: **(B)** Siemens 900 B, **(C)** Siemens 900C, and **(D)** Engström Erica. (From Viale et al.,[38] with permission.)

EXPIRATORY PRESSURE VALVES

Expiratory pressure valves regulate the level of airway pressure during spontaneous ventilation with CPAP, as well as during mechanical ventilation with PEEP. These valves are characterized as threshold, flow resistors, and balloon valves.[40,41]

Threshold Resistors

In theory, threshold resistors generate expiratory pressure (P) without associated flow resistance. Expiratory pressure in a threshold resistor results from a force (F), expressed in newtons (N), applied over a discrete surface area (SA), and expressed in square meters (m^2):

$$P \alpha F/SA \tag{1}$$

For example, a loading force of 10 newtons applied to a surface area of 0.01 m^2 generates a pressure of 1,000 N/m^2 ($\approx$ 10 cm H_2O). Exhaled gas passes freely through the completely open threshold resistor orifice until the balance of forces on opposite sides of the valve mechanism is disrupted.[41] At this point, the valve closes abruptly, preventing further gas loss from the airways and lungs.

Table 15–9. Desirable Characteristics of a Demand-Flow Valve CPAP System

Response time	Delay time from the onset of spontaneous inhalation to DFV opening and gas flow to patient (<0.2 sec)
Triggering pressure	1–2 cm H_2O below end-expiratory pressure (required airway pressure below the level of CPAP during spontaneous inhalation to initiate flow from the DFV)
Flow rate output	≥ 120 L/min during spontaneous inhalation; must be able to accelerate and decelerate flow rate on patient demand
CPAP range	0 ≥ 30 cm H_2O (upper limit has not been established)
Expiratory pressure valve	Low-resistance threshold resistor (e.g., Vital Signs, Hamilton, and Emerson)
Air/oxygen blender	High-flow output (≥ 120 L/min), directly related to flow rate output of DFV
Resistance characteristics of breathing circuit	Low flow-resistive components in the breathing circuit (e.g., humidifier, one-way valves, properly sized diameter tubing, avoidance of right-angle and narrow-bore endotracheal tube connections)

(From Banner and Smith,[53] with permission.)

Various mechanisms have been employed in the design of threshold resistors (Table 15–10); the following are examples of some commercially available types. The Emerson water column valve is a gravity-dependent device that uses the weight of a column of water to exert force over the surface area of a diaphragm. Expiratory pressure (level of CPAP) may be titrated by varying the amount of water (force) held in a column (Fig. 15-23).

The Hamilton threshold resistor (Hamilton Medical, Veolar, and Amadeus ventilators) produces expiratory pressure by relying on electromagnetic force, generated by a solenoid, and applied over the surface area of a diaphragm. With this device, force and, therefore, expiratory pressure, are proportional to the electric current supplied to the solenoid. By regulating the amount of current with a rheostat (control knob on ventilator panel), the level of CPAP is selected.

The Vital Signs valve produces expiratory pressure by employing flexed, coiled springs which exert force against a plastic disk. A *flexing,* rather than compressing, action of the springs appears to maintain constant force no matter how much the valve is open during exhalation; thus, force over surface area and expiratory pressure remain fairly constant (Fig. 15–24). The Vital Signs valves are available in preset pressure levels of 2.5, 5, 7.5, 10, 12.5, 15 and 20 cm H_2O.

In contrast, spring-loaded valves that rely on *compression* of a spring result in an increase in force when the spring is compressed as the valve opens during exhalation. When exhaled flow rate is high, the valve opens wider and spring compression increases. Marini et al.[43] found that spring-loaded valves with only one spring produce significant resistance to flow rate. Hence, such valves are not true threshold resistors.

Another type of threshold resistor found on the Bear BP 200 and Cub infant ventilators (Bear Medical) uses gas flow from a Venturi (jet pump) directed against a diaphragm. By regulating gas-flow rate into the Venturi, the backpressure of the Venturi, and thus the force over the surface area of the diaphragm, is controlled. Titrating gas-flow rate to the jet regulates the level of CPAP.

Flow Resistors

Flow-resistor expiratory pressure valves generate expiratory pressure by imposing an adjustable orifice resistance (R) to exhaled flow

Table 15–10. Expiratory Positive-Pressure Valves

Valve	Description
Threshold Resistors	
Non-gravity dependent	
Vital Signs	Flexion of multiple springs against a disk
Ambu	Compression of a single spring against a disk
Hamilton	Electromagnetically activated piston over a diaphragm
Instrumentation Industries	Magnetic attraction of a metal disk valve
Bourns BP 200, BEAR Cub, Ohmeda CPU-1, Puritan-Bennett 7200a	Venturi (jet pump) backpressure against a diaphragm
IMV Bird	Pressure-loaded diaphragm-disk mechanism
Gravity dependent	
Emerson	Water-column hydrostatic force over a diaphragm
Boehringer	Weighted-ball valve (force) over an orifice
Underwater valve	Hydrostatic force over the orifice of the exhalation tube
Flow resistor	
Screw-clamp	Variable orifice
Flow resistor-like devices	
Siemens 900B and 900C[a]	Hinged clamp scissor valve
Hybrid valves	
Balloon valves[b]	
Puritan-Bennett MA-1, MA-2, and BEAR 1, 2, and 5	Inflatable balloon (mushroom) valve
Babybird outflow valve	Variable orifice and diaphragm

[a] Although the Siemens expiratory pressure valve is Servo-controlled, it responds as a flow resistor, i.e., pressure drop across the valve increases as flow rate increases.[42–44]

[b] This design has characteristics of both threshold and flow resistors, although in theory it is a theshold resistor; flow resistance occurs primarily because of the limited opening area for exhalation.[41]

rate ($\dot{V}$). Expiratory pressure varies directly with resistance, or stated another way, inversely with the orifice size, assuming flow rate is constant:

$$P \alpha R\dot{V} \qquad (2)$$

This relationship is congruent only under laminar flow conditions and a given range of flow rates (Fig. 15–25). For example, if resistance is 10 cm H_2O/L/sec and exhaled flow rate is 1 L/sec, expiratory pressure = 10 cm H_2O. If the adjustable exhalation orifice is narrowed, greater resistance to flow rate results; thus, greater pressure (CPAP) is generated in the breathing circuit.

The expiratory pressure valve on the Siemens 900B and 900C ventilators is a Servo-controlled valve, but that does not preclude the valve from exhibiting flow resistor-like characteristics[42–44] (Fig. 15–26). With this device, a narrow diameter exhalation orifice is situated between a hinged clamp mechanism.

Hybrid Valves

Another type of expiratory pressure valve employs a pressurized inflatable balloon to obstruct the exhalation outlet. The balloon valve frequently is pressurized by a Venturi mechanism. By regulating the flow rate of gas supplied to

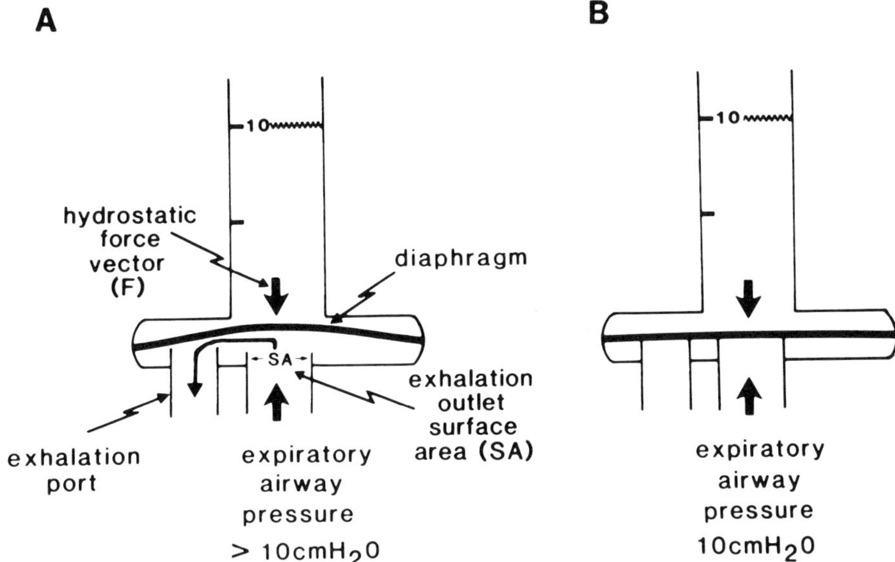

Fig. 15-23. A threshold resistor expiratory pressure valve (J. H. Emerson Company) generates expiratory positive-pressure (P) by exerting force (F) over a surface area (SA). Force is the critical factor; the imbalance of forces acting across the valve opens and closes the valve. At the beginning of exhalation **(A),** F exerted by the patient's expiratory airway pressure is greater than the hydrostatic F vector exerted by the water column; consequently, the diaphragm rises upwards and allows exhalation. At end-exhalation **(B),** the force generated by the decreasing airway pressure is not enough to counter the hydrostatic F, and the diaphragm descends, occluding the exhalation outlet. (From Banner et al.,[56] with permission.)

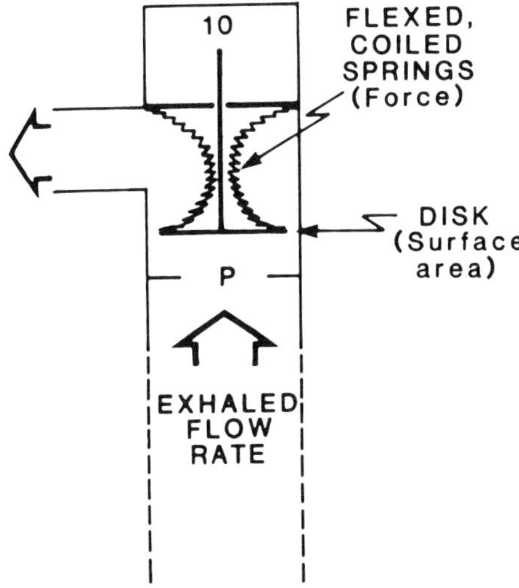

Fig. 15-24. Threshold resistor expiratory pressure valve (Vital Signs). (Low flow-resistant.) Expiratory positive-pressure (P) is generated through force (F), exerted by the *flexion* of multiple coiled springs against a plastic disk, i.e., exhalation outlet surface area (SA), (P α F/SA). Flexion, rather than compression, of the springs seems to allow F to remain constant as the disk is displaced away from the orifice during exhalation. Thus, near-constant P is maintained as the valve opens wider to accommodate higher exhaled flow rates. The orifice size of the valve is such that flow resistance is minimal.

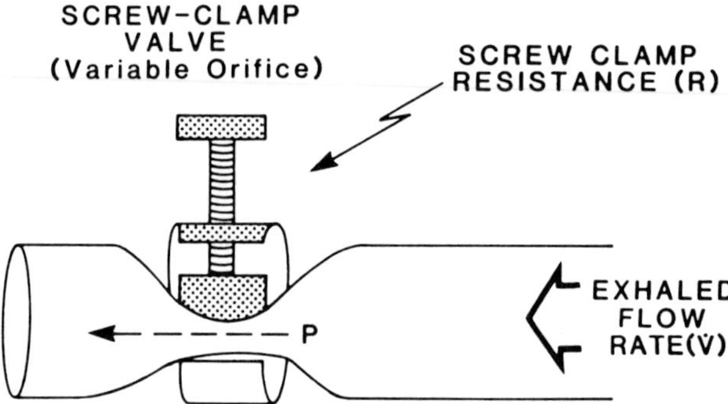

Fig. 15-25. A flow resistor (screw-clamp variable orifice) determines expiratory positive-pressure (P) by the product of resistance (R) and flow rate ($\dot{V}$) directed through the valve. (High flow-resistant.) R is regulated with the screw clamp and varies inversely with orifice size. The smaller the exhalation orifice, the greater the R and, thus, the greater the P (assuming constant flow rate) and vice versa. (From Banner et al.,[56] with permission.)

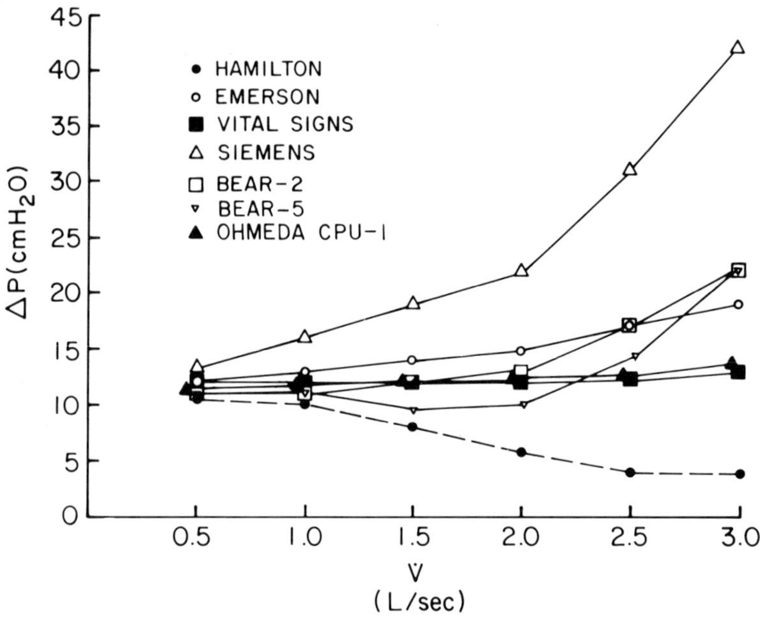

Fig. 15-26. Comparison of the flow-resistance characteristics of various expiratory positive-pressure valves. The pressure drop (ΔP) was measured across each valve set at 10 cm H_2O continuous positive airway pressure (CPAP) at incremental flow rates ($\dot{V}$). The greater the slope, the greater the resistance and vice versa. (Values are means.) At flow rates of ≥1 L/sec, the Siemens exhalation valve ΔP was significantly higher ($P < 0.05$), while the Hamilton threshold resistor ΔP was significantly lower than the ΔP of all other valves. Note: As flow rate increased, the ΔP values for all valves became more divergent. (From Banner,[44] with permission.)

the Venturi, one controls the loading pressure to the balloon and the resultant CPAP. Balloon valves have characteristics of both threshold and flow resistors. Although this valve was conceived as a threshold resistor, flow resistance occurs primarily because of the limited opening area of the balloon valve for exhalation.[41] Inflatable balloon valves generate expiratory pressure as a result of loading pressure applied to the balloon and the resistance characteristics of the valve (Fig. 15–27). Mathematically, these relationships may be stated as

$$P \alpha \text{ loading pressure} + R\dot{V} \qquad (3)$$

Ventilators that incorporate inflatable balloon expiratory pressure valves are the Puritan-Bennett MA-1 and MA-2 models, and the BEAR 1, 2, and 5 models.

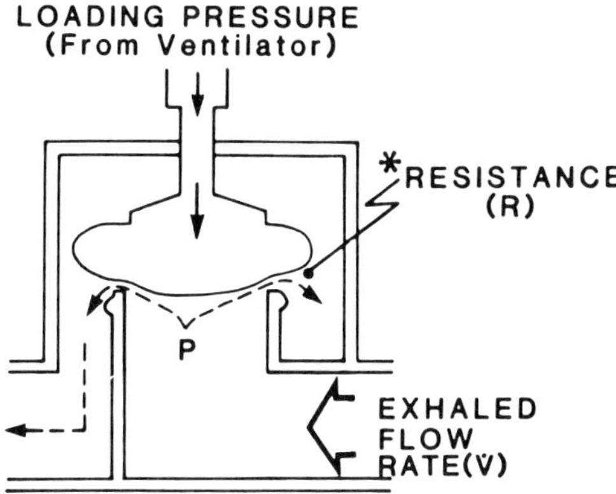

Fig. 15-27. Inflatable balloon expiratory pressure valve. (Moderate flow-resistant.) An inflatable balloon is pressurized by a loading pressure from the ventilator that is set by the operator. The exhalation orifice is thus obstructed and exhaled flow rate ($\dot{V}$) is opposed by the balloon-loading pressure. Exhaled $\dot{V}$ is directed through narrow openings between the bottom of the balloon and the valve seat, which give rise to resistance (R) to $\dot{V}$. Under these conditions, a small exhalation area (EA) for gas efflux occurs (similar to flow resistor). As R increases, expiratory positive-pressure (P) increases, assuming $\dot{V}$ is unchanged. Thus, P is proportional to the loading pressure in the balloon plus the product of R and $\dot{V}$.

The Babybird outflow valve (Babybird ventilator) regulates expiratory pressure by directing gas flow through an orifice against a diaphragm. The exhalation orifice can be positioned closer to or further away from the diaphragm which, in turn, acts to increase or decrease resistance to flow, respectively. Force is also exerted by the elastic recoil properties of the diaphragm over the exhalation orifice and directly affects the expiratory pressure generated. It is increased as the diaphragm is displaced upward when the exhalation orifice is positioned closer to the diaphragm in a fashion analogous to compression of a coiled spring. At flow rates of greater than approximately 30 L/min, expiratory pressure progressively increases, while at flow rates less than this amount, expiratory pressure is relatively stable. Therefore, this valve also has characteristics of both flow and threshold resistors. It was designed to be used at low flow rates (2 to 15 L/min) and for newborn patients. Because of its flow resistor characteristics at higher flow rates, it is not recommended for adult patients.

Resistance Characteristics

Theoretically, a threshold resistor should maintain a constant pressure regardless of variations in exhaled flow rate, as contrasted with a flow resistor, in which airway pressure deviations occur when the flow rate of gas through the CPAP system is changed.[44] In actuality, resistance to exhaled flow occurs with both types of valves.[42–46] As a result, pressure increases above the desired level when the exhaled flow rate and/or the continuous flow rate through the CPAP system increases. Thus, all valves are to some extent hybrid. When exhaled flow rate is high (as during coughing), excessive airway pressures can result (Fig. 15–28), potentially increasing the likelihood of barotrauma. Gal[47] has reported that intubated patients can generate peak exhaled flow rates up to 240 L/min during coughing.

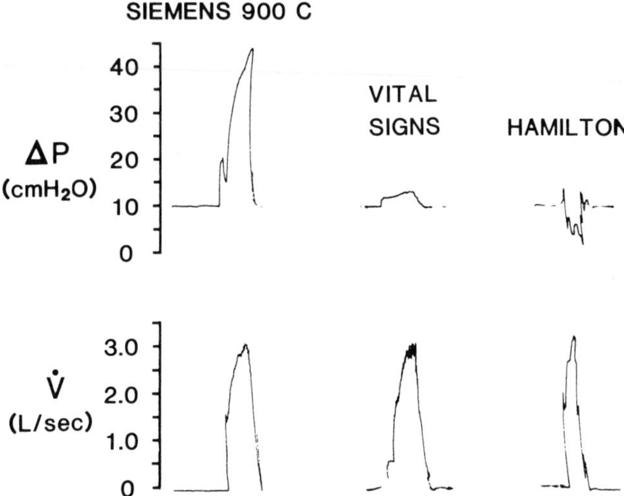

Fig. 15-28. Effects of a simulated cough with high- and low-resistance expiratory pressure valves. All valves were set to a CPAP of 10 cm H_2O when the flow rate ($\dot{V}$) was zero. The pressure drop (ΔP) across each valve was measured when a peak sinusoidal $\dot{V}$ of 3 L/sec (180 L/min) was suddenly directed through each valve, i.e., a simulated cough. Note that the ΔP was approximately 45 cm H_2O with the Siemens valve, approximately 12 cm H_2O with the Vital Signs valve, and approximately 5 cm H_2O with the lower resistant Hamilton valve. The Hamilton valve opens wider under conditions of a sudden high $\dot{V}$, as during coughing. Low-resistance expiratory pressure valves may lessen the incidence of pulmonary barotrauma, since acute increases in airway pressure during coughing do not occur.

When high-resistance valves are used, exhalation is no longer passive, and expiratory work of breathing and oxygen consumption increase. When high-resistance expiratory pressure valves are combined with poorly designed demand-flow valves (those with slow response time; substantial reduction in airway pressure to initiate flow during spontaneous inhalation; and no provision for instantaneous, high flow rate on demand), intolerably high resistance to flow and increased work of breathing result.

EFFECTS OF EXPIRATORY PRESSURE VALVE FLOW RESISTANCE ON INSPIRATORY WORK OF BREATHING

Resistance of the expiratory pressure valve affects the inspiratory positive airway pressure level and the work required to breathe against the external load of the CPAP system. A highly flow-resistant expiratory pressure valve leads to a greater decrease in airway pressure and, hence, greater work than a low flow-resistant one during spontaneous breathing (if all other factors are constant).[48,49]

For CPAP systems employing a continuous flow of gas, the generated pressure results from resistance to gas flowing through the orifice of the expiratory pressure valve [Eq. (2)]. During spontaneous inhalation, flow is diverted from the expiratory pressure valve to the lungs and airway pressure decreases. For example, a flow resistor valve with a resistance of 10 cm H_2O/L/sec creates an airway pressure of 10 cm H_2O with a continuous flow rate of 1 L/sec (60 L/min). If the patient inhales with a peak inspiratory flow rate of 0.75 L/sec (45 L/min), flow rate through the expiratory valve will decrease to 0.25 L/sec (15 L/min); and airway pressure decreases transiently from 10 to 2.5 cm H_2O. The work required to breathe against the external load of the CPAP system increases, since it is dependent on the change in airway pressure and VT:

$$W = \int P_{AW} \times V_T \quad (4)$$

Under these conditions, Ppl must decrease by a corresponding amount to generate appropriate changes in transpulmonary pressure.[49] The greater the change in transpulmonary pressure for a given tidal volume, the greater the patient's work of breathing (Fig. 15-29).

Unless attempts are made to decrease resistance to flow throughout the breathing circuit, work of breathing may become intolerable. This observation explains why CPAP and IMV have failed in the hands of some clinicians. Therefore, we recommend that all sources of flow resistance in the breathing circuit be minimized, and that only threshold resistor valves with low flow resistance be used to provide CPAP.

CONVENTIONAL AND MICROPROCESSOR-CONTROLLED VENTILATORS

Major advances in computer technology have occurred in recent years. Microprocessor computer and pneumatic circuit technologies have

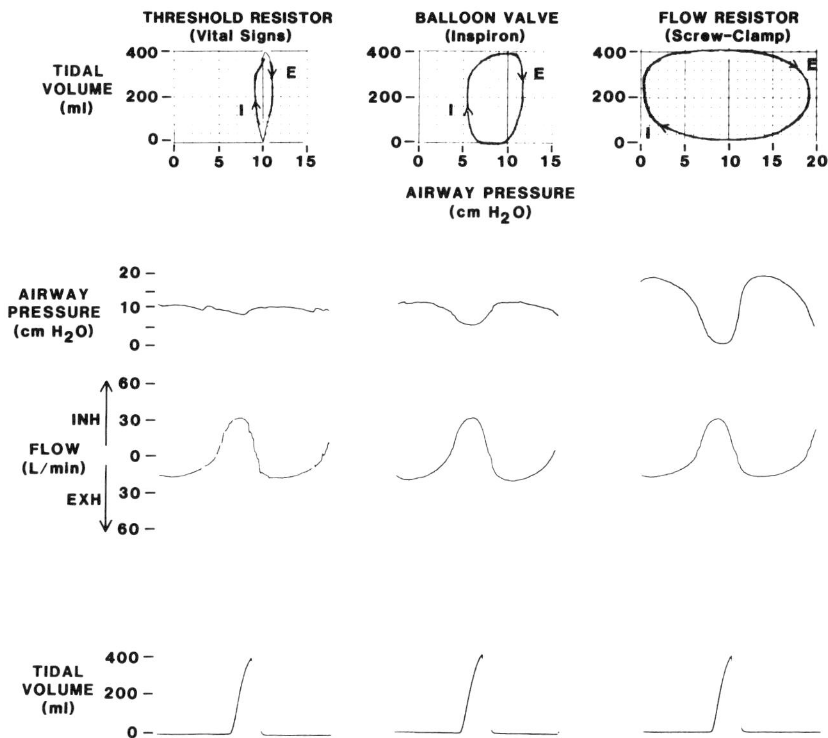

Fig. 15-29. Airway pressure, flow rate, and VT recordings for 3 types of expiratory pressure valves with an end-expiratory pressure of 10 cm H_2O. During all conditions, the peak inspiratory and expiratory flow rates, the I:E ratio, breathing frequency, spontaneous tidal volume, and the flow rate (40 L/min) directed through the CPAP breathing circuit were constant. Variations in airway pressure during inhalation (I) and exhalation (E) were directly proportional to flow resistance of valves. The circumscribed area within the pressure-volume loops represents the work required to breathe against the external load of the system (W). Since VT was constant, the greater the change in airway pressure, the greater the W. (From Banner et al.,[48] with permission.)

been combined to produce a new generation of mechanical ventilators, that is, microprocessor-controlled ventilators (see Ch. 3). Potential advantages of microprocessor control mechanisms are summarized in Table 15–11.

In the remainder of this chapter we compare the pressure, volume, and flow rate characteristics; ventilatory modalities; inspiratory flow waveforms; and monitoring capabilities of popular microprocessor- and nonmicroprocessor-controlled (conventional) ventilators (Table 15–12). The monitoring and alarm capabilities of both types of ventilators are listed in Table 15–13.

Table 15–11. Potential Advantages of Microprocessor-Controlled Ventilators

General versatility
- Capable of providing various modalities of mechanical and spontaneous positive-pressure ventilation
- Ability to ventilate with a variety of inspiratory flow waveforms
- Choice of cycling mechanisms
- Capability of being reprogrammed and upgraded, depending on current trends
- Ability to ventilate adult and pediatric patients

Monitoring capability
- Real-time monitoring of a variety of ventilatory parameters
- Ability to calculate and monitor lung-thorax compliance, airways resistance, minute exhaled ventilation
- Permits self-checking and cross-checking to ensure proper functioning of computer and pneumatic operation
- Computer memory permits the storage and retrieval of ventilation data for trend analysis

Computer-correction capability
- Allegedly able to perform automatic corrections to maintain the inspiratory flow rate, waveform, and as PIP increases due to changes in CLT and RAW
- Measured tidal and minute volumes corrected to BTPS
- Allegedly, volume losses in the ventilator breathing circuit secondary to compression may be calculated and/or compensated

Display and communications capability
- Computer-controlled LED indicating all current ventilatory parameters, alarms, and limits
- Communication with separate microcomputers available for the monitoring and storage of data

Repairs and maintenance
- System down time reduced due to the relative ease of diagnosing and troubleshooting ventilation programs and the minimal number of moving components in a microprocessor-controlled ventilator.
- Modular components facilitate repair

Inspiratory Flow Rate and Tidal Volume Characteristics

A problem with most conventional ventilators is that high PIP, secondary to decreased CLT and/or increased RAW, cause the inspiratory flow rate and waveforms to decay, resulting in decreased tidal volume delivery. The inspiratory flow rate can be *manually* increased to maintain the delivered VT in some cases. However, other ventilators may be unable to generate sufficient inspiratory flow rates and therefore fail to deliver an appropriate VT.

A ventilator capable of detecting high PIP and maintaining the preselected inspiratory flow waveform, flow rate, and VT is desirable. Microprocessor-controlled ventilators with properly operating feedback systems, in theory, accomplish this goal. In our experience, however, such is not the case.

To illustrate the point, conventional and microprocessor-controlled ventilators were compared (Puritan-Bennett Corp. and Bear Inter Med). Under identical conditions, the inspiratory flow rate and waveform of both types decayed. Thus, VT decreased as PIP increased with the microprocessor as well as the nonmicroprocessor-type ventilators (Fig. 15–30), although the decline was slightly less with the Puritan-Bennett 7200A than with its first generation counterpart, the conventional MA-1. Similar decreases in inspiratory flow rate and VT were noted comparing the BEAR II (conventional) and BEAR V (microprocessor-controlled) ventilators (Fig. 15–31). Other microprocessor-controlled ventilators we have tested responded in the same way. These observations are disappointing, to say the least.

Accuracy of Displayed Exhaled Tidal Volume

Exhaled VT is measured and displayed on microprocessor-controlled ventilators and most conventional ventilators. The accuracy of the displayed data has been questioned.[50] Location of the exhaled flow sensor in the ventilator breathing circuit appears to be the key factor

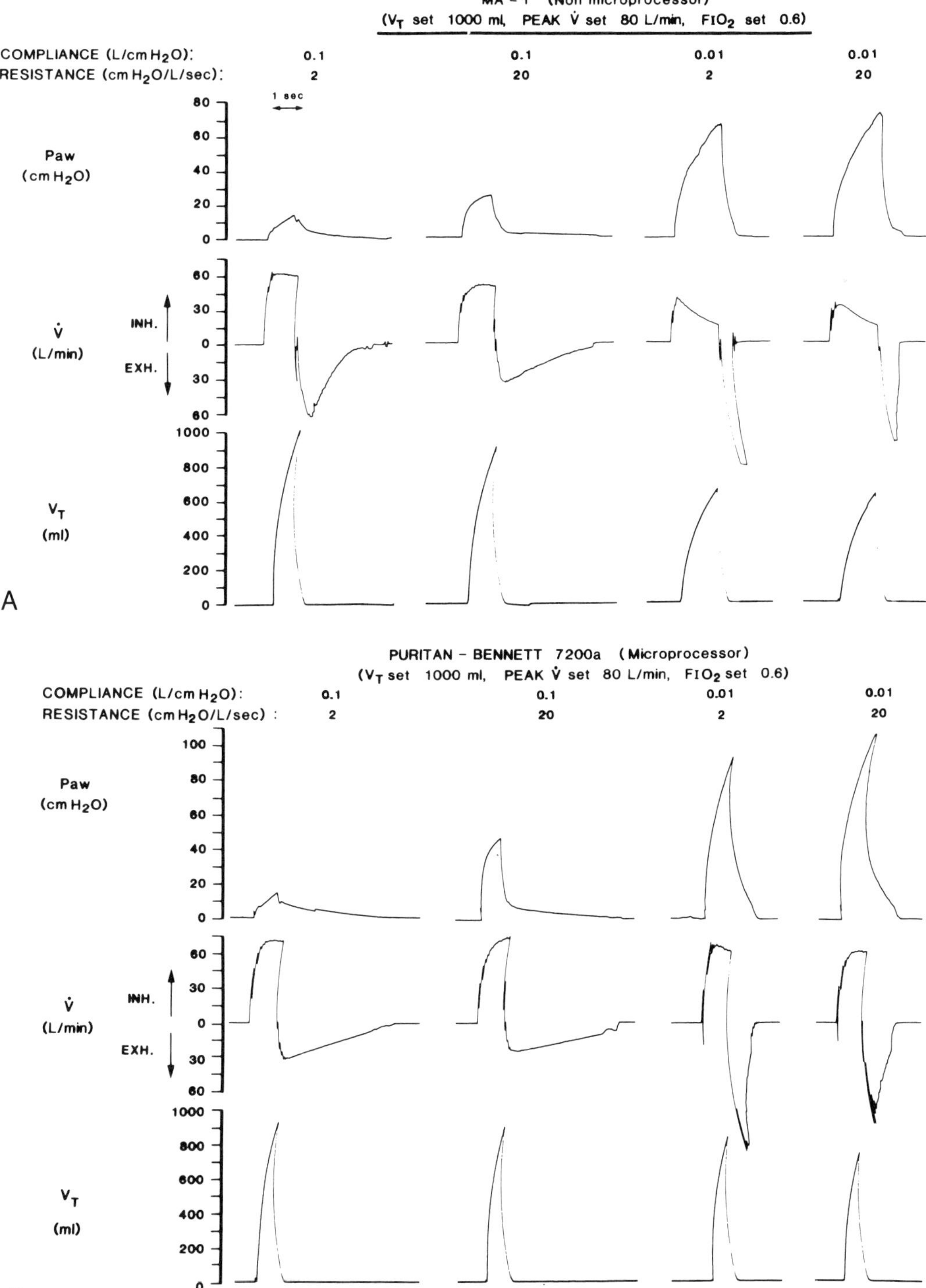

Fig. 15-30. Airway pressure (PAW), flow ($\dot{V}$), and tidal volume (VT) characteristics of the Puritan-Bennett MA-1 nonmicroprocessor type ventilator **(A)** and the 7200a microprocessor type ventilator **(B)** under conditions of varying compliance and resistance. Measurements were obtained between the ventilator Y piece and the endotracheal tube. Note the deterioration in the inspiratory flow rate and waveform, and hence VT as PIP increased. This effect was more pronounced with the MA-1 ventilator. Also note that the LED displayed values for VT are spuriously high on the 7200a ventilator under conditions of high PIP.

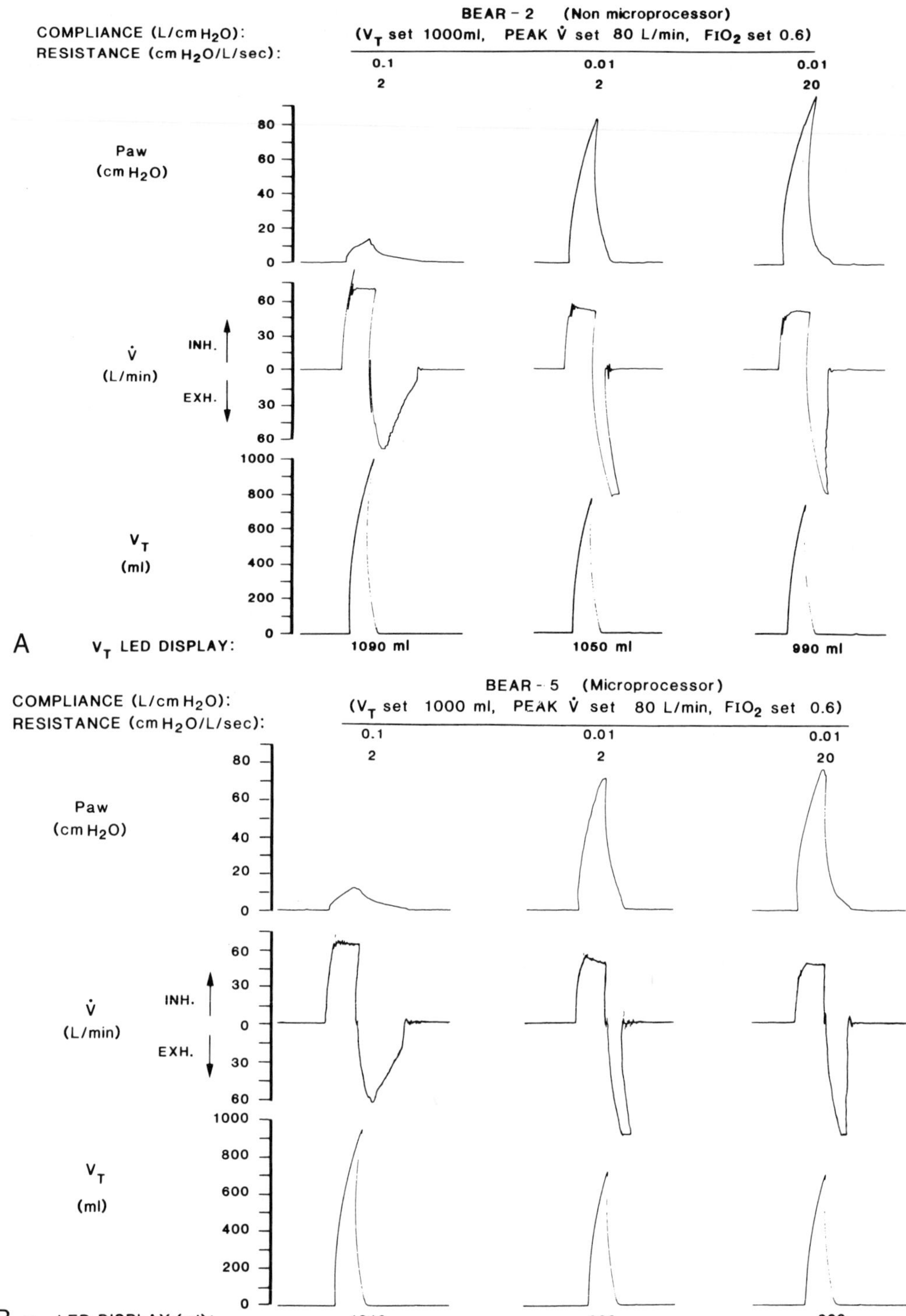

Fig. 15-31. Airway pressure (PAW), flow ($\dot{V}$), and tidal volume (V_T) characteristics of the Inter Med Bear 2 nonmicroprocessor-type ventilator **(A)** and the Bear 5 microprocessor type ventilator **(B)** under conditions of varying compliance and resistance. Measurements were obtained between the ventilator Y piece and the endotracheal tube. Note that the deteriorations in inspiratory flow rate and waveform, and hence V_T, as PIP increased are similar for both types of ventilators. Also note that the LED values for V_T are spuriously high on the Bear 2 and Bear 5 ventilators under conditions of high PIP.

affecting the validity of the measurement (Table 15–12). The exhaled flow sensor should be located between the ventilator Y piece and the endotracheal tube, as in the Hamilton Veolar ventilator (Fig. 15–32). However, on most ventilators it is positioned on the expiratory limb of the breathing circuit. Here the entire VT delivered by the ventilator, not that actually received by the patient, is measured. Under conditions of decreased CLT and/or high RAW, the higher PIP results in an increase of gas volume compressed in the breathing circuit, with correspondingly less delivered to the patient (Figs. 15–30 and 15–31). A flow sensor positioned on the expiratory limb of the breathing circuit will not reflect this change.

Microprocessor-Controlled Ventilators

Hamilton Veolar Ventilator

The Hamilton Veolar ventilator uses pneumatic and electrical power sources, and is a microprocessor-controlled, time-cycled, volume-limited, constant and nonconstant-flow generator (Fig. 15–33). CMV, AV, SIMV/IMV, EIP, CPAP, PSV, and MMV are available modes of ventilation. Constant, accelerating, decelerating, or sinusoidal inspiratory flow waveforms may be selected. Pressure support is available in the SIMV, spontaneous CPAP, and MMV modes. In addition, a backup mode of ventilation is available during the administration of SIMV, CPAP, PSV, and MMV. The operator chooses the rate, VT, percentage of inspiratory time, and inspiratory flow waveform during backup ventilation. When engaged, backup ventilation is activated if apnea occurs for 15 seconds or more, or if the measured exhaled minute volume drops to or below 1 L/min (Table 15–12).

Controls

Three clearly differentiated sections comprise the operating panel of the ventilator: controls, alarms, and monitoring sections. Standard, rotating type control knobs (potentiometer or "pots") and a keypad arrangement are employed to control the operation of the ventilator. A keypad system is used to operate the monitoring functions of the ventilator (Table 15–13). Small green LEDs are used throughout the operating panel. These LEDs are used to indicate active control knobs or push keys. On the basis of the ventilatory mode selected, different control knobs and keys are active. On the control section of the panel, ventilatory modes are selected by depressing the appropriate keys for at least two seconds. Ventilatory parameters are selected by regulating the rate, tidal volume percent cycle time, EIP, patient-trigger, CPAP, PSV, and FIO_2 control knobs. Several of the controls use dual knobs; a larger diameter control that is closer to the control panel and a smaller diameter knob that is closer to the operator. Percent inspiratory time and percent expiratory time are regulated with a dual control knob arrangement; one control positioned closer to the control panel affects the inspiratory time while a second control, positioned closer to the operator, affects expiratory time. The I:E ratio is adjustable for 1:4 to 4:1 using both controls; values falling outside this range activate an alarm. Peak inspiratory flow rate varies inversely with the percent inspiratory time setting (i.e., the shorter the inspiratory time, the greater the inspiratory flow rate, and vice versa). EIP time is set by separating the position settings of the percent inspiratory and percent expiratory time controls, that is, the greater the separation the longer the EIP time. An EIP is required for the ventilator to perform CLT and RAW calculations. These dual controls regulate the total respiratory cycle time (TCT), where TCT = 60 sec/rate.

Dual control knobs are also used for the CPAP-PSV controls. Rotation of the CPAP control activates the demand-flow system and pressurizes the exhalation valve to the desired level of CPAP. CPAP may be used with all ventilatory modes. The level of inspiratory PSV above the CPAP level is controlled by rotating the other control. An O_2 flush control allows 100 percent oxygen to be directed into the breathing circuit for as long as the operator depresses the control.

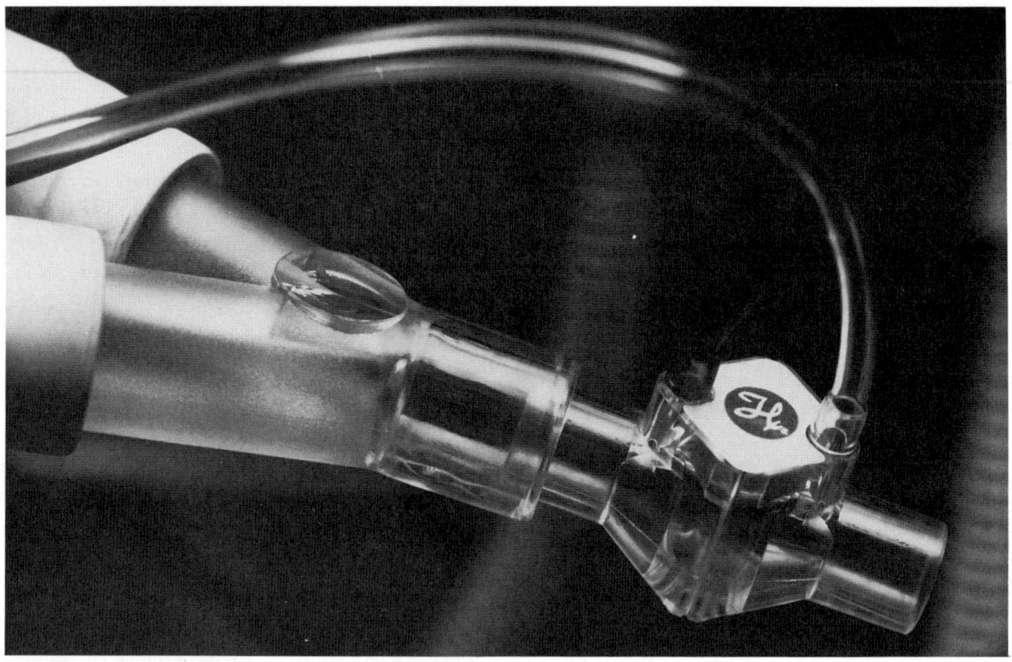

Fig. 15-32. Miniature pneumotachograph (Hamilton Veolar ventilator) correctly positioned between the ventilator Y piece and the endotracheal tube to measure exhaled tidal volume. (Courtesy of Hamilton Medical, Inc., Reno, NV.)

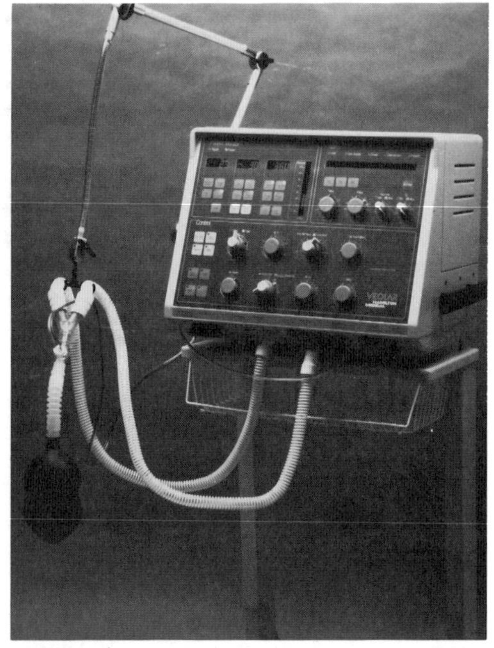

Fig. 15-33. Hamilton Veolar ventilator. (Courtesy of Hamilton Medical, Inc., Reno, NV.)

Operation

Mechanical inhalation and exhalation phases of gas flow are indicated in Figures 15–34 and 15–35. Electronic and pneumatic systems operate the ventilator. Two interrelated microprocessors control the electronic system: a front panel microprocessor and a control microprocessor. The two microprocessors monitor each other to ensure that each functions properly. The front panel microprocessor interprets all signals from the control panel and operates the displays and alarms. The control processor interprets signals from the front panel microprocessor and controls the delivery of gas to the patient.

The pneumatic system provides gas flow through the ventilator to the patient. Compressed air and oxygen are directed through filters to two precision regulators that reduce the air and oxygen source pressures to 18.5 psig. The regulated gases then pass to a mechanical blender or mixer to regulate F_{IO_2} (maximum flow rate output 90 L/min). Blended gas then enters a

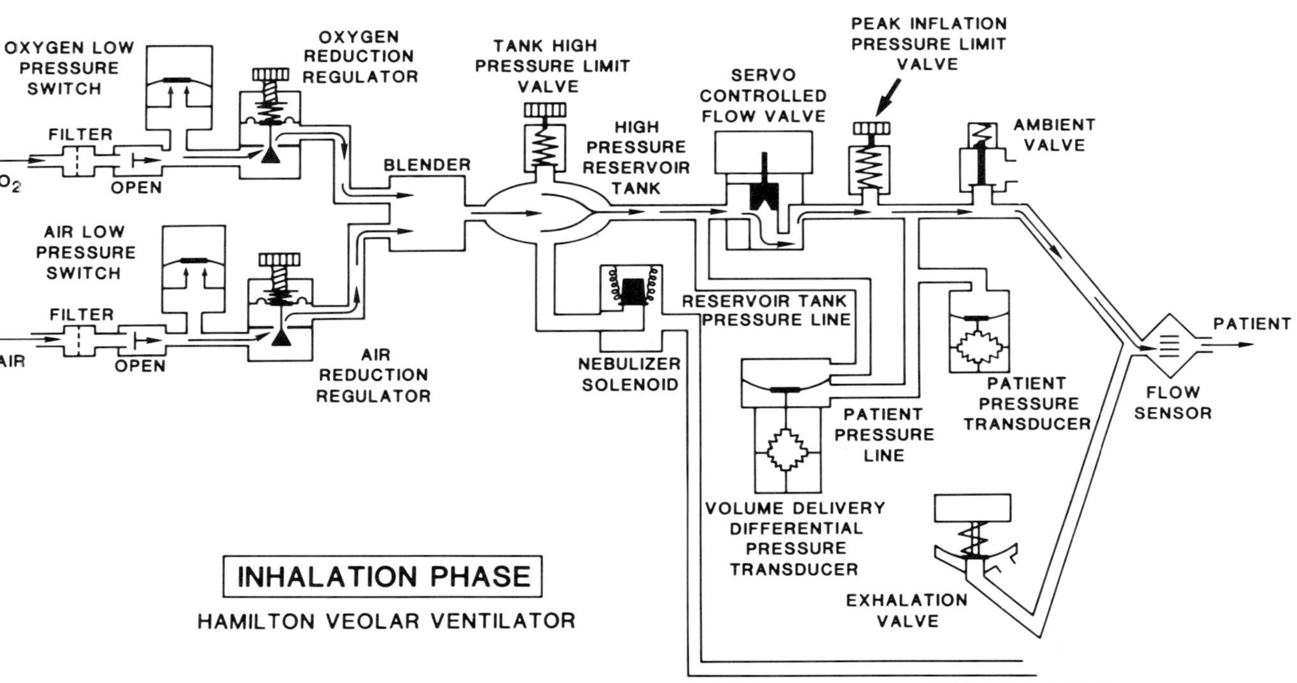

Fig. 15-34. Mechanical inhalation phase of the Hamilton Veolar ventilator.

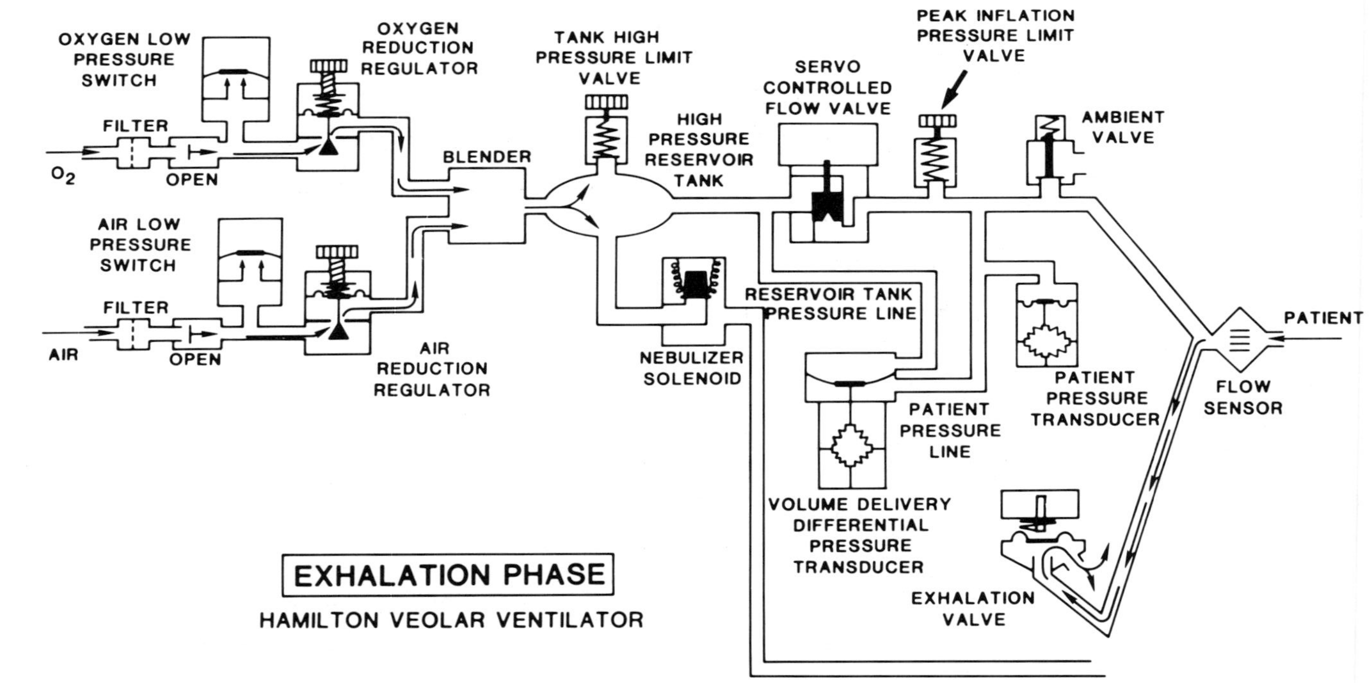

Fig. 15-35. Exhalation phase of the Hamilton Veolar ventilator.

7-L reservoir tank, and pressure in the reservoir is regulated at 350 cm H_2O (5 psig). The purpose of the reservoir is twofold: to ensure accurate F_{IO_2} delivery and secondly, to allow peak inspiratory flow rates during mechanical or spontaneous inhalation to exceed the flow rate capabilities of the air/oxygen blender (90 L/min).

Gas-flow rate to the patient during mechanical and spontaneous breathing is controlled by a high speed electrodynamic valve. The valve is opened or closed with an up-and-down motion, similar to a gate valve. As the valve opens during inhalation (mechanical or spontaneous), the height of an isosceles-triangle-shaped orifice progressively increases. Gas flows from the high pressure reservoir through the isosceles-triangle-shaped orifice to the inspiratory limb of the breathing circuit. The opening (height) is modulated by an electrodynamic motor, which oscillates similarly to the high-speed movement (vibration) of a loudspeaker. Electric current is passed through a coil connected to the triangular plunger by a shaft, producing a variable magnetic field at the apex of the valve housing. The magnitude of the electric current is altered by a microprocessor that compares (references) the preselected ventilatory parameters entered into its memory from the control panel to the actual gas-flow rate traversing the valve. The height of the triangular orifice is measured by a position sensor that provides a signal proportional to the square root of the orifice area. When the differential pressure across the valve is constant, the flow rate is proportional to the orifice area. By sensing the height of the triangular orifice and continually correcting variations in differential pressure, the ventilator delivers flow rates from 20 to 3,000 ml/sec in constant, sinusoidal, decelerating, or accelerating inspiratory flow waveforms.

An electronically controlled exhalation valve consists of a silicone rubber membrane that occludes the exhalation limb of the breathing circuit by the action of a linear motion electronic motor, similar to the inspiratory flow control valve. During mechanical inhalation, an electric current is passed through a coil, creating an electromagnetic field which forces an actuating shaft against the silicone rubber membrane, causing it to occlude the exhalation outlet. Passive exhalation occurs when the electric current switches off, eliminating the magnetic field. The weight of the rubber membrane and the actuating shaft is offset by a spring; thus minimizing valve resistance and allowing the exhalation valve to open.

This valve functions also as a threshold-resistor type expiratory pressure valve when CPAP is used (see under Threshold Resistors).

Inspiratory Flow Waveforms

Constant, sinusoidal, decelerating, and accelerating inspiratory flow waveforms may be selected during mechanical inhalation. Since the ventilator is time-cycled, inspiratory time and the I:E ratio do not change, while peak inspiratory flow rate varies when changing from a constant to one of the other flow waveforms.

A sinusoidal inspiratory flow waveform begins at zero flow rate, accelerates to peak flow rate, and then decelerates to zero flow rate. Assuming the same V_T and inspiratory time, the peak inspiratory flow rate is approximately 1.5 times greater as compared to using a constant inspiratory flow waveform.[51] A decelerating inspiratory flow waveform begins at a peak inspiratory flow rate and is followed by a linear deceleration to zero flow rate. An accelerating inspiratory flow waveform is the opposite, beginning at zero and then accelerating in a linear manner to peak inspiratory flow rate. Changing from a constant to either a decelerating or an accelerating inspiratory flow waveform causes the peak inspiratory flow rate to increase two times.[51] Changes in peak flow rate results in changes in peak inflation pressure, since pressure is proportional to flow rate times resistance.

Monitors, Alarms, and Safety Features

Monitoring of inspiratory and expiratory flow rate and V_T is provided by a miniature pneumotachograph positioned between the Y piece of

Table 15–12. Characteristics of Microprocessor and Nonmicroprocessor Ventilators

	Engström Erica	BEAR V	Hamilton Veolar	Bennett 7200a	Bird 6400 ST	Ohmeda CPU-1
Modalities of ventilation	CMV, AV, EIP, SIMV, MMV, PSV, CPAP	CMV, AV, Sigh, IMV/SIMV, PSV, MMV, CPAP, EIP	CMV, AV, IMV/SIMV, PSV, MMV, EIP, CPAP	CMV, AV, Sigh, IMV/SIMV, PSV, EIP, CPAP	CMV, AV, IMV/SIMV, PSV, CPAP, Sigh	CMV, AV, Sigh, IMV/SIMV, PSV, MMV, EIP, CPAP
Tidal volume (ml)	100–2,000	50–2,000	20–2,000	100–2,500	50–2,000	50–6,000
Peak mechanical, inspiratory flow rate (L/min)	20–120	5–150	0–180	10–120	10–120	5–120
Inspiratory flow waveforms	Accelerating constant, decelerating	Accelerating, constant, decelerating, sinusoidal	Accelerating, constant, decelerating, sinusoidal	Constant, decelerating, sinusoidal	Constant and decelerating	Constant
CPAP (cm H_2O)	1–30	1–50	1–50	1–45	1–30	1–30
Peak spontaneous inspiratory flow (L/min)	120	5–150	0–180	180	10–120	5–120
Inspiratory plateau (sec)	0–7	0–2	0–3	0–2	NA	0–1
Peak inflation pressures limit (cm H_2O)	0–120	0–150	0–110	10–120	0–140	5–100
Rate (BPM)	0.8–60	0–150	5–60 CMV 0.5–30 IMV	0.5–70	0–80	1–55
F_{IO_2}	0.21–1.0	0.21–1.0	0.21–1.0	0.21–1.0	Requires additional blender	Requires additional blender
Patient-triggering sensitivity (cm H_2O)	0.2–0.04 L/sec[a]	−0.5 to −5	OFF. −1 to −15	−0.5 to −20	−1 to −20	−0.8 to −1.5 (nonadjustable)
Cycling mechanism	Volume	Volume or time	Time	Volume	Volume	Time or pressure
Pressure support (cm H_2O)	1–30	1–72	1–50	1–70	1–50	1–30
Location of exhaled VT sensor	Distal to exhalation valve	Distal to exhalation valve	Y piece of breathing circuit	Proximal to exhalation valve	NA	Distal to exhalation valve
Classification and function of expiratory valve	Pneumatically powered	Pneumatically powered	Threshold resistor (diaphragm)	Threshold resistor (diaphragm)	Threshold resistor (diaphragm)	Threshold resistor (diaphragm)

[a] Cycled by flow rate.

the breathing circuit tubing and the endotracheal tube. Location of the flow sensor at the airway allows for accurate measurement of inhaled and exhaled tidal volume. The patient's exhaled volume only, and not the gas volume compressed in the breathing circuit, is measured (see under Accuracy of Displayed Exhaled Tidal Volume). An electronic transducer measures peak and mean airway pressures. Integration of the flow rate, VT, and PAW data allows the ventilator's microprocessor to determine lung-thorax compliance and airways resistance. Peak inflation pressures are indicated in real time with a vertical bar display. Peak inflation, mean, and end-

Siemens 900C	Bear 2	IMV-Bird	Emerson 3MV	Bennett MA-1	Hamilton Amadeus
CMV, AV, IMV/SIMV, PC, PSV, EIP, CPAP	CMV, AV, Sigh, IMV/SIMV, EIP, CPAP	IMV, CMV, CPAP	IMV, CMV, CPAP	CMV, AV, Sigh, IMV	CMV, AV, EIP, IMV/SIMV, PSV, CPAP
25–2,000	100–2,000	100–1,500	100–2,000	100–2,200	20–2,000
0–180	10–120	0–180	0–150	5–100	0–180
Accelerating, constant	Constant, decelerating	May be constant or decelerating	Sinusoidal	May be constant or decelerating	Constant, decelerating
1–50	1–50	1–35	1–50	NA (1–20 with optional value)	1–50
0–180	0–100	0–160	0–100 (with optional demand valve)	0–100 (with optional demand valve)	0–180
0–3.6	0–2	NA	NA	NA	0–3
16–120	0–120	110 nonadjustable	40–100	10–80	0–110
5–120 CMV 4–40 IMV	0.5–60	0.3–30	0.2–25	6–60	0.5–120
Requires additional blender	0.21–1.0	Requires additional blender	Requires additional blender	0.21–1.0	0.21–1.0
0 to −20	"Less-more"	NA	NA	−0.1 to −10	−1 to −10
Time	Volume	Time	Time	Volume	Time
1–100	NA	NA	NA	NA	1–100
Proximal to exhalation valve in expiratory limb	Distal to exhalation valve	NA	NA	NA	Y piece of breating circuit
Flow resistor-like (scissors)	Inflatable balloon	Threshold resistor (pneumatic poppet)	Threshold resistor (water-weighted diaphragm	Inflatable baloon	Threshold resistor (diaphragm)

expiratory pressures are indicated on LED displays. Other measured parameters are shown in Table 15–13.

Nonadjustable alarms include apnea (15 seconds), fail to cycle (20 seconds), patient disconnect (2 breaths), inhaled and exhaled tidal volume mismatch (3 breaths), flow rate out of range (greater than 180 LPM), and low compressed air and oxygen inlet pressures (less than 29 psig). Also, the ventilator automatically notifies the operator if the flow sensor is improperly oriented.

Table 15–13. Monitoring and Alarm Characteristics of Microprocessor and Nonmicroprocessor Ventilators

	Engström Erica	Bear V	Hamilton Veolar	Bennett 7200a	Bird 6400 ST	Ohmeda CPU-1
Exhaled tidal volume (ml)	Displayed only	Low alarm, mandatory (0.30–2,000) Low alarm, spontaneous (0.30–2,000)	Displayed but no alarms	Low alarm (0–2,500) High: NA	NA	Displayed and inadequate volume
Exhaled minute volume (L/min)	Low alarm (1–40) High alarm (1–40)	Low alarm (0.3–40) High alarm (1.0–80)	Low alarm (1–40) High alarm (1–40)	Low alarm (0–60) High: NA	NA	Low alarm (0–30) High: NA
Breath rate (BPM (L)	Apnea (30 sec or 15 sec) High: NA	Low alarm (3–150) High alarm (3–155)	Apnea (15 sec) High alarm (10–70)	Apnea (10–60 sec) High alarm (0–70)	Apnea (20 sec) High: NA	Apnea (15 sec) High: NA
CPAP (cmH_2O)	NA	Low alarm (0–50) High alarm (0–55)	Monitored and displayed only	Low alarm (0–45) High: NA	Low alarm (−20 to 30) High: NA	NA
Inspiratory time (sec)	NA	Low alarm (0.05–3.0) High alarm (0.1–3.2)	Monitored only	NA	Displayed but no alarms	NA
Inspiratory pressure (cmH_2O)	Low alarm (0–120) High alarm (0–120)	Low alarm (3–140) High alarm (3–140)	Low pressure (monitored only) High alarm (10–110)	Low alarm (3–99) High alarm (10–120)	Low alarm (Off–140) High alarm (0–140)	Low: NA High alarm (5–100)
F_{IO_2}	NA (optional)	NA	Low alarm (0.18–1.03) High alarm (0.18–1.03)	NA	NA	NA
Mean airway pressure ($\overline{P_{AW}}$)	NA	Low alarm (0–75) High alarm (0–75)	NA	Measured and displayed but no alarm	NA	NA
Compliance (ml/cmH_2O)	Yes	Yes	Yes	Optional	NA	Optional
Resistance (cm/L/sec)	Yes	Yes	Yes	Optional	NA	Optional
Flow rate (L/min)	NA	Graphics only	Yes	Optional	NA	NA

Siemens 900C	Bear II	IMV-bird	IMV Emerson	Bennett MA-1	Hamilton Amadeus
Displayed but no alarm	Low alarm (Off, 100–2,000) High: NA	NA	NA	Measured and displayed and low exhaled volume alarm	Measured and displayed but no alarms
Low alarm (0–37) High alarm (0–43)	NA	NA	NA	NA	Low alarm (0.2–50) High alarm (0.2–50)
Apnea (15 sec) High: NA	Apnea (2–20 sec) High alarm (10–80)	NA	NA	NA	Apnea (20 sec) High rate (30–130)
NA	Low alarm (3–50) High: NA	NA	Low alarm (5–25) High: NA	NA	Monitored and displayed only
NA	NA	NA	NA	NA	NA
Low: NA High alarm (16–120)	Low alarm (3–75) High alarm (0–120)	NA	Low alarm (0–90) High alarm (0–120)	Low: NA High alarm (20–80)	Low pressure (monitored only) High alarm (10–110)
Low alarm (18–90) High alarm (30–100)	NA	NA	Monitored only	NA	High alarm Low alarm
Measured but no alarm capability	NA	NA	NA	NA	NA
NA	NA	NA	NA	NA	Yes
NA	NA	NA	NA	NA	Yes
NA	NA	NA	NA	NA	Yes

In the event of an electrical and/or pneumatic power loss or malfunction, an audible dysfunction alarm is activated, all ventilatory functions cease, and a safety valve automatically opens the breathing circuit to room air so that the patient can ventilate spontaneously.

Hamilton Amadeus Ventilator

The Hamilton Amadeus ventilator uses pneumatic and electrical power sources, and is a microprocessor-controlled, time-cycled, constant and nonconstant flow generator (Fig. 15–36). CMV, AV, SIMV/IMV, CPAP, PSV, and EIP are available ventilatory modes. Pressure support is available in the SIMV and CPAP modes. Constant or decelerating inspiratory flow waveforms may be selected (Table 15–12).

Controls

The operating panel is partitioned into three sections: ventilator controls, patient monitors, and ventilator alarms. Standard rotating type control knobs (potentiometer or "pots") and a keypad arrangement are employed to control the operation of the ventilator and its alarms. Small green LED are used throughout the operating panel. These LED are used to indicate active control knobs or push keys. On the basis of the ventilatory mode selected, different control knobs and keys are active. On the control section of the panel, ventilatory modes are selected by depressing the appropriate keys for at least two seconds. Ventilatory parameters are selected by regulating the rate, V_T, percent cycle time, EIP, patient-trigger, CPAP, PSV, and F_{IO_2} control knobs. Several of the controls use dual knobs: a larger-diameter control that is closer to the control panel and a smaller diameter knob that is closer to the operator. Percent inspiratory time and percent expiratory time are regulated with a dual control knob arrangement; one control, positioned closer to the control panel, affects inspiratory time, while a second control, positioned closer to the operator, affects expiratory time. The I:E ratio is adjustable from 1:9 to 4:1 using both controls; values falling outside this range activate an alarm. Peak inspiratory flow rate varies inversely with the percent inspiratory time setting (i.e., the shorter the inspiratory time, the greater the inspiratory flow rate, and vice versa). EIP time is set by separating the position settings of the percent inspiratory and percent expiratory time controls (i.e., the greater the separation the longer the EIP time). An EIP is required for the ventilator to perform C_{LT} and R_{AW} calculations. These dual controls regulate the total respiratory cycle time (TCT), where TCT = 60 sec/rate. At SIMV rates less than 15 breaths/min, the TCT remains at 4 seconds. This prevents excessive inspiratory time when low SIMV rates are used.

Dual control knobs are also used for the CPAP-PSV controls. Rotation of the CPAP control activates the demand-flow system and pressurizes the exhalation valve to the desired level of CPAP. CPAP may be used with all ventilatory modes. The level of inspiratory PSV above the CPAP level is controlled by rotating the other control.

The ventilator provides gas flow for spontaneous inhalation in the SIMV/IMV and the CPAP modes. The operator selects a pressure below the baseline airway pressure that the patient must generate to trigger the ventilator "ON." In an attempt to overcome the lag time and reduce inspiratory work, the ventilator provides PSV at 10 cm H_2O for the first 50 msec of all spontaneously initiated breaths. Following this initial period, the preselected level of CPAP is maintained for the remainder of the breath.

Other control functions may be initiated by depressing specific keys on the keypad. An O_2 flush control allows a 5-minute interval of 100 percent oxygen when activated. A Cal O_2 control calibrates the oxygen sensor in the ventilator.

Operation

The ventilator consists of two separate but interconnected systems: the pneumatic flow system and an electronic control system. A schematic representation depicting the ventilator during mechanical inhalation and exhalation

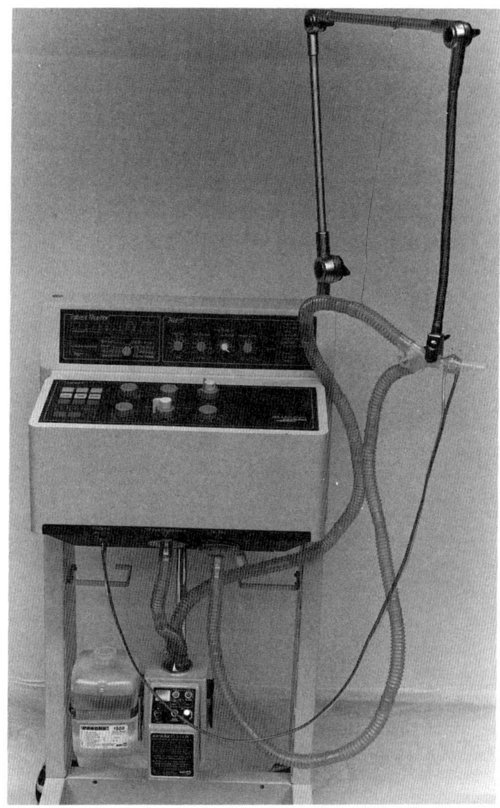

Fig. 15-36. Hamilton Amadeus ventilator. (Courtesy of Hamilton Medical, Inc., Reno, NV.)

phases is shown in Figures 15–37 and 15–38.

Three microprocessors control the operation of the ventilator: the control microprocessor, the oxygen microprocessor and the front panel microprocessor. The three microprocessors monitor one another to ensure that each functions properly. If aberrations in any of the microprocessors are detected, emergency backup procedures and alarms are activated.

The control microprocessor is responsible for the operation of a high speed electrodynamic valve that governs gas-flow rate to the patient during spontaneous and mechanical breathing. This valve, as well as the remaining pneumatic components found on the Amadeus ventilator, is identical to those incorporated into the Veolar ventilator (see under Hamilton Veolar Ventilator).

Compressed medical-grade air and oxygen, are directed into the ventilator. The oxygen blending system consists of two solenoid valves: one for air and one for oxygen. The oxygen microprocessor, which receives input data from a differential pressure transducer, opens and closes the solenoid valves to mix air and oxygen to the preselected oxygen concentration. The flow rate output from the blending system (90 L/min) is directed into a 7-L reservoir tank with the reservoir pressure at 350 cm H_2O. The pressurized reservoir allows the ventilator to generate peak inspiratory flow rates up to 180 L/min. A pressure relief valve (400 cm H_2O) prevents excessive pressures in the reservoir tank.

Inspiratory Flow Waveforms

Constant or decelerating inspiratory flow waveforms during mechanical inhalation may be selected. Normally, a constant flow waveform is provided. A decelerating inspiratory flow waveform is selected by turning "ON" an option switch on the rear panel of the ventilator. Higher peak inspiratory flow rates relative to the constant flow waveform occur, using the decelerating flow waveform. Initially, a high peak inspiratory flow rate occurs followed by a linear deceleration. When the flow rate decelerates to 33 percent of the peak flow rate, the preselected tidal volume will have been delivered. At this point the ventilator cycles "OFF."

Monitors, Alarms, and Safety Features

Monitoring of inhaled and exhaled flow rate and V_T is provided by a miniature pneumotachograph (flow sensor) positioned between the Y piece of the breathing circuit tubing and the endotracheal tubc. Location of the flow sensor in this position is preferred for accurate measurement of tidal and minute volume (see under Accuracy of Displayed Exhaled Tidal Volume).

On the patient monitoring section of the operating panel, an LED display exhibits one monitored parameter at a time. Selections are made

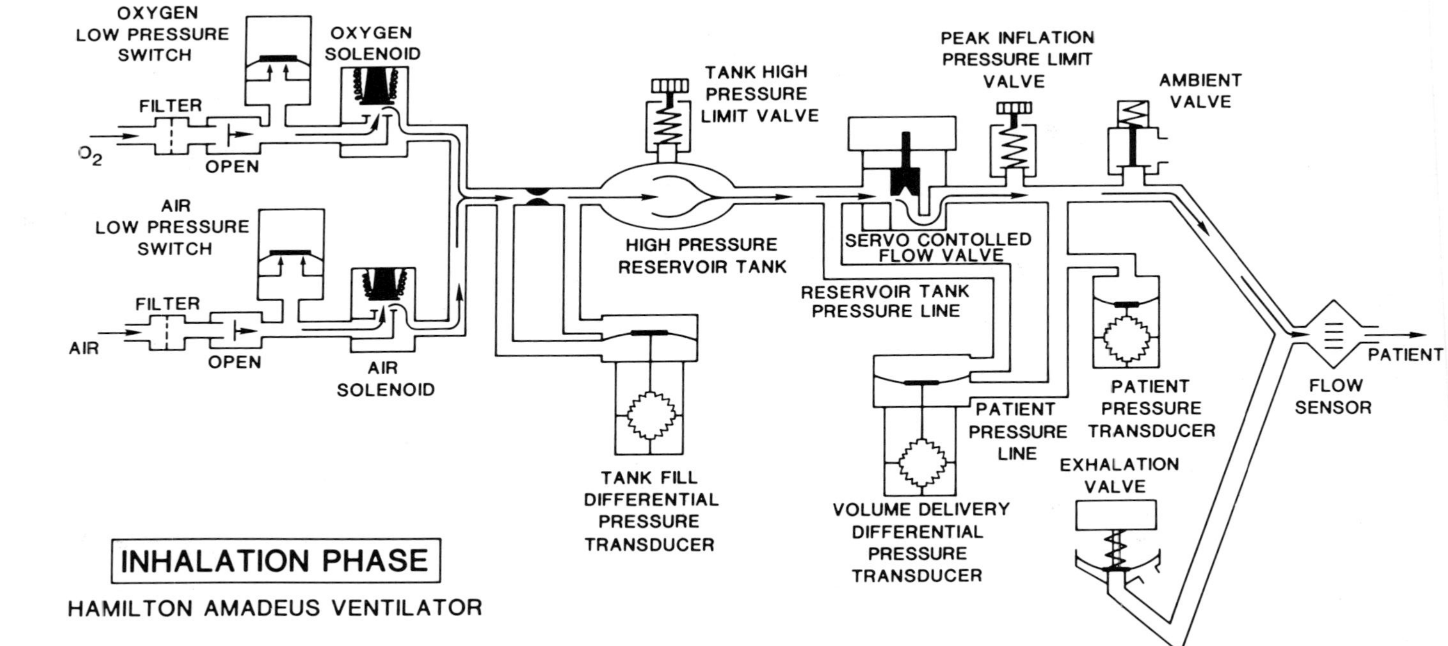

Fig. 15-37. Mechanical inhalation phase of the Hamilton Amadeus ventilator.

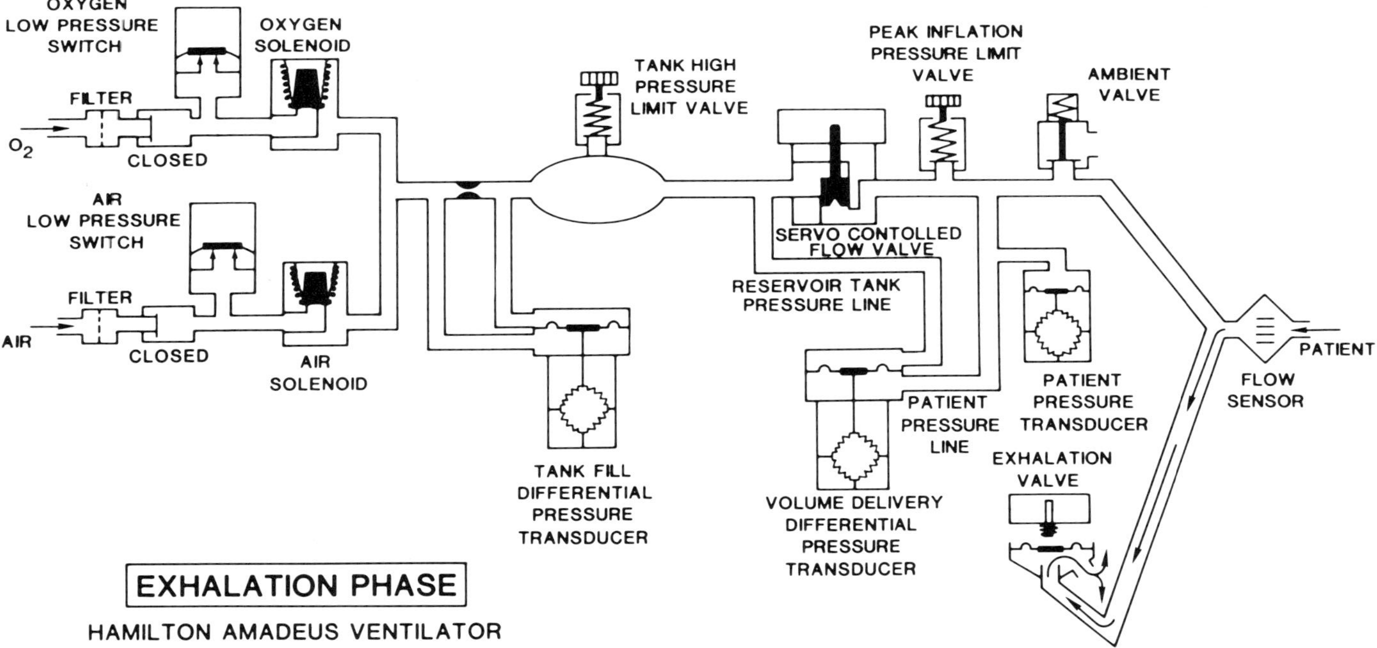

Fig. 15-38. Exhalation phase of the Hamilton Amadeus ventilator.

with an eight position switch and include rate (spontaneous and mechanical), O_2 percent, peak inspiratory flow rate (L/min), exhaled minute volume (L/min), exhaled VT (ml), CPAP (cm H_2O), RAW (cm H_2O/L/sec), and CLT (ml/cm H_2O). Peak inflation pressures are indicated in real time with a horizontal bar display. The bar is lighted for each 2 cm H_2O increase of pressure in the breathing circuit. A segment of the bar display remains lighted at the peak inflation pressure until the next positive-pressure breath.

The function of monitoring the patient, alerting personnel to alarm conditions, and instituting emergency safety procedures is assigned to the front panel microprocessor. Patient alarms, user alarms, power alarms, inoperative alarms, and gas supply alarms are provided.

Six patient alarms are available: four of the alarms are adjustable and two are nonadjustable. Adjustable alarms include high pressure, exhaled minute volume, O_2 percent, and high rate (see Table 15–13 for ranges). The apnea alarm is nonadjustable and activated when after 20 seconds no breathing is detected. A nonadjustable disconnect alarm is activated when the inhaled VT is less than one-half the preselected VT, or when the exhaled VT is less than one-eighth the preselected VT.

User alarms include the *turn flowsensor,* control settings, calibration, flow out of range, and fan filter systems. Violation of one or more of these systems results in audible and visual alarms. Alarm activation does not differentiate which *user* alarm has been violated. Under these conditions, the operator must ''troubleshoot'' the ventilator to ascertain the problem. *Turn flowsensor* alarm indicates that the flow sensor has been installed backward. A *control settings* alarm condition occurs when a control has been set improperly. The *flow out of range* alarm alerts the operator that the selected ventilator settings require a peak inspiratory flow rate in excess of 180 L/min. The *calibration* alarm signals a flowsensor or oxygen cell that fails the calibration procedure. A *fan filter* alarm alerts the operator of an occluded cooling fan filter. The *power alarm* indicates a loss of the external electrical power or that the ventilator has been plugged into an inappropriate voltage power source. The *inoperative alarm* is activated when aberrations in the functioning of any of the microprocessors or a failure of the electronic control systems is detected. In the event that both gas sources fail, *Power or Inoperative* alarms are activated. Under these conditions, the ventilator ceases to operate, and the exhalation valve and an antiasphyxia valve open the breathing circuit to room air, and audible and visual alarms also are activated.

Puritan-Bennett 7200a Ventilator

The Puritan-Bennett 7200a ventilator uses electrical and pneumatic power sources, and is a microprocessor-controlled, volume-cycled,

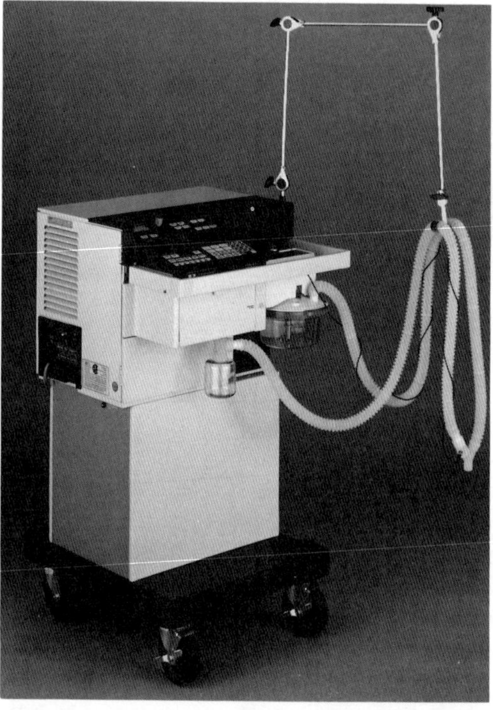

Fig. 15-39. Puritan-Bennett 7200a ventilator. (Courtesy of Puritan-Bennett Corp., Overland Park, KS.)

constant and nonconstant-flow generator (Fig. 15–39). CMV, AV, IMV/SIMV, EIP, CPAP, and PSV modes are available. Constant, decelerating, and sinusoidal inspiratory flow waveforms may be selected for mechanical inhalation (Table 15–12).

Controls

The operating panel is partitioned into three sections: ventilation settings, patient data, and ventilator status. All ventilatory settings are controlled by a keypad display board. The CPAP control is the only exception; a standard, rotating-type control knob attached to a regulator is used to set the level of CPAP. Alteration of ventilatory and monitoring parameters is accomplished by depressing the appropriate sequence of keys which is then entered into the microprocessor using the ENTER command. Entered or programmed values are then displayed in a message window. The operator may confirm the selection or correct entry errors by using the CLEAR command. If the ENTER command is not made, the proposed changes are not executed, and the previous values in the microprocessor are retained. This procedure prevents accidental changes in ventilatory and monitoring parameters. In addition, improper or impossible settings are not allowed and the computer immediately notifies the operator of an inappropriate entry.

The operator has control of the following ventilator functions: VT, rate, peak inspiratory flow rate, sensitivity (patient-triggering pressure), EIP, PSV, level of CPAP, and FIO_2. Other controls include a 100 percent oxygen suction key which delivers 100 percent oxygen for 2 minutes, as well as keys to switch a nebulizer "ON" or "OFF" and to control the delivery of a tidal or sigh volume breath manually. Sigh breaths may be given between 1 and 15 times per hour in sequences of 1, 2, or 3 sighs. The sigh volume and PIP are adjustable but may not be less than or exceed by a factor of 2 the previously programmed values for tidal volume and the peak inflation pressure.

Operation

Mechanical inhalation and exhalation phases of gas flow are indicated in Figure 15–40 and 15–41). The ventilator is composed of electropneumatic and electronic systems. After passing through filters, compressed air and oxygen are directed to 2 precision regulators to reduce air and oxygen source pressures to 10 psig (517 mmHg). Each gas then passes through a secondary filter, a flow transducer, and then to a proportional solenoid valve assembly. This valve assembly is comprised of two solenoid valves (one for air and one for O_2) coupled into a single unit. The two gases flow from the solenoid valve assembly into a common outlet leading to the breathing circuit. Each valve can be actuated to open stepwise to 5,000 discrete apertures (openings). Each aperture corresponds to a specific gas flow rate. A microprocessor controls the aperture positions of the solenoid valves and thus controls the FIO_2, VT, inspiratory flow rate, and inspiratory flow waveform during mechanical inhalation.

Measured/delivered inspiratory flow rates from the ventilator's flow sensors are referenced to the preselected inspiratory flow rates.

During CPAP and PSV modes, a microprocessor uses data from the ventilator's pressure transducers to regulate the opening of the two solenoid valves to provide the inspiratory flow rate needed to maintain the preselected airway pressure level.

At the onset of spontaneous inhalation when airway pressure decreases to the preselected pressure threshold (sensitivity patient-triggering pressure), a microprocessor instructs the proportional solenoid valves to open and provide demand flow. If the flow rate is too high, PAW will rise above the preselected CPAP setting, causing the microprocessor to reduce flow rate. Conversely, if PAW decreases too much during spontaneous inhalation, the microprocessor instructs the system to increase inspiratory flow rate (up to 180 L/min).

Continuous positive airway pressure is controlled by rotation of a control knob that activates a regulator to the desired level of airway pres-

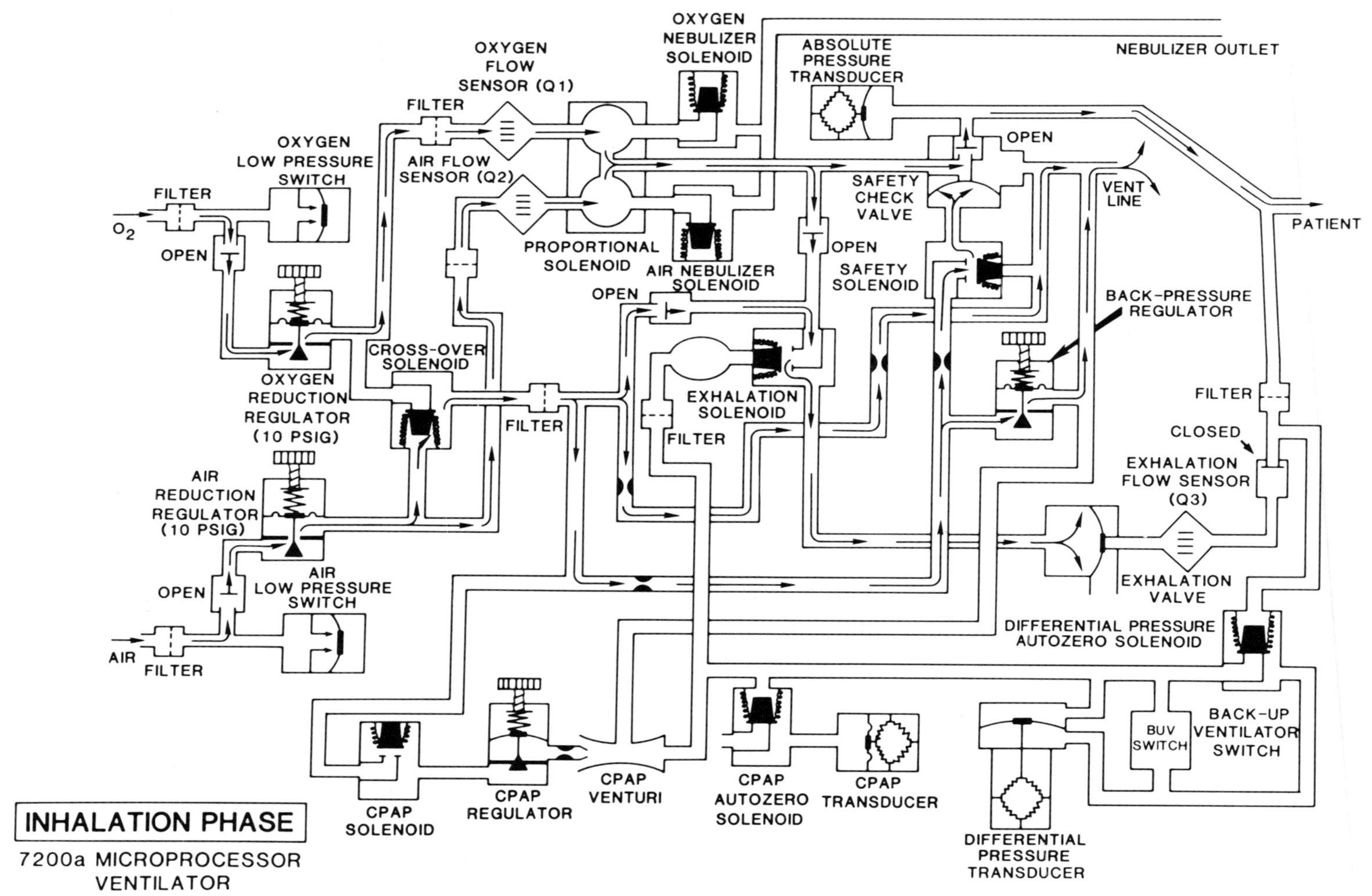

Fig. 15-40. Mechanical inhalation phase of the Puritan-Bennett 7200a ventilator.

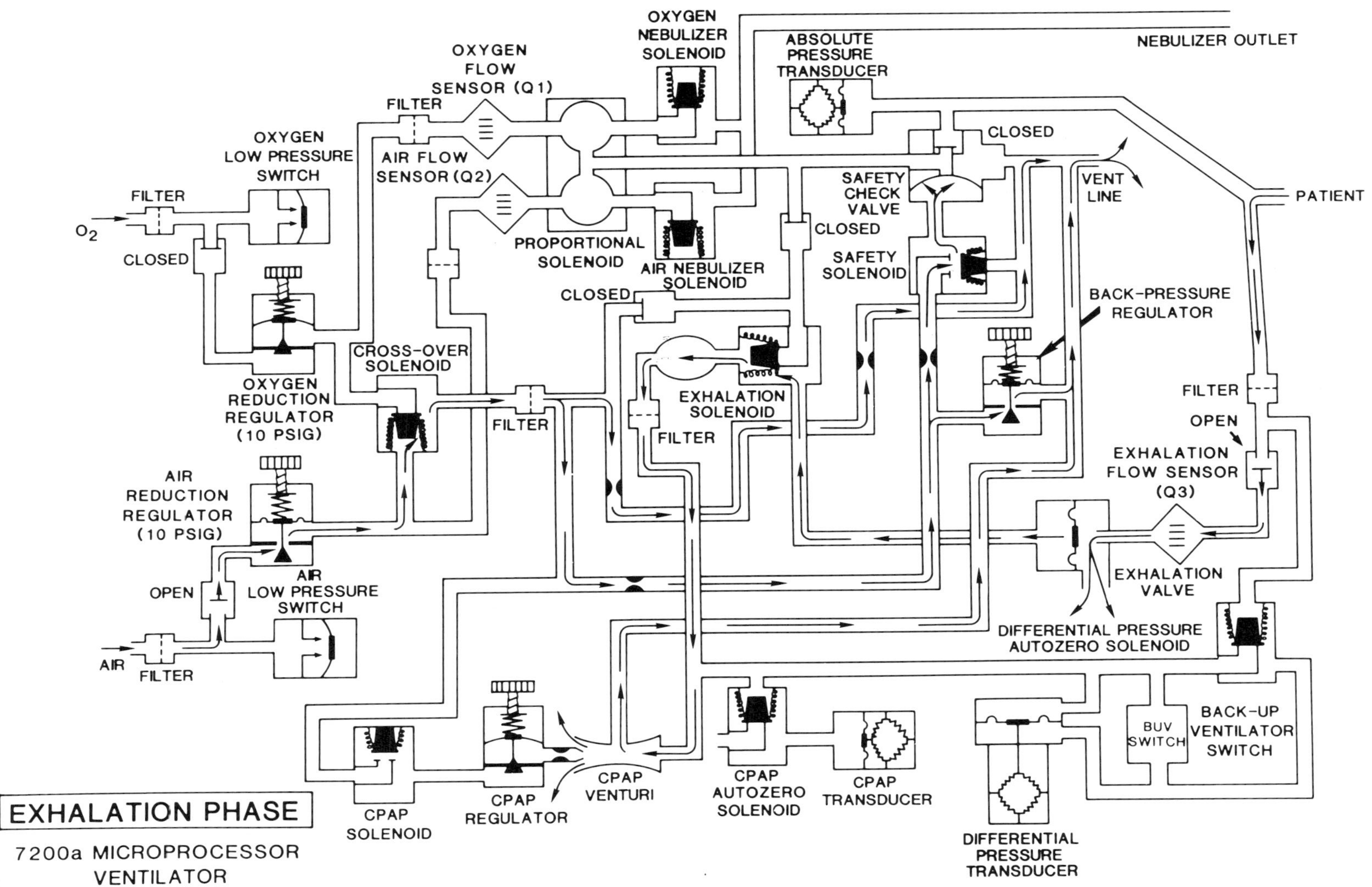

Fig. 15-41. Exhalation phase of the Puritan-Bennett 7200a ventilator.

sure. Metered gas flow rate from a Venturi is directed to the rear side of the diaphragm-type exhalation/CPAP valve, which functions as a threshold resistor. A nebulizer may be activated by depressing the appropriate key to deliver aerosols to the patient. Nebulizer operation is automatically terminated 30 minutes after activation.

Mechanical inhalation during CMV, AV, and SIMV is volume-cycled; VT, inspiratory flow rate, PIP and FIO_2 are programmed by the operator. When the ventilator detects apnea for a preselected period of time (adjustable from 10 to 60 seconds), ventilation is provided by the operator-determined parameters. A backup ventilation (BUV) mode is automatically provided by nonoperator-selected values for VT (500 ml), inspiratory flow rate (45 L/min), ventilator rate (12/min), PIP limit, and FIO_2 (1.0), and the original level of CPAP when the ventilator detects abnormalities in the control microprocessor or the electrical power source.

Inspiratory Flow Waveform

Constant, sinusoidal, and decelerating inspiratory flow waveforms may be selected during mechanical inhalation. Inspiratory time varies with changes in the inspiratory waveform (assuming the same tidal volume). As a result, PAW changes due to changes in the I:E ratio.[51]

A sinusoidal inspiratory flow waveform begins at a flow rate of 5 L/min, accelerates to a peak flow rate, and then decelerates to 5 L/min. Inspiratory time increases by approximately 50 percent, switching from a constant to a sinusoidal inspiratory flow waveform. Thus, PAW and the I:E ratio are affected. Similarly, when changing from a constant to a decelerating inspiratory flow waveform, initially a high peak inspiratory flow rate is delivered and then followed by a linear deceleration to 5 L/min. As a result, inspiratory time is approximately doubled and PAW and the I:E ratio increase.[51]

Monitors, Alarms, and Safety Features

Patient data are displayed on an analog gauge (airway pressure and exhaled volume) and LED windows. Exhaled VT is measured via a flow sensor located immediately proximal to the exhalation valve. Location of the flow sensor in this position may predispose to errors in measuring tidal and minute volumes (see under Accuracy of Displayed Exhaled Tidal Volume).

The 7200a ventilator also incorporates a number of monitoring and alarm systems of the ventilator's status. Each alarm triggers audible and visual signals when activated (Table 15–13). The high PIP or pressure limit and the low airway pressure alarms are considered critical and may not be disarmed. The operator has the option of using the remaining alarms which include: low PEEP/CPAP, low exhaled VT, low exhaled minute volume, and high respiratory rate.

The patient is constantly monitored for any occurrences of apnea. The apnea interval time range (seconds) is programmable. In the event the operator neglects to enter a value for the apnea time interval, the default value of 20 seconds is used. When apnea occurs, audible and visual alarms activate and the patient is automatically switched to the apnea ventilation mode.

A series of windows are provided displaying information of all ventilatory parameters, for example, PAW, PIP, CPAP, EIP or plateau pressure, rate, I:E ratio, exhaled VT, exhaled minute volume, and spontaneous exhaled minute volume. Optional software permits the calculation and monitoring of CLT and RAW.

Safety features include alarms for losses of electrical power and source gas. Loss of electrical power results in the cessation of all ventilator function, and automatically a safety valve opens the breathing circuit to room air to permit spontaneous ventilation. Fifteen seconds after electrical power is restored, the ventilator resumes operation. Restoration of electrical power activates the power on self-test (POST) system. Whenever power is interrupted and then restored, POST automatically runs to check the microprocessor electronics and other vital functions. If one source gas is lost, an automatic switch powers the ventilator with the other source gas, and ventilation is uninterrupted.

The microprocessor constantly monitors its own operation as well as all other critical ventilator functions. If any function falls outside the expected values, the ventilator ceases to operate and the patient is ventilated by a backup ventilator mode. BUV is not under microprocessor control and, in fact, has a separate power supply. When BUV is engaged, audible and visual alarms are activated, and a message, "do not use—run EST (extended self-test)" appears in the message display window. EST consists of an extensive battery of tests to verify proper operation of all functions of the ventilator (e.g., pressure and flow transducers, electrical system, check competence and compliance of breathing circuit). Failure of crucial tests renders the ventilator "nonfunctional." Failure of tests not considered to be critical may be bypassed and the ventilator may be used at the operator's risk. EST allows technicians to diagnose the sytem quickly so as to facilitate repair of the ventilator.

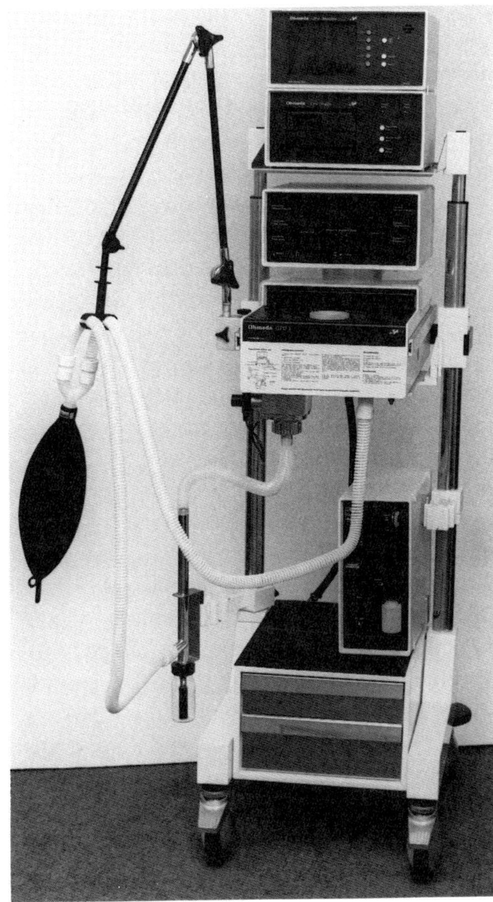

Fig. 15-42. Ohmeda CPU-1 ventilator. (Courtesy of Ohmeda, Columbia, MD.)

OHMEDA CPU-1 Ventilator

The Ohmeda CPU-1 ventilator uses pneumatic and electrical power sources and is a microprocessor-controlled, time- or pressure-cycled, and a constant-flow generator (Fig. 15–42). CMV, AV, IMV/SIMV, EIP, MMV, PSV, and CPAP are available ventilatory modes. Pressure support is available in any mode allowing spontaneous ventilation. A constant inspiratory flow waveform is applied during mechanical inhalation (Table 15–12).

Controls

The operating panel is divided into two sections: a control panel and a display panel. The control panel is protected by a sliding plexiglas shield. The operating controls are standard, rotating type control knobs attached to either a potentiometer ("pot") or a needle valve. Various ventilatory modes may be chosen with a selector switch. V_T is the product of inspiratory time (seconds) and inspiratory flow rate (ml/sec). For example, if the preselected inspiratory time was 2 seconds and the inspiratory flow rate 30 L/min (500 ml/sec), the ventilator is then programmed to eject a V_T of 1,000 ml. EIP is available during CMV, AV, IMV, and SIMV. CPAP is available in all ventilatory modes. PSV may be used as a stand-alone ventilatory mode or combined with SIMV and IMV. Ventilator cycling rate is determined by the expiratory time control. Rate may vary in the SIMV mode (see below, under Operation). The PIP limit is set by rotating the bezel of the airway pressure manometer. The operator simply aligns a red dot with the maximum pressure desired. This control also serves to determine the cycling pressure of the ventilator when in the pressure-cycled mode. Sigh breaths may be given automatically after 100 mechanical breaths or manually by switching on a sigh control knob. Sigh breaths may be administered singly or in multiples of three. Sigh volume may be either 1.5 or 2 times the preselected tidal volume. Controls for the number and volume of sigh breaths are regulated by adjusting dual inline package (DIP, ON or OFF) switches located on the rear panel of the ventilator. A decal on the side of the plexiglas control panel cover lists the function of each DIP switch. An inspiratory effort control sets the amount of pressure below the baseline airway pressure that the patient must generate at the onset of inhalation in order to trigger the ventilator "ON" (used during AV and SIMV).

Operation

Mechanical inhalation and exhalation phases of gas flow are indicated in Figures 15–43 and 15–44. Mechanical breaths are delivered when the electronic timing system opens a solenoid valve and directs blended gas (from an external air-oxygen blender) to a flow control system. A flow regulator stabilizes the incoming pressure and the flow rate control regulates the gas flow rate to the patient. Mechanical inhalation terminates when the preselected inspiratory time elapses (time-cycled). A microprocessor adjusts that operation of the ventilator to accommodate the mode selection made by the operator. In the Control/IMV mode, the ventilator is a time-cycled, constant flow generator capable of permitting spontaneous breathing with or without CPAP. Ventilator rate is determined by the formula 60/(inspiratory time + plateau time + expiratory time). In the SIMV mode, expiratory time is variable even though a preselected value is entered on the control panel. At the conclusion of the preselected expiratory time period, the microprocessor insures that there is no spontaneous inspiratory or expiratory flow from the patient. If no flow is detected, the mandated breath is provided. If flow is detected, the expiratory phase may automatically be extended for up to 3 seconds. With the cessation of flow after 3 seconds, a 1-second "triggering window" is activated. If the patient initiates inhalation during this window, the ventilator delivers an SIMV breath. Thus, the SIMV rate cannot be accurately predicted and may vary slightly from minute to minute.

The MMV mode is similar to the SIMV mode. As the operator switches from SIMV into MMV, the processor stores in memory the values of expiratory, inspiratory, and EIP times, as well as the synchronization "window" time currently in use. The microprocessor is then allowed to raise or lower expiratory time as required in order to maintain the minimum minute volume selected on the display panel. The CPU-1 simply adjusts the SIMV rate to sustain the operator selected minimum minute volume (see under Mandatory Minute Volume).

The CPU-1 allows the patient to initiate mechanically delivered breaths in the Assist/Control mode. To ensure adequate exhalation time, the microprocessor will not allow the patient to trigger the ventilator "ON" for 0.6 seconds following the end of mechanical inhalation. If no inspiratory effort is detected, the ventilator reverts to time-cycled operation. In the pressure-cycled mode, the ventilator-delivered mechanical breath is terminated by the maximum pressure setting, with rate controlled primarily by the patient's inspiratory effort or by the expiratory time setting. Three seconds is the maximum inspiratory time allowed with the ventilator in the pressure-cycled mode. If it is not possible to achieve the preselected cycling pressure (e.g., due to a leak in the breathing circuit), the ventilator will limit the mechanical inspiratory phase to 3 seconds.

Spontaneous breathing with CPAP is accommodated by a demand-flow valve. A decrease

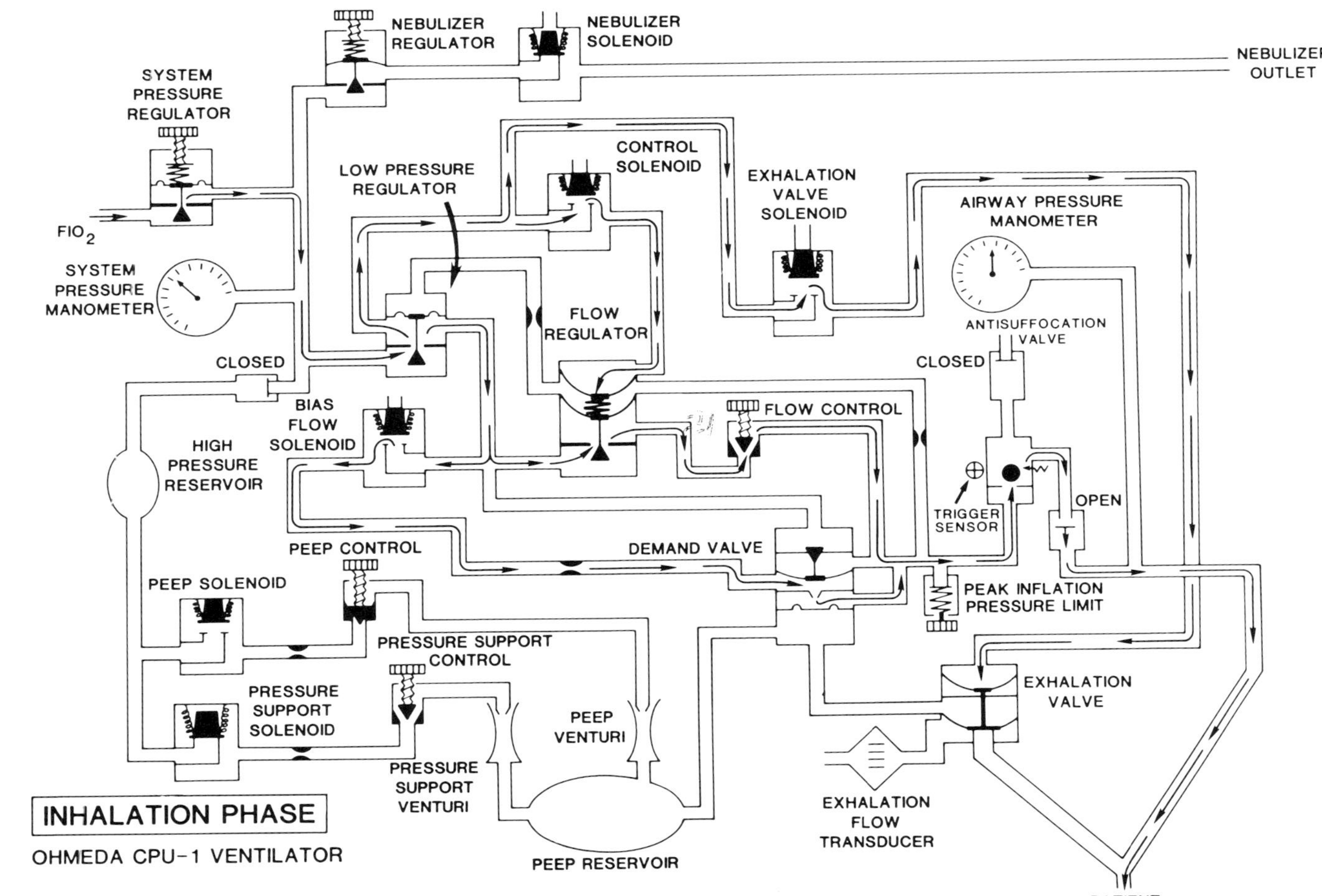

Fig. 15-43. Mechanical inhalation phase of the Ohmeda CPU-1 ventilator.

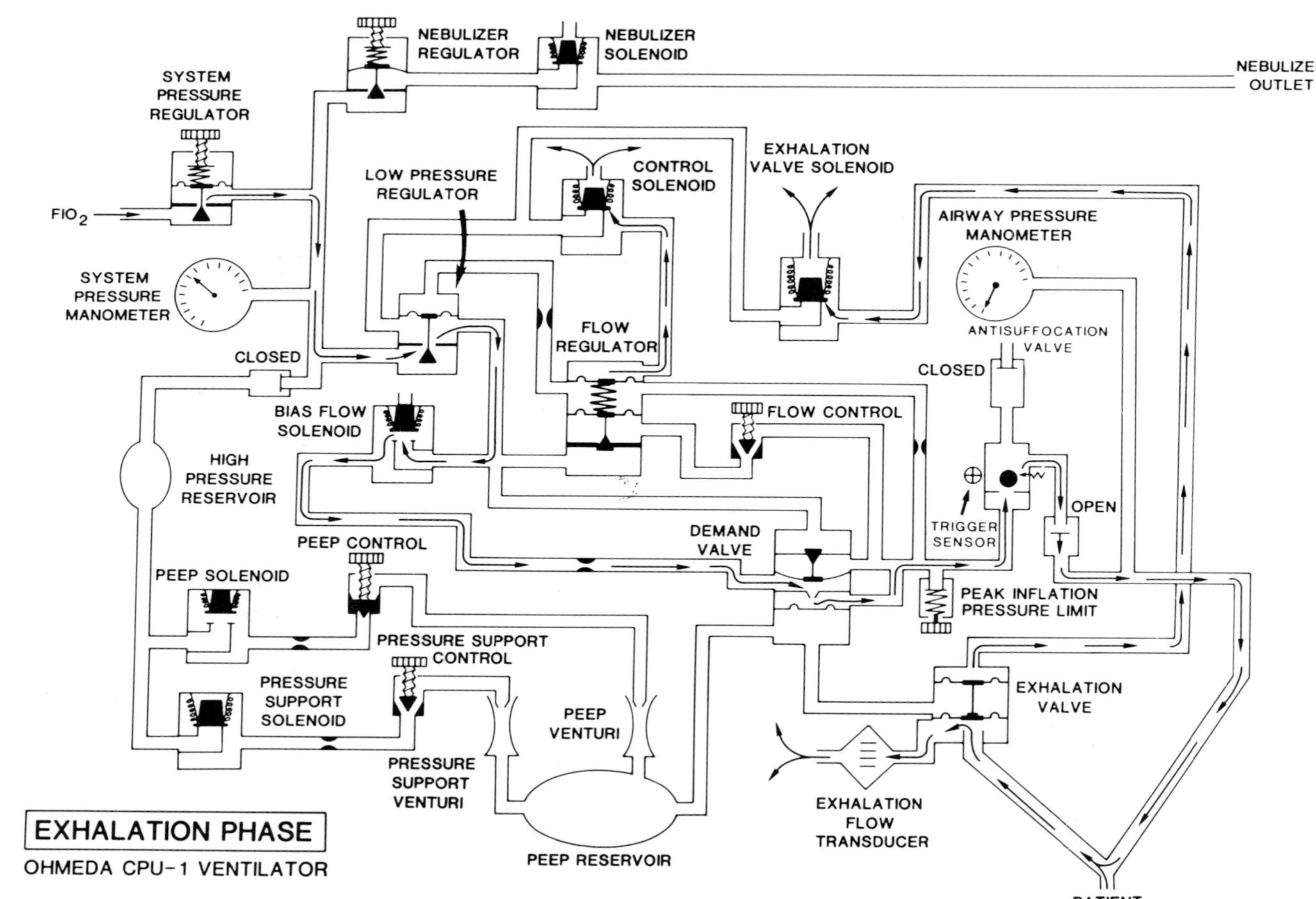

Fig. 15-44. Exhalation phase of the Ohmeda CPU-1 ventilator.

in PAW below the selected CPAP level results in the onset of flow from the demand-flow valve. The level of CPAP is controlled by the rotation of the control knob. Metered gas-flow rate from a Venturi is directed to the rear side of the diaphragm-type exhalation/CPAP valve, which functions as a threshold resistor.

Pressure support ventilation may be included with any mode allowing spontaneous breathing. During PSV, the ventilator establishes immediately an 80 L/min peak flow rate until the PSV pressure level is reached. Flow rate is then decelerated, while maintaining the PSV pressure level. The PSV breath is terminated at the point of zero flow or after one second elapses.

Monitors, Alarms, and Safety Features

The CPU-1 ventilator monitors exhaled tidal and minute volume via a flow sensor located distal to the exhalation valve. Location of the flow sensor in this position in the breathing circuit may predispose to errors in measuring tidal and minute volumes (see under Accuracy of Displayed Exhaled Tidal Volume). Data from this sensor are presented on the display panel as tidal and minute volume, and ventilator frequency. One side of the display panel indicates the preselected minute and tidal volume, ventilator frequency, and I:E ratio. The other side of the panel is relegated to monitoring and alarm functions. An optional monitor is available for expanded monitoring capabilities (Table 15-13).

Four primary patient alarms are available: apnea, maximum airway pressure, minimum minute volume, and inadequate tidal volume. The apnea alarm sequence begins when after 15 seconds no breath is detected by the expiratory flow sensor. A visual alarm is activated, and the patient receives a mechanical breath based on the preselected settings. If no breath is detected for another 15-second period, both audible and visual alarms are activated and the patient is mechanically ventilated based on the preselected settings. Under these conditions, a microprocessor will automatically choose an expiratory time corresponding to an I:E ratio of 1:3. This condition is aborted when the operator depresses the Alarm Reset button. Patient disconnection from the breathing circuit resulting in loss of airway pressure and exhaled flow, also activates the apnea alarm.

The maximum airway pressure alarm functions on a delayed basis. The first time the peak inflation pressure limit is violated, a visual alarm is activated and the exhalation valve opens. A second consecutive violation of the peak inflation pressure limit results in a similar response. When three consecutive peak inflation pressure limit violations occur, audible and visual alarms are activated. This delayed alarm feature precludes the nuisance of frequent PIP limit violations as occurs during coughing. The alarm is automatically inactivated when the ventilator is in the pressure-cycled mode.

The minimum minute volume alarm limit is set with a control on the display panel. If the combined spontaneous and mandatory minute volume fall below the preselected minimum minute volume limit, then visual and audible alarms are activated.

The inadequate tidal volume alarm limit is set with a control on the display panel. If the volume falls below the preselected limit, then visual and audible alarms are activated. The inadequate tidal volume alarm is an optional alarm system that monitors the patient's spontaneous tidal volume. To use this alarm, the operator must depress two DIP switches on the rear of the panel of the ventilator. The first switch activates or deactivates the alarm, while the second switch is used to select the threshold value that will activate the alarm (threshold values may be 25 percent or 37 percent of preselected ventilator tidal volume). When activated, the microprocessor monitors five spontaneous breaths. If the average value of those five breaths falls below the threshold value, or four consecutive breaths fall below the threshold value, the ventilator treats the condition as apnea (i.e., the apnea sequence detailed above is initiated).

Loss of pneumatic power activates an audible alarm. An antisuffocation valve automatically opens the breathing circuit to room air to allow spontaneous breathing. Loss of electrical power or pneumatic system failure (other than demand valve failure) activates visual and audible alarms. All electronic and pneumatic operations stop; however, the patient is allowed to breathe on CPAP.

Bird 6400ST Ventilator

The Bird 6400ST ventilator uses pneumatic and electrical power sources and is controlled by microprocessor electronics, and is a volume-cycled, constant, and nonconstant-flow generator (Fig. 15-45). CMV, AV, IMV/SIMV, PSV, and CPAP are available modes of ventilation. PSV is available for use in the IMV/SIMV and CPAP modes. Constant and decelerating inspiratory flow waveforms may be selected (Table 15-12).

Controls

Two clearly differentiated sections comprise the operation panel of the ventilator: ventilator controls and the alarms/monitoring sections. Standard rotating type control knobs (potentiometer or "pots") are employed to control the operation of the ventilator.

Ventilatory parameters are selected with the following controls: VT, ventilator rate, peak inspiratory flow rate, patient-triggering sensitivity pressure, CPAP, and pressure support. Other controls include mode selector, high PIP limit, low PIP alarm, low CPAP alarm, low inspiratory VT alarm, and push buttons to activate the ventilator's sigh mechanism and provide a manual inhalation. An air-oxygen blender is required since no oxygen mixing mechanism is provided in the ventilator.

The mode-selector switch has two functions: choice of the ventilator mode and the inspiratory flow waveform. When activated, a sigh mechanism enables the ventilator to deliver a sigh breath at 1.5 times the preselected tidal volume every 100 mechanical breaths. The sigh volume is delivered using the peak inspiratory flow rate and flow waveform settings preselected on the ventilator. A manual breath may be given at any time except during a control breath or during the mandatory expiratory phase. VT, inspiratory flow waveform, and the peak inspiratory flow rate of the manual breath are the same as the preselected values.

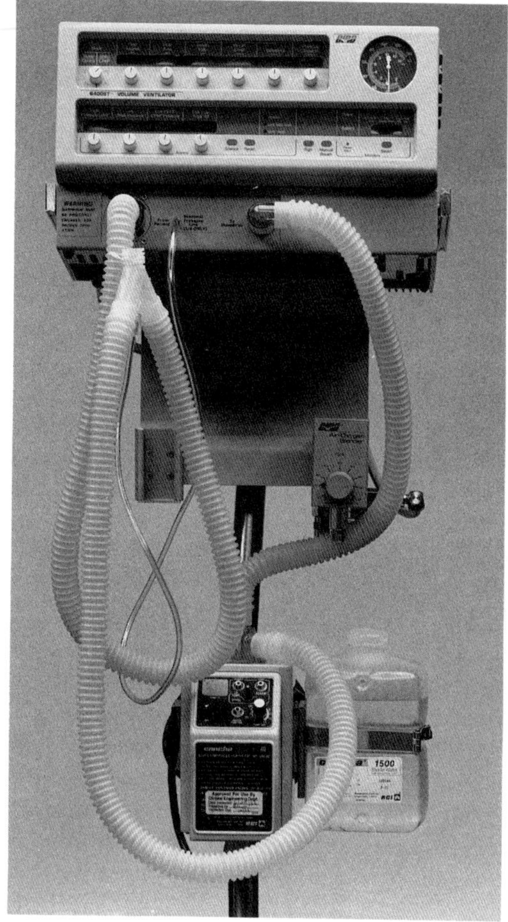

Fig. 15-45. Bird 6400 ST ventilator. (Courtesy of Bird Products Corp., Palm Springs, CA.)

Operation

Mechanical inhalation and exhalation phases of gas flow are indicated in Figures 15-46 and 15-47. The ventilator's pneumatic system is electronically controlled by two microprocessors: the main microprocessor controls functions

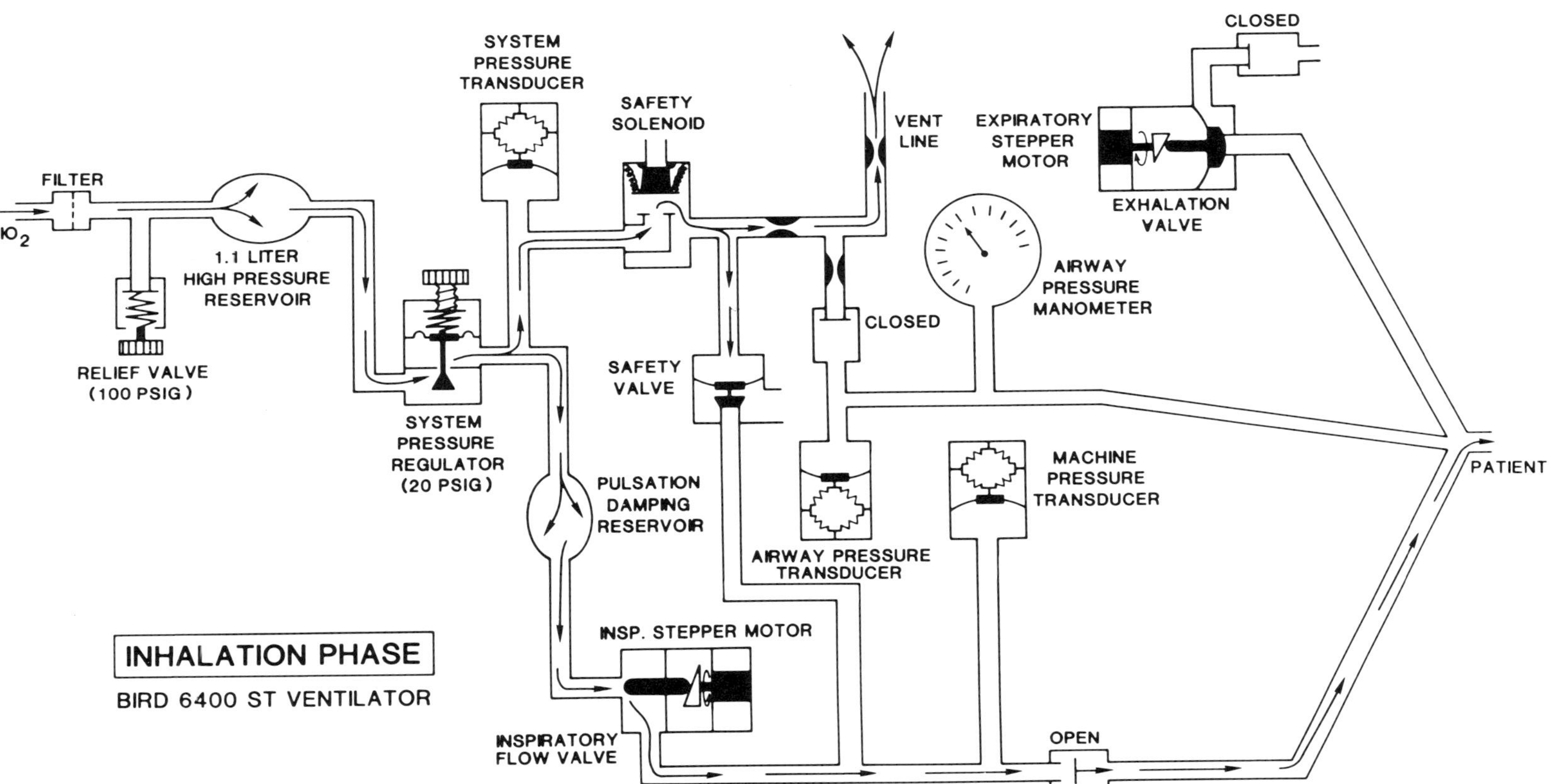

Fig. 15-46. Mechanical inhalation phase of the Bird 6400 ST ventilator.

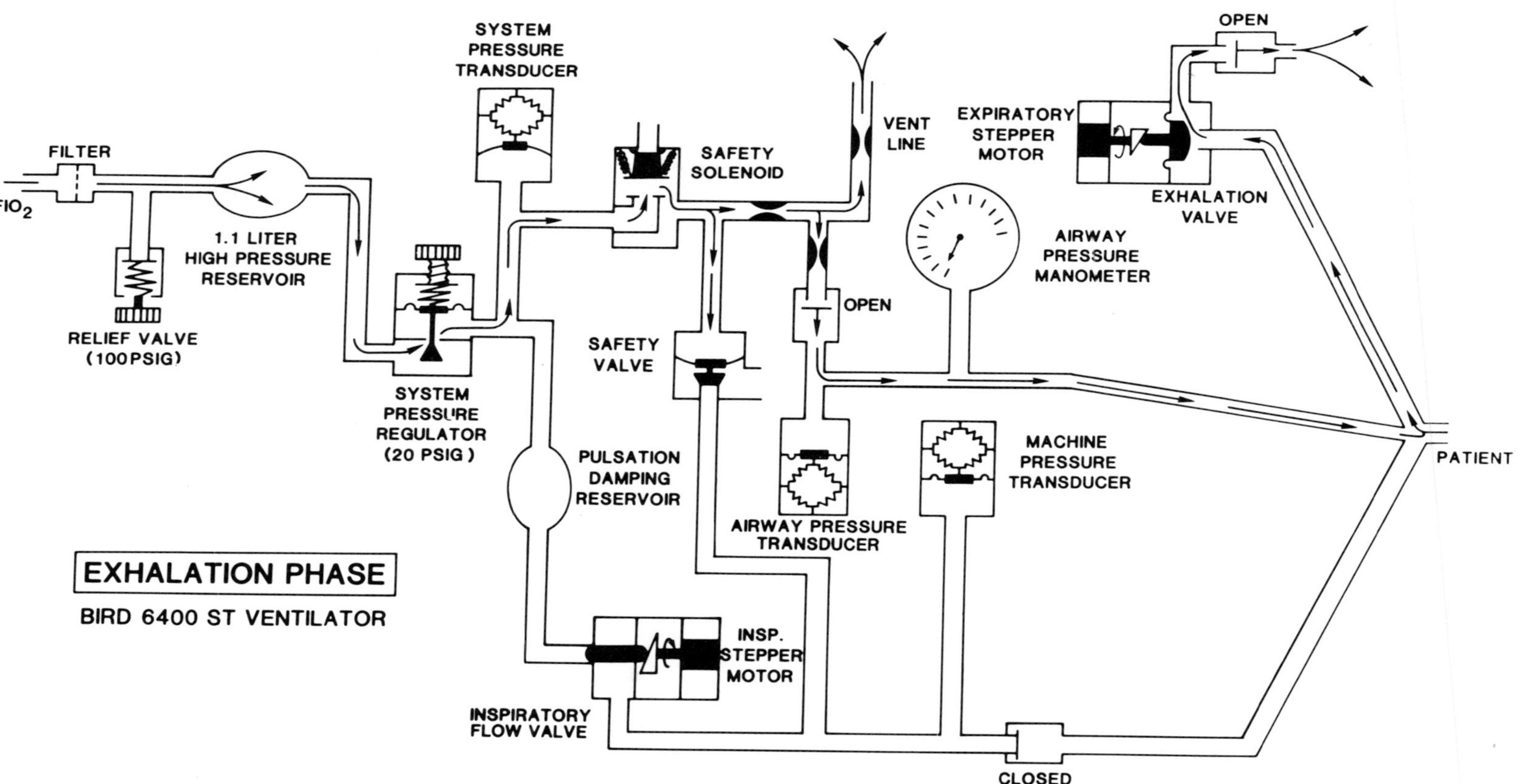

Fig. 15-47. Exhalation phases of the Birt 6400 ST ventilator.

such as breath rate timing, VT control, and the monitoring of patient alarm systems. The movement of the inspiratory flow control valve and the exhalation valve are directed by the second microprocessor.

The inspiratory flow control valve and the exhalation valves are both defined as *electromechanical* valves. These valves convert rotary motion into linear motion. Electric signals from the microprocessor control a motor that rotates a shaft in each valve. Rotation of the shaft occurs as a series of steps. Each step opens or closes a poppet-type orifice to a calibrated distance. Resolution of gas-flow rate through the inspiratory flow control valve orifice is claimed to be 1 L/min per rotational step. The relationship between valve position and inspiratory flow rate is programmed into memory. This information allows the microprocessor to operate the inspiratory flow control valve in a preprogrammed sequence to deliver the preselected VT, peak inspiratory flow rate, and flow waveform.

To provide spontaneous breathing, the microprocessor relies on information obtained from the airway pressure transducer. As airway pressure decreases at the onset of spontaneous inhalation, the microprocessor opens the inspiratory flow control valve to maintain the preselected level of CPAP. The microprocessor then regulates the inspiratory flow rate to meet the patient's demand to maintain the preselected level of CPAP. As the inspiratory gas-flow rate approaches zero, the inhalation phase ends, and exhalation at the preselected level of CPAP occurs. Pressure support breaths are provided in essentially the same manner. In the PSV mode, the microprocessor regulates the inspiratory flow control valve to maintain the preselected level of PSV.

Inspiratory Flow Waveforms

Constant or decelerating inspiratory flow waveforms may be selected using the Mode Control knob. When a constant inspiratory flow waveform is selected, the inspiratory flow rate is delivered at a constant rate according to the peak flow rate setting. When the decelerating waveform is selected, the inspiratory flow rate peaks at the onset of mechanical inhalation at a value equal to the preselected peak flow rate setting and then decelerates to 50 percent of the peak flow rate setting at the conclusion of the mechanical breath.

Monitors, Alarms, and Safety Features

Expiratory flow rate and VT are not measured with this ventilator. No electronic flow transducer is used to monitor gas-flow rate in the breathing circuit. Displayed values for tidal and minute volumes are calculated by using the settings of VT and ventilator rate. Consequently, these values do not reflect the patient's true tidal and minute volume.

Airway pressure is measured at the Y piece of the ventilator breathing circuit and is displayed on a standard, aneroid type pressure gauge. A high PIP limit control regulates the maximum pressure generated in the breathing circuit during mechanical inhalation. Violation of this limit aborts the inhalation phase, opens the exhalation valve, and activates visual and audible alarms. If airway pressure returns to baseline within three seconds, the alarms reset; if not, the alarms persist. The microprocessor automatically adjusts the PIP alarm limit to a value of 50 percent greater than the preselected value during the delivery of a sigh breath. Under no circumstances may the peak inflation pressure exceed 140 cm H_2O.

The low peak pressure and the low CPAP alarms monitor for leaks in the breathing circuit and disconnection of the patient from the ventilator. The low inspiratory VT alarm is active in both the spontaneous and mechanical ventilation modes. If no spontaneous or mechanical breath is detected for a period of 20 seconds, visual and audible apnea alarms are activated (Table 15-13).

In the event of loss of electrical or pneumatic power, the ventilator enters into the "Vent Inop" condition. Under these circumstances, the patient is allowed to breathe room air via an intake safety valve (Fig. 15-47). Electrical power for transport situations may be provided via a DC input receptacle on the rear panel of the ventilator. The ventilator may be connected to a 12-V power supply for operation.

Bear V Ventilator

The Bear V ventilator uses pneumatic and electrical power sources, and is microprocessor-controlled, volume- or time-cycled, and a constant or nonconstant-flow generator (Fig. 15-48). CMV, AV, EIP, IMV/SIMV, MMV, PSV, and CPAP are available ventilatory modes. PSV is available in the SIMV, AV, and CPAP modes (Table 15-12). Constant, accelerating, decelerating or sinusoidal inspiratory flow waveforms may be selected.

Controls

Two differentiated sections comprise the operating panel of the ventilator: ventilator controls and the CRT monitor/control sections. All controls are based on a keypad-type entry system. Selections are made by depressing the key corresponding to the desired ventilator function. A numeric keypad permits entry of ventilator parameters. Current values for each parameter are displayed above the numeric keypad. The operator can change a value by touching the appropriate keys. When the display indicates the new desired value, the ENTER command must be depressed to delete the previous value from memory and insert the new one. The newly entered value is then displayed in a window next to the ventilator function. This serves as visual confirmation that the change has been made.

Mode and parameter keys comprise the ventilator controls. CMV, AV-CMV, MMV (so-called augmented minute ventilation), IMV/SIMV, CPAP, and TIME CYCLE are the ventilator mode keys. The parameter keys include V_T, ventilator rate, peak inspiratory flow rate, percentage of oxygen, CPAP, EIP, patient-triggering sensitivity (assist sensitivity), PSV, MMV, inspiratory time, continuous flow, pressure relief (PIP limit), sigh rate, and volume controls, and the numeric keypad. Keys for manual V_T, sigh, panel lock, and a key to provide 100 percent oxygen are included. Finally, keys to select the four inspiratory flow waveforms are designated.

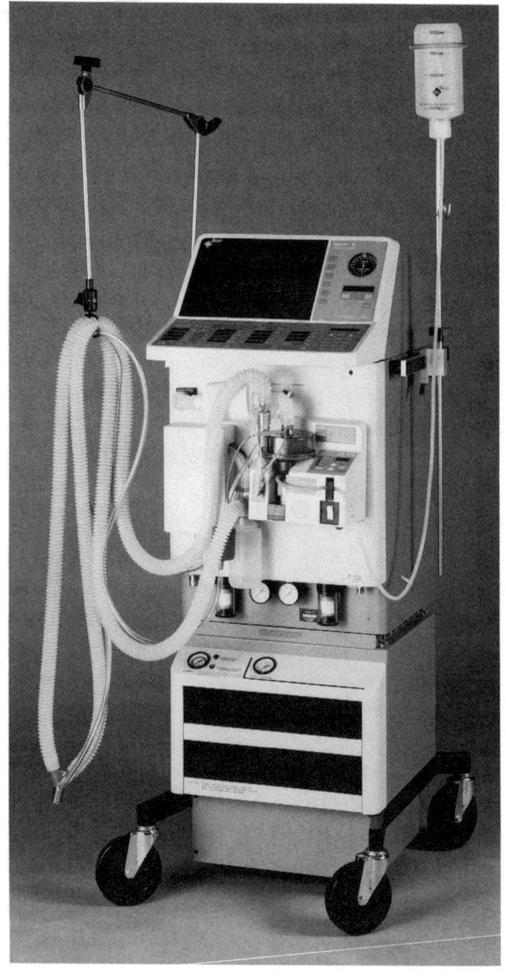

Fig. 15-48. Bear 5 ventilator. (Courtesy of Bear Inter Med, Riverside, CA.)

The CRT monitor/control section of the operating panel consists of a multicolored high resolution CRT monitor capable of displaying alphanumeric, airway pressure, and inspiratory-expiratory flow waveform data. Control keys to silence and reset alarms and to test the system are provided. In addition, a set of six vertically aligned keys are available for selecting alarms, graphics, and other data for display on the CRT monitor.

Operation

Mechanical inhalation and exhalation phases for gas flow are indicated in Figures 15-49 and 15-50. Precision regulators reduce air and oxygen source gases to approximately 18 psig. A connection allows the output from the air regulator to control the output of the oxygen regulator. This pressure "relay" system insures that both regulators have identical output pressure. Any variation at the air regulator is immediately matched at the oxygen regulator. Accuracy of the oxygen blending system is maintained with this design.

Internal function of the Bear V is primarily dependent upon three "stepper motor" and valve combinations. Stepper motors are small electric motors that rotate a shaft in a series of discrete steps. When linked to a valve, each step opens or closes the valve slightly. Information such as the open position, the closed position, the number of steps between open and closed, and the change in flow rate, pressure, or percent of each step is programmed into computer memory. The three stepper motors are used to control the F_{IO_2}, inspiratory flow rate, and PIP.

Regulated air and oxygen are blended by a stepper motor-controlled dual orifice valve. The computer verifies the function of the system with each F_{IO_2} change. Verification is achieved by checking the closed position, counting the steps to the open position, and checking the open position. If all is in order, the computer counts the steps to the position which delivers the preselected F_{IO_2}. Blended gas then fills a rigid tank reservoir, which in turn allows high peak inspiratory flow rates to be delivered. The tank reservoir also serves to reduce the response time for the onset of flow during spontaneous inhalation on CPAP.

A valve delivers blended gas to the inspiratory flow rate stepper motor control valve, the pressure relief (PIP limit) valve, and a purge/bleed valve. The purge/bleed valve directs a low flow rate of gas through an airway pressure sensing line to prevent migration of water into the ventilator. All flow to the patient is controlled by the inspiratory flow rate stepper motor control valve. Flow from the valve passes through a flow conditioner and then through a vortex-type flow transducer. Inspiratory flow continues until the preselected tidal volume has been measured. Inspiratory flow rate is also regulated by a feedback loop. Ideally, in a closed loop feedback system when incongruencies between measured and preselected values occur, a microprocessor should instruct the system to modify its output. In this ventilator, if the measured/delivered inspiratory flow rate is less than the preselected value, flow rate should be increased appropriately. The operator's manual states: "The internal flow transducer measures the actual flow output from the valve and transmits the measured value back. . . . If the actual value is less than desired, the flow command is increased." However, in actual practice, this does not seem to operate as described (see under Inspiratory Flow Rate and Tidal Volume Characteristics).

During exhalation, the stepper motor flow control valve directs a continuous flow rate of 5 L/min through the breathing circuit. It is contended that the continuous flow rate improves the responsiveness of demand flow system.

The exhalation valve is powered by a Venturi. A stepper motor alters the output pressure generated by the Venturi by varying the orifice size of the Venturi. During mechanical inhalation, the microprocessor maintains pressure in the exhalation valve at 20 cm H_2O above the peak inflation pressure. When the ventilator cycles "OFF," pressure in the exhalation valve returns to ambient pressure or the preselected level of CPAP.

A transducer provides continuous data of airway pressure readings. These data are used for

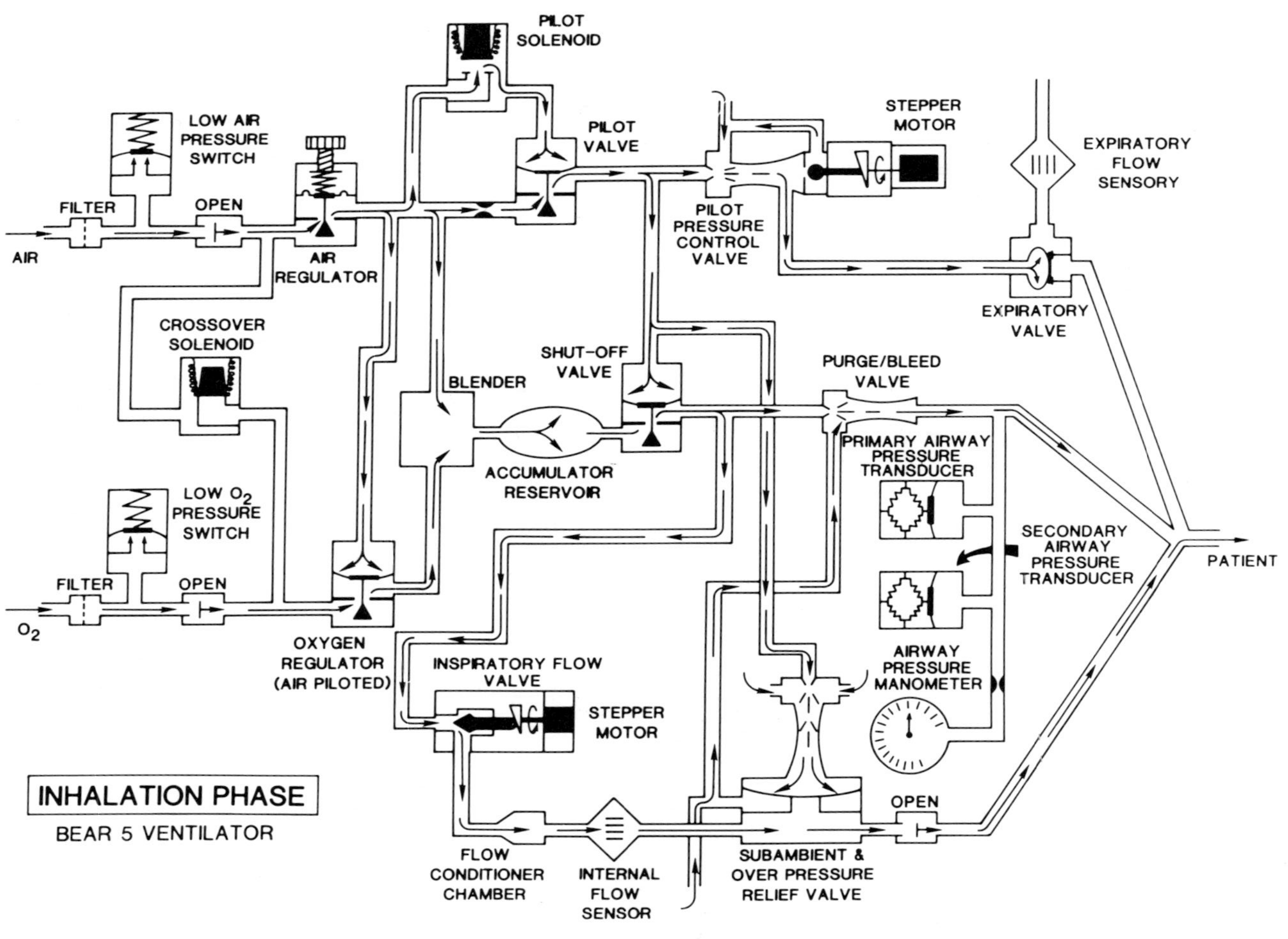

Fig. 15-49. Mechanical inhalation phase of the Bear 5 ventilator.

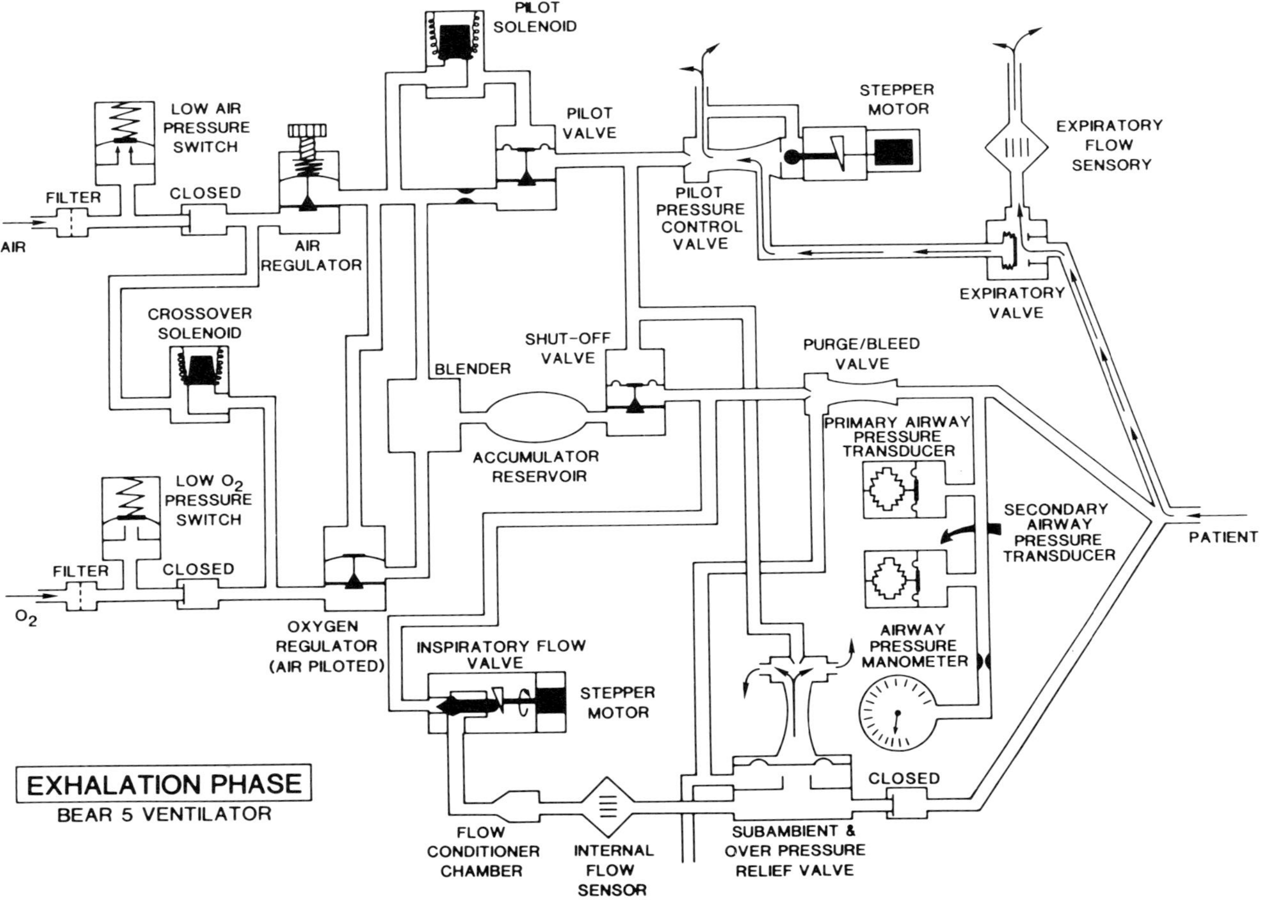

Fig. 15-50. Exhalation phase of the Bear 5 ventilator.

various ventilator functions: assist-sensitivity (patient-triggering pressure), pressure relief (PIP limit), mean airway pressure monitoring, CPAP, PSV, and spontaneous breathing. A second transducer monitors the function of the first. Data from both transducers must agree by ±6 cm H_2O or a "ventilator inoperative" condition occurs.

Spontaneous breathing is allowed in the SIMV/IMV and CPAP modes. If the patient's inspiratory effort reduces the baseline airway pressure by 0.5 cm H_2O, the stepper motor inspiratory flow rate control valve will deliver gas-flow rate to the patient on demand (up to 120 L/min).

Inspiratory Flow Waveforms

Constant, sinusoidal, decelerating, and accelerating inspiratory flow waveforms may be selected during mechanical inhalation. When the inspiratory flow waveform is changed, the peak inspiratory flow rate and the VT are unaffected; however, inspiratory time, $\overline{\text{PAW}}$, and I:E ratio vary.[51]

A sinusoidal inspiratory flow waveform starts at zero flow rate, accelerates to peak flow rate, and then decelerates to zero flow rate. Inspiratory time using this waveform is approximately 50 percent longer than for a constant inspiratory flow waveform at the same peak flow rate and VT settings. As a result, increases in the I:E ratio and mean airway pressure occur.[51]

A decelerating inspiratory flow waveform starts immediately at peak rate and is followed by a linear deceleration to 50 percent of the peak flow rate. The accelerating flow waveform is the opposite; peak flow rate starts at 50 percent of the peak inspiratory flow rate followed by a linear acceleration to the peak flow rate. Both flow waveforms increase inspiratory time by approximately 50 percent that of a constant flow waveform with the same peak inspiratory flow rate and tidal volumes. This results in increases in I:E ratio and mean airway pressure.[51]

Monitors, Alarms, and Safety Features

Inspiratory and expiratory flow sensors allow the Bear V to monitor all phases of ventilation. Airway pressure is monitored with an aneroid manometer and two pressure transducers. Integration of data allows the ventilator to monitor: rate, inspiratory time, I:E ratio, peak and mean airway pressures, CPAP, and exhaled tidal and minute volume. Exhaled volumes are measured via a flow sensor located distal to the exhalation valve. Location of the flow sensor in this position may predispose to spuriously high values for tidal and minute volumes (see under Accuracy of Displayed Exhaled Tidal Volume).

A number of adjustable alarms are available. With the exception of I:E ratio and exhaled VT, each monitored parameter has high and low alarm ranges that may be set. Alarms can be disabled by entering a value of 0 on the control panel for a particular alarm. Alarms include: low, mandatory, and spontaneous exhaled tidal volume; exhaled minute volume; breath rate; inspiratory time; I:E ratio; PIP; mean airway pressure; and CPAP. The operator may also select a high inflation pressure alarm for the sigh breaths (Table 15-13).

Calculation and display of CLT and airways resistance are provided on the Bear V. Nonadjustable alarms alert the operator to low air or oxygen inlet pressures and electrical power loss or mechanical failure (Vent-Inop).

Compliance Compensation

Potentially, a useful feature to compensate for the portion of ventilator delivered tidal volume compressed in the breathing circuit tubing during mechanical inhalation is *compliance compensation.* To use this feature, the operator determines the compliance factor of the breathing circuit and then enters it into the microprocessor. When engaged, inspiratory time is held constant, but the peak flow rate from the ventilator is increased appropriately. Since inspiratory time times inspiratory flow rate equals tidal volume, a larger tidal volume is delivered or added to the preselected tidal volume in order to compensate for volume compressed in the tubing. The increase in peak flow rate is the product of the compliance factor of the breathing circuit and the initial peak inflation pressure.

Engström Erica IV Ventilator

The Enström Erica IV ventilator uses pneumatic and electrical power sources, and is a microprocessor-controlled, volume-cycled, constant and nonconstant flow generator (Fig. 15-51). Constant, accelerating, and decelerating inspiratory flow waveforms are available. CMV, AV, AV/CMV, EIP, SIMV, MMV (so-called extended mandatory minute volume), CPAP and PSV (so-called inspiratory assist) are available modes of ventilation. PSV is available for use in the SIMV, MMV, and CPAP modes (Table 15-12).

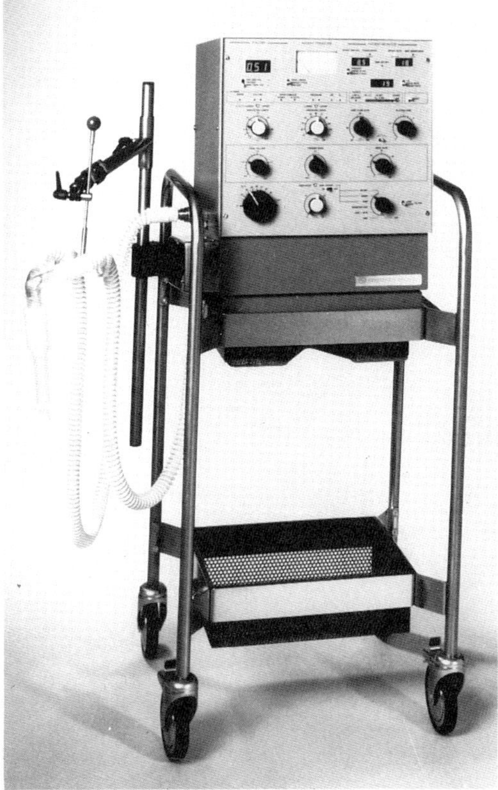

Fig. 15-51. Engström Erica IV ventilator. (Courtesy of Gambro Engström, Lincolnshire, IL.)

Controls

Ventilatory parameters are selected and monitored on the operating panel. Standard rotating type control knobs (potentiometers or "pots") and multiposition toggle switches are employed to control the operation of the ventilator. Controls include V_T, rate, patient-triggering pressure, CPAP, F_{IO_2}, inspiratory flow rate, waveform selection, and I:E ratio. The I:E ratio ranges are 1:3, 1:2, 1:1, 2:1, or 3:1.

The mechanical inhalation phase may contain "dynamic" and "static" phases. The dynamic phase, when the preselected V_T is delivered, is regulated by the inspiratory flow rate control. The static or EIP phase is regulated by the I:E ratio control (greater the I:E ratio setting, the greater the EIP time). EIP may not be applied during SIMV, MMV, or PSV.

A seven position control knob allows ventilatory mode selection, including: OFF, CMV, CMV + SIGH, assisted CMV, SIMV, extended MMV, and spontaneous. Inspiratory assist (PSV) may be engaged for the last three modes only. Sigh breaths can be provided but in the CMV mode only. A sigh is delivered after 100 controlled breaths at a volume twice the preselected tidal volume.

Operation

Mechanical inhalation and exhalation phases of gas flow are indicated in Figures 15-52 and 15-53). Compressed air and oxygen are filtered and regulated to identical pressures prior to entering the air-oxygen mixing system. The mixing system incorporates a dual needle valve

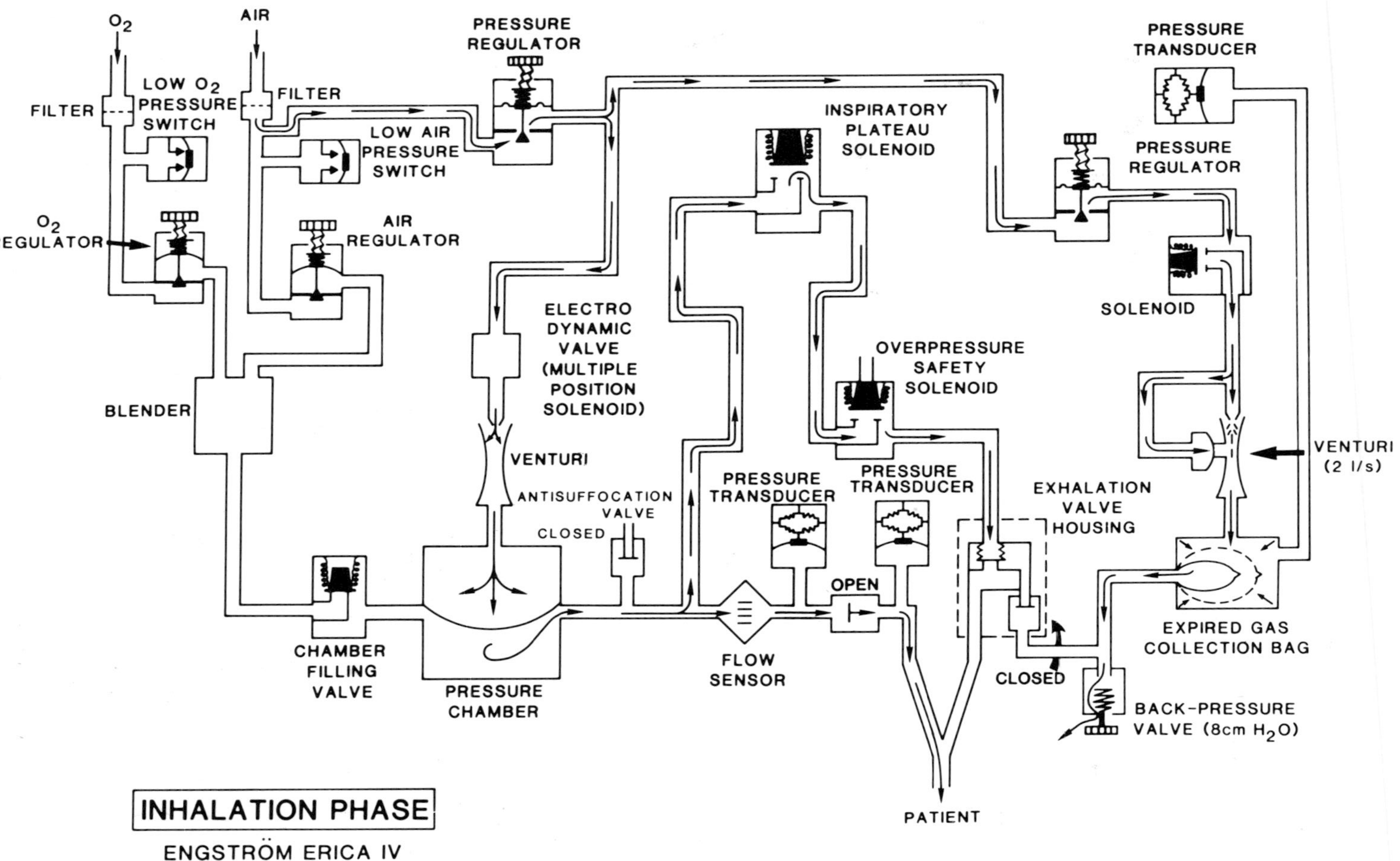

Fig. 15-52. Mechanical inhalation phase of the Erica IV ventilator.

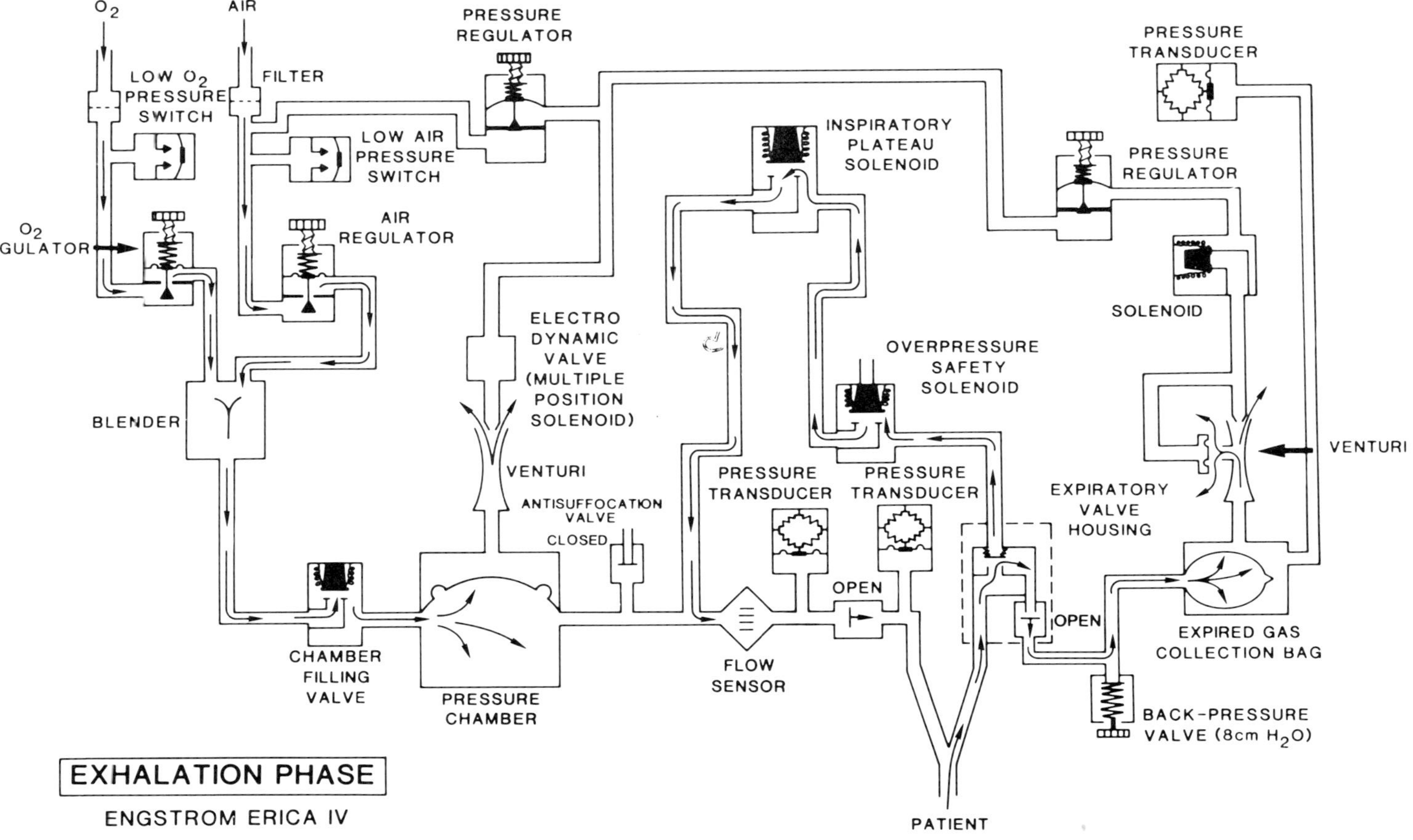

Fig. 15-53. Exhalation phase of the Erica IV ventilator.

mechanism. Blended gas then passes through a filling valve and into the patient side of a pressure chamber. The pressure chamber is a large vessel divided into patient and ventilator sides by a diaphragm. It functions similarly to a bellows. Pressure generated on the ventilator side collapses the diaphragm ejecting the preselected tidal volume to the patient. Overfilling of the chamber is prevented by a filling valve which diverts gas flow as soon as the pressure chamber is full. Should the valve malfunction, a relief valve located in the diaphragm prevents overfilling.

The mechanical inspiratory phase begins with a patient-triggered breath (AV and SIMV modes) or as the result of electronic timing (CMV and SIMV modes). A Venturi device is activated that directs flow and thus pressurizes the ventilator side of the pressure chamber. The output pressure from the Venturi is regulated by a microprocessor-operated electrodynamic valve. By regulating the drive pressure to the Venturi jet, the inspiratory flow rate and inspiratory flow waveform are controlled. Gas-flow rate continues until the preselected VT, as measured by a flow sensor, is delivered. Gas-flow rate from a Venturi varies inversely with PIP. Decrease in CLT and/or increased RAW precipitate high peak inflation pressures, leading to decreased inspiratory flow rate output and a prolongation of inspiratory time, similar to the MA-I ventilator (Fig. 15-30).

Spontaneous breathing with or without CPAP may be used. During spontaneous inhalation, the patient inhales from the pressure chamber. When CPAP is applied, an inflatable balloon type exhalation valve is pressurized commensurate to the desired level of CPAP.

The ventilator uses four pressure transducers to control and monitor operation. A differential pressure transducer distal to the pressure chamber is used to measure inhaled volume. Two pressure transducers measure airway pressure; data are directed to an airway pressure manometer and to a microprocessor that controls ventilator operation. A fourth transducer is used to assess exhaled volume; the exhaled volume measuring system is a bag-in-a-bottle apparatus. During exhalation, the exhaled tidal volume is directed into a rubber bag contained within a rigid chamber. Subsequently, during the inhalation phase exhaled volume is emptied from the bag by applying a constant flow rate into the bottle, collapsing the bag. The emptying time is derived from the pressure transducer and the exhaled volume is calculated from the emptying time.

During mechanical inhalation, the inflatable balloon exhalation valve is pressurized closed. Pressure is maintained in the valve to produce an EIP, after which the valve depressurizes and airway pressure returns to baseline pressure. Pressurization and depressurization of the exhalation valve are governed by the opening and closing of two solenoid valves.

Inspiratory Flow Waveforms

A three-way selector switch permits selection of constant, accelerating, or decelerating inspiratory flow waveforms. However, as the operator's manual states, the actual flow waveform that results in the patient's airways depends on many parameters, in particular, the patient's CLT and RAW. With a constant inspiratory flow waveform, for example, when high PIP are generated as a result of decreased CLT and/or increased RAW, there is a decay (deceleration) in the inspiratory flow rate and waveform, similar to the MA-1 ventilator (Fig. 15-30).

Monitoring, Alarms, and Safety Features

The previously described exhaled volume monitoring system, coupled with the airway pressure transducer, allows the ventilator to monitor exhaled tidal and minute volume (spontaneous and mandatory), breathing frequency (spontaneous and mandatory), lung-thorax compliance, and airway resistance. Airway pressure is displayed via the analog gauge.

Patient alarms include high- and low-minute volume and high and low airway pressure. Interlocking controls prevent the operator from selecting a high limit value lower than the low limit and vice-versa. The patient is also monitored for apnea. If no exhaled gas is detected for 30 seconds, visual and audible alarms are activated. If the ventilator rate is set greater than 10 breaths/min, the apnea interval is reduced automatically to 15 seconds. Other alarms alert the operator to electrical power loss, disconnection, and loss of air or oxygen pressure sources (Table 15-13).

Conventional Ventilators (Non-Micropressor Controlled)

Siemens 900C

The Siemens 900C ventilator uses pneumatic and electrical power sources and is an electronically controlled, time-cycled, constant- and non-constant-flow generator (Fig. 15-54). Manipulation of the ventilator's "working pressure" control enables the system to function as a constant pressure generator. CMV, AV, SIMV, PSV, EIP, pressure control (PC), and CPAP are available modes of ventilation. Constant or accelerating inspiratory flow waveforms may be selected during mechanical inhalation. PSV can be used in conjunction with SIMV and CPAP (Table 15-12).

Controls

Standard rotating-type control knobs (potentiometer or "pots") are employed to control most of the operations of the ventilator. Ventilatory controls include: working pressure, minute volume, ventilator rate, SIMV rate, percent inspiratory time, pause time (EIP), inspiratory pressure (for PSV and PC modes), CPAP, PIP limit, and patient-triggering sensitivity pressure. Ventilatory mode is determined by an eight-position rotary knob. Three special function buttons allow an inspiratory pause, an expiratory

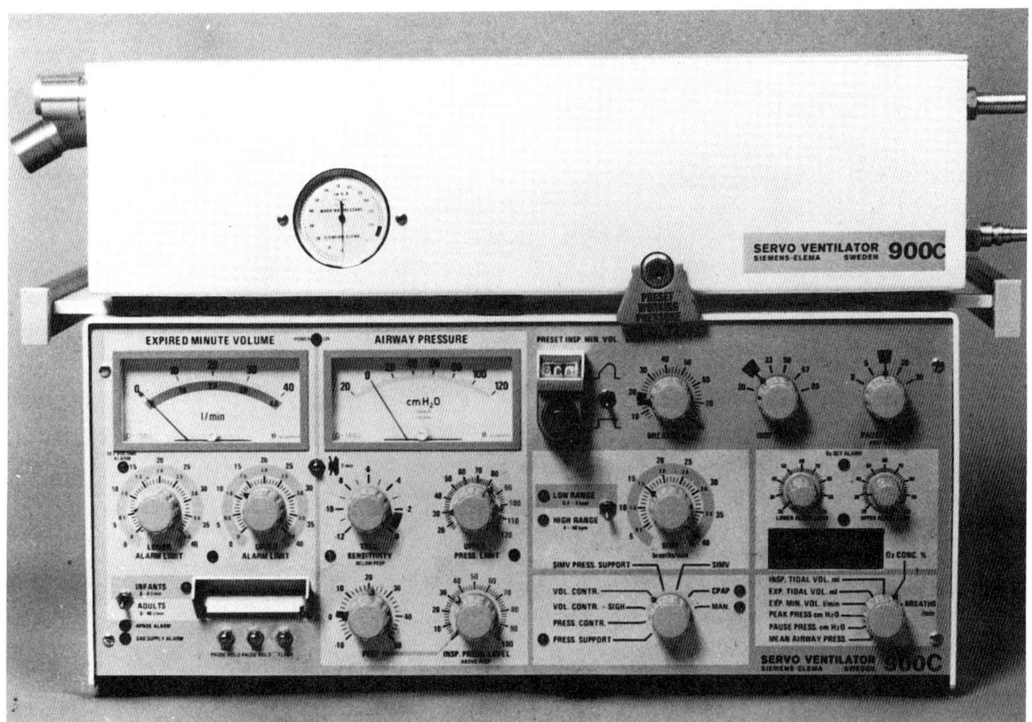

Fig. 15-54. Siemens 900C ventilator. (Courtesy of Siemens-Elema Ventilator Systems, Schaumberg, IL.)

pause, or a gas-flush mode. In the pause functions, the ventilator will remain in the selected mode with both inspiratory and expiratory valves closed, for as long as the button is depressed. The flush mode opens both valves, allowing a continuous flow of gas through the circuit. This maneuver replaces all gas in the reservoir in a matter of seconds and is useful for changing FIO_2 rapidly.

In the PC mode, at the onset of mechanical inhalation, airway pressure rises immediately to the preselected level. The ventilator rate can be ventilator-controlled or patient-triggered "ON"; the ventilator cycles "OFF" when a preselected inspiratory time elapses. Resultant tidal volume depends on inspiratory time, change in airway pressure, CLT, and RAW. A decelerating inspiratory flow waveform is applied during mechanical inhalation with the ventilator set in the PC mode.

Operation

Mechanical inhalation and exhalation phases of gas flow are indicated in Figures 15-55 and 15-56. Compressed gases from an oxygen blender (external to the ventilator and purchased separately) enter the ventilator and fill a bellows. Pressure in the bellows (working pressure) is maintained by adjusting a series of springs against two metal plates. The springs and plates provide a constant squeezing action on the bellows in order to maintain the preselected working pressure. When full, the bellows actuates a flow refill valve, which stops flow from the blender. Removal of gas from the bellows, as during mechanical or spontaneous inhalation, opens the valve and allows the bellows to refill.

Electronic timing initiates mechanical inhalation whenever the patient is unable to "trigger" the ventilator "ON." Patient-initiated inhalation occurs when the patient's inspiratory effort lowers the baseline airway pressure to the preselected setting on the SENSITIVITY control.

The inspiratory flow control valve is comprised of a step motor that actuates a lever arm of a hinged clamp device that pinches a silicone rubber tube. The scissors-like opening and closing movement of the valve against the tube occurs as a series of discrete steps controlled by the step motor. From the closed position, each step opening increases the gas-flow rate by approximately 10 percent. The valve can be opened from the closed position in as little as 0.1 second, or at a rate of 480 steps/sec. As inhalation begins, the valve opens to allow the predetermined flow rate. Gas flow is then directed through an inspiratory flow transducer where the rate of flow is measured. The measured and predetermined flow rates are compared, and the valve is opened or closed accordingly to produce the desired flow rate. This design is referred to as a *closed feedback (Servo) loop*. The Siemens company was the first to use this concept, hence the name Servo Ventilator.

The expiratory valve is also a scissors-like valve. It is electronically controlled and is either open during exhalation or closed during mechanical inhalation. During exhalation, gas-flow rate is directed through an expiratory flow transducer, which monitors exhaled tidal volume, and then through an open expiratory valve.

During CPAP, the opening and closing of the inspiratory valve is regulated by signals from pressure transducers. During spontaneous breathing, the inspiratory scissor valve opens appropriately to provide the requisite gas-flow rate to meet the patient's inspiratory demand and maintain the preselected level of CPAP. The expiratory scissor valve also receives input from a pressure transducer. The level of expiratory pressure is controlled by closing the valve when exhaled flow has reached a minimal level and the preselected expiratory pressure is reached.

Inspiratory Flow Waveforms

Constant or accelerating inspiratory flow waveforms may be selected during CMV, AV, and SIMV. Since the ventilator is time-cycled, the peak inspiratory flow rate increases by a factor of 1.5 times when the flow waveform

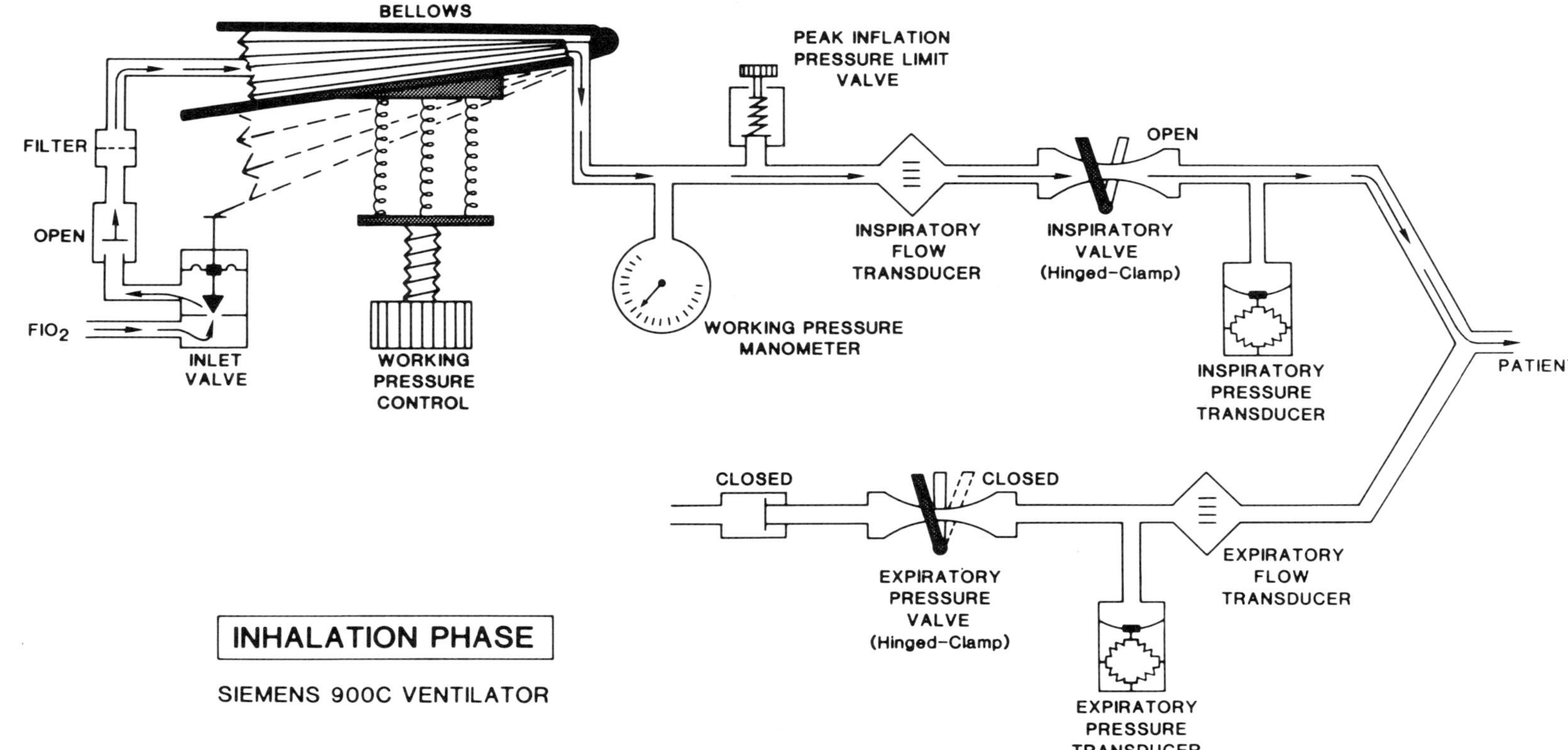

Fig. 15-55. Mechanical inhalation phase of the Siemens 900C ventilator.

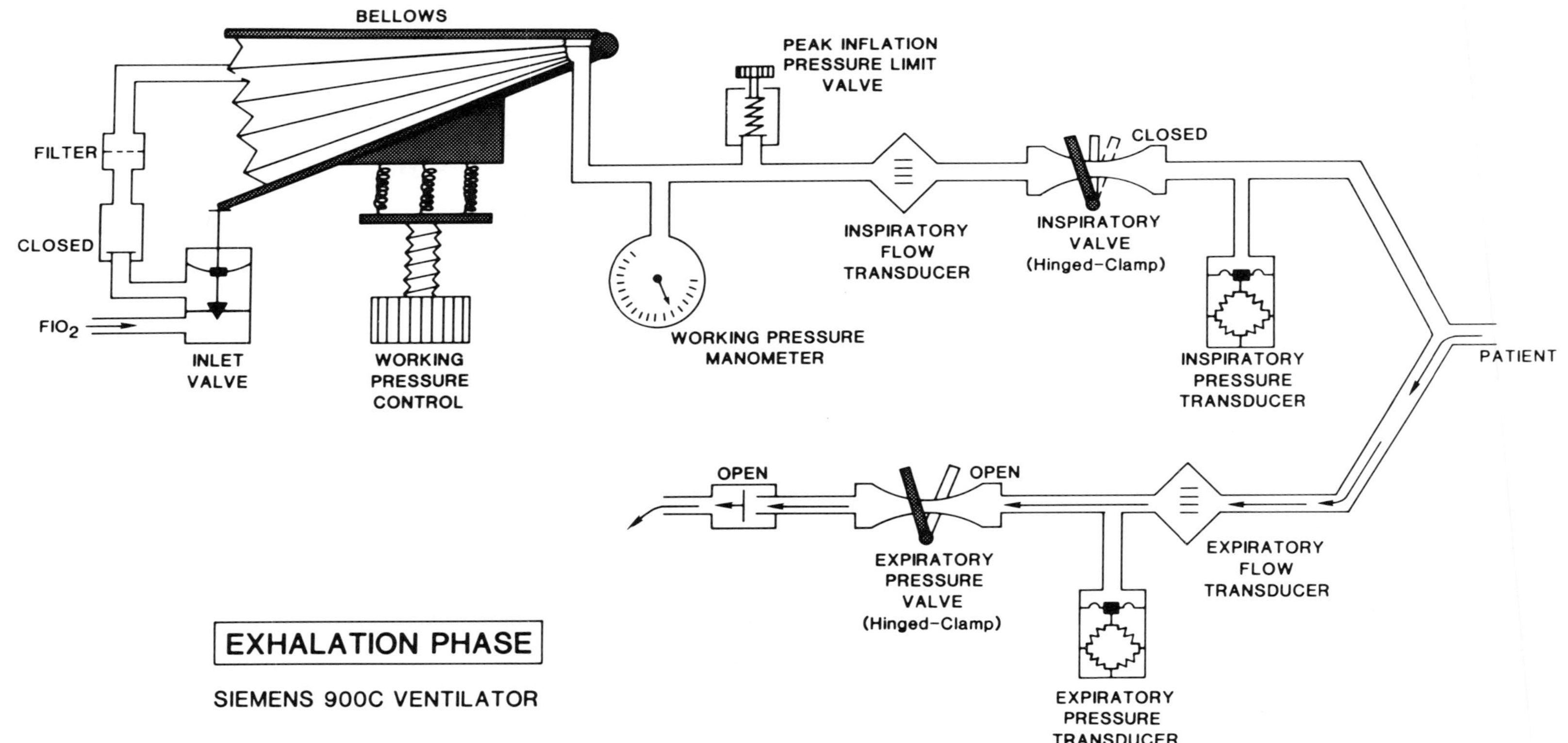

Fig. 15-56. Exhalation phase of the Siemens 900C ventilator.

is changed from constant to accelerating. The increase in flow rate is required to deliver the same preselected tidal volume.[51]

Since pressure is proportional to flow rate times resistance, increases in peak inspiratory flow rate will result in increases in PIP. Increases in mean airway pressure may also occur, since mean pressure is the integration of airway pressure over time.

A decelerating inspiratory flow waveform may also be applied in the PSV and PC modes or when a low working pressure is set with an appropriate setting for inspiratory time. Tidal volume is variable when any of these modes are used.

Monitors, Alarms, and Safety Features

Because exhaled flow rate and VT are measured on the exhalation limb of the breathing circuit, spuriously high values for VT may be displayed (see under Accuracy of Displayed Exhaled Tidal Volume). Airway pressure information is provided by inspiratory and expiratory pressure transducers. An analog display of airway pressure changes, as well as an LED display, are incorporated on the Siemens 900C. Monitored airway pressures include: PIP, EIP pressure, and mean airway pressure.

Operator adjustable alarms include high minute volume, low minute volume, high oxygen percent, low oxygen percent, and high airway pressure. The patient is constantly monitored for apnea; if no exhaled flow is measured at the expiratory flow sensor for fifteen seconds, visual and audible alarms are activated. The apnea alarm is the primary ventilator disconnect alarm (Table 15-13).

In the event of electrical power loss, an alarm is sounded, all ventilator functions cease, and all valves in the ventilator revert to the OPEN position. This allows constant, high flow of gas through the circuit, and permits the patient to breathe spontaneously. However, under these conditions, approximately 15 cm H_2O pressure may be generated in the breathing circuit and applied to the patient.

IMVbird Ventilator

The IMVbird ventilator is a pneumatically-powered and controlled, time-cycled, nonconstant-flow generator (Fig. 15-57), with CMV, IMV, and CPAP as available modes of ventilation. Its small size and modest gas consumption make it an ideal transport ventilator, as well as an ICU ventilator (Table 15-12) (see Ch. 8).

Controls

Standard rotating-type control knobs attached to needle valves are employed to control the operation of the ventilator. Ventilator controls include: inspiratory time, expiratory time, inspiratory flow rate, and CPAP. Other controls include a master switch (ON/OFF), which should not be turned off while the ventilator is in use since it terminates all gas power to the ventilator; a manual push-button, which allows the operator to provide manual breaths up to 5 seconds long; an auxiliary nebulizer control used to augment humidification during spontaneous breathing; and an inspiratory flow deceleration control. This latter control allows the operator to preselect an airway pressure at which the ventilator reduces inspiratory flow rate, thereby producing a decelerating inspiratory flow waveform. Inspiratory flow deceleration is accomplished by the venting of gas to the atmosphere, resulting in a reduction in inspiratory flow rate and hence, tidal volume. Tidal volume may be restored by increasing inspiratory time.

Operation

Mechanical inhalation and exhalation phases of gas flow are indicated in Figures 15-58 and 15-59. Compressed gases from an externally mounted air/oxygen blender enter the ventilator. Gas is then directed to a normally open pneumatic cartridge—the *master cartridge*—which provides control for the delivery of mechanical tidal volumes. During the mechanical inhalation

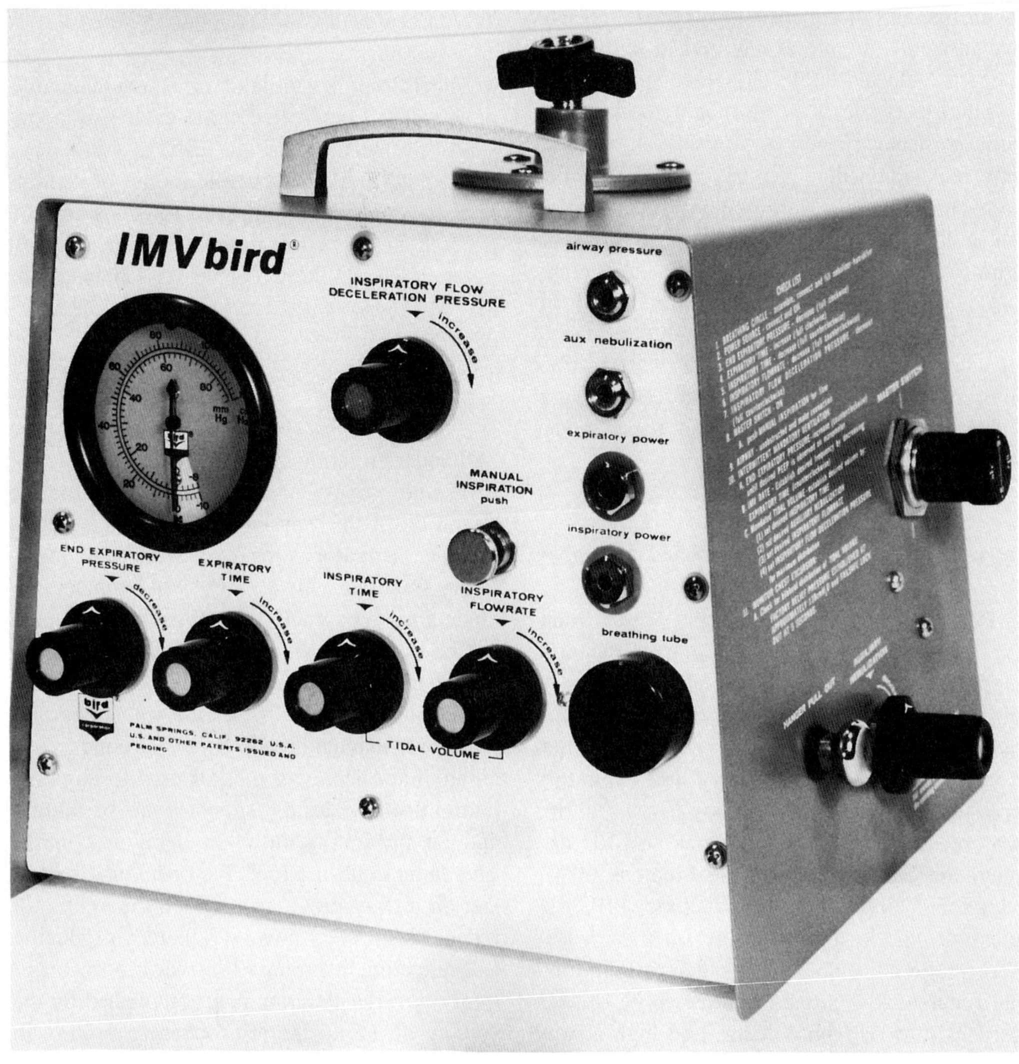

Fig. 15-57. IMVbird ventilator. (Courtesy of Bird Products Corp., Palm Springs, CA.)

phase, the master cartridge delivers blended gas at a pressure of 50 psig to a timing circuit, the inspiratory service socket (exhalation valve and nebulizer), through the flow deceleration cartridge, to the master Venturi and finally, to an inspiratory flow acceleration cartridge. Inspiratory time is a function of the time required for a sufficient amount of gas to go through the inspiratory time control valve to terminate the inspiratory flow rate from the master cartridge. Inspiratory flow rate is regulated by the position of the inspiratory flow rate control and is also affected by the PIP during mechanical inhalation. Decreases in CLT and increases in RAW result in high PIP. During mechanical inhalation, pressure in the breathing circuit increases as well as at the outflow port of the master Venturi, causing a reduction in flow entrainment and thus, inspiratory flow rate. An inspiratory flow accelerator cartridge is incorporated to help compensate for reductions in flow rate. At an airway pressure of approximately 40 cm H_2O, the flow accelerator cartridge automatically directs gas-flow rate to a second jet in the master

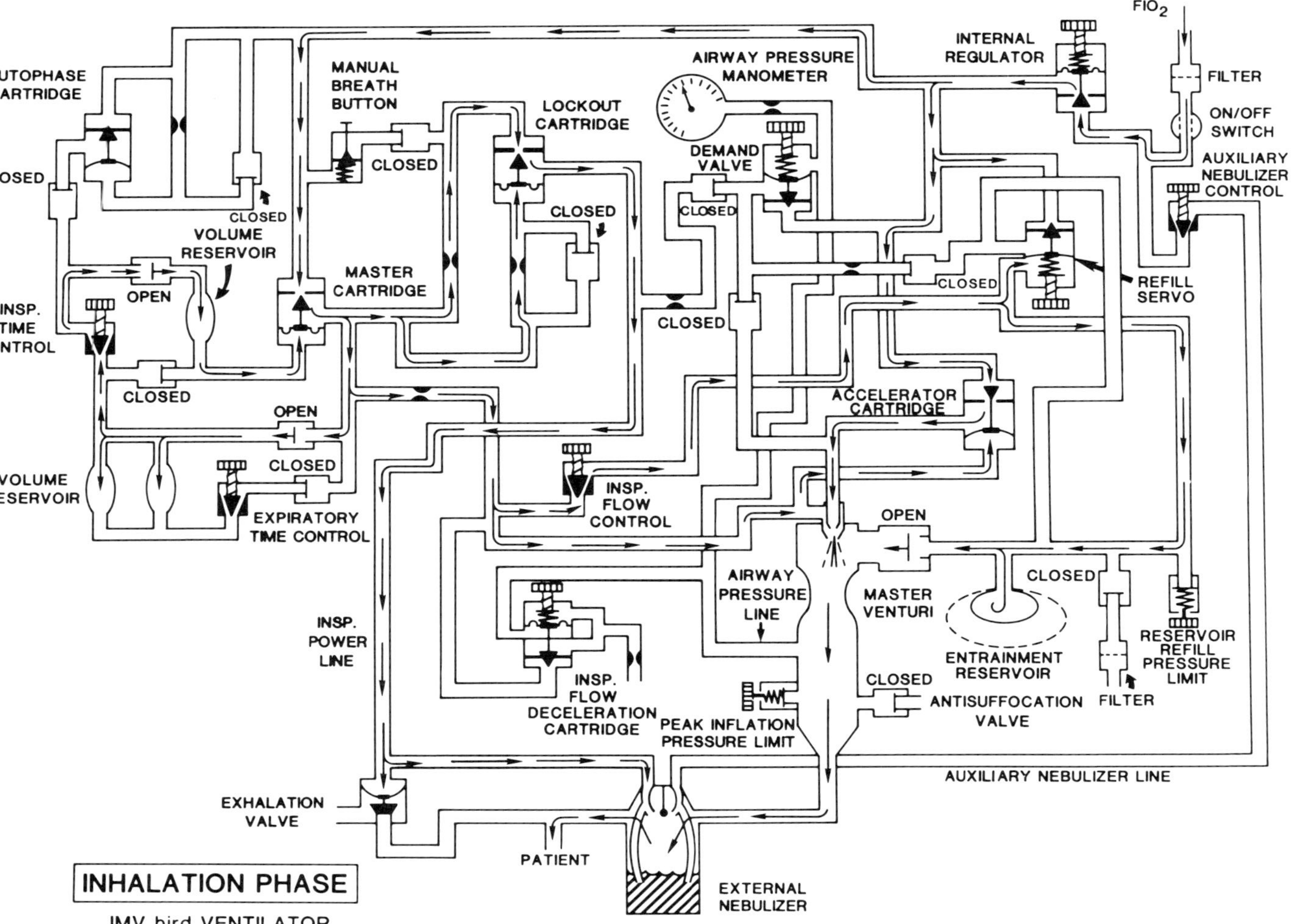

Fig. 15-58. Mechanical inhalation phase of the IMVbird ventilator.

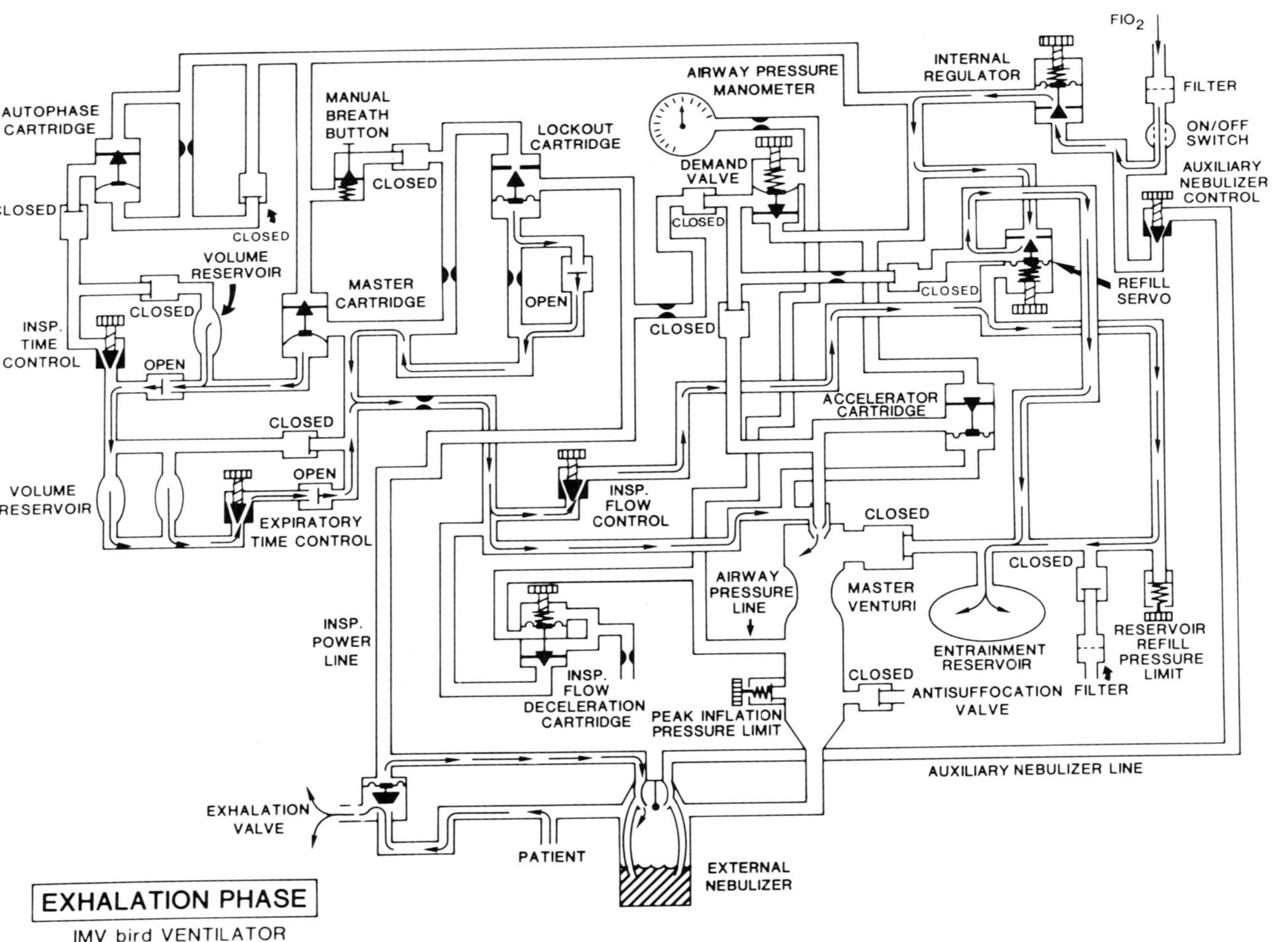

Fig. 15-59. Exhalation phases of the IMVbird ventilator.

Venturi in an attempt to maintain the preselected inspiratory flow rate.

The gas trapped in the timing circuit during the inspiratory phase must be allowed to escape before the master cartridge initiates another mechanical breath. The expiratory time control regulates the rate of escape of gas from the timing circuit and thus controls the rate of the ventilator. Rates as high as 30 breaths/min and as low as 1 breath every 3 minutes are possible.

Gas-flow rate for spontaneous breathing results when the airway pressure falls below the preselected level of CPAP, at which time a demand-flow valve delivers blended gas to the master Venturi (see under Demand-Flow CPAP). The further the airway pressure falls below the level of CPAP, the greater the flow rate from the demand-flow valve.

The preselected FiO_2 is maintained constant by a reservoir and refill Servo cartridge system. As the Venturi entrains blended gas from the reservoir, the refill Servo acts like a demand-flow valve and restores the reservoir to full capacity.

Monitors, Alarms, and Safety Features

The IMVbird offers no patient monitoring capability other than the standard airway pressure manometer. The continuous monitoring of critical patient parameters can only be accomplished by using separately purchased monitoring devices.

The ventilator does have several safety features, however. An inspiratory time lockout cartridge automatically terminates mechanical inhalation when the inspiratory time exceeds 5 seconds. An audible alarm is activated on newer models of this ventilator when the inspiratory time lockout cartridge terminates mechanical inhalation. The alarm and lockout cartridge automatically reset at the termination of the prolonged mechanical inhalation. An audible alarm is activated when either the compressed air or oxygen drive pressure has decreased at 40 psig or less. An antisuffocation valve allows the patient to breathe room air in the event of system failure or loss of source gas. Finally, an internal pressure relief valve limits pressure in the breathing circuit to 110 cm H_2O (Table 15-13).

Emerson 3MV Ventilator

The Emerson 3MV ventilator uses pneumatic and electrical power sources. It is a time-cycled, volume-limited, nonconstant-flow generator (Fig. 15-60) with three available modes of ventilation: CMV, IMV, and CPAP. A sinusoidal

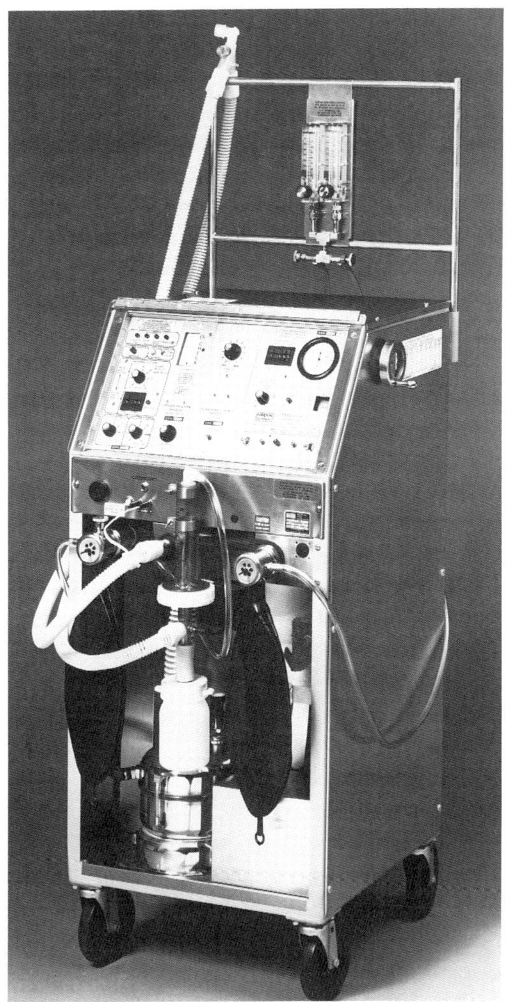

Fig. 15-60. Emerson 3MV ventilator. (Courtesy of J. H. Emerson Co., Cambridge, MA.)

inspiratory flow waveform is applied during mechanical inhalation (Table 15-12).

Controls

Standard rotating-type control knobs (potentiometers or "pots") and toggle switches control the operation of the ventilator. Mechanically delivered tidal volume is adjusted by the rotation of a crank that moves a linkage to alter the stroke volume of a piston. A window displays the preselected tidal volume. Ventilator rate is controlled by adjusting the total cycle time control. An inspiratory time (seconds) control regulates the duration of V_T delivery. The preselected inspiratory time, in conjunction with the expiratory time must not exceed the total cycle time setting because in the event of such an occurrence, the ventilator will not cycle properly. The inspiratory time control also regulates the peak inspiratory flow rate during mechanical inhalation. The shorter the inspiratory time, the greater the peak flow rate and vice versa. The main power toggle switch is used to switch "ON" or "OFF" all electric functions, while a "pump switch" activates only the piston pump mechanism. The humidifier and alarm systems are independent of the piston pump mechanism. A push-button control allows the operator to deliver a manually controlled tidal volume. Humidity output is regulated by a humidifier output control knob, which also monitors the temperature of the water in the humidifier and thus, the water vapor output. LEDs indicate the ON/OFF status of the main power and piston pump switches, and the status of the humidifier function, and when the piston is in motion during mechanical inhalation.

Operation

Mechanical inhalation and exhalation phases of gas flow are indicated in Figures 15-61 and 15-62. Two flowmeters, one for compressed air and the other for oxygen, are adjusted appropriately to regulate the F_{IO_2} and provide a sufficient flow rate of gas into the ventilator for the preselected MMV, and to satisfy the patient's spontaneous minute volume. An air-oxygen blender may be used in place of the flowmeters. When a blender is used, two flowmeters are attached to it; one flowmeter regulates gas flow rate to a reservoir bag for the piston pump, while the second provides gas-flow rate to another reservoir bag for spontaneous breathing. Excessive flow rates directed to the reservoir bag for the piston pump are vented to the atmosphere via a pressure popoff valve, which prevents overpressurization of the reservoir bag. Should the reservoir bag become overpressurized, the exhalation valve will also become pressurized, resulting in inadvertent CPAP.

At preselected intervals, a timer activates an electric motor which rotates a wheel. A piston is connected off-center to the wheel, and as a result, a reciprocal movement of the piston occurs. Because of the off-center configuration of the piston on the rotating wheel, a sinusoidal inspiratory flow waveform results. Three microswitches are positioned around the rotating wheel. Each controls the movement of the piston during the inhalation and exhalation phases. The microswitches are activated "ON" and "OFF" as the wheel rotates. An inspiratory microswitch is activated at the start of mechanical inhalation, causing voltage to be sent to the electric motor for a finite period of time. The inspiratory time control raises or lowers the voltage, and thus shortens or lengthens inspiratory time, respectively. As the piston strokes upward, a small amount of gas pressurizes the exhalation valve to the closed position. As the wheel continues to rotate, a second microswitch is activated which defines the expiratory time interval. As the piston descends, fresh gas is drawn from the reservoir bag for the subsequent mechanical breath. The third microswitch stops the motor with the piston near the bottom, ready for the next cycle.

The patient may breathe spontaneously from a reservoir bag supplied by a continuous flow rate of gas. A demand-flow valve in place of the reservoir bag may be used to provide gas flow for spontaneous breathing. Improper ad-

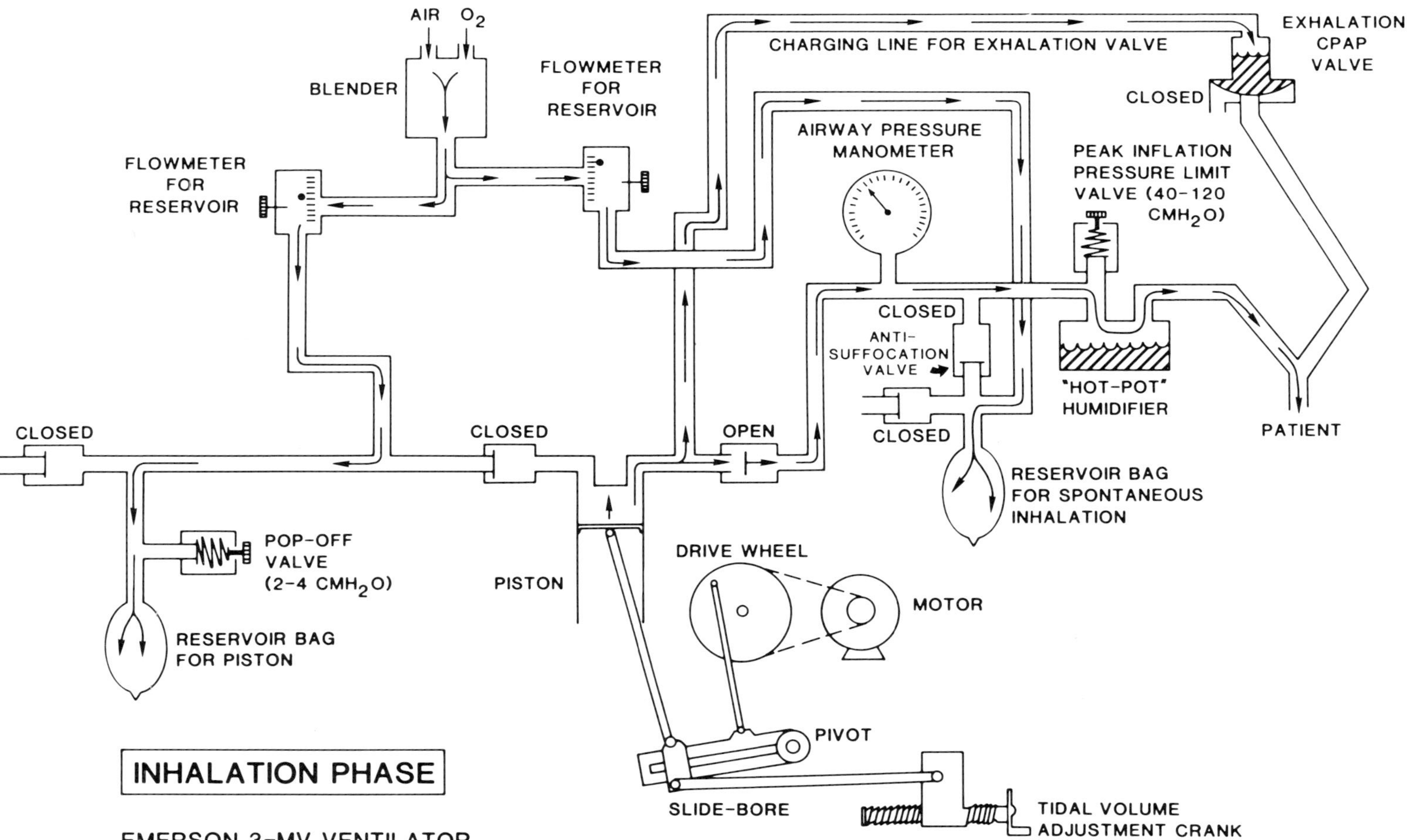

Fig. 15-61. Mechanical inhalation phase of the Emerson 3MV ventilator.

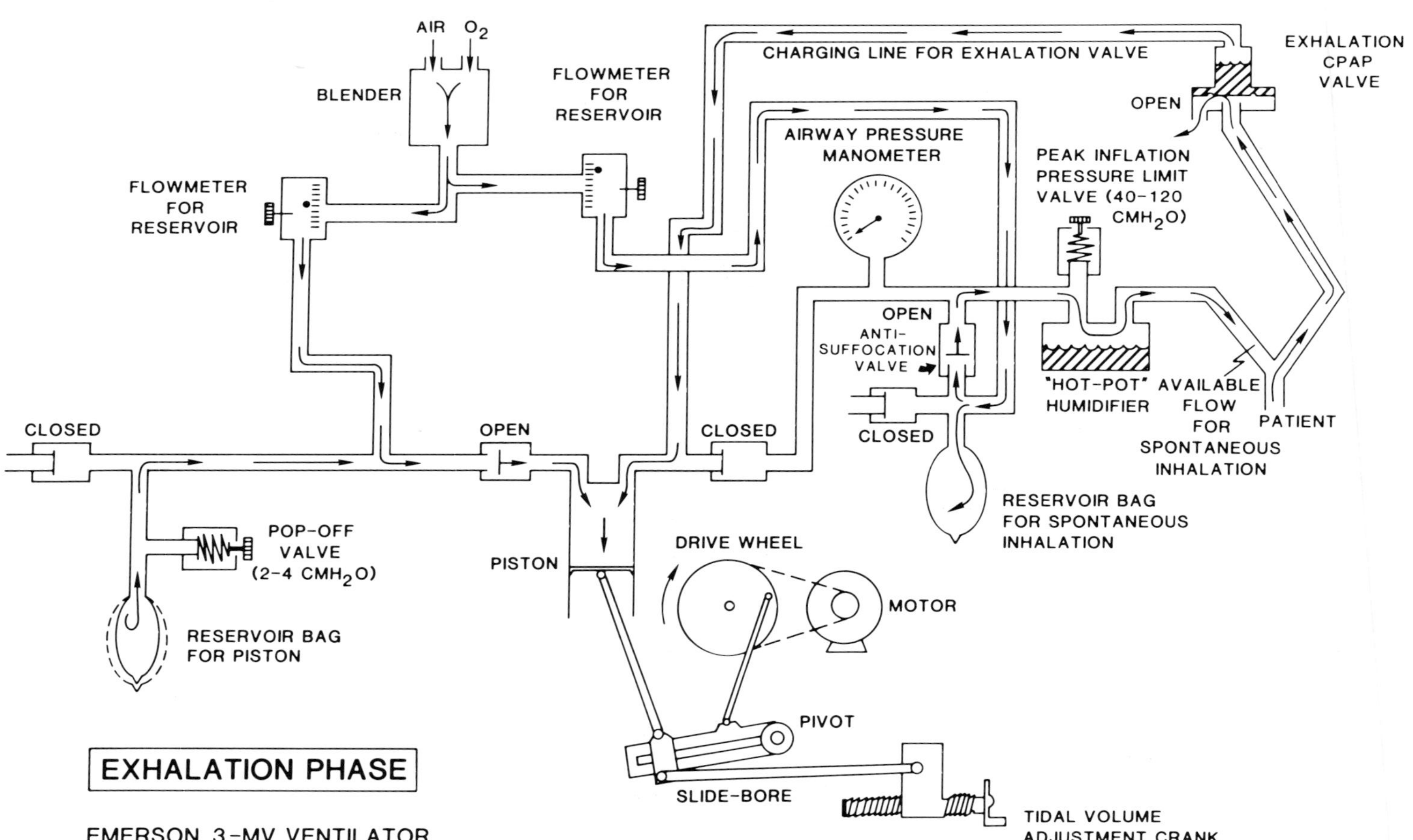

Fig. 15-62. Exhalation phase of the Emerson 3MV ventilator.

justment of the demand flow valve can lead to excessive peak inflation pressures and exaggerated tidal volumes during mechanical inhalation. CPAP is controlled by regulating the level of water in a threshold resistor-type expiratory pressure valve; that is, the greater the level of water, the greater the level of CPAP, and vice versa.

Monitors, Alarms, and Safety Features

A standard aneroid manometer is used to display airway pressure values. An alarm/monitor module is an optional piece of equipment that monitors loss of CPAP, high PIP, and failure to cycle (Table 15-13). Violation of any preselected alarms activates visual and audible alarms. Emergency air inlet valves on the two reservoir bags allow the patient to breathe spontaneously in the event of gas power failure. Excess peak inflation pressures are limited by adjusting the spring-loaded, pressure relief valve mounted on the humidifier.

Bear 2 Ventilator

The Bear 2 ventilator uses pneumatic and electrical power sources, and is an electronically controlled, volume-cycled, constant- and nonconstant-flow generator (Fig. 15-63). CMV, AV, EIP, IMV/SIMV, and CPAP are the available modes of ventilation on this ventilator. Constant or decelerating inspiratory flow waveforms may be applied during mechanical inhalation (Table 15-12).

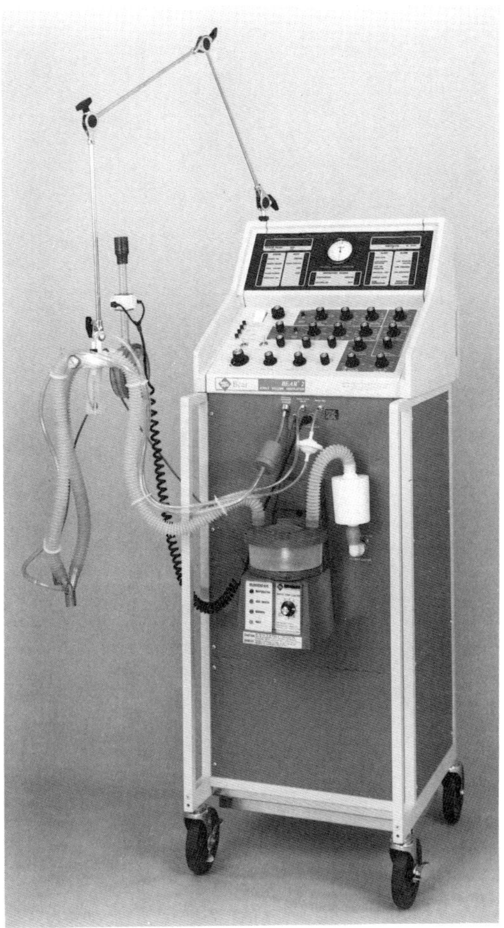

Fig. 15-63. Bear 2 ventilator. (Courtesy of Bear Inter Med, Riverside, CA.)

Controls

Two clearly separate sections comprise the operating panel of the ventilator: ventilator controls and alarm section. Primary ventilator controls include: V_T, ventilator rate, PIP limit, peak inspiratory flow rate, inspiratory pause (EIP), F_{IO_2}, CPAP/PEEP, and a four-position rotating knob mode selector control. Other controls include the master ON/OFF power switch, patient-triggering sensitivity (range: less to more), and push buttons that allow either a manually controlled V_T or sigh volume. Sighs are regulated with controls for sigh rate, sigh volume, and sigh peak inflation pressure limit. The multi-sigh control selector permits sighs to be delivered as one, two, or three sigh sequences.

Operation

Mechanical inhalation and exhalation phases of gas flow are indicated in Figures 15-64 and 15-65. A mechanical tidal volume is delivered

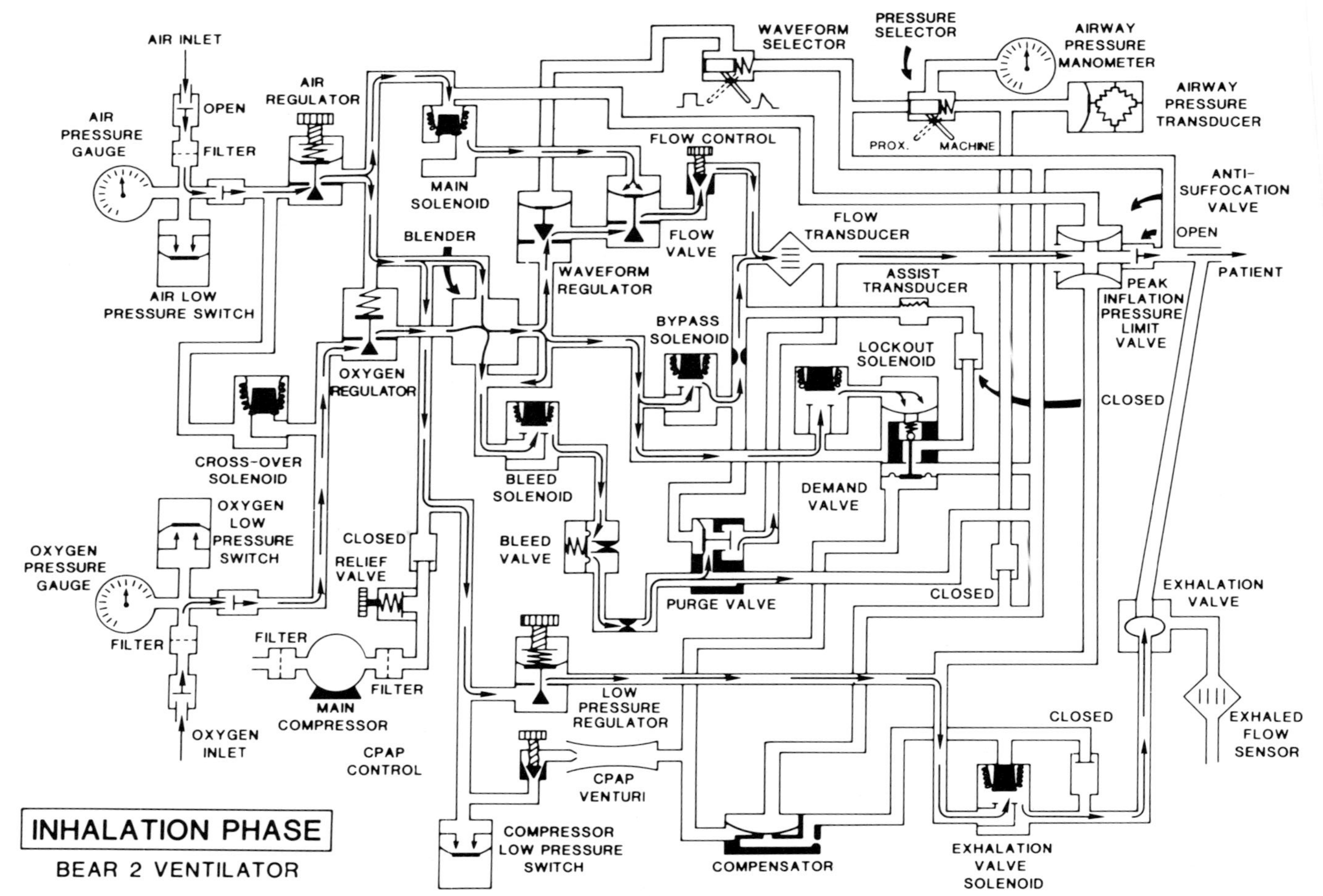

Fig. 15-64. Mechanical inhalation phase of the Bear 2 ventilator.

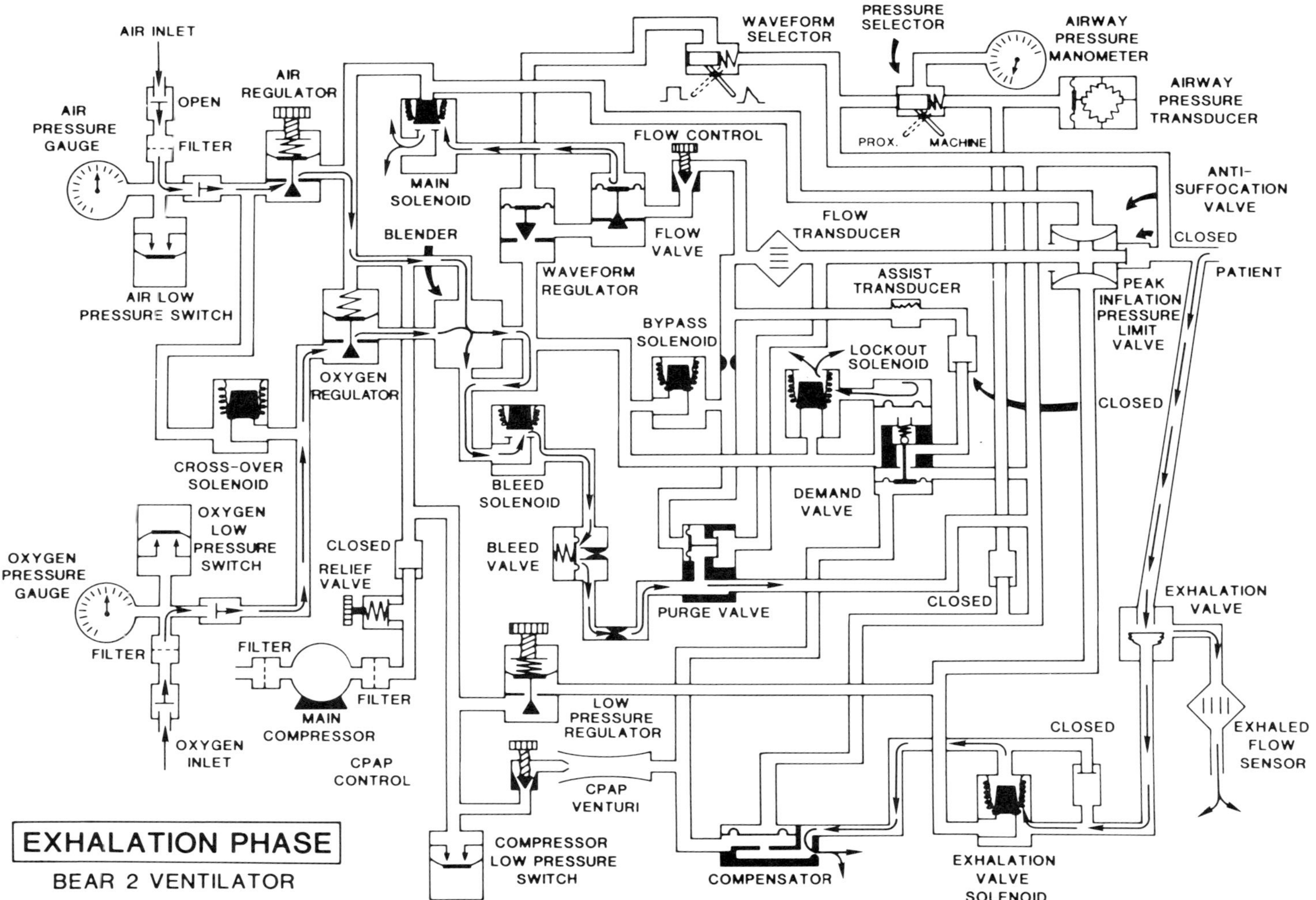

Fig. 15-65. Exhalation phase of the Bear 2 ventilator.

when the electronic timing system opens the main solenoid valve, which pressurizes the exhalation valve and directs gas flow to the peak inspiratory flow rate control valve. Gas flow then passes through the internal flow transducer and on to the patient. Gas-flow rate to the patient continues until the preselected tidal volume has passed the flow transducer, at which time the ventilator cycles OFF. Normally, a constant inspiratory flow waveform is applied; however, if the patient breathing circuit pressure reaches approximately 120 cm H_2O, a waveform regulator can decelerate the flow rate by approximately 50 percent.

A patient-triggered or assisted breath begins when the patient's spontaneous effort lowers airway pressure by approximately 1 to 2 cm H_2O below baseline pressure, at which time gas flow passes through the "assist" transducer, which in turn sends the signal to initiate a mechanical inhalation. The remainder of the breath delivery sequence is identical to that described above.

SIMV breaths are delivered in a manner similar to patient-triggered breaths. The SIMV rate is divided into one minute increments to produce the total cycle time, which becomes the timing window. For example, if the SIMV rate was 6/min, the total cycle time is 10 seconds; therefore, every 10 seconds, a timing window appears. If the patient initiates a breath during the timing window, the SIMV breath is provided. All other patient-initiated breaths for the remainder of total cycle time are spontaneous breaths with gas flow coming from a demand flow valve. If no spontaneous inspiratory effort is detected during the timing window, a mechanical breath is delivered.

The demand-flow valve provides gas flow for spontaneous breathing with or without CPAP. As mentioned previously, gas flow is provided on demand when airway pressure decreases to 1 cm H_2O below baseline pressure at the onset of inhalation. CPAP is provided by the pressurization of an inflatable balloon-type expiratory pressure valve.

Monitors, Alarms, and Safety Features

Exhaled tidal volume is measured with a vortex-type flow transducer located distal to the exhalation valve. Values are displayed on an LED. This type of an arrangement may predispose to errors in measuring tidal and minute volume (see under Accuracy of Displayed Exhaled Tidal Volume). A standard, aneroid type airway pressure manometer is used to indicate airway pressure values. I:E ratio, respiratory rate, and gas temperature are also displayed on LEDs. Lights indicating the status of several functions are displayed: power on, minute volume, tidal volume, alarm silence, nebulizer on, and mode choice. Another light illuminates with each breath indicating the delivery mode: spontaneous, controlled, assisted, or sigh.

A number of other alarms and alerts are also included. Continuous visual and audible alarms result when violations in the alarm limits occur. Alert parameters include high ventilatory rate, low air and oxygen pressure, PIP limit, I:E ratio, and temperature. Alarm settings include low exhaled tidal volume, low inspiratory airway pressure, low PEEP/CPAP, apnea, and a ventilator inoperative condition indication (Table 15-13).

Safety features include a mechanical pressure-relief valve, which is used to relieve airway pressure in the event of electronic failure or a kink in the expiratory limb of the breathing circuit. Loss of electrical power or a ventilator inoperative condition opens an air inlet valve to allow spontaneous breathing from room air.

Puritan-Bennett MA-1 Ventilator

The Puritan-Bennett MA-1 ventilator uses pneumatic and electrical power sources, and is an electronically controlled, volume cycled, constant-flow generator (Fig. 15-66). CMV and AV are available modes of ventilation. Positive end-expiratory pressure can be applied with an optional attachment. IMV and CPAP may be

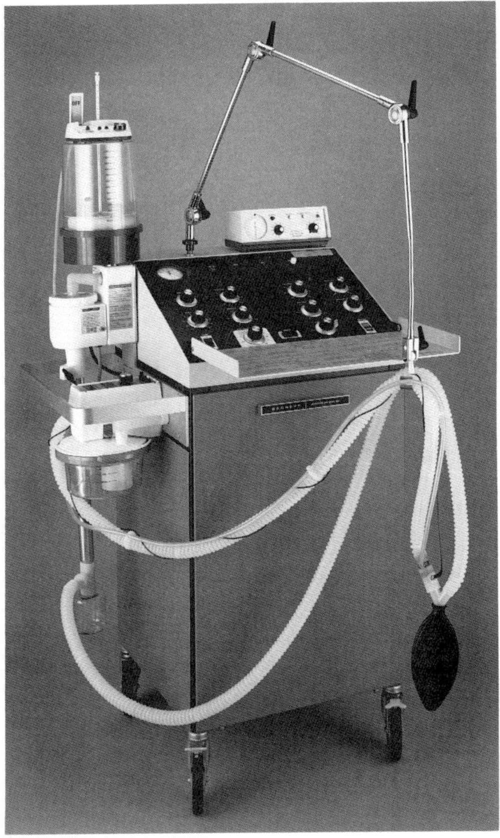

Fig. 15-66. Puritan-Bennett MA-1 ventilator. (Courtesy of Puritan-Bennett Corp., Overland Park, KS.)

applied with modifications to the ventilator. A constant inspiratory flow waveform is applied during mechanical inhalation under conditions of low peak inflation pressures (Fig. 15-30 and Table 15-12).

Controls

Standard, rotating-type control knobs (potentiometers or "pots") control the operation of the ventilator. Ventilator controls include V_T, PIP limit, ventilator rate, peak inspiratory flow rate, patient-triggering sensitivity pressure, F_IO_2, sigh volume, and sigh peak inflation pressure. Sigh volume and sigh pressure limit controls are adjusted separately from the V_T and PIP limit settings. Other controls include: a power switch (ON/OFF), a nebulizer switch (ON/OFF), an expiratory resistance control, and two push buttons: one for a manually delivered tidal volume, the second for sigh volume.

Aerosolized medications may be administered via a nebulizer in the breathing circuit. The nebulizer is powered by a nonadjustable flow rate of gas. The expiratory resistance control regulates the rate at which the exhalation valve depressurizes, resulting in the retardation of flow and tidal volume from the lungs during exhalation.

Operation

Mechanical inhalation and exhalation phases of gas flow are indicated in Figures 15-67 and 15-68. The MA-1 ventilator employs a double circuit drive mechanism. A compressor in the ventilator directs gas-flow rate to a Venturi device which, in turn, compresses a bellows. Tidal volume is defined when the signal from the tidal volume control equals the signal generated by a pulley-actuated "pot" located on the bellows.

Electronic timing or sufficient patient inspiratory triggering effort, as defined by the sensitivity control, initiates mechanical inhalation by opening the main solenoid valve. Gas pressure from the compressor is then directed to the exhalation valve to pressurize it shut and to the peak inspiratory flow rate control valve. Rotation of the peak inspiratory flow rate control moves a series of calibrated orifices in front of the nozzle of the Venturi. Gas-flow rate is then directed to compress the bellows and eject the tidal volume. Venturi flow rate output, however, varies inversely with airway pressure. The result is significant inspiratory flow deceleration as PIP rises (Fig. 15-30). At the end of mechanical inhalation, the main solenoid valve closes, the exhalation valve depressurizes, allowing passive exhalation, and the bellows falls and refills.

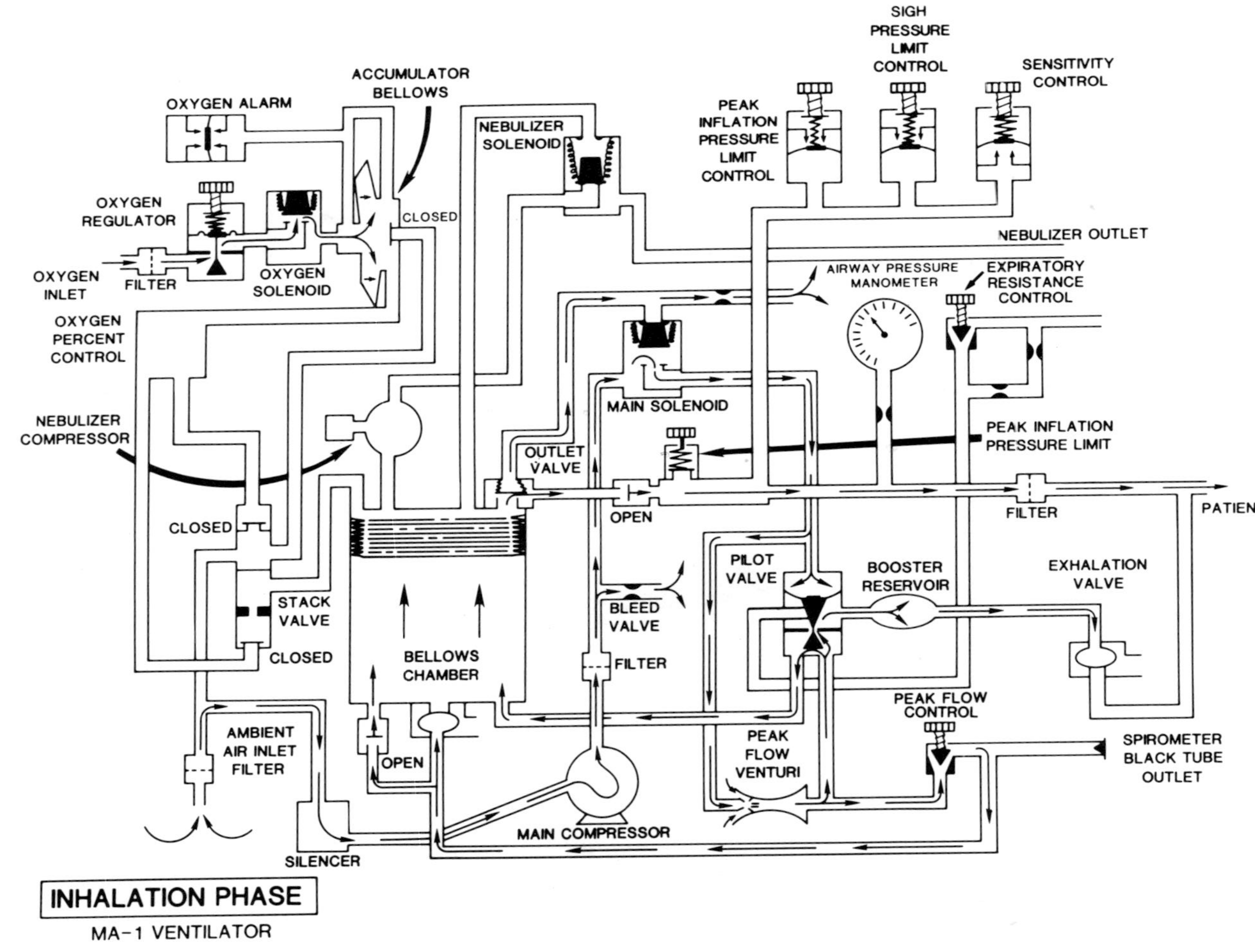

Fig. 15-67. Mechanical inhalation phase of the Puritan-Bennett MA-1 ventilator.

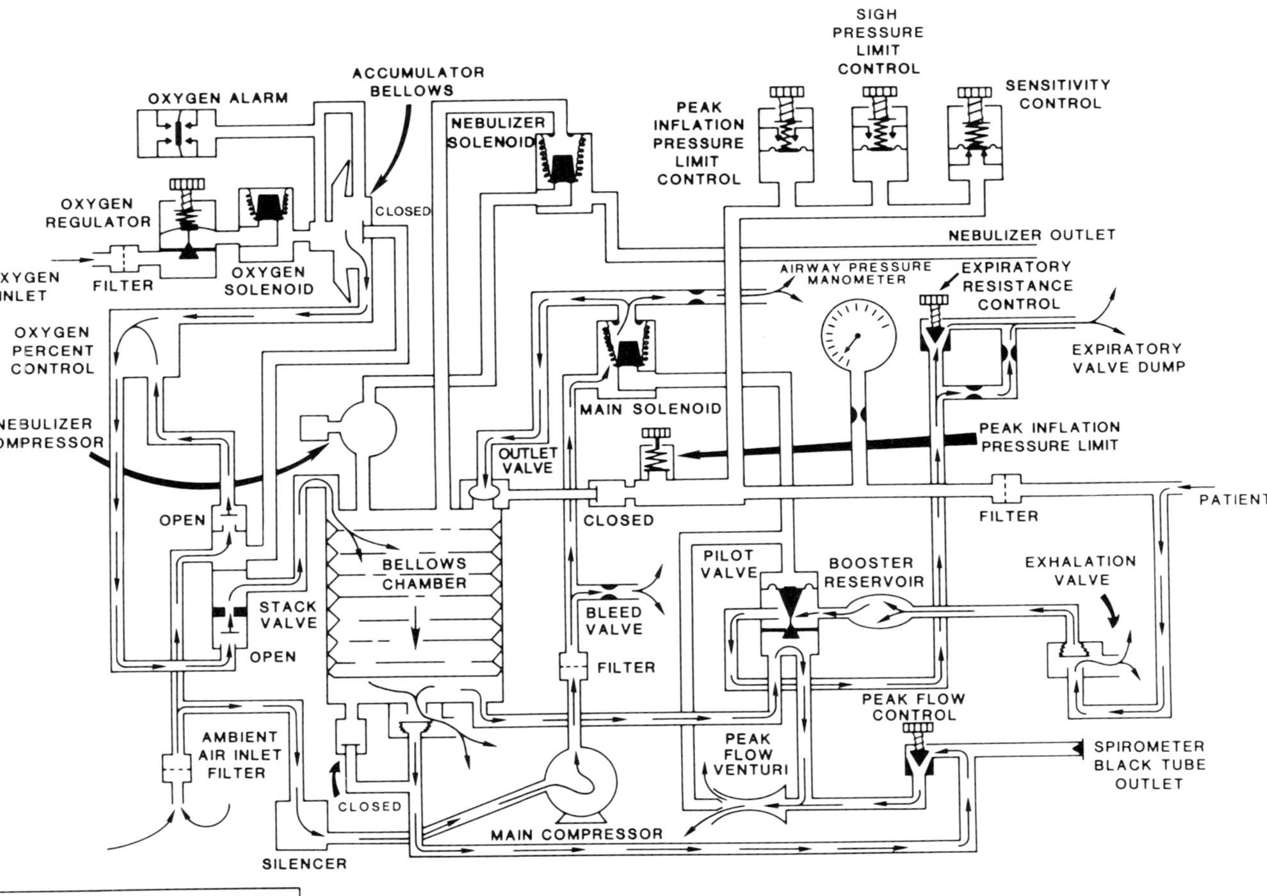

Fig. 15-68. Exhalation phase of the Puritan-Bennett MA-1 ventilator.

Monitors, Alarms, and Safety Features

A standard aneroid manometer is used to display airway pressure values. Ventilator function is monitored by a series of small lights at the top of the control panel. An amber light indicates patient-initiated breaths and an adjacent red light with an audible alarm warns of high peak inflation pressures. If the I:E ratio is in excess of 1:1, a red warning light is illuminated. A white light signals the delivery of a sigh breath. If the operator attempts to provide an FIO_2 greater than 0.21 without attaching a compressed oxygen high pressure source to power the ventilator, a red light is activated and an audible alarm sounds. Attachment of any high pressure source gas results in the illumination of a green light, which then inactivates the visual and audible alarms.

Exhaled VT is measured distal to the exhalation valve. A concertina bag-type spirometer captures exhaled gas volume. Displacement of the concertina bag reflects exhaled tidal volume. This type of device may predispose to errors in measuring tidal and minute volume (see under Accuracy of Displayed Exhaled Tidal Volumes). An alarm on the spirometer alerts the operator of low exhaled tidal volumes, a condition generally resulting from a disconnection or a leak in the breathing circuit (Table 15-13).

Neonatal/Infant Ventilators

Originally, newborn ventilators were modifications of adult ventilators. Designed to be pressure- or volume-cycled, adult ventilators had compliant, large-bore tubing breathing circuits with significant compressible volume and dead space which, when used with neonates, could predispose to rebreathing. CMV or AV were the modes of ventilation provided with these ventilators. Also, the response time to patient-trigger the ventilator "ON" while in the AV mode was too slow to accommodate the rapid breathing rates of infants, and CMV was not appropriate for awake patients. Consequently, such ventilators and modes of positive-pressure ventilation were of limited success when applied to newborn patients. Thus, a new breed of mechanical ventilators, as well as a new philosophy for ventilating newborns were needed.

During the early 1970s, continuous-flow time-cycled ventilators were proposed as an alternative. The approach allowed newborns to breathe spontaneously as desired between ventilator controlled breaths (IMV). Inspiratory and expiratory times could be controlled and PIP limited.[13,14] During the same period, Gregory et al.[52] described the beneficial effects of using a continuous flow CPAP system to treat infants with hyaline membrane disease (HMD). Because of the significantly higher survival rate of the patients treated with CPAP, Gregory's approach to ventilating newborns was regarded as a quantum leap forward, and CPAP also was incorporated into newborn ventilator design.

Tidal volume delivery with a time-cycled, continuous flow newborn ventilator is provided by intermittently occluding the expiratory limb of the breathing circuit. By regulating the gas-flow rate through the breathing circuit and the inspiratory time (exhalation valve occlusion time), VT is controlled. For example, if the continuous flow rate was 133 ml/sec (8 L/min) and the inspiratory or exhalation valve occlusion time was 0.2 seconds, the VT would equal approximately 27 ml.

Newborn ventilators employ various methods that occlude the expiratory limb of the breathing circuit. The Babybird ventilator uses gas-flow rate from a Venturi directed against a diaphragm positioned to occlude the expiratory limb. At regular preset intervals (i.e., the IMV rate), and for a controlled period of inspiratory time, gas-flow rate from the Venturi pushes against the diaphragm and occludes the expiratory limb. The Bear BP 200 ventilator uses an electronic solenoid valve placed in the expiratory limb of the breathing circuit. During the inhalation phase (IMV), the valve closes; as a result, continuous gas-flow rate is diverted into the infant's lungs. Occlusion of the expiratory limb is abrupt, thereby creating a constant inspiratory flow waveform. The Bear Cub ventilator uses a Venturi device that directs gas flow to diaphragm-type exhalation valve. At the onset of inhalation, the solenoid valve opens and gas flow pushes the diaphragm exhalation valve so as to occlude the expiratory limb of the breathing circuit; as a result, gas flow is diverted to the patient.

Alarm and safety mechanisms in newborn ventilators are of utmost importance. Critical ventilatory parameters that require continuous surveillance are: high PIP limit, low pressure in the breathing circuit, disconnection of the patient from the breathing circuit, excessive inspiratory time, insufficient expiratory time, ventilatory rate, low compressed air and oxygen inlet pressures, loss of pneumatic and electrical power, loss of CPAP and ventilator inoperative conditions. It is essential to maintain the preselected peak and mean airway pressures and level of CPAP, as well as minute ventilation. Newborn ventilators should be capable of monitoring continuously the aforementioned parameters.

First- and Second-Generation Ventilators

First-generaton newborn ventilators were relatively simple in design and inexpensive. A potential shortcoming was that the ventilators had no built-in electronic monitoring functions. As technology evolved, a second generation of ventilators employed electronic and pneumatic systems and more sophisticated monitoring capabilities. Relative to first-generation ventilators, the second generation of newborn ventilators are easier to operate and provide more information regarding ventilatory status. Rather than describe a variety of first- and second-generation of newborn ventilators, an example of each type is presented. The Babybird and the Bear Cub ventilators are typical of first- and second-generation newborn ventilators, respectively.

Bird Products Corporation Babybird Ventilator

The Babybird ventilator is a pneumatically powered, constant-flow generator that is time-cycled and pressure-limited (Fig. 15-69). CMV, IMV, and CPAP are available modes of ventilation. A decelerating inspiratory flow waveform results when airway pressure is limited (see under Pressure Limited, Time-Cycled Mechanical Ventilation).

Controls

Standard rotating-type control knobs are employed to control the operation of the ventilator. A mode-selector knob changes the ventilator from providing continuous flow with or without CPAP to providing IMV or CMV with or without CPAP. CPAP is regulated with a variable orifice diaphragm type expiratory pressure valve (see under Hybrid Valves). The flow rate control regulates the gas-flow rate directed through the breathing circuit that is available for spontaneous breathing during CPAP and for mandatory breathing during IMV. A Bourdon-type flow rate gauge is used to regulate flow rate in L/min. In the IMV mode, minute volume is determined by setting the inspiratory time, expiratory time, and inspiratory flow-rate controls. Inspiratory time (seconds) times inspiratory flow rate (ml/sec) equals V_T, and since expiratory time affects the rate of the ventilator, then V_T times rate equals minute volume. Should the ventilator be pressure-limited during mechanical inhalation, tidal and minute volume may be less than the product of inspiratory flow rate and inspiratory time.

The PIP limit control, called the inspiratory relief pressure control, regulates the maximum PIP during mechanical inhalation (IMV). By

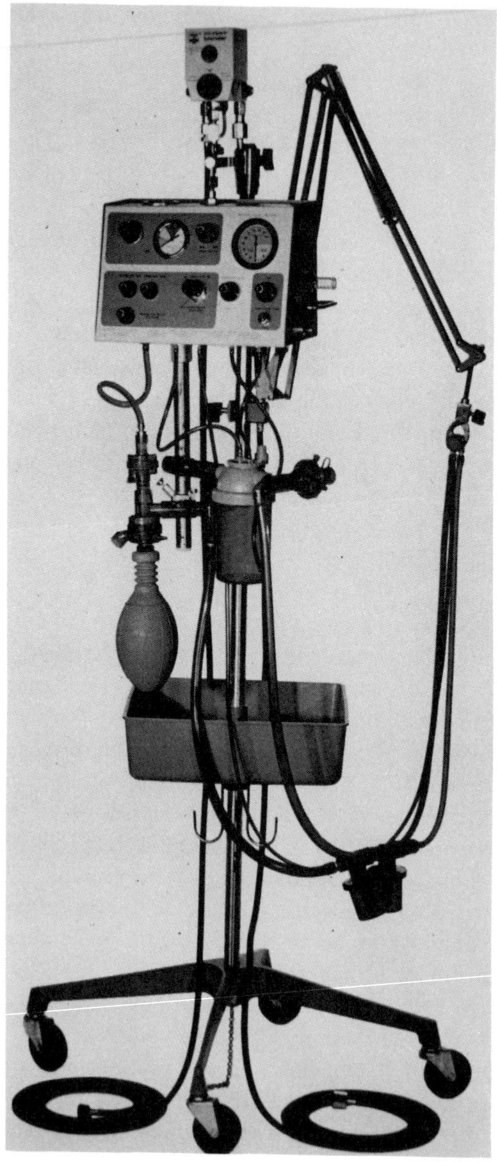

Fig. 15-69. Babybird ventilator. (Courtesy of Bird Products Corp., Palm Springs, CA.)

regulating this and the inspiratory time control, pressure limited, time-cycled ventilation may be applied.

The expiratory time control adjusts duration of exhalation and hence the rate at which the ventilator cycles. Measurement of the rate requires a stopwatch or external monitor to quantify the rate.

The F_{IO_2} is adjusted by an air-oxygen blender that is external to the ventilator. Peak flow rate capability from the blender is 95 to 120 L/min depending upon the F_{IO_2} setting; however, the ventilator reduces the system flow rate from 0 to 30 L/min. Compressed air and oxygen source gas pressures must be 35 to 55 psig with a maximum pressure difference between gases no greater than 20 psig. Should the pressure differential be greater than 20 psig, an audible alarm on the blender is activated. Under these circumstances, the source gas with the higher pressure enters the ventilator. If the total output pressure from the air-oxygen blender falls below the 35 psig, the ventilator will "lock" in the inspiratory phase. Thus, the inspiratory time limit control should be preset to limit inspiratory time to an appropriate period (e.g., twice the preselected inspiratory time) should the ventilator inadvertently lock "ON."

The nebulization control regulates gas flow rate to a nebulizer and is set to control the humidity output of the nebulizer. Many have opted to replace the nebulizer with heated humidification systems.

An expiratory flow gradient control regulates the gas-flow rate to a Venturi device positioned so that the entrainment port on the Venturi is attached to the expiratory limb of the breathing circuit. When operating, the Venturi decreases expiratory flow resistance by evacuating gas from that limb of the breathing circuit. Because the Venturi device decreases pressure and the CPAP control increases pressure in the breathing circuit, the controls for both may be set to the preselected level of CPAP.

Operation

Mechanical inhalation and exhalation phases of gas flow are indicated on Figures 15-70 and 15-71. The ventilator provides a predetermined mixture of air and oxygen delivered to the patient through a low compressible volume tubing system. The infant inhales and exhales freely until the ventilator cycling component is activated, at which time the exhalation valve closes in

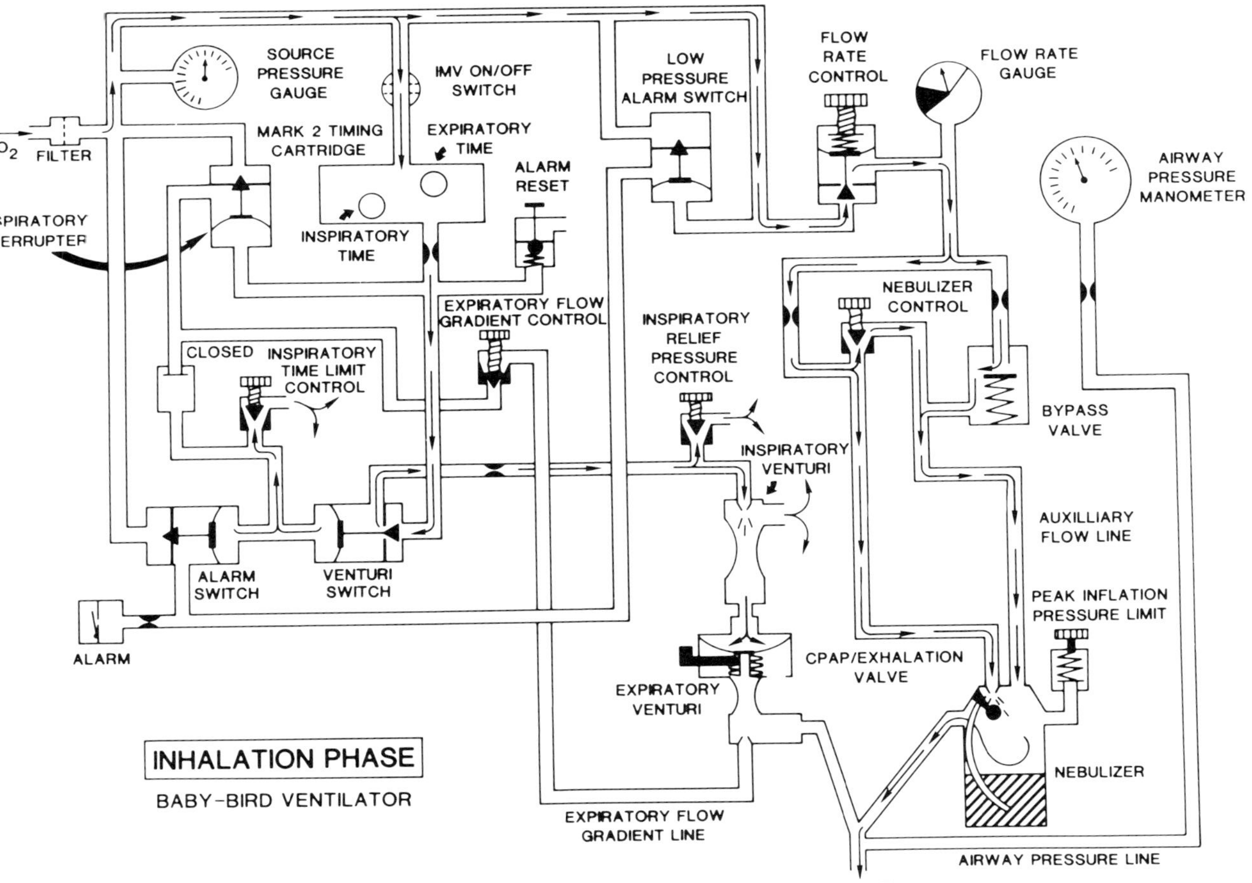

Fig. 15-70. Mechanical inhalation phase of the Babybird ventilator.

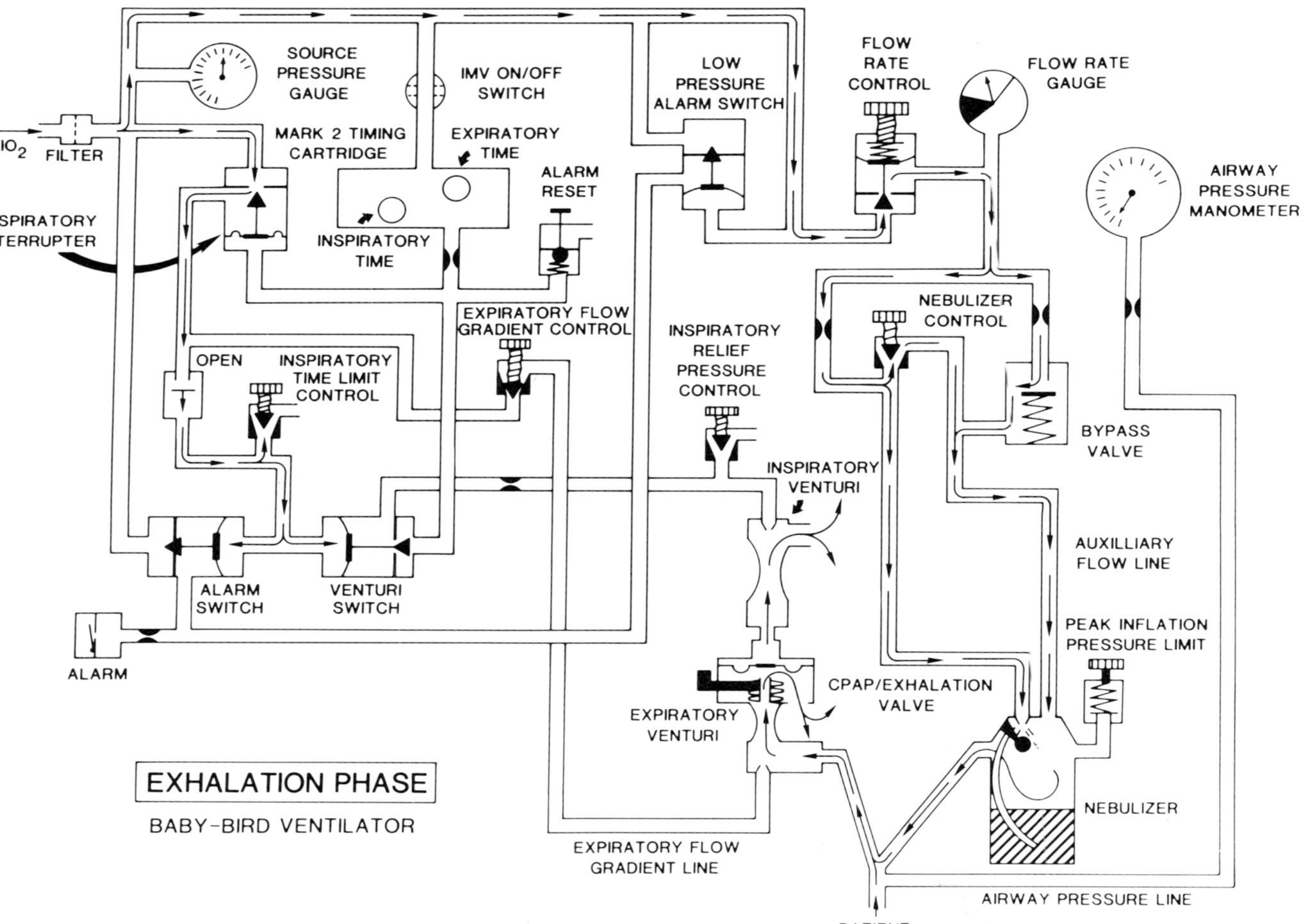

Fig. 15-71. Exhalation phase of the Babybird ventilator.

order to divert the continuous gas-flow rate, under pressure, into the patient's lungs.

During exhalation, the exhalation valve opens, passive exhalation occurs, and airway pressure decreases to the baseline pressure (CPAP or ambient pressure). Continuous gas flow "carries" the patient's exhaled gas through the variable orifice CPAP valve. The expiratory flow gradient control, which activates a Venturi mechanism, facilitates exhalation.

A Mark 2 timing device (Bird) inside the ventilator is used to control inspiratory and expiratory times. A self-inflating bag is attached to the breathing circuit and may be used for resuscitation should the ventilator fail. F_IO_2 is 0.21 from the self-inflating bag; a connector on the bag allows oxygen to be directed into it in order to raise the F_IO_2.

Monitors, Alarms, and Safety Features

A standard aneroid-type manometer displays airway pressure. The inspiratory time limit control is a safety mechanism which controls the maximum period of time that pressure is maintained in the breathing circuit during mandatory ventilation should the inspiratory time control fail. When this situation occurs, the inspiratory time limit control opens the exhalation valve after the preselected inspiratory time limit period elapses. Under these conditions, an audible alarm is activated. The ventilator remains in the exhalation phase until the Reset button is pushed to restart the cycling mechanism.

A pressure-relief valve in the breathing circuit serves as a backup to the inspiratory pressure relief mechanism built into the ventilator. A low-input pressure (audible) alarm is activated when the driving pressure in the ventilator is less than 43 psig. Specific characteristics of the Babybird ventilator are listed in Table 15-14).

Table 15–14. Specific Characteristics of the Babybird Ventilator

Item	Minimum	Maximum
Rate (BPM)	4.2	100
Volume (ml)	3	500
Flow rate (L/min)	0	30
Pressure (cm H_2O)	0	81
F_IO_2	0.21	1.0
Inspiratory time (sec)	0.3	10
CPAP (cm H_2O)	1	20
I:E ratio	1:0.5	1:9.9
Compressible volume (ml/cm H_2O)	0.815	—
Size (inches)	27 × 60	—
Weight (lb)	40	—
Power source	Pneumatic	—

(From Babybird Operators Manual: Bird Products Corporation, Palm Springs, CA, 1987, with permission.)

Bear Cub Ventilator

The Bear Cub newborn ventilator uses electrical and pneumatic power sources, and is an electronically controlled, time-cycled, pressure-limited, constant flow generator (Fig. 15-72). CMV, IMV, and CPAP are available modes of ventilation. A decelerating inspiratory flow waveform results when airway pressure is limited (see under Pressure Limited, Time-cycled Mechanical Ventilation).

Controls

Standard, rotating type control knobs are employed to control the operation of the ventilator. A multiposition control knob labeled MODE allows the ventilator to provide continuous flow with or without CPAP, and CMV/IMV with or without CPAP. A position labeled LAMP/BATTERY TEST may be chosen to test the visual displays and battery systems for integrity. CPAP is controlled with a threshold resistor-type expiratory pressure valve (pressure α force/surface area). Gas-flow rate from a Venturi (force) is directed against the diaphragm (surface area). The level of CPAP is controlled by regulating the flow rate to the Venturi (the greater the flow rate the greater level of CPAP, and vice versa). The patient is allowed to breathe spontaneously as desired on CPAP from the continuous gas-flow rate directed through the breathing circuit. Gas-flow rate is regulated by a Thorpe tube flowmeter in liters per minute. The CMV/IMV control activates all ventilator related controls and alarms for mechanical ventilation. Flow rate, inspiratory time, ventilator

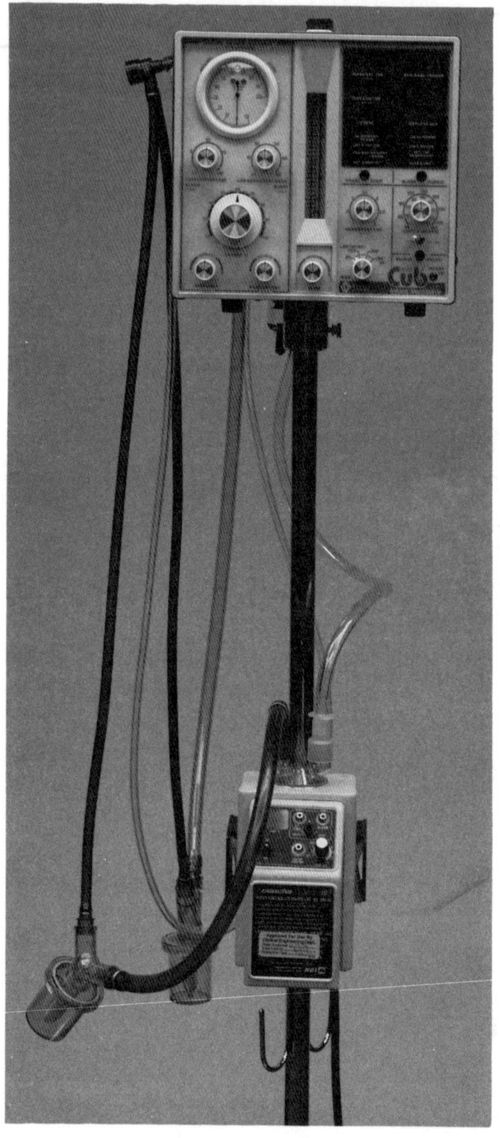

Fig. 15-72. Bear Cub infant ventilator. (Courtesy of Bear Inter Med, Riverside, CA.)

rate, and PIP limit, as well as the level of CPAP and F_{IO_2} are regulated during CMV and/or IMV. Tidal and minute volume are controlled by regulating the inspiratory flow rate, inspiratory time, and ventilator rate controls (identical to the Babybird). Should the peak pressure limit be reached before inspiratory time is complete, V_T will be less than the product of inspiratory flow rate and inspiratory time. Under these circumstances, V_T = change in airway pressure × C_{LT}, and minute volume = V_T × ventilator rate. The ventilator rate control regulates the number of mandatory breaths per minute.

The inspiratory time control regulates the duration of time the ventilator is "ON" during the IMV breath. Adjustable from 0.1 to 3 seconds, inspiratory time is set to provide the proper excursion of the chest in a reasonable period of time. If the inspiratory time is set for too long a period so that it does not provide a minimum of 0.25 seconds for exhalation, a rate/time incompatibility indicator flashes, and the ventilator will cycle to exhalation.

The PIP limit control is used to regulate the maximum pressure generated during mechanical inhalation. The pressure limit is adjustable from 0 to 72 cm H_2O. A secondary pressure limit preset by the manufacturer is set at approximately 90 cm H_2O. In addition, a tertiary pressure limit control is located on the rear side of the ventilator. The oxygen percent control regulates the percentage of oxygen from 21 to 100 percent as long as the source gas pressures are stable.

Operation

Mechanical inhalation and exhalation phases of gas flow are indicated in Figures 15-73 and 15-74. During mechanical inhalation, a solenoid valve opens and gas flow from the pressure limit control is directed through a metering valve to pressurize the exhalation valve closed, causing gas flow to be diverted to the patient. The pressure loading the exhalation valve is equal to the preselected pressure limit. Any excess pressure generated during mechanical inhalation is vented past the exhalation valve. Proximal airway pressure is indicated on an aneroid manometer and monitored by a transducer for electronic calculations. A continuous flow rate of 0.2 L/min of blended gas is purged through the proximal airway pressure measuring line into the breathing circuit to prevent moisture contamination of the manometer and transducer.

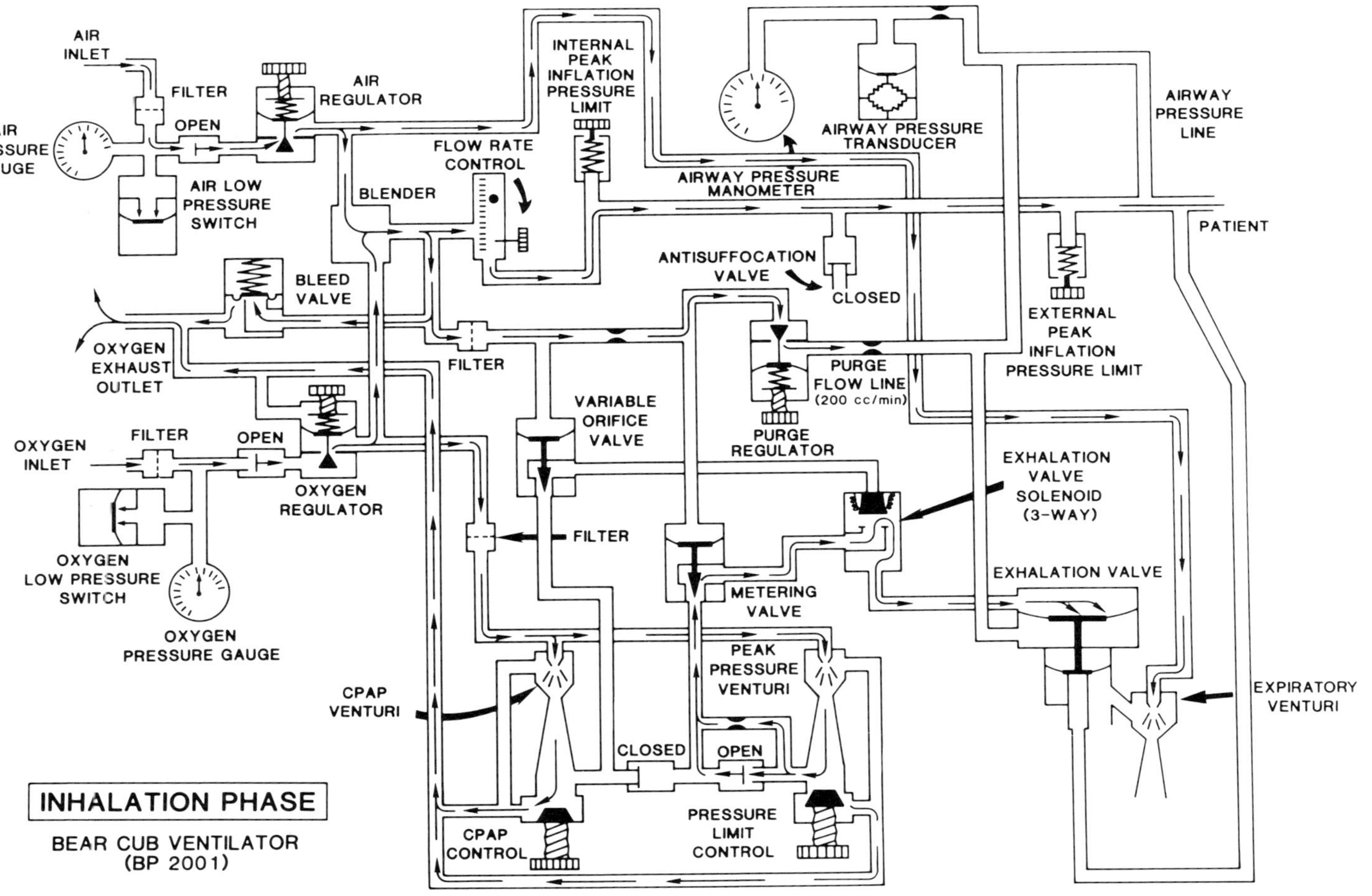

Fig. 15-73. Mechanical inhalation phase of the Bear Cub ventilator.

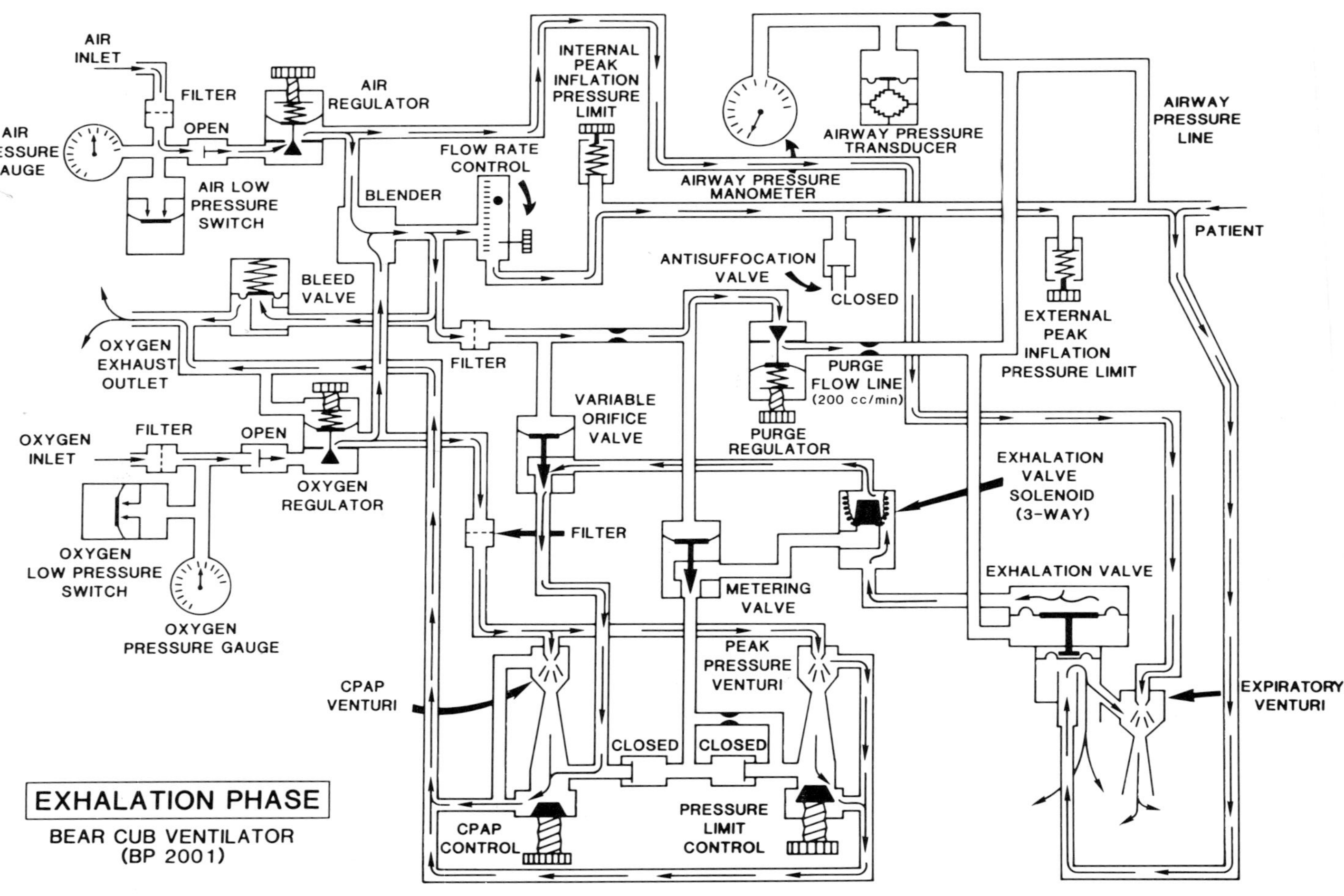

Fig. 15-74. Exhalation phase of the Bear Cub ventilator.

During exhalation, the solenoid valve closes, causing the exhalation valve to depressurize to ambient pressure (unless the CPAP control is activated) and open, allowing passive exhalation. If CPAP is used, the exhalation valve is pressured to the desired level of CPAP (by previously described mechanism). A fixed-flow jet Venturi device creates subambient pressure in the exhalation valve assembly (0 to −2 cm H_2O), depending on the pressure developed by the continuous circuit flow rate. This mechanism helps minimize breathing circuit resistance, and is balanced with the CPAP control to establish the desired expiratory pressure. A subambient inspiratory relief valve permits spontaneous breathing from room air if ventilator malfunction occurs. An inspiratory effort of −2 cm H_2O is required to open this valve.

Monitors, Alarms, and Safety Features

A standard aneroid-type manometer displays airway pressure. An electronic transducer also measures airway pressure for a series of pressure alarm functions. Inlet pressure gauges indicate air and oxygen inlet pressure from 0 to 100 psig. The normal operating range is 35 to 75 psig for air and oxygen. Both gauges are located on the rear panel of the ventilator.

Five multicolored LEDs indicate essential ventilatory parameters: (1) Mean airway pressure (cm H_2O) (displayed in green) indicates the average airway pressure over the inhalation and exhalation phases; (2) inspiratory time (seconds) (displayed in red) indicates the preselected inspiratory time period; (3) exhalation time (seconds) (displayed in red) indicates the period of time allotted to the exhalation phase; (4) ventilator rate (breaths/min) (displayed in amber) indicates the preselected ventilator rate; and (5) I:E ratio (displayed in red) indicates the inhalation-to-exhalation time ratio. At I:E ratios greater than 3:1, the digital display starts blinking and activates an audible alarm, indicating that the Excessive Inverse I:E Ratio function has been violated.

A series of alarm indicators are activated when abnormalities occur. A loss of PEEP/CPAP alarm, adjustable from 0 to 20 cm H_2O, activates visual and audible alarms when the level of CPAP drops below the preselected level. This alarm mechanism also establishes the prolonged inspiratory pressure alarm threshold. The threshold is automatically set at 10 cm H_2O above the loss of CPAP alarm control setting. If the airway pressure during mechanical inhalation remains above the threshold pressure for greater than 3.5 seconds, the prolonged inspiratory pressure alarm, adjustable from 0 to 50 cm H_2O, activates visual and audible alarms. A low inspiratory pressure alarm is activated if during mechanical inhalation the airway pressure fails to exceed the preselected low inspiratory pressure alarm value. The ventilator inoperative alarm monitors six alarm conditions: fail to cycle, electrical power failure/power disconnect, panel control malfunction, prolonged solenoid "ON" time, high/low inspiratory time, and timing circuit failure. In addition, alert indicators for low air and oxygen input pressures, rate/time incompatibility, and alarm silence are available.

All alarm functions except rate/time incompatibility and alarm silence must be reset by depressing a push button after correction. Audible alarms may be silenced by depressing another button. Specific characteristics of the Bear Cub ventilator are listed in Table 15-15.

Table 15–15. Specific Characteristics of the Bear Cub Ventilator

Item	Minimum	Maximum
Rate (BPM)	1	150
Volume (ml)	5	1,500
Flow rate (L/min)	3	30
Pressure (cm H_2O)	0	72
Time (sec)	0.1	3
FIO_2	0.21	1.0
CPAP (cmH_2O)	1	20
I:E ratio	1:0.8	1:9.9
Compressible volume (ml/cm H_2O)	0.12	0.25
Size (inches)	10 × 10 × 14	—
Weight (lb)	27	—
Power sources	Pneumatic and electrical	

(From Model 2001 Instruction Manual No. 5000–10220 and Maintenance Manual No. 5000–12033. Bear Medical Systems, Inc., Riverside CA, 1985, with permission.)

REFERENCES

1. Dammann JF, McAslan TC: Optimal flow pattern for mechanical ventilation of the lungs. Crit Care Med 5:128, 1977
2. Banner MJ, Lampotang S: Clinical use of inspiratory and expiratory flow waveforms. p. 139. In Kacmarek RM, Stoller JK (eds): Current Respiratory Care. BC Decker, Philadelphia, 1988
3. Bergman MA: Fourier analysis of effects of varying pressure waveforms in electrical lung analogues. Acta Anaesthesiol Scand 28:174, 1984
4. Jansson L, Jonson B: A theoretical study of flow patterns of ventilators. Scand J Respir Dis 55:237, 1972
5. Al-Saady N, Bennett ED: Decelerating inspiratory flow waveform improves lung mechanics and gas exchange in patients on intermittent positive-pressure ventilation. Intensive Care Med 11:68, 1985
6. Baker AB, Colliss JE, Cowie RW: Effects of varying inspiratory flow waveform and time in intermittent positive-pressure ventilation. II. Various physiologic variables. Br J Anaesth 49:1221, 1977
7. Johansson H, Lofstrom JB: Effects on breathing mechanics and gas exchange of different inspiratory gas flow patterns during anaesthesia. Acta Anaesthesiol Scand 19:8, 1975
8. Ashbaugh D, Bigelow D, Petty T, et al: Acute respiratory distress in adults. Lancet 2:319, 1967
9. Kirby RR: Mechanical ventilation in acute respiratory failure: facts, fiction, and fallacies. p. 51. In Gallagher TJ (ed): Advances in Anesthesia. Year Book Medical Publishers, Chicago, 1984
10. Froese AB, Bryan AC: Effects of anesthesia and paralysis on diaphragmatic mechanics in man. Anesthesiology 41:242, 1974
11. Downs JB, Mitchell LA: Pulmonary effects of ventilatory pattern following cardiopulmonary bypass. Crit Care Med 4:295, 1976
12. Murphy EJ, Downs JB: Ventilator induced ventilation-perfusion mismatching. p. 345. In Abstracts of Scientific Papers. 1976 ASA Annual Meeting. American Society of Anesthesiologists, Park Ridge, IL, 1976
13. Kirby RR, Robison E, Schulz J: A new pediatric volume ventilator. Anesth Analg 50:553, 1971
14. Kirby RR, Robison E, Schulz J: Continuous flow ventilation as an alternative to assisted or controlled ventilation in infants. Anesth Analg 51:871, 1972
15. Downs JB, Klein EF, Desautels DA, et al: Intermittent mandatory ventilation, a new approach to weaning patients from mechanical ventilators. Chest 64:331, 1973
16. Kirby RR, Downs JB, Civetta JM: High level positive end-expiratory pressure (PEEP) in acute respiratory insufficiency. Chest 67:156, 1975
17. Kirby RR, Perry JC, Calderwood HW: Cardiorespiratory effects of high positive end-expiratory pressure. Anesthesiology 42:533, 1975
18. Poulton TJ, Downs JB: Humidification of rapidly flowing gas. Crit Care Med 9:59, 1981
19. Downs JB: Ventilatory pressure and modes of ventilation in acute respiratory failure. Respir Care 28:586, 1983
20. Shapiro BA, Harrison RA, Walton JR: Intermittent demand ventilation: a new technique for supporting ventilation in critically ill patients. Respir Care 21:521, 1976
21. Hasten RW, Downs JB, Heenan TJ: A comparison of synchronized and nonsynchronized intermittent mandatory ventilation. Respir Care 25:554, 1980
22. Heenan TJ, Downs JB, Douglas ME: Intermittent mandatory ventilation—is synchronization important? Chest 77:598, 1980
23. Hewlett AM, Platt AS, Terry VG: Mandatory minute volume. A new concept in weaning from mechanical ventilators. Anesth Analg 32:163, 1977
24. Forette TL, Cairo JM: Mandatory minute volume: a conceptual approach. Curr Rev Respir Crit Care 10:163, 1988
25. Fulerham SF: Effect of mechanical ventilation with end-inspiratory pause on blood gas exchange. Anesth Analg 55:122, 1976
26. Reynolds EOR: Pressure waveform and ventilator settings for mechanical ventilation in severe hyaline membrane disease. p. 1. In Bourns Educational Series ES1. Little, Brown, Boston, 1977
27. MacIntyre N: Respiratory function during pressure support ventilation. Chest 89:677, 1986
28. MacIntyre N: Pressure support ventilation. Respir Care 31:189, 1986
29. Prakash O, Maiji S: Cardiopulmonary response to inspiratory pressure support during spontaneous ventilation vs. conventional ventilation. Chest 83:403, 1985
30. Black JW, Grover BS: A hazard of pressure support ventilation. Chest 93:333, 1988
31. Downs JB: New modes of ventilatory assistance. Chest 90:626, 1986
32. Gibney RTN, Wilson RS, Pontoppidan H: Com-

parison of work of breathing on high gas flow and demand valve continuous positive airway pressure systems. Chest 82:692, 1982
33. Cox D, Niblett DJ: Studies on continuous positive airway pressure breathing systems. Br J Anaesth 56:905, 1984
34. Op't Holt TB, Hall MW, Bass JB, et al: Comparison of changes in airway pressure (CPAP) between demand valve and continuous flow devices. Respir Care 27:1200, 1982
35. Gjerde GE, Katz JA, Kramer RW: Inspiratory work and airway pressure with continuous positive airway pressure delivery systems. Crit Care Med 12:272, 1984
36. Henry WC, West GA, Wilson RS: A comparison of the oxygen cost of breathing between a continuous flow CPAP system and a demand-flow CPAP system. Respir Care 28:1273, 1983
37. Kirby RR: Continuous positive airway pressure; to breathe or not to breathe. Anesthesiology 65:578, 1985
38. Viale JP, Annat G, Bertrand O: Additional work in intubated patients breathing with continuous positive airway pressure systems. Anesthesiology 63:536, 1985
39. Kacmarek RM: The role of pressure support in reducing work of breathing. Respir Care 33:99, 1988
40. Kacmarek RM, Dimar S, Reynolds J, et al: Technical aspects of positive end-expiratory pressure (PEEP): 1. Physics of PEEP devices. Respir Care 27:1478, 1982
41. Kirby RR: Positive airway pressure: system design and clinical application. p. G1. In Shoemaker WC (ed): Critical Care: State of the Art. Vol. 6. Society of Critical Care Medicine, Fullerton, CA, 1985
42. Banner MJ, Lampotang S, Boysen PG, et al: Resistance of expiratory positive-pressure valves. Chest 94:893, 1988
43. Marini J, Culver BH, Kirk W: Flow resistance of exhalation valves and positive end expiratory pressure devices used in mechanical ventilation. Am Rev Respir Dis 131:850, 1985
44. Banner MJ: Expiratory positive-pressure valves: flow resistance and work of breathing. Respir Care 32:431, 1987
45. Hall JR, Rendleman DC, Downs JB: PEEP devices: Flow dependent increases in airway pressure (abstract). Crit Care Med 6:100, 1978
46. Nunn JF: Applied Respiratory Physiology. 2nd Ed. p. 100. Butterworths, London, 1977
47. Gal TJ: Effects of endotracheal tube intubation on normal cough performance. Anesthesiology 52:324, 1980
48. Banner MJ, Downs JB, Kirby RR, et al: Effects of expiratory flow resistance on inspiratory work of breathing. Chest 93:795, 1988
49. Pinsky MR, Hrehocik D, Culpepper JA, et al: Flow resistance of expiratory positive-pressure systems. Chest 94:788, 1988
50. Gammage GW, Banner MJ, Blanch PB, et al: Ventilator displayed tidal volume—what you see may not be what you get. Crit Care Med 16:454, 1988
51. Spearman CB, Sanders HG: The new generation of mechanical ventilators. Respir Care 32:403, 1987
52. Gregory GA, Kitterman JA, Phibbs RH, et al: Treatment of the idiopathic respiratory distress syndrome with continuous positive airway pressure. N Engl J Med 284:1333, 1971
53. Banner MJ, Smith RA: Mechanical ventilation. p. 1173. In Civetta JM, Taylor RW, Kirby RR (eds): Critical Care. JB Lippincott, Philadelphia, 1988
54. Kirby RP, Desautels DA, Smith RA: Mechanical ventilation. p. 556. In Burton GG, Hodgkin JE (eds): Respiratory Care. 2nd Ed. JB Lippincott, Philadelphia, 1984
55. Fiastro et al: Chest 93:499, 1988
56. Banner MJ, Lampotang S, Boysen PG, et al: Flow resistance of expiratory positive-pressure value systems. Chest 90:212, 1986

16

Equipment Safety for a Changing Standard of Care

Robert B. Spooner

The medical community has made recent major advances in setting standards of care that improve patient safety in critical care mechanical ventilation and the administration of inhalation anesthesia. This surge of awareness, however, has been under way for quite a few years without fanfare. The most significant of these recent advances are specifications (and even regulations) for monitors and alarms to be used with mechanical ventilation. The use of the monitors and alarms are the result of investigations and studies of mishaps that could be compared with the then current standard of care, acceptance of electrical and electronic equipment in the operating room, development of new monitoring equipment, and legal pressure associated with malpractice suits. Acceptance of these changes has been difficult and slow because of increased costs, the reluctance to learn about and to use new technologies, and the independent nature of practitioners in the art of anesthesia and ventilatory support.

ECRI, formerly Emergency Care Research Institute, Inc., whose mission is management of technology in health care, has been involved in this process since its early days. Over 10 years ago, it made a major commitment to improving the safety and performance of ventilatory and anesthesia equipment. Since then, it has continued to make many contributions to this process. Most of these improvements come as a result of our published hazards and evaluations, which are useful to the hospital members in our Health Devices program and to the manufacturers of the equipment involved. Our focus is on correction of equipment, design deficiencies, and operating problems and improvement of patient safety. Our 2,500 hospital members report problems to us, and our solution to each, usually worked out with the equipment manufacturer, contributes to improving the standard of care for patients. Our continuing investigations of ventilatory and anesthesia accidents and incidents often result in hazard reports for correction of problems of general concern to our other members.

A comparative product evaluation provides the best opportunity to bring together all of the information available on a particular kind of device, to devise criteria and test methods for testing all available models, and to determine how well each performs under both hazardous and normal conditions. By choosing criteria that eliminate hazards or reduce their effects, we can search for "a little extra," rather than just meeting minimum standards, from each device being tested. We then give highest ratings to units that best meet the demands. Subsequently, when the next upgrade in the standard of care occurs, hospitals that have purchased the preferred units are already in compliance.

An important part of our efforts, begun in the mid-1970s, was our publication of *Health Devices Alerts* (HDA), which, among other things, provides medical-device hazard and recall information, including ventilation-related equipment. Most recently, the HDA database has been augmented by ECRI-enhanced Food and Drug Administration (FDA) databases on medical device problems; all are available online through Dialog Information Services. These databases of problems and hazards are the inverse of a standard of care and tell us where an improvement is needed in that standard.

PULMONARY RESUSCITATORS

ECRI's earliest evaluation of ventilatory devices was of manually operated pulmonary resuscitators. It was published in 1972 in the first issue of *Health Devices*.[1] Although it involved one of the simplest types of ventilatory equipment, there were many problems and performance criteria to address. One criterion was delivering an adequate tidal volume at a rapid enough rate for proper oxygenation and gas exchange. Another was achieving a good mask seal so that most of the tidal volume delivered went to the patient, rather than leaking into the atmosphere.

Although delivery of a high oxygen concentration was a criterion, most uses of manual resuscitators, at the time, were under emergency conditions in the field with no oxygen available. Even so, a number of resuscitator evaluations published around that time focused on oxygen delivery as the determining factor in selecting one unit over another. ECRI considered other factors more important; of 18 resuscitators tested, 9 proved unacceptable or totally ineffective. Three units were listed in the highest group of acceptable models and they have continued to improve, as shown by our last evaluation in 1979.

In the totally ineffective group were the units in Figure 16-1. For example, one unit had a mouthpiece that was difficult to seal and an accompanying nose clamp that was too weak to seal nasal passages. There was no nonrebreathing or exhalation valve, so the mouthpiece had to be removed from the patient for exhalation. Considerable force on the mask was required for even a slow inhalation and this downward force on the patient was likely to occlude the pharynx. All the unacceptable units were ultimately withdrawn from the market, making emergency resuscitations much safer.

Infant resuscitators were evaluated in 1973[2] following a protocol similar to that used for adult units, but adjusted for infant conditions, such as higher breathing rates and lower volumes. By this time, totally ineffective units were off the market and all units tested could deliver adequate volumes at room temperature. However, one unit could not easily be compressed at frigid temperatures and certainly could not be compressed rapidly.

Another unit was the subject of a hazard report after its nonrebreathing valve permitted continuing high airway and patient lung pressure to develop with only 12 L/min of supplementary oxygen flow. Therefore, it was not submitted for the evaluation and was withdrawn from the market until a new valve was introduced. One of the infant units had an adequate oxygen reservoir and delivered a high oxygen concentration,

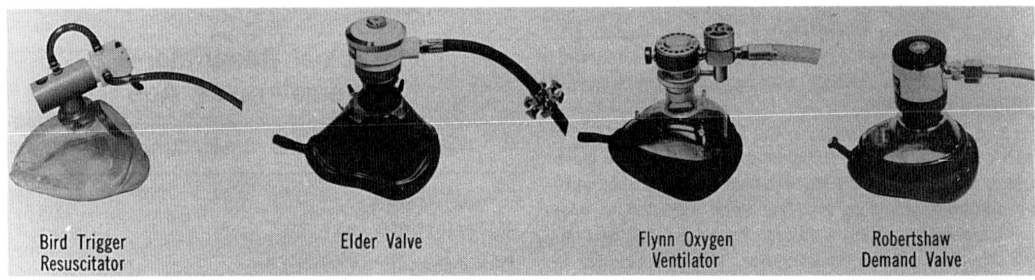

Fig. 16-1. Totally ineffective pulmonary resuscitators. (Courtesy of ECRI, Plymouth Meeting, PA.)

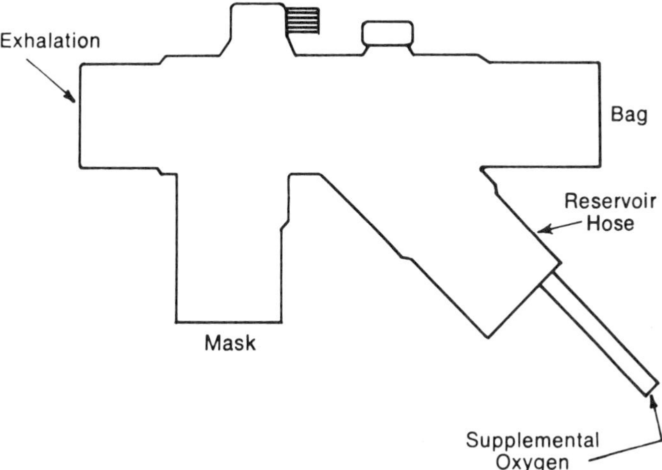

Fig. 16-2. Arrangement of identical 22-mm fittings. (Courtesy of ECRI, Plymouth Meeting, PA.)

but the oxygen reservoir fitting repeatedly disconnected from the unit.

An updated study of adult and infant resuscitators in 1974[3] found many of them modified and improved. The unit with the stiff bag was now available with a silicone rubber bag and excellent "feel." More units were able to deliver high oxygen concentrations, but a panel of clinicians were evenly split on whether 60 percent was adequate or whether manufacturers should continue striving for 100 percent. On the other hand, these clinicians agreed that the possibility of misconnections was hazardous. Four of the 12 units were rated unacceptable because of such misconnection possibilities. One actually had four fittings on the nonrebreathing valve (Fig. 16-2), all of which were 22-mm male fittings with the potential for multiple misconnections.

In our most recent evaluation of reusable manual resuscitators in 1979,[4] 14 units were rated acceptable with various advantages and disadvantages for consideration in the selection of a unit. The remaining two were acceptable only conditionally. One with a capped oxygen inlet required an experienced user to match oxygen flow with patient delivery (Fig. 16-3); the other, with a low stroke volume, required that large patients be intubated.

Currently, disposable resuscitators have taken over a large part of the market and have brought along both old and new problems, as shown by an evaluation in 1989.[5] Performance at low temperatures is not always satisfactory because of materials used for some of the bags. Only two other manufacturers did not seem to have learned from earlier experience. One was making a bellows-type unit; the other had a valve design that would leak with slow bag compression causing gas to bypass the patient.

Gas-powered resuscitators, evaluated in 1974,[6] are often used by emergency groups such as ambulance units. Only manually controlled

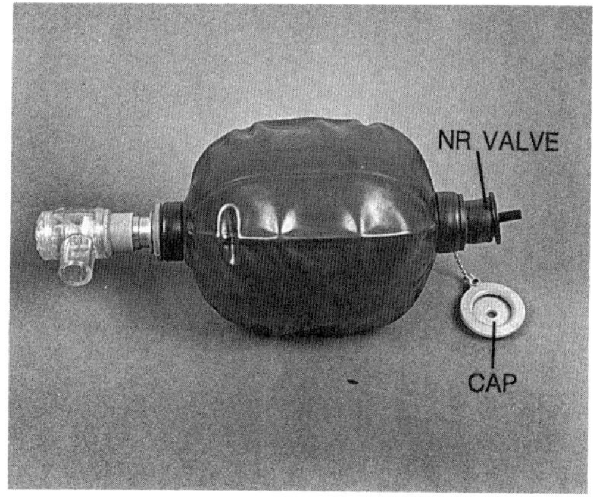

Fig. 16-3. Resuscitator with capped oxygen inlet. (Courtesy of ECRI, Plymouth Meeting, PA.)

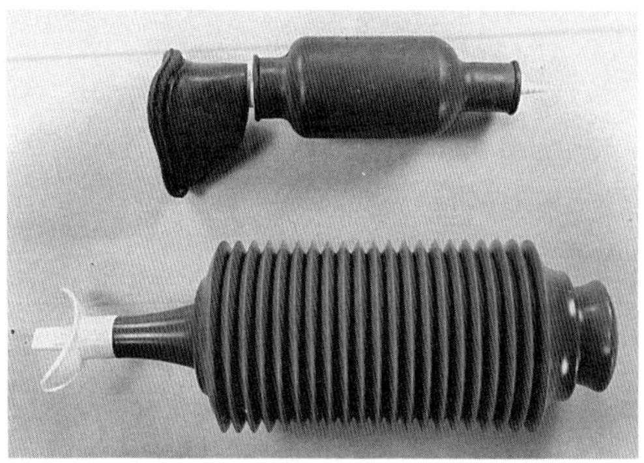

Fig. 16-4. Oxygen-powered resuscitators with masks. (Courtesy of ECRI, Plymouth Meeting, PA.)

units were considered because only they can be used in cardiopulmonary resuscitation (CPR). Pressure-cycled resuscitators cannot be used for this application. Most of these devices have a secondary mode of operation for patients who can breathe spontaneously—a demand valve mode that delivers a breath in proportion to a patient's inspiratory efforts, or an inhalator mode to supply a constant flow of oxygen to the mask.

Gas-powered resuscitators are small devices (Fig. 16-4). They must be connected to a source of pressurized oxygen for both power and breathing. Three of the units tested delivered

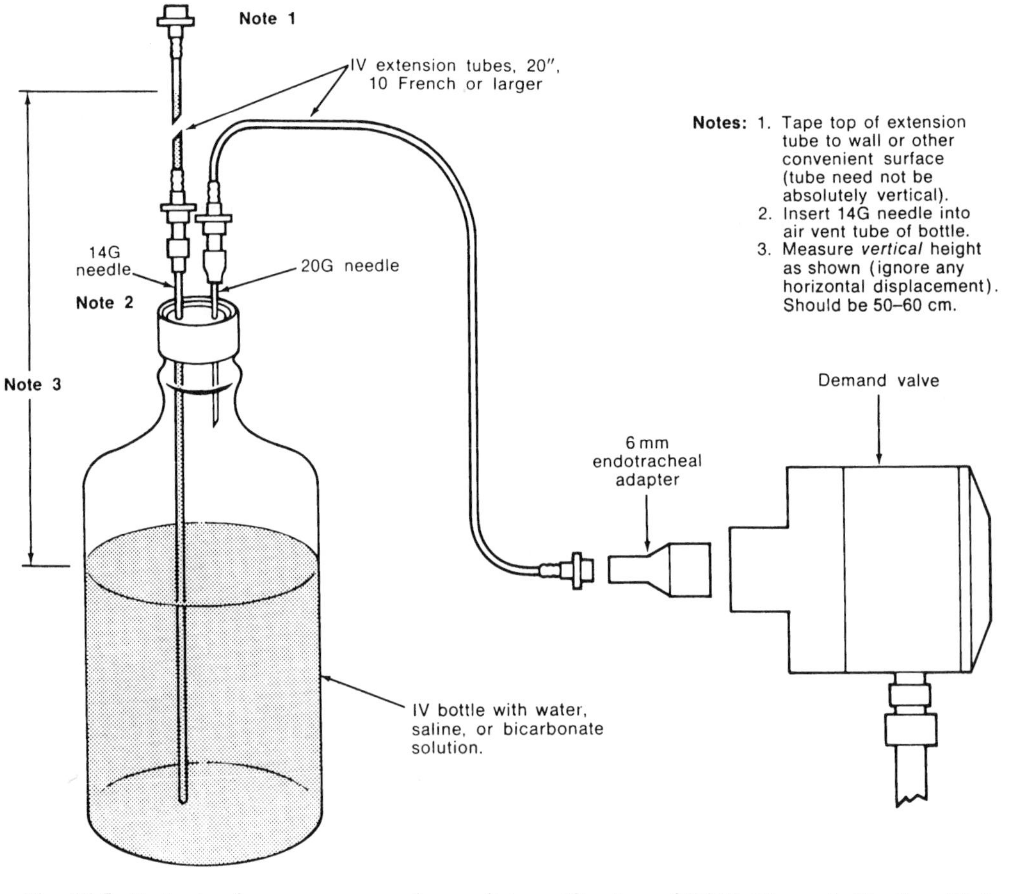

Fig. 16-5. Test setup for oxygen-powered resuscitators. (Courtesy of ECRI, Plymouth Meeting, PA.)

100 percent oxygen; the other used a Venturi arrangement to deliver an oxygen-air mixture. One of the units originally submitted could be misassembled by simply inverting its valve. The problem was corrected by the manufacturer, and a new unit was resubmitted for testing.

These resuscitators are vulnerable to rough handling and inadequate maintenance. Damage can go undetected until a malfunction occurs. This problem was reported by member hospitals and, in 1976, we published a hazard report[7] about damage to a thin rubber diaphragm that regulates the pressure at which airway pressure is relieved.

In an update of the original evaluation, reported in 1978,[8] seven units failed updated safety criteria or ability to deliver 100 percent oxygen and were rated only conditionally acceptable. Some did not limit pressure to 60 cm H_2O. Some could be misassembled, and two could not be put back in operation after attempts of 5-second duration to clear vomitus. Conditions for the acceptable use of those units prone to clogging varied from having a second unit available to using the unit only on intubated patients. On other units, the condition for acceptable use was pre-use testing on a balloon or a test lung. As effective as these units were for emergency use, they required care in operation and maintenance. A test unit for maximum airway pressure, which can be made from components readily available in a hospital, is shown in Figure 16-5. An additional need was a check on whether units were complying with revised guidelines for CPR that, among other specifications, required lower inspiratory flow rates.

Typical of problems with gas-powered resuscitators was a hazard report published in 1985[9] in which cleaning and sterilization of a unit, but without pre-use testing, resulted in an inoperative valve during a resuscitation. The user-replaceable valve had deteriorated during repeated processing and was not checked and replaced by a knowledgeable person. Continuing problems of this type led to another hazard report in 1988[10] that recommended further care, including placing all of these resuscitators on a routine inspection and preventive maintenance schedule. Subsequently, procedures were described for such a program.[11]

INTUBATION EQUIPMENT

Since tracheal intubation is an essential part of ventilation and begins with a laryngoscope, we evaluated the latter equipment in 1976.[12] Included were 12 units made of metal or plastic and arranged for direct illumination by bulbs at the blade tips or light pipes from sources in the handles. All of the units were rated acceptable, although problems with bulbs and sockets were identified. The bulbs could remain lighted even though, in some cases, they were within a fraction of a turn of falling out and into a patient's airway. With one combination, the bulb lit before it was screwed into the socket. Since nothing could be done about poorly standardized bulbs and sockets, we recommended a pre-use test for bulb tightness and operation for at least 10 seconds as a check that the battery output does not drop.

In 1978, we evaluated oropharyngeal airways and cuffed tracheal tubes.[13] We rated 14 of the oropharyngeal units acceptable, but one was not recommended for general use because it was intended for mouth-to-airway resuscitation. Another was rated unacceptable because it could be occluded by a strong bite.

The tracheal tubes were tested for various properties, but especially for cuff pressure on the trachea and stiffness where they exerted pressure on arytenoid cartilages. Both of these characteristics have potential for damage to patient airways. Cuff-tracheal pressure was measured with Knowlson-Bassett tubes between the inflated cuff and a simulated trachea after leakage stopped. Arytenoid pressure was measured on an anatomical model arranged for measuring the force required to pull the tracheal tube away from the arytenoids.

Our data showed considerable differences between tubes. Although we could not draw a line between damage and no damage, because of different uses and durations of use, we did group tubes according to results and did not recommend the low-volume high-pressure tubes. A liquid-filled cuff tube was also not recommended because it could not seal the trachea.

Even cuffless pediatric tracheal tubes, as simple as they are, cause problems.[14] When the adapters are lubricated with a substance, such as lidocaine jelly, for easy insertion in the tube, the jelly is likely to form a film over the hole at the end that goes into the tube. Although this film has little strength when applied, the tube may not be used immediately and instead is saved for another patient later on. This delay gives the film time to dry, giving it strength. If the tube is not tested for patency, for example by a probe that breaks through it, leaving jagged edges, (Fig. 16-6) it will remain occluded at breathing circuit pressures and ventilation will be impossible.

Suction catheters are necessary for airway maintenance, but may also inflict damage to the tracheal mucosa. We evaluated these devices in 1977[15] after first conducting a short research project in cooperation with a local hospital. Hospital personnel suctioned 40 patients using an instrumented system. We measured the necessary pressure level for successful suctioning and related it to a viscoelastic measurement made on a sample of the mucus removed. The entire range of mucus samples encountered could be successfully suctioned with up to 150 mmHg suction level. This is about the level where mucosal damage had been reported to begin. Our catheter testing began somewhat above that point. With the suction system occluded, we set the suction source at 200 mmHg in order to preclude reaching any higher level.

The 21 evaluated units were distributed in 3 groups as a result of our testing. Five were in the preferred group because they had large multiple eyes for low risk of tissue attachment, but good suctioning efficiency, and would easily rotate in a tracheal tube. Twelve were not recommended, in particular, one because its control permitted too much flow through the catheter when it was not supposed to be suctioning. The control end of this catheter is the top unit in Figure 16-7. The others had only single-eyed whistle tips and could attach to the mucosa if the end hole was occluded.

This study provided data for an evaluation of tracheal suction sources in 1977.[16] We were looking for units with vacuum regulators capable of limiting suction to 150 mmHg, but able to give 20 L/min air-flow rate without the vacuum level falling below 120 mmHg. These values are required for use with a typical adult catheter.

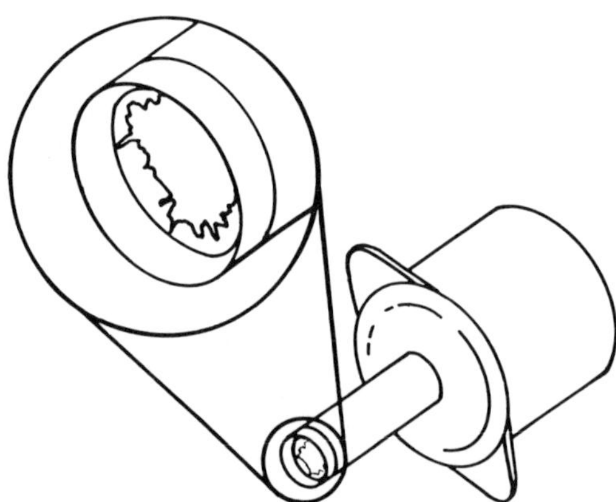

Fig. 16-6. Schematic enlargement of adapter end showing occluding film near the patient end of a tracheal tube adaptor. (Courtesy of ECRI, Plymouth Meeting, PA.)

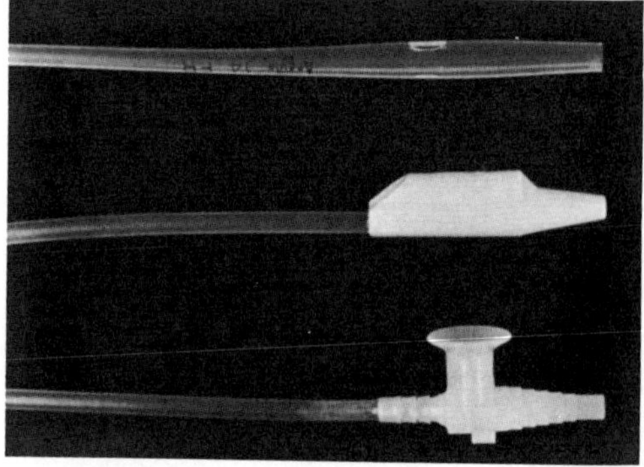

Fig. 16-7. Thumb control openings on suction catheters. (Courtesy of ECRI, Plymouth Meeting, PA.)

Of 18 candidates for tracheal suctioning, none was able to meet the requirement; all had inefficient regulating devices. With a suitable external regulator (Fig. 16-8), two met the requirement and another 10 approached it; the remaining six were not recommended for the application.

INSPIRATORY GAS MONITORS AND ALARMS

The predominant cause of the anesthesia- and ventilation-related accidents we investigated from 1977 to 1979 was hypoxia, which typically

Upgrade Your Portable Suction Source

Difficult tracheal suctioning requires equipment with higher capacity components than those we found in the evaluated suction sources. Hospital personnel can upgrade an inadequate unit with a capable pump by assembling standard components as shown in the diagram.

• *Pump:* Use one from a Conditionally Acceptable tracheal/emergency suction source. You can attach a bracket to the base to support the other components.

• *Regulator and gauge:* A typical wall regulator, such as the Chemetron Regu-Gage, Foregger Tracheal Suction Regulator, or Ohio Intermittent Suction unit, is satisfactory. We tried these because we had them on hand, but others may do equally well.

• *Valve:* The valve should have one pump inlet and two suction outlets, relatively large ports (at least ¼") to insure an adequate air flow rate, a convenient handle that is easy to turn, and two positions, fixed by handle stops, to be labeled *EMERGENCY* and *TRACHEAL*. In each handle position, the switch should connect one outlet to the inlet and vent the other outlet to the room.

• *Collection bottles:* Use standard bottles that have built-in overflow protection, large bore tubing without sharp corners, and threaded fittings that allow rigid attachment of the bottle cap to the regulator or mounting bracket. Bottles may then be unscrewed from the firmly supported caps for quick emptying.

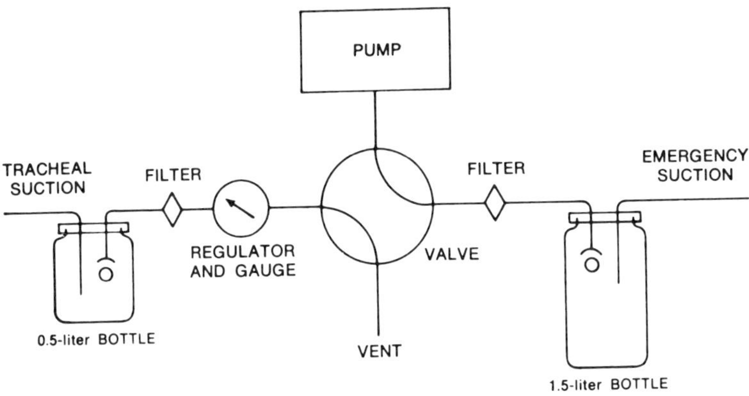

• *Extension tubing:* Connections between the completed unit and the suction catheter *(TRACHEAL)* and suction tip *(EMERGENCY)* should be thick-walled suction tubing with at least a 9/32" inside diameter. For convenience, attach the suction tip to a coiled extension tube and store them in a plastic bag, instantly ready for use.

See *HEALTH DEVICES*, Vol. 1, pp. 183 ff for suction machine inspection procedures. Apply the updated performance criteria included in the present evaluation.

Fig. 16-8. Recommended regulator installation. (Courtesy of ECRI, Plymouth Meeting, PA.)

led to coma and serious injury or death. In each case, we found that no oxygen monitor had been used during anesthesia, even though ECRI's earlier evaluation of seven continuous oxygen monitoring units[17] found all of them acceptable. At the time, respiratory care personnel used these monitors for periodic checks of intensive care unit (ICU) ventilator systems. Many users, however, considered them unreliable and had to learn that maintenance was a necessary part of these monitors' use. The instruments must be checked for proper operation and batteries or sensors replaced (Fig. 16-9).

To improve the situation, we stated in 1978[18] that use of an oxygen monitor should be mandatory every time a gaseous anesthetic is administered. We added instructions for a pre-use performance check of the oxygen monitor and its low-oxygen-concentration alarm. Later, when we again evaluated oxygen monitors,[19] we found them to be reliable, although still in need of significant maintenance. We did fault all of the test units for not incorporating an interlock that would automatically enable the monitor whenever the anesthesia unit or ventilator was turned on.

Monitoring of other ventilatory gases began to increase as clinical mass spectrometers came into use. However, the most important of these gases, carbon dioxide, was not monitored rapidly enough by the usual time-sharing models. What was needed was a dedicated capnograph, so waveforms could be analyzed and alarms generated without waiting for the system to first check other patients. Dedicated infrared units improved in capability and reliability, so that by 1986 ECRI completed an evaluation[20] of available CO_2 monitors. Of the 13 units tested, 7 were capnometers and 6 were capnographs. All of the capnometers could be connected to monitors or recorders to display waveforms, such as the waveform for end-tidal carbon dioxide ($ETCO_2$) in Figure 16-10. All passed our accuracy and response-time tests (with no inhalation anesthetics) and qualitatively detected CO_2 within 30 seconds of being turned on. They were ready to perform an important analytical function. However, sampling systems gave many problems. Some could be reversed, water and secretions interfered with flow and fouled cuvettes, and liquid traps were not effective.

To take advantage of the capabilities of these monitors and to avoid operating problems, users must exercise proper bronchial hygiene for the patient and position the sampling tube in the breathing circuit to minimize liquid entry.

Although we evaluated 13 units, only 6 received acceptable ratings. One unit was top-

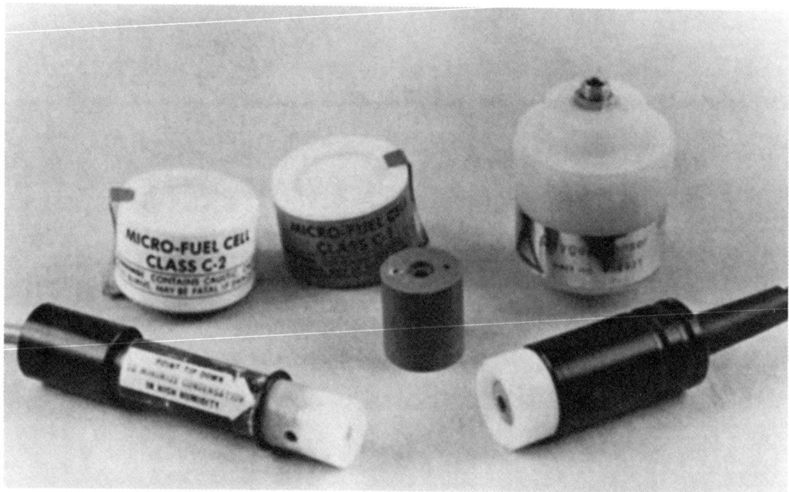

Fig. 16-9. Oxygen sensors for breathing gas monitors. (Courtesy of ECRI, Plymouth Meeting, PA.)

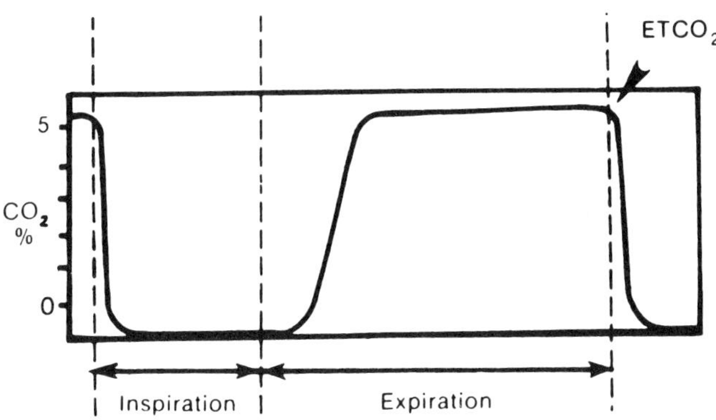

Fig. 16-10. Typical capnograph waveform. (Courtesy of ECRI, Plymouth Meeting, PA.)

rated because of its built-in CO_2 waveform display, among other features. It thus produced more vital information about ventilation conditions than would be obtained from an end-tidal monitor.

VENTILATORS

In 1979,[21] we published our evaluation of anesthesia ventilators after finding them all conditionally acceptable at best. The condition was that they be equipped with exhaled volume monitors to determine the volume actually delivered to the patient and then exhaled. None was so equipped. The highest ranking was given to the ventilator with an automatically activated low-pressure (disconnection) alarm with adjustable pressure levels that made it less susceptible to errors caused by backpressure. The second highest ranking was given to a unit with an integral alarm, but with only one set pressure level.

All but one of the test units were of the falling bellows type (the bellows descended to refill during exhalation). The other was an ascending bellows unit, with a useful characteristic of failing to rise and refill if there was a disconnection or leak larger than the gas inflow rate; thus flagging the problem. The other units, under the same conditions, had enough weight to fall and draw in air through the opening to refill. Their only indication of a leak was development of a "negative" airway pressure during the refill process.

After reports of barotrauma with ascending bellows ventilators, we published a hazard report in 1988.[22] A problem with these ventilators is that the bellows is typically collapsed before it is ready to be used and must be filled. Filling should be accomplished before it begins to cycle. Otherwise, especially if the flush control is actuated, a high gas flow may be injected into the circuit during the inspiratory phase when it cannot go to the ventilator. It can only flow to the patient, where pressure increases up to the maximum possible in the ventilator.

For this first ventilator evaluation, as is our frequent practice when there are no published standards specifying what we believed to be certain essential features, we gave higher ratings to the units that at least included them. And, since none was able to detect breathing circuit leaks, we advocated pre-use checks each time a ventilator was used.

Our first evaluation of critical care ventilators was in 1982[23] when we tested six units under simulated patient-use conditions. All could ventilate patients successfully, although some had more modes of ventilation than others. All were acceptable, but two were acceptable only under specified conditions. One required an antiasphyxia device so that a patient who could breathe spontaneously would be able to breathe air in the event of a power failure; the other lacked a ventilation alarm package.

With the growing practice of sending stabilized patients home with their ventilators, we evaluated home care ventilators in 1988.[24] Although these units do not have to be as sophisticated as critical care ventilators, they have their own special requirements and problems. If oxygen is required, continuous monitoring should be provided. Remote alarms are usually needed and should follow our 1986 recommendation[25] that the alarm unit should monitor its own connection to the ventilator. Remote alarm units are pictured in Figure 16-11. No one unit was equipped for all of the special problems related to home care use, so each was rated conditionally acceptable (i.e., that the ventilator should have the necessary features for anticipated service).

With new modes of ventilation coming into use, we listened to problems expressed about intermittent mandatory ventilation (IMV) and continuous positive airway pressure (CPAP) ventilation. The test ventilators used various methods, such as demand valves to aid the patient's spontaneous breathing in these modes, and patients had to exert more effort with some ventilators than with others. To measure the added work of breathing with a ventilator, we simulated an active lung that could inhale a breath at a set rate and determined the added inspiratory work expended on each ventilator from a pressure waveform, as in Figure 16-12. Thus, we could compare the different units to see why some were poor and others better.

From previous investigations, we knew that power-line conducted interference and air-transmitted electromagnetic interference could affect the operation of medical equipment. Two of the ventilators, we found, could be affected through their electronic circuitry when there were power line fluctuations.

The electromagnetic interference problem in more sophisticated ventilators was even more of a concern in our later evaluation of five microprocessor-controlled ventilators in 1989.[26] These units have a vastly increased capacity for monitoring ventilatory variables, both inspiratory and expiratory. Any mode of operation can be provided by the proper software.

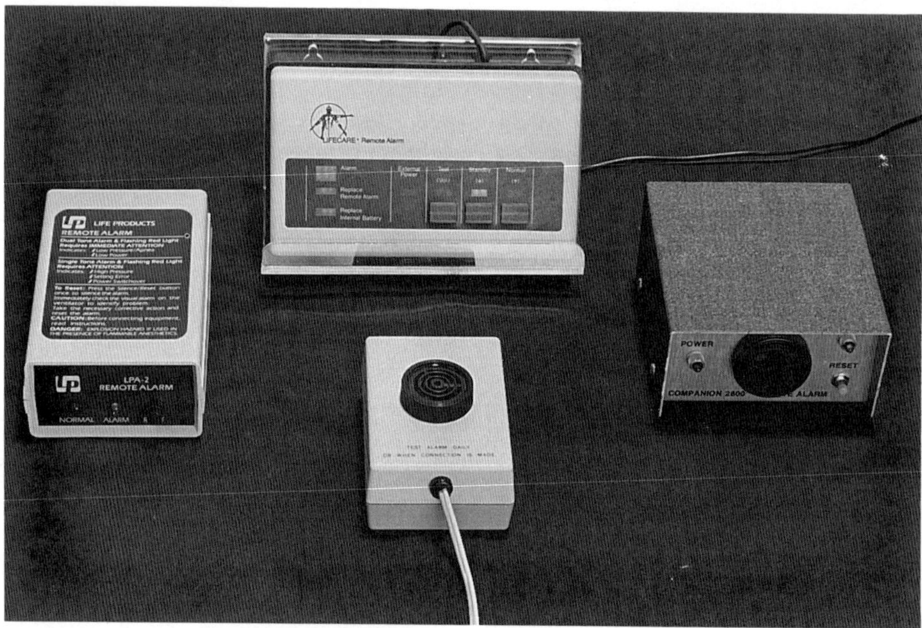

Fig. 16-11. Remote alarm units. Clockwise from left: Aequitron, Lifecare, Puritan-Bennett, Bear. (Courtesy of ECRI, Plymouth Meeting, PA.)

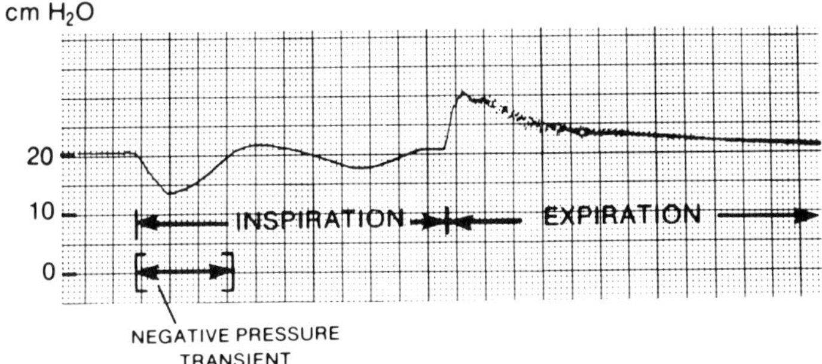

Fig. 16-12. Pressure waveform during spontaneous breathing with CPAP. (Courtesy of ECRI, Plymouth Meeting, PA.)

Pre-use checks are carried out automatically on start-up, and additional checks are performed regularly during operation. Problems found during checking are reported for diagnostic use. Yet, all of this capability comes at the expense of more susceptibility to electrical disturbances, such as power line transients and electrostatic discharges (ESD) from external sources. For example, the performance of only one of the ventilators was unaffected by ESD, although its monitor display was affected. All of the units were able to resume operation after power interruptions of 10 cycles and 10 seconds. Line transients had no effect on ventilation.

With the proliferation of new breathing modes came new, more complex modes for spontaneously breathing patients. A new test apparatus interconnected with a computer was developed to perform more thorough tests and to include newer modes, such as pressure support ventilation. Although clinical requirements had not been specified for these methods, the results with different ventilators were compared. Two of the ventilators offered continuous-flow breathing systems, which were studied to determine how much flow was needed to alleviate the patient's work.

The net result of the evaluation was to point out that all of the new ventilators are very powerful devices. However, they are also very complex and can be confusing and difficult to learn to use. Much depends on how "user-friendly" each is as a result of human factors, control, and software design.

VENTILATION MONITORS

Our first evaluations of ventilators found that they differed considerably with respect to their monitoring capabilities. Early ones used pressure gauges, later, alarms were added. Since machine ventilation did not permit direct hand sensing of the loss of pressure accompanying a disconnection, low-pressure alarms were devised. However, in our first evaluation of ventilation alarms in 1981,[27] we looked for units with low-pressure alarms that would interlock with a ventilator to provide disconnection alarms. The monitors should also alarm with high or continuing positive pressure. The preferred unit had all of these features to some degree. Exhaled volume monitors, although useful in critical care ventilation, were unreliable in the operating room because of electrosurgical unit interference.

This inability to discriminate between leaks, disconnections with backpressure, and other sources of reduced pressure had long been a problem with these units. A hazard report in 1981[28] found troubles in both equipment and operation of low-pressure alarms. In the first, a low-pressure ventilation alarm failed to activate at the set pressure because of a faulty pressure switch. However, the malfunction had not been detected in an equipment check. Although we could not dictate choice of a more reliable pressure switch, we did recommend daily pre-use checks and a quarterly maintenance program for these units to find malfunctions as they occured.

A similar problem in 1989[29] involved pressure switches in alarms of an anesthesia ventilator. In this case, the malfunction was immediately apparent on inspection of the interior of the ventilator. The pressure switches had actually separated (Fig. 16-13). Further investigation revealed that the wrong formulation of Loctite had been put on the threads of the pressure adjustment screw; it had attacked the plastic switch housing, and the weakened housing had broken under spring pressure. The manufacturer reported that the screws would hold their adjustments and that Loctite was unnecessary.

Another hazard, reported in 1983,[30] concerned the operation of low-pressure alarms which, if set to alarm at pressures too far below the peak inspiratory pressure, could prevent a pressure drop in the breathing circuit from falling below the alarm point (Fig. 16-14). Some commercial units had alarm points factory-set below such a point. Other units, with adjustable alarms, were regularly found to have been user-set to a value that was too low to sound. We recommend reviewing and following the manufacturer's setup procedures and replacing units with low factory-set alarms with more acceptable alarms.

Our later review of the disconnection problem in 1984[31] showed that breathing circuit discon-

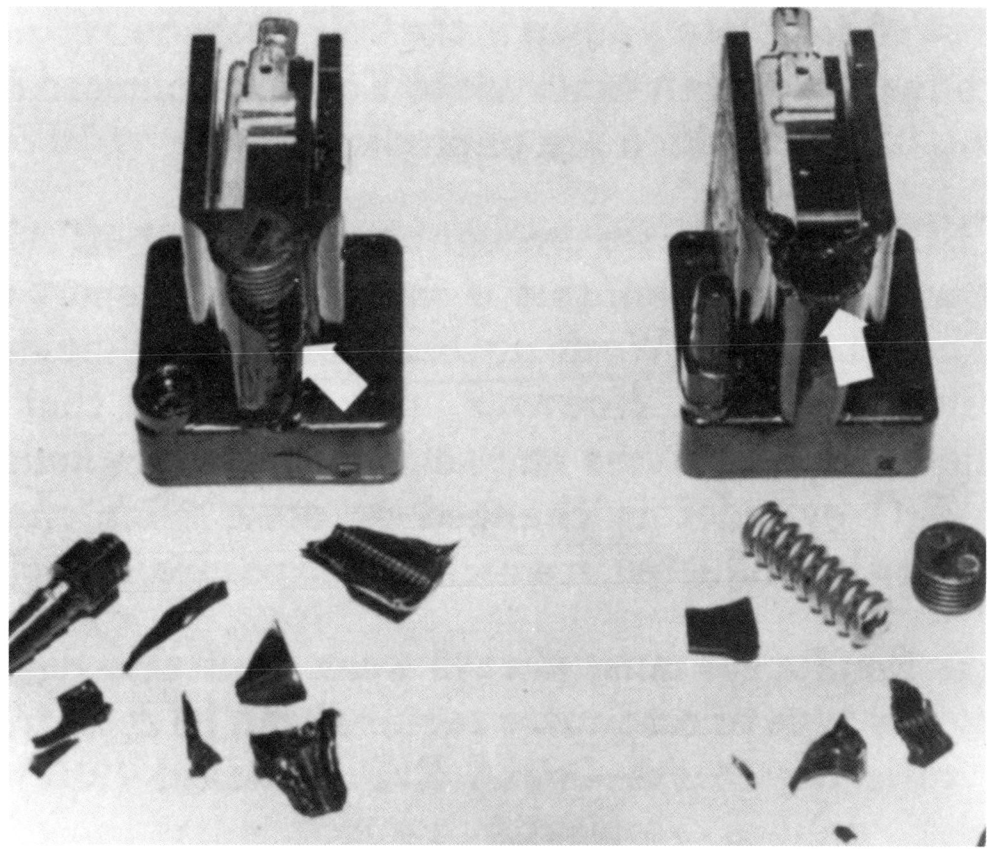

Fig. 16-13. Damaged pressure switches from Loctite. (Courtesy of ECRI, Plymouth Meeting, PA.)

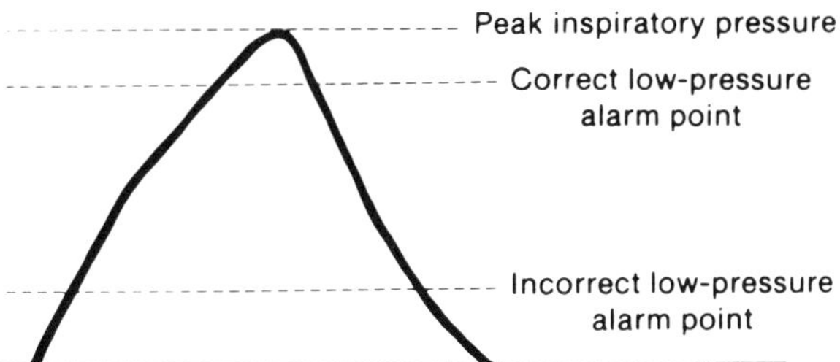

Fig. 16-14. Proper and improper alarm point setting of low-pressure alarm. (Courtesy of ECRI, Plymouth Meeting, PA.)

nections would continue to occur until there were major changes in the concepts of circuit design. Until then, breathing circuit integrity would have to be protected by acceptable exhaled CO_2 and exhaled-volume monitors that were already available. For applications where connections must remain tight, such as fresh gas hoses, we recommended locking fittings, as shown in Figure 16-15. However, we found that only two such fittings were available, and they were seldom used.

BREATHING CIRCUITS AND HUMIDIFIERS

During a 1979 evaluation of disposable anesthesia breathing circuits,[32] we identified many problems of leaks and disconnections and noted that special care is needed during inspection before use. These circuits were also very easily ignited (i.e., by an electrosurgical unit pencil) and would separate and burn with an intensive flame whether carrying oxygen or an oxygen/nitrous oxide mixture (Fig. 16-16). Therefore, special care was necessary when sources of ignition were used near these circuits. In early 1980,[33] we gave further warnings of the dangers of fire during head and neck surgery.

Excessive breathing circuit temperatures were also considered during our evaluation of heated humidifiers.[34] We found inadequate monitoring and inadequate control of gas temperature, as well as temperature overshoot (Fig. 16-17), when flow rates were increased. The duration of the overshoot was greatest for units with large reservoirs of water heated to temperatures sufficient to ensure adequate temperature and

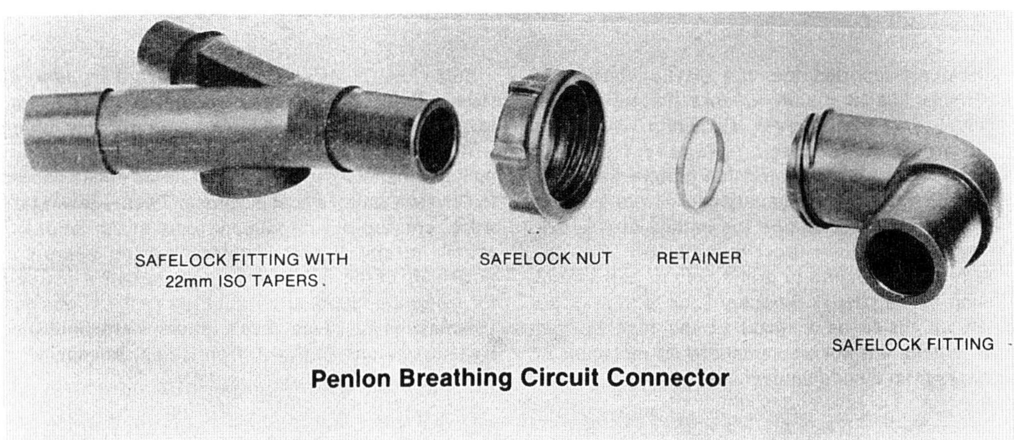

Fig. 16-15. Locking fittings for breathing circuits. (Courtesy of ECRI, Plymouth Meeting, PA.)

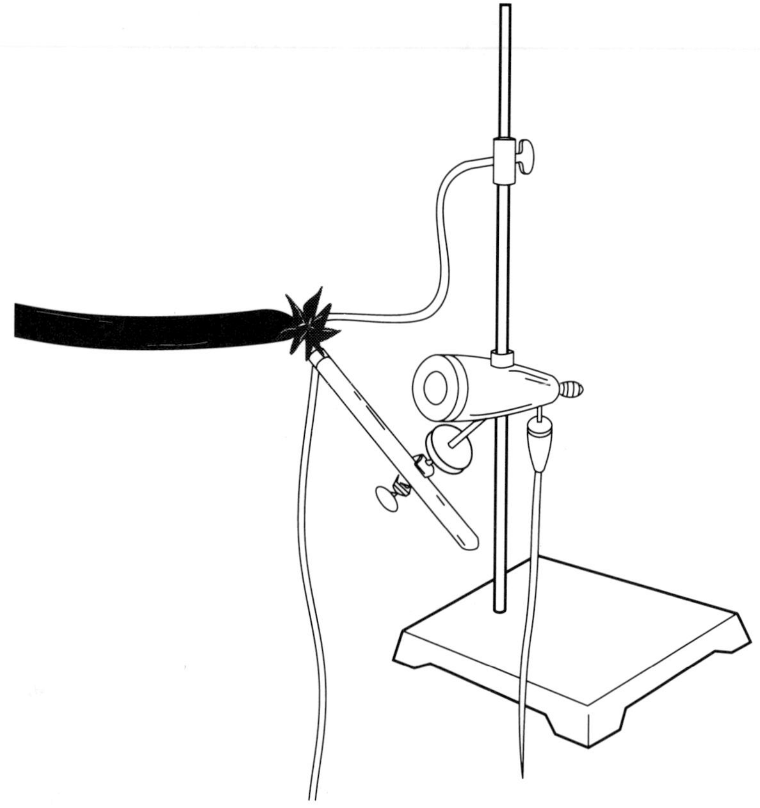

Fig. 16-16. Breathing circuit ignited by electrosurgical spark. (Courtesy of ECRI, Plymouth Meeting, PA.)

humidity at the end of a long inspiratory hose. Consequently, for acceptance, we recommended that there should always be a temperature monitor and alarm, with its sensor at the patient connection of the breathing circuit. Later, in 1981, we recommended the pre-use test protocol shown in Figure 16-18 for heated humidifiers.[35]

One of the highest-rated humidifiers was a unit that divided the heating process between the humidifier and the inspiratory limb of the breathing circuit. This division meant that the water in the humidifier never had to get much above the desired patient input temperature. Heating in the inspiratory line was only sufficient to maintain the temperature by balancing heat losses. Thus, there should be no temperature overshoot and no rainout in the inspiratory line. Finally, even this system had its hazards as more and more different heated circuit systems came into use. For example, in 1989,[36] the problem of excessive heating and melting or charring of inspiratory hoses caused by using wires not specified for the control unit or wires that are bunched together, especially in disposable circuits, was reviewed. The best protection to warn of such a hazard is a low expired-volume monitor that can detect a leak caused by melting plastic.

In our most recent heated humidifier evaluation in 1987,[37] all the units tested had temperature monitors and alarms for breathing circuit use at the patient input. All of the units were acceptable; however, the one with the largest water reservoir also failed the temperature overshoot test and was not recommended.

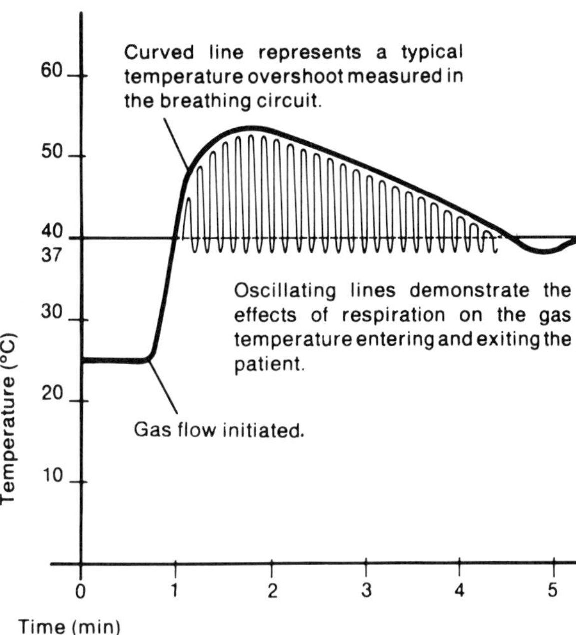

Fig. 16-17. Temperature overshoot with flow increase. (Courtesy of ECRI, Plymouth Meeting, PA.)

Pre-Use Checks of Heated Humidifiers

We recommend that the respiratory therapy or other user department conduct regular pre-use checks of heated humidifiers and their accessories. However, we do not recommend pre-use checks with a lung simulator for two reasons. Such checks compromise the sterility of the humidifying chamber and the patient circuit unless the system is connected to the patient very soon after the checks. However, if this is done, the hot start-up can be hazardous. It can result in an excessive patient inspiratory temperature, especially at high flow rates (heat loss in the inspiratory hose at high flow rates is less than the loss at low flows because the gas spends less time in the hose). Interruption of ventilation to correct a problem can also result in a hot start-up.

We recommend first assembling sterile patient circuit and humidifier components on a ventilator that is already at the bedside. Pre-use checks are then performed with the equipment connected to the patient, rather than to a lung simulator.

Visual Checks

Examine the unit for the general physical condition of both reusable and disposable components (this includes checking for loose, frayed, or taped line cords and plugs). Tubing and connectors should fit tightly without kinks or leaks. Examine humidity chambers as closely as possible to determine if the airway through them is occluded.

Assembly Checks

While assembling the unit, follow the manufacturer's procedure to check all alarms, including those for omission of the sensor and low water level.

Perform a system leak test after the humidifier has been included in the system (*e.g.*, compare exhaled tidal volume with delivered tidal volume).

Filling

Fill the humidifier with sterile distilled water to the full level. Avoid hot water to prevent a hot start-up; warm water, however, will shorten the warm-up time.

Warm-up

Warm-up time varies between units from one to 30 minutes. Be sure you know the warm-up time for your unit and check the patient inspiratory temperature frequently during this period. [Consult the operator's manual for specified warm-up time or base your estimate on experience.] Look for condensation in the inspiratory hose to confirm output.

If the temperature rapidly approaches the desired temperature, reduce the heater control to avoid temperature overshoot and watch for a slower approach. If the equilibrium temperature is too low, increase it in small increments, again to avoid an overshoot. Confirm that the system responds to these control changes.

By following this pre-use procedure, ventilation will begin safely and you will avoid a hot start-up.

Fig. 16-18. Pre-use check procedure for heated humidifier. (Courtesy of ECRI, Plymouth Meeting, PA.)

ANESTHESIA SYSTEMS

By the end of 1980, we published our first evaluation of six anesthesia units from six manufacturers.[38] We found that some new units were already well ahead of the requirements of the 1979 ANSI Z79 standard. The top ratings were given to units that would not deliver less than a preset concentration of oxygen (about 30 percent). Some other advanced features that were in our performance criteria and that were used to give higher ratings are summarized in Table 16-1. One of the manufacturers had a checklist on the front panel of its unit (Fig. 16-19). However, none of the units had an automatic interlock for enabling the oxygen monitor.

By our second evaluation of anesthesia systems in 1988,[39] all but two of the American manufacturers had stopped manufacturing gas machines and systems. One foreign system, based on a critical care ventilator that was adapted for anesthesia gases and vapors, was also evaluated, but with suitable modifications in criteria and test methods (Fig. 16-20). Legal liability and requirements for monitoring and other safety devices had increased to the point that only the "strongest" manufacturers could survive. The net result was that all of these modern systems could safely deliver general anesthesia after following pre-use checklists in their operating manuals.

Pre-use Checklist

In 1982, we recognized the need for a comprehensive pre-use checklist for use on anesthesia systems analogous to a pilot's preflight checklist. Since no manufacturer had developed one for general use, we proposed, tested, and published our own checklist,[40] that could be used with any basic machine. Our aim was to include tests that would detect all of the malfunctions that our investigations of patient injuries and deaths had disclosed. All that was lacking was a check of vaporizer output that would catch unreasonably high output. Our one-page checklist was revised in 1984[41] (almost 2 years before the issuance of the FDA checklist, which was less complete), with the addition of a rapid check for vaporizer output using the oxygen analyzer after its calibration check at 100 percent oxygen. The checklist was printed on a small card (Fig. 16-21) and distributed by ECRI on request. Monitoring of anesthetic gases still was not available; even mass spectrometer systems could not do it continuously.

Our checklist identified grossly excessive output from flowmeter-controlled vaporizers with valve malfunctions or improper piping connections, problems that ECRI had investigated,[42–46] which put these vaporizers in disfavor. The checklist also helped to find excessive output from concentration-calibrated flowmeters, a hazard that our experience[47–49] showed always seemed to occur when such a vaporizer had been removed from its machine and was not tested after recalibration. This updated checklist is still available on request without charge.

Table 16–1. Advanced Features of Top-Rated Anesthesia Systems

A vaporizer selector device that prevents the use of more than one vaporizer at a time
An on–off control that activates monitors and alarms (especially the oxygen monitor) when gas was turned on
A pre-use checklist for testing the unit before connection to a patient

CURRENT SITUATION

Many of the devices and features we sought, which were available first as add-on components, are now incorporated in complete integrated anesthesia and ventilator systems. This is especially important because of the increase in monitoring and alarms brought on by more and more specific and stringent requirements of regulations and standards of care. This is shown clearly by our most recent evaluations of current models of anesthesia and ventilator systems. Some of these essential features are realized only in integrated systems, so the old

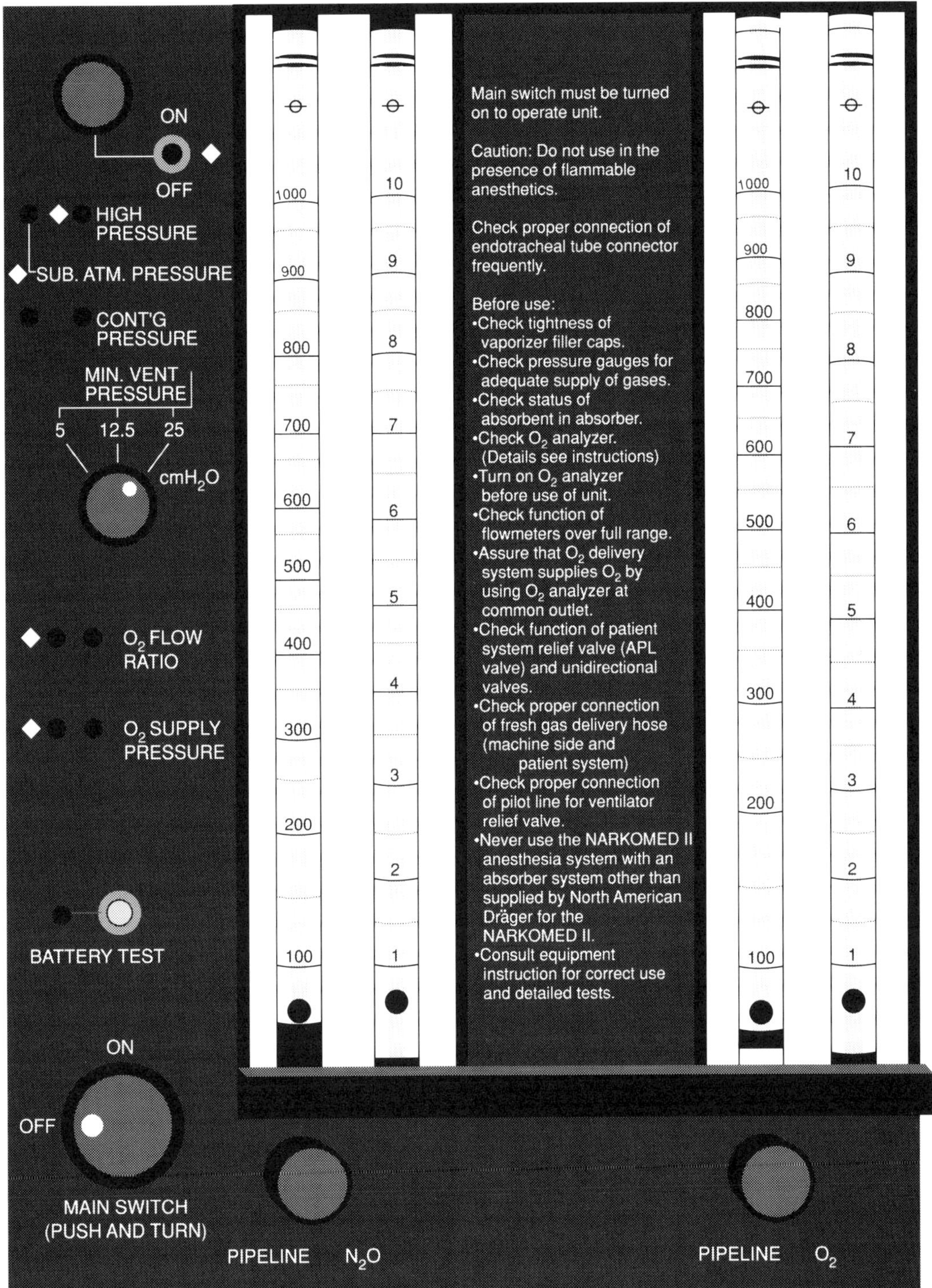

Fig. 16-19. Anesthesia unit with checklist on front panel. (Courtesy of ECRI, Plymouth Meeting, PA.)

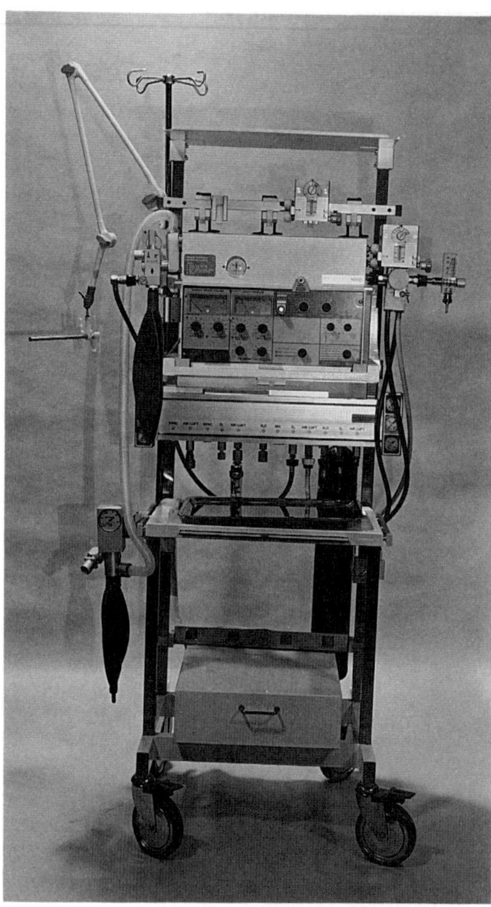

Fig. 16-20. Critical care ventilator adapted for administration of anesthesia. (Courtesy of ECRI, Plymouth Meeting, PA.)

approach of a piecemeal collection of components from various manufacturers does not result in an optimum system by today's standards. On the other hand, the integrated systems we reported on do have growth potential; missing parts of the ideal system can be incorporated as they are developed, in some cases by a software change. We recommend that all anesthesia and respiratory care departments have plans for rapidly replacing inadequate equipment with such integrated systems.

CONCLUSION

ECRI clearly has contributed significantly to these important safety developments and, in turn, appreciates the contributions and responsiveness of both clinicians and manufacturers that have participated in this process. We will continue to contribute to patient safety by investigating accidents and incidents with such equipment, evaluating new equipment, developing training materials, and participating in development of standards for equipment in the United States and around the world.

EDITOR'S NOTE

An individual who contemplates the purchase of any respiratory care equipment, from endotracheal tubes to mechanical ventilators, may have a difficult time sorting out the merits and deficiencies of the items to be considered. At least a dozen different types of mechanical ventilators are commonly used in the United States and many more types are used abroad. They range from relatively unsophisticated, inexpensive, but reliable types to those representing state-of-the-art technology (and prices to match). Over 20 pulse oximeters are currently offered with widely differing capabilities. At least as many endotracheal and tracheotomy tubes are available. Almost all feature high volume, low pressure cuffs and are constructed of nontissue toxic materials. But are they similar in performance? Unfortunately, for the consumer, a skilled salesperson can make even an inferior product appear to be a top-of-the-line performer. What then can one do when the decision to purchase must be made?

The author of this chapter, Dr. Robert Spooner, is employed by ECRI, an organization best described as a not-for-profit, consumer-oriented, testing group that evaluates medical equipment. For almost two decades, they have placed heavy emphasis on comparative analyses of most of

Pre-Use Checklist for Anesthesia Units (Machines and Accessories)

To be performed daily.
Items marked with a * should be performed before each case.

* ☐ 1. **Controls off**
  Has anything been left on? Sniff! If gas has been leaking through a vaporizer all night, there may be significant initial concentration of vapor due to condensed liquid anesthetic in the piping manifold.

* ☐ 2. **Cylinder contents sufficient**
  Turn on each cylinder and check its contents gauge for adequate pressure. Is there sufficient oxygen to operate the ventilator in an emergency? Turn all cylinders off, or pipeline fluctuations may gradually use up reserve supplies.

☐ 3. **Oxygen supply failure**
Turn on the oxygen analyzer in STANDBY or ON mode for later test. Turn on flows of both oxygen and nitrous oxide. Then disconnect the oxygen hose. Confirm nitrous oxide flow decrease or cessation and alarm (if so equipped) indicating proper operation of the oxygen supply failure device (failsafe).

☐ 4. **Pipeline supplies**
When reattaching the oxygen hose, check that all fittings hold firmly, that no leaking gases can be heard, and that the hoses are arranged properly to prevent occlusion. Check pipeline pressure gauges (if so equipped) for proper pressure (50-55 psig). [Test oxygen flow during the Ventilator test, Item 13.]

☐ 5. **Controls, gas flow**
Confirm that all gas flow rates are easy to adjust accurately and that floats do not stick. Press the flush control and confirm that the reservoir bag fills quickly.

* ☐ 6. **Vaporizers filled**
  Examine fluid levels in vaporizers that might be used, fill carefully with the correct agent to the proper level, and record the amount. Since it may be necessary to change anesthetics during the course of a procedure, the reserve vaporizer should also be filled and ready. Be sure all vaporizers are tightly capped and off before leak testing (Item 7). If the patient may be sensitive to the agent in an unused vaporizer, do not include it in the following leak test.

☐ 7. **Leak test, machine** (if no manufacturer-specified test)
Attach a pressure gauge to the common outlet in place of the fresh gas hose and set the oxygen flow so that it indicates a steady 30 cm H_2O. Less than 30 mL/min inflow should be required to compensate for leakage. If such a low flow cannot be set, use the manufacturer's recommended leak test. Turn on vaporizers individually with oxygen flowing through them if they are to be included in the leak test. Remove the gauge, replace the fresh gas hose, and verify that all vaporizers are off.

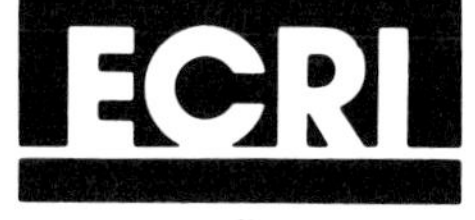

5200 BUTLER PIKE
PLYMOUTH MEETING, PA 19462

A

Fig. 16-21. ECRI pre-use checklist for anesthesia systems. (Courtesy of ECRI, Plymouth Meeting, PA.) (Figure continues.)

☐ 8. **Oxygen and vaporizer check**

Confirm the oxygen analyzer battery condition (if so equipped). Calibrate the sensor with air, then install in the fresh gas flow line and check at 100% oxygen. With the oxygen analyzer set at 100%, turn on the vaporizer and check for decreases in the oxygen concentration while increasing the vaporizer control in 1% steps. Turn off the vaporizer, set the gas flow for 50% oxygen, and check for that reading (this also checks flowmeters). Note how rapidly the indication changes. Compare these observations with the manufacturer's recommendations on need for maintenance. Adjust, in turn, the high- and low-oxygen alarms to the indicated concentration to confirm proper alarm actuation. Leave the low-oxygen alarm at 20% or higher.

• ☐ 9. **Absorber**

Be sure the absorbent has been changed recently and that its color indicates adequate capacity for the next procedure. Confirm that the bypass valve (if so equipped) is shut.

• ☐ 10. **Patient circuit assembly**

Confirm that the patient circuit is properly assembled and that hoses are wrung-on tightly.

• ☐ 11. **Patient circuit leak test** (if no manufacturer-specified test)

Occlude the reservoir bag fitting (or roll up bag and hold it to prevent inflation), shut off the pressure-limiting (pop-off) valve, and measure the oxygen flow rate that will sustain a pressure of 30 cm H_2O. It should not exceed 150 mL/min. Tighten the absorber seals, drain plug, and other possible sources or replace the bag and hoses to reduce leakage. Continue until it is within specification.

• ☐ 12. **Patient circuit flow**

Attach a simple lung simulator to simulate patient ventilation. Fill and compress the reservoir bag while checking for proper operation of one-way valves. Confirm that the lung is insufflated and empties with both forcible and gentle compression. Confirm that the pressure-limiting (pop-off) valve can be adjusted for various pressure levels in the patient circuit during simulated ventilation.

• ☐ 13. **Ventilator and alarm**

Turn on the ventilator (with appropriate fresh gas flow and settings) and the ventilation (disconnect) alarm and confirm that the simulated lung is ventilated as intended. Also confirm that the oxygen flow rate does not fall more than 10% on inspiration. Disconnect the lung and note if the alarm is activated after proper delay. Confirm battery condition, if so equipped. Perform a leak test per manufacturer's method. Turn off the ventilator and open the pressure-limiting valve.

☐ 14. **Scavenging system**

Confirm proper connection of the scavenging system and that an active system has the manufacturer-specified suction flow rate. Alternatively, with a gas flow of 8 L/min oxygen, put the oxygen sensor at the overflow release point of the scavenging system and check that the oxygen analyzer does not indicate over 21%. Replace the oxygen sensor.

• ☐ 15. **Controls off**

Note completion of tests on the Anesthesia Record.

Completion of this safety check ensures that more common equipment items have been tested for the most important types of failures. However, equivalent safety checks should be performed on drugs to ensure that they are properly marked and mixed, and on any other equipment that may be used.

B

Fig. 16-21. (*Figure continued*).

the devices described in the preceding pages. Their careful analytical and objective approach, with meticulous attention to detail, has contributed without question to improved patient safety and better quality products. Manufacturers whose products are "zinged" by an ECRI report are seldom happy, but they can never claim bias or an unfair approach. Most importantly, the would-be purchaser can use the published information as an important part of his or her personal assessment before signing on the dotted line. This chapter presents a historical resumé of ECRI's major forays into the respiratory care and anesthesia equipment field. His obvious, but understated pride with respect to ECRI's role shows, as well it should. This is an organization whose accomplishments and contributions should be known to every reader.

REFERENCES

All references are to ECRI's journal, *Health Devices*. No individual authors are named in these reports.

1. Evaluation: Manually operated resuscitators. 1:13, 1972
2. Evaluation: Manually operated infant resuscitators. 2:240, 1973
3. Evaluation: Manually operated resuscitators. 3:164, 1974
4. Evaluation: Manual resuscitators. 8:133, 1979
5. Evaluation: Disposable manual resuscitators. 18:231, 1989
6. Evaluation: Oxygen-powered resuscitators. 3:207, 1974
7. Hazard: Demand valve resuscitators. 5:145, 1976
8. Evaluation: Gas-powered resuscitators. 8:24, 1978
9. Hazard: Elder demand valve resuscitator. 14:438, 1985
10. Hazard: Gas-powered resuscitators. 17:352, 1988
11. Inspection and preventive maintenance procedure: Pulmonary resuscitators (gas-powered). 17:348, 1988
12. Evaluation: Intubation laryngoscopes. 5:283, 1976
13. Evaluation: Artificial airways. 7:67, 1978
14. Hazard: Unusual occlusion of small tracheal tubes. 17:379, 1988
15. Evaluation: Suction catheters. 6:132, 1977
16. Evaluation: Portable suction sources. 7:119, 1978
17. Evaluation: Portable oxygen analyzers. 1:203, 1972
18. Oxygen analyzers and anesthesia machines. 7:147, 1978
19. Evaluation: Oxygen analyzers for breathing circuits, 12:183, 1983
20. Evaluation: Carbon dioxide monitors. 15:255, 1986
21. Evaluation: Anesthesia ventilators. 8:151, 1979
22. Hazard: Barotrauma from anesthesia ventilators. 17:354, 1988
23. Evaluation: Critical care ventilators. 11:264, 1982
24. Evaluation: Portable volume ventilators. 17:107, 1988
25. Remote alarms for ventilators and other life-support equipment. 15:323, 1986
26. Evaluation: Microprocessor-controlled third-generation critical care ventilators. 18:59, 1989
27. Evaluation: Ventilation alarms. 10:204, 1981
28. Hazard: Bunn model 65 ventilation alarm. 11:72, 1981
29. Hazard: Damage to plastic components from Loctite. 18:288, 1989
30. Hazard: Low-pressure alarms for sensing ventilator disconnects. 12:260, 1983
31. Hazard update: Patient circuit disconnections. 13:108, 1984
32. Evaluation: Disposable anesthesia patient circuits. 9:3, 1979
33. Hazard: Fires during surgery of the head and neck area. 9:50, 1979
34. Evaluation: Heated humidifiers. 9:167, 1980
35. Pre-use checks of heated humidifiers. 10:122, 1981
36. Hazard: Heated wires can melt disposable breathing circuits. 18:174, 1989
37. Evaluation: Heated humidifiers. 16:223, 1987
38. Evaluation: Anesthesia units. 10:31, 1980
39. Evaluation: Anesthesia systems. 17:3, 1988
40. Avoiding anesthesia mishaps through pre-use checks. 11:201, 1982
41. Update: Pre-use checklist for anesthesia units. 13:324, 1984
42. Puritan-Bennett models 705 and 710 anesthesia units. 12:264, 1983

43. Hazard update: Foregger 705 anesthesia units. 13:263, 1984
44. Hazard: Crossed copper kettle vaporizer connections in Foregger anesthesia machines. 13:322, 1984
45. Hazard: Anesthesia units with a flowmeter-controlled vaporizer. 15:336, 1986
46. Hazard: Pre-use anesthesia check fails to find faults. 17:274, 1988
47. Hazard: Water in halothane vaporizers. 14:326, 1985
48. Hazard: Vaporizer leak with Mapleson breathing circuits. 15:344, 1986
49. Hazard: Concentration-calibrated vaporizers. 16:112, 1987

Index

Page numbers followed by an f refer to figures; those followed by a t refer to tables

B

D

E

F

G

H

I

J

K

L

M

N

O

P

Q

R

S

T

U

V

W

Z